PSYCHOTROPIC
DRUG
DIRECTORY
2007

THE PROFESSIONALS' POCKET
HANDBOOK AND AIDE MEMOIRE

PSYCHOTROPIC
DRUG
DIRECTORY
2007

THE PROFESSIONALS' POCKET HANDBOOK AND AIDE MEMOIRE

STEPHEN BAZIRE

HEALTHCOMM UK Ltd

Mental Health UK, a subsidiary of HealthComm UK Limited, Suite 3.1,
36 Upperkirkgate, Aberdeen AB10 1BA

British Library Cataloguing-in-Publication Data
A catalogue record is available for this book

First published 2007
Reprinted 2008

ISBN-10   0-9549193-8-6
ISBN-13   978-0-9549193-8-2

Printed in Malta by Gutenberg Press Limited, Tarxien, Malta

CONTENTS

INTRODUCTION   ix

CHAPTER 1: DRUG TREATMENT OPTIONS IN PSYCHIATRIC ILLNESS   1

1.1	Acute psychiatric emergency	1	
1.2	Aggression	6	
1.3	Agoraphobia	8	
1.4	Alcohol dependence and abuse	9	
1.5	Alcohol withdrawal syndrome	14	
1.6	Anxiety disorder	17	
1.7	Attention deficit hyperactivity disorder	23	
1.8	Autistic disorder	27	
1.9	Benzodiazepine dependence and withdrawal	30	
1.10	Bipolar mood disorder	32	
1.10.1	Prophylaxis and maintenance	33	
1.10.2	Mania and hypomania	40	
1.10.3	Bipolar depression	47	

1.10.4	Rapid-cycling bipolar disorder	51
1.11	Borderline personality disorder	53
1.12	Catatonia	56
1.13	Dementia	57
1.13.1	Management of dementia and BPSD	58
1.13.2	Prophylaxis and prevention	66
1.14	Depression	68
1.15	Dysthymia	93
1.16	Eating disorders	95
1.16.1	Anorexia nervosa	95
1.16.2	Bulimia nervosa	97
1.16.3	Binge-eating disorder	99
1.17	Epilepsy	100
1.17.1	Status epilepticus	110
1.18	Insomnia	113
1.19	Narcolepsy	118

1.20	Obsessive-compulsive disorder	120
1.21	Panic disorder	125
1.22	Post-traumatic stress disorder	129
1.23	Psychosis and schizophrenia	133
1.24	Seasonal affective disorder	161
1.25	Self-injurious behaviour	163
1.26	Sexual deviancy disorders	164
1.27	Social anxiety	166
1.28	Tourette's syndrome	169
1.29	Trichotillomania	172
1.30	Caffeinism	173
1.31	Electroconvulsive therapy	174

CHAPTER 2: SELECTING DRUGS, DOSES AND PREPARATIONS   179

2.1	Relative side-effects of:	
2.1.1	Hypnotics	179
2.1.2	Antidepressants	180
2.1.3	Antidepressants — pharmacokinetics and receptor effects	182
2.1.4	Antipsychotics	184
2.1.5	Antipsychotics — pharmacokinetics and receptor effects	186
2.1.6	Anxiolytics	188

2.2	Switching or discontinuing psychotropics	189
2.2.1	Antipsychotics	190
2.2.1.1	General advice	191
2.2.1.2	Specific drug switches	192
2.2.1.3	Antipsychotic dose equivalents	196
2.2.1.4	Post-switching antipsychotic issues	198
2.2.2	Benzodiazepines	198

2.2.3	Anticholinergics	199
2.2.4	Drugs of abuse	199
2.2.5	Antidepressants	199
2.3	Weight changes	208
2.3.1	Antipsychotics	208
2.3.2	Antidepressants	209
2.3.3	Mood stabilisers	211
2.3.4	Benzodiazepines	211
2.3.5	Anticonvulsants	211
2.3.6	Other drugs	212

CHAPTER 3: PSYCHOTROPICS IN PROBLEM AREAS   209

3.1	Breast-feeding	213
3.1.1	Antipsychotics	214
3.1.2	Antidepressants	215
3.1.3	Anxiolytics and hypnotics	218

3.1.4	Anticonvulsants	218
3.1.5	Others	220
3.2	Cardiovascular disease	221
3.2.1	Antipsychotics	222

3.2.2	Antidepressants	224
3.2.3	Anxiolytics and hypnotics	226
3.2.4	Anticonvulsants	226
3.2.5	Others	227

3.3	Diabetes	229	3.5.2	Antidepressants	239	3.7.5	Others	252
3.3.1	Antipsychotics	230	3.5.3	Others	239	3.8	Pregnancy	253
3.3.2	Antidepressants	231	3.6	Hepatic impairment	241	3.8.1	Antipsychotics	256
3.3.3	Anxiolytics and		3.6.1	Antipsychotics	242	3.8.2	Antidepressants	258
	hypnotics	232	3.6.2	Antidepressants	242	3.8.3	Anxiolytics and	
3.3.4	Anticonvulsants	232	3.6.3	Anxiolytics and			hypnotics	261
3.3.5	Others	233		hypnotics	243	3.8.4	Anticonvulsants	262
3.4	Epilepsy	234	3.6.4	Anticonvulsants	244	3.8.5	Others	267
3.4.1	Antipsychotics	234	3.6.5	Others	245	3.9	Renal impairment	270
3.4.2	Antidepressants	235	3.7	Old age	246	3.9.1	Antipsychotics	271
3.4.3	Anxiolytics and		3.7.1	Antipsychotics	247	3.9.2	Antidepressants	271
	hypnotics	236	3.7.2	Antidepressants	248	3.9.3	Anxiolytics and	
3.4.4	Others	236	3.7.3	Anxiolytics and			hypnotics	272
3.5	Glaucoma	238		hypnotics	250	3.9.4	Anticonvulsants	273
3.5.1	Antipsychotics	239	3.7.4	Anticonvulsants	251	3.9.5	Others	274

CHAPTER 4: DRUG INTERACTIONS 275

4.1	Anxiolytics and		4.3.3.1	Duloxetine	307	4.6.1	Acamprosate	349
	hypnotics	275	4.3.3.2	Mianserin	308	4.6.2	Anticholinergics	349
4.1.1	Benzodiazepines	275	4.3.3.3	Mirtazapine	308	4.6.3	Anticholinesterases	350
4.1.2	Buspirone	278	4.3.3.4	Moclobemide	309	4.6.3.1	Donepezil	350
4.1.3	Chloral hydrate	279	4.3.3.5	Reboxetine	311	4.6.3.2	Galantamine	350
4.1.4	Zaleplon	280	4.3.3.6	Trazodone	311	4.6.3.3	Rivastigmine	351
4.1.5	Zolpidem	280	4.3.3.7	Tryptophan	312	4.6.4	Atomoxetine	351
4.1.6	Zopiclone	281	4.3.3.8	Venlafaxine	312	4.6.5	Buprenorphine	351
4.2	Antipsychotics	281	4.3.3.9	St John's wort	313	4.6.6	Bupropion	352
4.2.1	General antipsychotics	281	4.3.4	MAOIs	316	4.6.7	Clomethiazole	353
4.2.2	Aripiprazole	285	4.4	Lithium	321	4.6.8	Disulfiram	353
4.2.3	Clozapine	285	4.5	Anticonvulsants	326	4.6.9	Memantine	354
4.2.4	Olanzapine	288	4.5.1	Carbamazepine	326	4.6.10	Methadone	355
4.2.5	Quetiapine	290	4.5.2	Ethosuximide	332	4.6.11	Methylphenidate	356
4.2.6	Risperidone	290	4.5.3	Gabapentin	332	4.6.12	Modafinil	357
4.2.7	Sertindole	291	4.5.4	Lamotrigine	332	4.6.13	Sodium oxybate	358
4.2.8	Ziprasidone	292	4.5.5	Levetiracetam	334	4.7	Non-prescribed drugs	358
4.2.9	Zotepine	293	4.5.6	Oxcarbazepine	334	4.7.1	Alcohol	358
4.3	Antidepressants	293	4.5.7	Phenobarbital and		4.7.2	Cannabis	361
4.3.1	Tricyclic anti-			primidone	336	4.7.3	Cocaine	361
	depressants	293	4.5.8	Phenytoin	338	4.7.4	Smoking	362
4.3.2	SSRIs	297	4.5.9	Piracetam	345	4.8	Cytochrome P450	
4.3.2.1	Citalopram/		4.5.10	Pregabalin	345		drug metabolism	363
	escitalopram	297	4.5.11	Tiagabine	345	4.8.1	CYP1A2	364
4.3.2.2	Fluoxetine	299	4.5.12	Topiramate	346	4.8.2	CYP2B6	365
4.3.2.3	Fluvoxamine	301	4.5.13	Valproate	346	4.8.3	CYP2C9	366
4.3.2.4	Paroxetine	304	4.5.14	Vigabatrin	348	4.8.4	CYP2C19	367
4.3.2.5	Sertraline	305	4.5.15	Zonisamide	348	4.8.5	CYP2D6	368
4.3.3	Other antidepressants	307	4.6	Other drugs	349	4.8.6	CYP3A3/4	370

CHAPTER 5: DRUG-INDUCED PSYCHIATRIC DISORDERS 373

5.1	Agitation, anxiety and		5.5	Depression	377	5.8.2	Akathisia	386
	nervousness	373	5.6	Hallucinations	380	5.8.3	Dystonias	387
5.2	Aggression	374	5.7	Mania, hypomania or		5.8.4	Dyskinesias	388
5.3	Behavioural changes	374		euphoria	381	5.8.5	Other movement	
5.4	Delirium and		5.8	Movement disorders	384		disorders	389
	confusion	375	5.8.1	Pseudoparkinsonism	385	5.8.5.1	Catatonia	389

Contents

5.8.5.2 *Choreas*	389	
5.8.5.3 *Tics*	389	
5.9.	Neuroleptic malignant syndrome	390
5.10	Obsessive-compulsive symptoms	391

5.11	Panic disorder	392
5.12	Paranoid or schizo-phrenic-like psychoses	392
5.13	Seizures	396
5.14	Serotonin syndrome	399
5.15	Sleep problems	401

5.15.1	Sleep disturbances	401
5.15.2	Vivid dreams and nightmares	402

CHAPTER 6: MANAGEMENT OF SIDE-EFFECTS

403

6.1	Anticholinergic and related side-effects	404
	~ blurred vision	404
	~ constipation	
	~ dry mouth	404
	~ urinary retention	404
	~ urinary hesitancy	404
	~ urinary incon-tinence	405
6.2	Cardiac effects	405
	~ hypertension	405
	~ hypotension	405
	~ postural hypo-tension	405
	~ QTc prolongation	406
	~ tachycardia	406
6.3	Central adverse effects	406
	~ delirium	406
	~ depression	407
	~ drowsiness	407
	~ dysphoria	407
	~ fatigue	407
	~ hypomania	407
	~ insomnia	407
	~ nausea	408
	~ nocturnal enuresis	408
	~ OCD	408
	~ panic	409
	~ sedation	409
	~ seizures	409
6.4	Endocrine effects	409
	~ diabetes insipidus	409

	~ diabetes mellitus	409
	~ hepatotoxicity	410
	~ hyperammonaemia	410
	~ hypercholesterol	410
	~ hyperglycaemia	410
	~ hyperlipidaemia	411
	~ hyperprolactinaemia	411
	~ hyperthyroidism	412
	~ hyponatraemia	412
	~ hypothyroidism	413
	~ polyuria	413
	~ renal impairment	413
	~ weight gain	414
6.5	Movement disorders	418
	~ blepharospasm	418
	~ dysphagia	418
	~ laryngospasm	418
	~ EPSE, akathisia	418
	~ EPSE, dyskinesias	420
	~ EPSE, Parkinsonism	422
	~ EPSE, dystonia	423
	~ myoclonus	424
	~ restless legs	424
	~ bruxism	425
6.6	Neuroleptic malignant syndrome	425
6.7	Serotonin syndrome	427
6.8	Sexual side-effects	428
	~ libido	429
	~ arousal	429
	~ anorgasmia	430
	~ ejaculation problems	432

	~ priapism	433
6.9	Others, side-effects	433
	~ abnormal dreams and nightmares	433
	~ alopecia	433
	~ anorexia	433
	~ ataxia	433
	~ bleeding	434
	~ blood dyscrasias	434
	~ gastric irritation or nausea	434
	~ glaucoma	434
	~ hair loss	435
	~ hypersalivation	435
	~ incontinence	435
	~ jaundice	435
	~ jitteriness or agitation	435
	~ mastalgia	435
	~ megaloblastic anaemia	435
	~ oedema	435
	~ osteopenia	435
	~ pain at site of injection	436
	~ photosensitivity	436
	~ raised LFTs	436
	~ rash	436
	~ siallorhoea	436
	~ sweating	438
	~ tremor	438
	~ vomiting	438

CHAPTER 7: MISCELLANEOUS INFORMATION

439

7.1	New psychotropic drugs expected	439
7.2	Laboratory tests	440

	~ urea and electrolytes	440
	~ renal function	441

	~ liver function tests	441
	~ blood	442
	~ miscellaneous	442

INDEX AND ABBREVIATIONS

445

INTRODUCTION

Why the *Psychotropic Drug Directory* (*PDD*) *2007*? Well, the title tries to describe the contents, and how you should use them. The 'directory' part is because the book contains general principles, lists, issues, advice and references to help you make decisions but then directs you where to go to get the further information you might need, since it would be virtually impossible to convey all the subtleties of a research paper, case report or review in a couple of lines. I have, for instance, added well over 1250 new references to the text in this edition. If I spent a couple of hours thoroughly reading and analysing each and every paper, I'd never be able to finish the book and would have to give up the day job, before it gives up on me. So, you really should check papers before making important decisions. I would be hugely grateful for any advice or tips about papers that I may have taken at face value and inadvertently missed the errors, hidden bias or multiple publication.

It may be worth pointing out that this book is an entirely independent publication. There is no commercial sponsorship, support or influence on the content, which remains entirely my own work.

How to use the book...

The *PDD 2007* is arranged in a problem-solving way to aid optimum medication use:

- *Chapter one*: select a mental health problem needing medication management and consider the pharmacological options from the BNF, combination and unlicensed lists.
- *Chapter two* aids choosing a drug and dose, where a choice exists or is necessary.
- *Chapter three* aids drug choice in a compromised patient.
- *Chapter four* allows checking for drug–drug interactions.
- *Chapter five* is an important check that the mental health problem isn't drug-induced.
- *Chapter six* helps to guide you where a drug works, but side-effects limit effectiveness.
- *Chapter seven* has got some snippets of information I couldn't think where else to put.

A minimum level of knowledge is assumed and information given should be followed up in the appropriate sources when time allows. References, where quoted, are either of good recent review articles, or, of specific information.

Further information can be obtained by referring to the main paper or papers cited and also to the reference sections of those main papers. Lists and references are as comprehensive as viable but could never claim to be fully complete, nor could this book ever be as comprehensive as a MedLine or PsychLit search on a chosen topic. The listing of a drug use in this book does not in any way imply that it is licensed or safe for this use, and all information is presented in good faith. Throughout, I have tried to be as objective as possible. It must be up to the reader to make up his or her own mind on a topic, but I hope that the statements and references will have pointed you in the right direction and the time saved in looking papers up will allow more thought. It is inevitable that some papers are from specialist journals but, where possible, I have always quoted more accessible journals in preference. If the only paper published on the use of a drug is from an obscure or ancient source this may well indicate the status of the paper. Also, perhaps, I'll endeavour to remind readers of their ethical duty and responsibility (blindingly obvious statement) to include service-users' aspirations when choosing unlicensed and novel therapies.

Changes to this edition

Updates have been made to all chapters, as well as an entirely new chapter on managing drug-induced side-effects. Bipolar mood disorder has been grouped as one condition (maintenance, mania, depression, rapid-cycling) in *Chapter one*.

Acknowledgements

Writing and continually updating a book such as this is a tremendous challenge and drain on my stamina and enthusiasm. Subsequently, the continued help, encouragement, constructive criticism and advice I have received from colleagues and correspondents throughout the world has always been utterly invaluable, not to mention very rewarding. It is wonderful to know that the book has helped improve the pharmaceutical care of many people with mental health needs. I would thus like to thank all the people I have thanked in previous editions, the many members of the UK Psychiatric Pharmacy Group who have conveyed continued enthusiasm, encouragement and support, and all those people I have met at conferences and talks or who have written to me. Thanks as ever must go to my pharmacy staff and colleagues in the trust for continuing to tolerate and humour me and being the reason I'm a 'Stakhanovite', and special thanks to the University of East Anglia's fab new School of Pharmacy for the honour. I also wish to thank the many people who have fed back on the book's contents and/or spotted ambiguities in the quarter of a million words, including Stephen Griffiths, Simon Walpole, Marian Coyne, Vanessa Bate, Jane Wright, Sunny Sanjeev Sharm, Laura Regan, Sarah Harris, Simon Howe, Kiran Hewitt, Jenny Lawrence, Roman Montanari, Andrea Goodenough, Roger Ingham, Père Datthe, Mo Gilmour, Yashmi Jogessar, Sharif Shazia, Dr R Pyatt and Caroline Parker, though I've doubtless forgotten a few people (so sorry if that's you). Thanks also to John Tams, Virgin Radio and Richard Thompson for the company; to Kirsty, Andy, Dawn, Paula and David for being challenging; to my old mate Paul Woods; Judy and Wendy in the library; my parents and my godmother Kate Baxter for continuing to show interest, and Jill, Rosie and Chris for steering clear of my study. And finally, a big hello to all student nurses called Bazire doing their mental health placement in Birmingham in 2007.

Stephen Bazire *BPharm, FRPharmS, DipPsychPharm, MCMHP*
Chief Pharmacist, Norfolk and Waveney Mental Health Partnership NHS Trust,
Hellesdon Hospital, Norwich NR6 5BE
Honorary Professor, School of Chemistry and Pharmacy,
University of East Anglia, Norwich
England
E-mail: steve.bazire@nwmhp.nhs.uk
Website for service users: www.nwmhp.nhs.uk/pharmacy
UKPPG website: www.ukppg.org.uk
Declaration of interests: www.ukppg.org.uk/committee.html

January, 2007

DRUG TREATMENT OPTIONS IN PSYCHIATRIC ILLNESS

This chapter lists medicines which are indicated for, or have been used in, the conditions listed and the author would welcome suggestions for further inclusions. References should be consulted for fuller details of non-approved uses. In some cases, drugs not available in the UK have been included as possible options if available and for non-UK readers.

Drugs are classified as follows:

BNF listed

BNF listed drugs are listed in the *British National Formulary* and licensed in the UK for that condition. See the appropriate section in the BNF for a review of a drug's role in therapy and its prescribing details. Much information provided here is in addition to that in the standard texts.

+ Combinations

The combinations section includes some combinations that have been used, but carry the risks of additive side-effects and interactions.

● Unlicensed/some efficacy

This section includes drugs of some clinical efficacy (eg. RCTs) or are strategies which can be used, but where no product licence exists.

■ Unlicensed/possible efficacy

This section includes drugs of minor or unproven importance or efficacy. No product licence exists.

◆ Others

This section includes drugs tried, but where no significant data exists since the original reports. The lack of positive follow-up data suggests a lack of efficacy although, if you know otherwise, the author would like to hear.

✻ No efficacy

Drugs in this section are not thought to be of clinical use.

Information in these last four categories is given to provide help once all recognised and evidence-based treatments have been tried. These classifications are to some extent arbitrary, and the information is based on data presently available.

It is the prescriber's responsibility to ensure that all precautions are taken when prescribing a drug for an unlicensed use.

1.1 ACUTE PSYCHIATRIC EMERGENCY (APE) including RAPID TRANQUILLISATION
see Aggression (*1.2*), Mania and hypomania (*1.10.2*) and Psychosis and schizophrenia (*1.23*)

Violent patients (usually either schizophrenic, manic or substance abusers) present a risk to themselves and others. Swift, safe and effective treatment is often needed. Rapid tranquillisation (RT), is the term used to define the procedure of giving varying amounts of antipsychotic medication, usually with benzodiazepines, over brief intervals of time to control agitated, threatening and potentially destructive patients.

Routes: IV administration is generally quicker-acting than IM, which is often little quicker than oral drugs (especially if concentrated liquids or melt-in-the-mouth tablets are used) and allows physical restraint to be removed more quickly. IV drug use does, however, carry additional dangers and the IM route should generally be the preferred choice except in exceptional circumstances. IM absorption will be more rapid in an active patient than a quiet one. Parenteral (IV/IM) doses generally have a higher potency than oral doses, so 'when required' or regular doses prescribed as 'IM/PO' are entirely inappropriate. All 'PRN' doses should be checked daily to ensure maximum doses are not being exceeded. Benzodiazepines are generally safe by (slow) injection, but antipsychotics can be fatal in moderate doses in drug-naïve people.

Doses: The need for high doses of antipsychotics is unnecessary, as violent patients respond to standard doses and higher doses may, in fact, be less effective, eg. inducing akathisia. Use of concomitant benzodiazepines is safer and more effective than using high doses of antipsychotics as monotherapy.

Conditions: Manic patients may respond well to benzodiazepines, with antipsychotics as adjuncts. Schizophrenic patients usually respond best to antipsychotics, with benzodiazepines as adjuncts. In substance misuse, benzodiazepines and antipsychotics may be effective, but more studies are needed.

General principles of the management of acute psychiatric emergency (APE) (eg. Pilowsky et al, Br J Psychiatry 1992;**160**:31–5 and NICE)

1. Obtain a drug history and carry out a physical examination if possible. Unless known previous exposure to psychotropics, use doses at the lower end of the ranges.
2. Antipsychotics in combination with benzo-diazepines are preferred.
3. Parenteral administration is generally the quickest and most reliable route, but should be reserved **only** for when the patient cannot be persuaded to take drugs orally.
4. No anticholinergics should be used as this may confuse the clinical picture.
5. Switch to oral doses as soon as possible.
6. Check bp, pulse and temperature frequently.
7. Although APE can be carried out in the community, great care is needed and it is not recommended.

Potential complications of (particularly older) antipsychotics in APE:

1. Cardiovascular complications and sudden death — drugs causing QTc prolongation are contraindicated in patients with pre-existing cardiac problems, and care is needed in adrenaline-driven excited patients.
2. Respiratory depression.
3. Extrapyramidal symptoms, especially acute dystonia (may occur in 10–30% of patients within the first 24 hours and later in up to 50% of young males). Akathisia should be considered if agitation occurs, worsens or recurs after antipsychotics have achieved

adequate behavioural control, as it may be drug-induced and exacerbate the disturbed behaviour (see Chapter 6.5).

4. Acute hypotension (minimised if the patient can lie down) can occur, especially with phenothiazines and in the elderly.
5. Seizures, especially in non-compliant epileptics.
6. Mega-colon (rare), heatstroke, aspiration.
7. Neuroleptic malignant syndrome — see Chapter 6.6 for risk factors. Close observation of temperature should be carried out, especially in early stages. Check CPK.
8. Local bruising, pain or extravasations (common, in up to 30% patients).
9. A depot given inadvertently into a vein may be rapidly fatal.
10. Disinhibition may occur with benzodiazepines, especially in people with poor impulse control or impulsivity, high-potency drugs, young or older age, with developmental disabilities and/or pre-existing CNS damage (review by Paton, Psychiatr Bull 2002;**26**:460–2) but remains controversial and probably over-rated (controlled study showing no effect: Rothschild et al, J Clin Psychopharmacol 2000;**20**:7–11; review by Paton, Psychiatr Bull 2002;**26**:460–2 noting the actual incidence may be as low as perhaps < 1%).
11. In patients already taking antipsychotics, additional acute doses may reach toxic levels.

Reviews: * Use of BDZs and antipsychotics in emergency departments (Rund et al, J Emerg Med 2006;**31**:317–24), reappraisal of current options (concludes that parenteral BDZs should now be the mainstay of treatment: McAllister-Williams and Ferrier, Br J Psychiatry 2001;**179**:485–9).

BNF listed

Drugs in this section are licensed for emergency, short-term or adjunct therapy of, eg. acute psychosis, mania, anxiety or exacerbations of chronic psychosis, violent or impulsive behaviour, psychomotor agitation and excitement, or violent or dangerously impulsive behaviour.

ANTIPSYCHOTICS
Chlorpromazine

Chlorpromazine injection should be given

by deep IM injection only, at 25–50 mg every 6–8 hours, with a lower dose (up to 25 mg eight-hourly) in the elderly. The IM injection is 2–4 times as potent, on a mg for mg basis, as oral chlorpromazine, and so prescriptions for '100 mg po/im' are entirely inappropriate and potentially dangerous. It can cause hypotension, has been associated with sudden death and is not recommended.

Haloperidol (see also combinations)

Haloperidol can be used at BNF doses, eg. up to 18 mg/d by injection. There have been some concerns about QTc prolongation potential; in the major study (Reilly et al, Lancet 2000;**355**:1048–52) QTc prolongation with haloperidol was only just short of significance and there were case reports of torsades de pointes. The IV route in acutely disturbed patients is thus, at best, controversial, and should be avoided unless essential. Akathisia may exacerbate disturbed behaviour.

Olanzapine IM *

A number of studies (eg. Wright et al, Am J Psychiatry 2001;**158**:1149–51; n=270, Wright et al, Schizophr Res 2001;**49**[Suppl 1]:250–1; n=270, RCT, p/c, d/b, Breier et al, Arch Gen Psychiatry 2002;**59**:441–8) have shown olanzapine IM 10 mg to be at least as effective as haloperidol 7.5 mg IM in acute agitation in schizophrenia, with a possibly slightly quicker onset of action (eg. at 30 minutes), no QT prolongation and significantly fewer EPS, including dystonia and akathisia (n=311, RCT, p/c, Wright et al, Can J Psychiatry 2003;**48**:716–21, MS; review by Smith, EBMH 2003;**6**:27, noting that the response is in line with what you would expect from other antipsychotics). Cochrane is critical of the supporting literature, noting the manufacturer's involvement, poor and incomplete reporting and the borderline ethical nature of the trials (s=4, n=769, Belgamwar and Fenton, Cochrane Database Syst Rev 2005;**2**:CD003729). The following recommendations are based on Lilly's first year's experience, more recent data and the outcomes of some off-licence use:

- Olanzapine intramuscular can be used to rapidly control agitation and disturbed behaviours in patients with schizophrenia or manic episodes when oral therapy is inappropriate.
- The maximum combined daily dose of oral and intramuscular olanzapine is 20 mg.
- The initial dose of olanzapine intramuscular is 10 mg as a single injection (use lower doses in elderly patients and those with renal or hepatic impairment).
- A maximum of three injections of olanzapine intramuscular may be administered in 24 hours, and a minimum of two hours should elapse between the first and any second injection.
- Olanzapine IM is intended for short-term use only, for up to a maximum of three consecutive days.
- Olanzapine 'Velotabs' produce a plasma level profile similar to oral tablets. IM peak plasma levels are five times higher than oral, peaking after a few minutes. Aggressive oral dosing strategies (eg. up to 40 mg/d) appear reasonably well-tolerated and effective in controlling acutely agitated people with a variety of diagnoses (n=148, RCT, p/c, 4/7, Baker et al, J Clin Psychopharmacol 2003;**23**:342–8, MS; comment by Citrome, EBMH 2004;**7**:12).
- There is no safety data on giving benzodiazepines IM simultaneously with IM olanzapine. Benzodiazepines should only be given an hour after olanzapine IM.

Review: use in acute agitation (Wagstaff et al, CNS Drugs 2005;**19**:147–64).

Risperidone

See combinations.

Trifluoperazine

This is licensed as an adjunct therapy.

Zuclopenthixol acetate (Clopixol Acuphase®)

Clopixol Acuphase® (Lundbeck) can be given at a dose of 50–150 mg stat, then repeated after 2–3 days (maximum every 1–2 days) after the first injection. The maximum cumulative dose is 400 mg per 'course', ie. four injections or over two weeks, whichever comes first. The maximum single dose in the elderly is 100 mg. While zuclopenthixol acetate appears as effective as haloperidol in APE, sedation at four hours may be greater and there is an advantage of the need for fewer injections (McNulty and Pelosi, *EBMH* 1998;1:56). The onset of action is at about eight hours (peaking at about 36 hours; see psychosis *1.23*), and so should only be used when initial control has been established with other agents. Several reviews have suggested that more data is needed to prove an advantage over standard therapies (Gibson *et al*, *Cochrane Database Syst Rev* 2004;3:CD000525). Care is needed with Acuphase® to avoid it being given into a vein of a struggling or over-active patient.

BENZODIAZEPINES
(see also combinations)

Diazepam (see also combinations)

The recommended dose of diazepam is 10mg IV or IM, repeated after not less than four hours. IV infusion is possible. IV diazepam is much more consistently absorbed than IM which, in turn, is little faster than oral and slower than the rectal route. If the IV route is used, it is strongly recommended to be into the large vein of the antecubital fossa with the patient, if possible, in a supine position to minimise the incidence of hypotension. The maximum IV dose is 5mg per minute. Mechanical ventilation and flumazenil should be available in case of respiratory depression, as hypoxic drive can be affected. Diazepam has a long half-life and active metabolites, and so accumulation and toxic delirium (especially in the elderly or hepatic impairment) must be avoided by use of decreased doses later on. A wide safety margin makes diazepam and lorazepam the drugs of choice.

Lorazepam (see also combinations)

Lorazepam is usually given by the IV route into a larger vein. IM absorption is as slow as oral administration, but more rapid in an active patient and IM generally carries less risk than IV. Lorazepam injection may be diluted 50:50 with water or normal saline pre-injection. The dose in acute anxiety is 0.025–0.05mg/kg (1.75–3.5mg for a 70kg person), repeated six-hourly. Some services use 0.5–2mg PO/IM every 1–2 hours until symptoms are controlled, omitting

doses when excessive sedation occurs. This can be a highly effective therapy. Caution is needed in renal and hepatic impairment and in the elderly, where a lower dose may be needed. Lorazepam does not accumulate with repeated doses or in hepatic impairment; distinct advantages over diazepam. Short-term lorazepam infusion has caused deterioration, possibly due to propylene glycol, a component of lorazepam intravenous formulations (n=1, Cawley, *Pharmacother* 2001;21:1140–4).

● Unlicensed/some efficacy

Clomethiazole (chlormethiazole)
See SPC for doses for other indications.

Clonazepam
Clonazepam is licensed only for status epilepticus in all its clinical forms, but can be used as an alternative to diazepam and lorazepam, although slower-acting. The dose is 1mg (1ml) by slow (1mg per 30 seconds) IV injection, which is strongly recommended to be into the large vein of the antecubital fossa with the patient in a supine position, if possible, to minimise the incidence of hypotension. Care is needed in the elderly and caution in chronic pulmonary insufficiency.

+ Combinations

Combinations of antipsychotics and benzodiazepines are highly effective and generally allow lower doses of both to be used. Patients receiving only a single drug in APE at first are more likely to need second injections (Pilowski *et al*, *Br J Psychiatry* 1992;160:831–5) and a recent review concluded that combinations of an atypical and a BDZ are optimal due to the lower incidence of EPS (s=11, n=701, Yildiz *et al*, *Emerg Med J* 2003;20:339–46).

Antipsychotic + benzodiazepine (see also separate drugs) *

This combination is widely and strongly recommended, as the drugs act synergistically, reducing the amount of each drug (particularly the antipsychotic) required. The effect of the combination is rapid and predictable and the patient is less likely to require a second injection. **Lorazepam** is the most widely used benzodiazepine, with 2mg IM plus haloperidol IM 5mg being significantly better than lorazepam alone after 60–180 minutes in one APE study (n=98, RCT, Battaglia et al, Am J Emerg Med 1997;**15**:335–40). No serious adverse effects occurred in either treatment group (n=20, d/b, Bieniek et al, Pharmacotherapy 1998;**18**:57–62). **Diazepam** 10mg IM/IV is a suitable alternative. There is now accumulating evidence for the combined use of **risperidone** and lorazepam. In acute psychotic agitation, oral risperidone 2mg plus lorazepam 2mg was as effective and as well-tolerated as haloperidol 5mg IM plus lorazepam 2mg IM over two hours (n=83+79, RCT, s/b, Currier et al, J Clin Psychiatry 2004;**65**:386–94). IM lorazepam alone was as effective as lorazepam IM plus either risperidone or haloperidol (both oral) in acute agitation and/or psychosis, although the combination therapy was numerically superior (n=30, RCT, d/b, d/b, Veser et al, J Psychiatr Pract 2006;**12**:103–8). Oral risperidone can be used effectively as an alternative to IM antipsychotics, eg. risperidone liquid 2mg plus oral lorazepam 2mg was shown to be as effective in psychotic agitation as haloperidol 5mg IM plus lorazepam 2mg IM, but with less complications (n=30, Currier and Simpson, J Clin Psychiatry 2001;**62**:153–7). In another trial, where patients were given a choice of oral risperidone (2mg) plus oral lorazepam (2–2.5mg) or standard IM antipsychotics, with or without lorazepam, most chose oral, which was more successful at two hours and significantly non-inferior with fewer side-effects (n=226, open, Lejeune et al, Int Clin Psychopharmacol 2004;**19**:259–69). Risperidone 2–6mg/d was also superior and much better tolerated than oral zuclopenthixol (20–50mg/d) when combined with lorazepam in acute psychosis (n=75, open, 14/7, Hovens et al, J Psychopharmacol 2005;**19**:51–7). The fast-dissolving risperidone tablet formulation may useful to ensure administration, although the peak plasma levels occur at 1.4–1.8 hours (the same as tablets).

Antipsychotic + antihistamine *

In a recent trial of lorazepam IM 4mg vs. haloperidol 10mg IM plus promethazine 25–50mg, 96% patients in each group were 'tranquil or asleep' after four hours, but 76% were asleep with HAL-PRO mix compared with only 45% with lorazepam IM monotherapy, concluding that both were equally effective but the combination was slightly quicker (n=200, RCT, Alexander et al, Br J Psychiatry 2004;**185**:63–9; favourable comment by McAllister-Williams, EBMH 2005;**8**:7).

■ Unlicensed/possible efficacy

Amylobarbital/amobarbital sodium
Great care is needed if used in APE. The IM route should be preferred. If IV must be used, the vial should be diluted and injected slowly (maximum 50mg/min) to prevent sudden respiratory depression. It is contraindicated in marked hepatic impairment.

Midazolam
Midazolam may be useful for short-term sedation, with a quick onset and off-set. IM can be used but IV is too dangerous in non-specialist mental health settings due to the potential for respiratory depression. Oral sprays may provide an alternative route of administration. 2.5–10mg IM/IV may be rapidly effective (6–20 minutes) in controlling acute agitation (eg. report by Bond et al, Am J Psychiatry 1989;**146**:925–6), repeated every 20 minutes up to 20mg per sedation event (Australian Psychotropic Guidelines, 5th edn, 2003) and monitored for at least four hours after the last dose. In a pragmatic real-world trial, with a simple end-point and only 1% drop-outs, IM midazolam was superior to haloperidol plus promethazine at 20 and 40 minutes in aggressive or agitated emergency room patients, with few side-effects (n=301, RCT, TREC-CG, BMJ 2003;**317**:708–13; comment by Waraich, EBMH 2004;**7**:42). Midazolam IM 5mg was as effective as, and much quicker acting than, lorazepam IM 2mg or haloperidol IM 5mg in acute agitation, but the effects were shorter-lived (82 minutes vs 217 minutes vs 126 minutes respectively; n=111, RCT, d/b, Nobay et al, Acad Emerg Med 2004;**11**:744–9).

Paraldehyde
Paraldehyde infusion should **only** be carried out in specialist centres, as it needs intensive care facilities.

Valproate

While valproate loading may have an antimanic effect over 48–72 hours, it has no detectable effect when given IV over 120 minutes (n=7, open, Phroloiv et al, J Clin Psychiatry 2004;**65**:68–70). See entry under mania (1.10.2).

Ziprasidone IM (not UK)

Available in some European countries, the IM formulation is effective in doses of 10mg IM every two hours or 20mg IM every four hours. The maximum dose is 40mg/day (Daniel et al, Psychopharmacol 2001;**155**: 128–34). Although lorazepam may be given at the same time, the two must not be mixed in the same syringe due to compatibility issues. If long-term therapy is required, oral should replace intramuscular administration as soon as possible.

1.2 AGGRESSION

see also Acute psychiatric emergency (1.1), Borderline personality disorder (1.11) and Self-injurious behaviour (1.25)

Aggression is considered to be behaviour accompanied by verbal or physical threats which, if carried out, would cause harm to others, self or property. It can include situational (provoked), non-situational (unprovoked), passive, physical or interictal (especially in temporal lobe epilepsy). Aggression is not a diagnosis in itself, but as well as being potentially drug-induced (through either intoxication or withdrawal), can be considered a symptom of many conditions, including dementia, personality disorders, PTSD, PMS, trauma, etc, or as an expression of a variety of emotional or behavioural motivations. Low GABA levels and low serotonin levels in various parts of the brain are associated with aggressive behaviour, and enhanced norepinephrine and dopamine levels in the brain are associated with increased aggression.

Role of drugs

Drugs may be useful in helping control some cases where suppression of aggression is considered important on safety grounds.
Reviews: pharmacotherapy (Brieden et al, Pharmacopsychiatry 2002;**35**:83–9), general (Hughes, Psychiatr Serv 1999;**50**:1135–7).

Lithium

Most studies with lithium have involved aggression in patients with learning disabilities and a two-month trial at 0.6–1.0mmol/L may be justified in patients unmanageable by environmental factors. Lithium has been shown to reduce aggression and the frequency of episodes in learning disabilities (eg. Langee, Am J Ment Retard 1990;**94**:448–52), reducing impulsive aggression in patients with organic brain damage, brain damaged individuals (Bellus et al, Brain Inj 1996;**10**:849–60) and in two trials in children with aggression or conduct disorder, albeit poorly tolerated (n=50, RCT, d/b, p/c, Campbell et al, J Am Acad Child Adolesc Psychiatry 1995;**34**:445–53; n=86, RCT, d/b, p/c, Malone et al, Arch Gen Psychiatry 2000;**57**:649–54). Lithium may exert an effect via several mechanisms, eg. enhancement of serotonin but the potential adverse consequences of sudden discontinuation (accidental or deliberate) should be considered.

+ Combinations

Fluvoxamine + antipsychotics

An aggressive schizophrenic improved when fluvoxamine 100mg/d was added to risperidone 8mg/d (n=1, Silver and Kushnir, Am J Psychiatry 1998;**155**:1298).

■ Unlicensed/some efficacy

Antipsychotics

Evidence for the efficacy of antipsychotics in aggression is suggestive rather than conclusive, as a clinical effect is difficult to quantify. It may be that raised dopamine levels are associated with aggression (Pabis and Stanislav, Ann Pharmacother 1996;**30**:278–87), in which case dopamine-blocking drugs may have some rationale. Use of higher doses of antipsychotics are generally considered to be effective only via a sedating effect. A number of drugs have been used. An analysis of 19 studies suggested that **risperidone** is useful for treating aggression in a range of behavioural disorders, agitation and dementia (s=19, De Deyn and Buitelaar, Eur Psychiatry 2006;**21**:21–8). It may be particularly useful at lower dose, eg. it was effective under several measures for severe, primary aggressive behaviour in adolescents admitted to hospital with disruptive behaviours compounded by sub-average cognitive abilities (n = 38, RCT, p/c, 6/52, Buitelaar et al, J Clin Psychiatry 2001;**62**:239–48; review by Young, EBMH 2002;**5**:11). **Clozapine** is not easy to use but reduced seclusion and restraint rates in aggressive, psychotic in-patients over 12 months, the effect not related to sedation (n = 137, Chengappa et al, Schizophr Res 2002;**53**:1–6). Short-term use of clozapine for aggression in an adolescent with autistic disorder has been reported (n = 1, Chen et al, J Clin Psychiatry 2001;**62**:479–80).

Benzodiazepines

Benzodiazepines are reported to be effective in episodic behavioural disorders by aborting aggression in the prodromal stage. Lorazepam has been used in resistant aggression in dementia, with 1.5–3mg/d effective orally over several years in some patients (Fritz and Stewart, Am J Psychiatry 1990;**147**:1250), as has 1–2mg lorazepam IV (d/b, Salzman et al, J Clin Psychiatry 1991;**52**:177–80). Use should normally be limited to only a few weeks to minimise the incidence of disinhibition or paradoxical reactions (review by Paton, Psychiatr Bull 2002;**26**:460–2, although the actual incidence may only be < 1%) and the problems of dependence, withdrawal and sedation.

Valproate

Valproate may exert an effect by correcting any abnormally low GABA levels, and a review of 17 studies (none d/b or p/c) indicated valproate has a promising but unproven anti-aggressive effect (n = 164, Lindenmayer and Kotsaftis, J Clin Psychiatry 2000;**61**:123–8). Two open studies have shown valproate effective for impulsive aggressive behaviour in people with personality disorders (n = 10, open, Kavoussi and Coccaro, J Clin Psychiatry 1998;**59**:676–80), and in adults with learning disabilities (n = 28, Ruedrich et al, J Intellect Disabil Res 1999;**43**:105–11). Blood levels above 50mcg/ml seemed most effective.

Reviews: management of agitation and aggression in the elderly (Parks-Veal, Consultant Pharm 1999;**14**:557–60).

■ Unlicensed/possible efficacy

Beta-blockers

Beta-blockers have been reported to help control aggression in learning disabilities (review, Am J Mental Retard 1990;**95**:110–9), autism, schizophrenia and in intermittent explosive disorders eg. pindolol 40–60mg/d (n = 11, d/b, c/o, 6/52, Greendyke and Kanter, J Clin Psychiatry 1986;**47**:423–6). However, they have fallen out of use, not least because of the potential effects on bp and heart-rate (review by Haspel, Harv Rev Psychiatry 1995;**2**:274–81).

Buspirone

Several old studies (eg. Ratey et al, J Clin Psychiatry 1991;**52**:159–62) and case reports (eg. Quiason et al, J Am Acad Child Adolesc Psychiatry 1991;**30**:1026), showed some bene-ficial effect. A three-month trial at 30mg/d seems necessary, and a transient worsening may occur initially (n=20, 3/12, Stanislav et al, J Clin Psychopharmacol 1994;**14**:126–30).

Carbamazepine

Data for the use of carbamazepine in aggression is largely anecdotal and historic, based on the proposed association between aggression and TLE or other EEG abnormalities, but one trial showed 600mg/d to reduce aggressive behaviour with schizophrenia (d/b, RCT, 15/52, Neppe, J Clin Psychiatry 1983;**44**:326–31). It has also been used in paroxysmal behaviour disorder and the elderly demented (n=51, RCT, 6/52, Tariot et al, Am J Psychiatry 1998; **155**:54–61). Beware of an interaction with any concomitant antipsychotics.

Clonidine

In an open study, 150–400mcg/d reduced aggressiveness in 88% of destructive children (n = 17, Kemph et al, J Am Acad Child Adolesc Psychiatry 1993;**32**:577–81), who noted some increases in CSF GABA levels.

Cyproterone

Cyproterone 200mg/d over one month has been successful in several cases (Thibaut et al, Br J Psychiatry 1991;**159**:298–9; Thibaut and Colonna, Am J Psychiatry 1992;**149**:411), but is difficult to use and presents many problems (Byrne et al, Br J Psychiatry 1992;**160**:282–3).

Estrogens (estrogens)

See dementia (1.13).

Gabapentin

Gabapentin has been used in episodic agitation in severely mentally ill patients (n = 11, 6/12, Megna et al, Ann Pharmacother 2002;**36**:12–6). See also dementia (1.13).

Lamotrigine

See dementia (1.13).

Oxcarbazepine *

Oxcarbazepine has improved a variety of measures of impulsive aggressiveness (n = 48[c = 45], RCT, d/b, p/c, 4–10/52, Mattes, J Clin Psychopharmacol 2005;**25**:575–9).

Phenytoin

A prison in-mate trial showed that 300 mg/d phenytoin reduces impulsive aggressive acts but not premeditated attacks (n = 60, d/b, p/c, Barratt et al, J Clin Psychopharmacol 1997; **17**:341–9).

SSRIs

The use of SSRIs may be rational if low serotonin levels associated with aggression can be corrected. Aggression in learning disabilities may also be associated with unrecognised mood disorders, eg. depression. **Citalopram** may be useful, as 20–60 mg/d significantly reduced aggressive incidents with no deterioration or significant side-effects (n = 15, d/b, c/o, 24/52, Vartiainen, Acta Psychiatr Scand 1995;**91**:348–61), and up to 40 mg/d reduced impulsive aggression in children, adolescents (n = 12, open, 6/52, Armentos and Lewis, J Am Acad Child Adolesc Psych 2002;**41**:522–9) and adults (n = 25, open, 8/52, Reist et al, J Clin Psychiatry 2003;**64**:81–5). A similar effect has been suggested with **sertraline** 50–200 mg/d (open, Kavoussi et al, J Clin Psychiatry 1994;**55**:137–41; n = 1, Campbell and Duffy, J Clin Psychiatry 1994;**56**:123–4). There is a case report and study of uncontrollable aggressive outbursts and anger attacks (secondary to stroke), unresponsive to other antidepressants

and antipsychotics, responding rapidly to **fluoxetine** 20 mg/d (Weinman and Ruskin, Am J Psychiatry 1994;**151**:1839; Fava et al, Am J Psychiatry 1993;**150**:1158–63). SSRIs have been used successfully for dementia and chronic aggression after head injury (n = 3, Kim et al, Pharmacother 2001;**21**:498–501).

Vitamins

Nutritional supplements (containing vitamins, minerals and fatty acids) caused dramatic reductions in antisocial behaviour and violent incidents of young offenders within just two weeks (n = 231, RCT, p/c, Gesch et al, Br J Psychiatry 2002;**181**:22–8; complimentary comment by Benton, EBMH 2003;**6**:41).

◆ Others

Other drugs tried include **dexamfetamine** (Cherek et al, Psychopharm 1986;**88**:381–6), the synthetic progestogen **medroxyprogesterone** (n = 3, O'Connor and Baker, Acta Psychiatr Scand 1983;**67**:399–403), **trazodone** (eg. n = 1, Mashiko et al, Psychiatry Clin Neurosci 1996;**50**:133–6) and **tricyclics** (mentioned in Acta Psychiatr Scand 1988;**78**:188–90).

1.3 AGORAPHOBIA

see also Anxiety disorder (1.6), Panic disorder (1.21) and Social anxiety (1.27)

Agoraphobia, an anxiety disorder, is an overwhelming and disabling anxiety provoked by being alone or in places where escape might be difficult or embarrassing and so these situations are avoided. Panic attacks may accompany the phobia and depression may be present in up to a half of patients. A connection with serotonin deficiency has been shown.

Role of drugs

Drug treatment may be effective in many patients, with psychotherapy being an essential component of the treatment package for many. A meta-analysis of 54 published studies has shown that symptoms are improved by tricyclics and high potency benzodiazepines and, although there may be a short-term deterioration, this usually turns to a longer term improvement. The best long-term benefit is from exposure therapy, particularly combined with antidepressants. There is a weak but significant placebo response in drug trials.

Reviews: SSRIs in panic and agoraphobia (Bakker et al, Int Clin Psychopharmacol 2000;15[Suppl 2]:S25–S30).

BNF listed

Citalopram

Citalopram is licensed in the UK for the symptoms of panic disorder, with or without agoraphobia. The dose is 10mg/d for a week, increasing to 20–30mg/d, with a maximum of 60mg/d. The maximal effect may take three months to develop. See panic disorder (1.21).

Escitalopram

Escitalopram is licensed in the UK for the symptoms of panic disorder, with or without agoraphobia (see also 1.21). The dose is 5mg/d for the first week, then 10mg/d (maximum 20mg/d). The maximal effect may take three months to develop.

Paroxetine

Paroxetine is licensed in the UK for the symptoms and prevention of relapse of panic disorder, with or without agoraphobia. It may be less likely to produce 'jitteriness' than tricyclics (n=326, naturalistic, Toni et al, Pharmacopsychiatry 2000; 33:121–31). See panic disorder (1.21).

• Unlicensed/some efficacy

Benzodiazepines

Alprazolam (n=69, 3.5 years, Kilic et al, Psychother Psychosom 1997;66:175–8) and **diazepam** have been used and shown to help, particularly with anxiety symptoms. **Clonazepam** 1–2mg/d has also shown significant efficacy (n=24, RCT, p/c, 6/52, Valenca et al, Arq Neuropsiquiatr 2000;58:1025–9; n=413, RCT, p/c, 16/52, Rosenbaum et al, J Clin Psychopharmacol 1997;17:390–400).

MAOIs

Phenelzine has been studied in agoraphobia with panic attacks and shown to be highly effective at doses of up to 45mg/d (eg. Buigues and Vallejo, J Clin Psychiatry 1987;48:55–9).

Tricyclics

While SSRIs are now first choice, up to 70% may respond to tricyclics, but with 30% dropping out due to side-effects. 20% may worsen, with an increase in panic attacks. **Clomipramine**, at doses up to 300mg/d, has been shown to be effective (n=108, d/b, p/c, 8/52, Johnson et al, Arch Gen Psychiatry 1988;45:453–9), with a continuous improvement shown over many weeks. Doses as low as 75mg/d may be effective (n=17, open, 8/52, Gloger et al, J Clin Psychopharmacol 1989;9:28–32). A relationship between plasma levels and response has been proposed. See also panic (1.21).

■ Unlicensed/possible efficacy

Buspirone

Buspirone has been shown to be well-tolerated and enhance the effect of CBT in panic disorder with agoraphobia (n=41, d/b, 68/52, Cottraux et al, Br J Psychiatry 1995;167:635–41), although a subsequent naturalistic study was unable to replicate this long-term effect (Bouvard et al, Psychother Psychosom 1997;66:27–32).

◆ Others

Other drugs tried include **trazodone** at up to 300mg/d (n=11, Mavissakalian et al, Am J Psychiatry 1987;144:785–7) and **valproate** (Roy-Byrne et al, J Clin Psychiatry 1989;50[Suppl]:S44–S48).

1.4 ALCOHOL DEPENDENCE AND ABUSE

see also Alcohol withdrawal syndrome (1.5)

Symptoms

The main diagnostic symptoms of alcohol dependence are of a primacy of drinking over other activities, increased tolerance of alcohol, symptoms of repeated withdrawal, stereotyped pattern of drinking, compulsion to drink and relief drinking.

Risk factors

Some risk factors for alcohol abuse or being an alcohol-dependent drinker include:

1. Occupation, eg. brewers, reps, doctors, alcohol retailers.
2. Genetics (up to 30–40% influence).

3. Marital/social problems, eg. work.
4. Personality, eg. high anxiety levels.
5. Psychopaths and criminals, eg. taking alcohol before criminal events.
6. Psychiatric illness, eg. depression, phobia, etc.
7. Use for hypnotic or analgesic purposes.
8. Adverse childhood or adolescent experiences, eg. prenatal alcohol exposure (n = 433, Baer et al, Arch Gen Psychiatry 2003;**60**:377–85).
9. Parental misuse of alcohol (n = 2427, Lieb et al, Psychol Med 2002;**32**:63–78).
10. Sweet taste preference (n = 122, Kranzler et al, Am J Psychiatry 2001;**158**:813–5).
11. Following Norwich City FC.

The body metabolises approximately one unit of alcohol per hour (varies between individuals) and peak levels occur one hour after the drink is consumed. One unit gives a man an alcohol blood level of about 15 mg/100 ml and a woman about 20 mg/100 ml. Absorption is rapid with low volume drinks, eg. spirits and slower with higher volumes, eg. beer. Alcohol consumption of 7.7–12.9 units per week is associated with the lowest mortality in men (White, J Clin Epidemiol 1999;**52**:967–75, review by Caan, EBMH 2000; **3**:61), a finding now often quoted in bars throughout the world.

Role of drugs *

Pharmacological treatment can play its part in an overall plan. Any vitamin deficiency needs correcting (see AWS, 1.5). Other drugs may be useful to treat associated psychiatric morbidity, such as withdrawal, affective disorders, suicidal thoughts and hallucinations. In the longer term, disulfiram, naltrexone and acamprosate may have roles to play. **Acamprosate** has a good evidence base, is superior to placebo and is useful as part of a therapeutic approach targeted at achieving abstinence. **Naltrexone** has a good evidence base, is superior to placebo, may be more useful for programmes aimed at controlled consumption, and may be useful with cognitive bahvioural interventions (Garbutt et al, JAMA 1999;**281**:1318–25, 61 refs; reviewed in EBMH 2000;**3**:15). **Disulfiram** probably has limited efficacy. There is no real evidence for lithium or the SSRIs. Combinations of these drugs may be useful but the evidence base is not robust due to the difficulty of carrying out these types of study, eg. high drop-out rates.

Reviews: * pharmacotherapy (Mann, CNS Drugs 2004;**18**:485–504; Anton, J Clin Psychiatry 2001;**62**[Suppl 20]:S11–S17), management of Korsakoffs (Smith and Hillman, Adv Psychiatr Treat 1999;**5**:271–8), recent advances (Swift, N Engl J Med 1999;**340**:1482–90, 99 refs; Garbutt et al, JAMA 1999;**281**:1318–25), haematological changes in alcohol dependence (Drummond and Ghodse, Adv Psychiatr Treat 1999;**5**:366–75, 30 refs), GP review and options (Feeney and Nutt, Prescriber 2000;**11**:21–30; Drug Ther Bull 2000;**38**:60–4, 31 refs).

BNF listed

Acamprosate *

Acamprosate is licensed in some countries for abstinence maintenance therapy for up to one year in motivated alcohol-dependent patients. It is a GABA analogue and may act to reduce the severity and frequency of relapse by enhancing GABA inhibitory neurotransmission and antagonising glutamate excitation by antagonising mGluR5 receptors (De Witte et al, CNS Drugs 2005;**19**:517–37; glutamate receptors increase in chronic alcohol dependency), reducing intake via reduced reward, possibly restoring normal activity of glutaminergic neurons (which become overexcited by alcohol) and reducing craving (n = 29, p/c, 6/52, Weinstein et al, Addict Biol 2003;**8**:229–32). It takes about seven days to reach therapeutic levels and so should be started soon after detoxification (eg. n = 296, RCT, d/b, p/c, 26/52, Gual and Legert, Alcohol Alcohol 2001;**36**:413–8). Continued alcohol consumption negates the therapeutic effect, but occasional lapses do not necessarily do this. Many RCTs have shown clinical effect and a large meta-analysis concluded that acamprosate has a significant beneficial effect in enhancing abstinence in recently detoxified alcohol-dependent individuals (s = 20, n = 4087, Mann et al, Alcohol Clin Exp Res 2004;**28**:51–63) and as part of a therapeutic approach targeted at achieving abstinence (s = 33, Carmen et al, Addiction 2004;**99**:811–28), but there appear to be no predictors of the likelihood of efficacy (s = 7, n = 1485, RCT, p/c, Verheul et al, Psychopharmacol (Berl) 2005;**178**:167–73). Overall, acamprosate is well-tolerated, its efficacy may be enhanced by the addition of disulfiram, may be effective as an adjunct to psychosocial and behavioural therapies (including counselling) and can be considered a promising first-line pharmacological therapy for the maintenance of abstinence in detoxified alcohol dependent patients. It is certainly not a miracle 'cure' for repeatedly failed detoxification patients, and should be combined with continued counselling.

Reviews: * general (Boothby and Doering, *Clin Ther* 2005;**2**7:695–714; Overman et al, *Ann Pharmacother* 2003;**37**:1090–9; Anon, *Drugs* 2002;**3**:13–8; Mason, *J Clin Psychiatry* 2001;**62**[Suppl 20], S42–48), clinical pharmacokinetics (Siavin et al, *Clin Pharmacokinet* 1998;**35**:331–45, 44 refs), mode of action (De Witte et al, *CNS Drugs* 2005;**19**:517–37; Zornoza et al, *CNS Drug Rev* 2003;**9**:359–74).

Disulfiram *

Disulfiram acts as a negative reinforcer for abstinence via the potential for an adversive disulfiram-alcohol interaction, ie. an adversive/conditioning and maintenance therapy in alcoholics. It irreversibly inhibits ALDH (hepatic Aldehyde-NAD reductase) leading to accumulation of acetaldehyde from incomplete alcohol metabolism (Petersen, *Acta Psychiatr Scand* 1992;**369**[Suppl]:S7–S13, see also 4.7.1). A review of 24 studies published from 1967–1995 implied that while disulfiram can reduce total alcohol consumption, studies are poor, patient selection variable and compliance low. Maximum benefit occurs with supervised treatment (Hughes and Cook, *Addiction* 1997; **92**:381–95). Disulfiram seems superior to naltrexone in relapse prevention although

craving was lower with the naltrexone arm (n = 100 [c = 97], RCT, open, one year; De Sousa and De Sousa, *Alcohol Alcohol* 2004;**39**:528–31). One review suggested that the incidence of adverse reactions between alcohol and disulfiram may be as low as 28% (n = 33, retrospective, Mueser et al, *Am J Addict* 2003; **12**:242–52). Some published advice tends to underestimate doses needed so it is suggested to start with a loading dose of 400mg/d, with 365mg/d the average dose used. Disulfiram (200mg/d) may be effective in some adolescents (16–19 years) (n = 26, RCT, d/b, p/c, 3/12, Niederhofer and Staffen, *Drug Alcohol Rev* 2003;**22**:295–7). 'Antabuse®' (Alpharma) tablets are dispersible and so can be given as a liquid in a supervised setting (eg. with relatives, neighbours, clinics etc, *Alcohol Alcoholism* 1986, **21**:385–88). It can also be given as a twice-a-week dose (ie. daily dose x 7 divided by 2), as the enzyme block is irreversible and the clinical effect lasts about 7–10 days.

Reviews: general studies *Br J Psychiatry* 1992; **161**:84–9; *Acta Psychiatr Scand* 1992, **86**[Suppl 369] and compliance improvement, eg. implants, incentives, contracts, patient information, etc, *Alcohol Clin Exp Res* 1992;**16**:1035–41), efficacy (Hughes and Cook, *Addiction* 1997; **92**:381–95).

B vitamins

Vitamin deficiency occurs after chronic alcohol abuse, is due to inadequate diet, impaired absorption, increased metabolic demand and impaired utilisation. Thiamine (B_1) maintenance may be necessary to help reverse the mental confusion secondary to thiamine deficiency (Wernicke's syndrome) (*Lancet* 1990;ii:912–13) but possibly only about 10–20mg is absorbed

---

Disulfiram test dose

A test dose is now considered dangerous due to the risks involved and because the mode of action is via a conditioning process. If considered necessary, wait five days after starting treatment for full enzyme block to occur.
1. Give 10–15ml of 95% alcohol (or 15–25ml spirits).
2. Reaction should start in 5–15 minutes.
3. Repeat in 30 minutes if no reaction. Reaction shows as flushed face, tachycardia, nausea, vomiting, fall in blood pressure. (Have crash box plus personnel available.)
Usual cause of no reaction is too low a dose of disulfiram. Bronchospasm has also been reported (Beri et al, *Br Med J* 1993;**306**:396).

from each oral dose, via a saturable mechanism. See AWS 1.5.

Review: Cook and Thomson (*Br J Hosp Med* 1997;**57**:461–5).

+ Combinations

Acamprosate + disulfiram

In one study, alcoholics were randomised over one year to placebo or acamprosate, and could request additional disulfiram. Disulfiram improved the effectiveness of acamprosate, but a high drop-out did not allow full analysis (n = 118, RCT, Besson et al, *Alcohol Clin Exp Res* 1998;**22**:573–9).

Acamprosate + naltrexone

Combined naltrexone and acamprosate were slightly superior to monotherapy and significantly superior to placebo for time to first drink and time to relapse (n = 160, RCT, d/b, p/c, 12/52, Kiefer et al, *Arch Gen Psychiatry* 2003;**60**:92–9; see also review by Mason of two independent d/b studies: *Eur Neuropsychopharmacol* 2003;**13**:469–75).

Naltrexone + disulfiram *

In a four-arm study, active medication produced lower craving and improved abstinence, but combining naltrexone and disulfiram had no advantage over either agent individually (n = 254, RCT, p/c, 12/52, Petrakis et al, *Biol Psychiatry* 2005;**57**:1128–37).

Ondansetron + naltrexone

A small study indicated the combination was superior to placebo for self-reported drinking and other measures (n = 20, RCT, d/b, 8/52, Ait-Daoud et al, *Alcohol Clin Exp Res* 2001; **25**:847–9).

• Unlicensed/some efficacy

Carbamazepine

A significant long-term effect has been shown on time to first drink and survival rates (n = 29, RCT, 12/12, Mueller et al, *Alcohol Clin Exp Res* 1997;**21**:86–92).

Naltrexone *

Naltrexone has been well studied and may have significant efficacy in alcohol dependence, but the evidence remains contradictory, particularly recently. A systematic analysis concluded that naltrexone is more useful in programmes geared to controlling consumption (s = 33, Carmen et al, *Addiction* 2004; **99**:811–28), possibly because it seems to have little effect on reducing alcohol sampling by abstinent alcoholics, but has a significant effect on reducing subsequent drinking by somehow breaking the desire for the next drink. This may possibly be through blocking the pleasure (or 'high') caused by alcohol and reducing alcohol-seeking behaviour (Volpicelli et al, *Am J Psychiatry* 1995;**152**:613–5), or reduced craving for alcohol (n = 43, O'Malley et al, *Am J Psychiatry* 1996;**153**:281–3). The efficacy may be enhanced by limited psychosocial interventions (n = 111, RCT, p/c, 12/52, Morris et al, *Addiction* 2001;**96**:1565–73), CBT (n = 131, RCT, Anton et al, *Am J Psychiatry* 1999;**156**:1758–64; reviewed by Chick, *EBMH* 2000;**3**:75), medical advice (n = 107, RCT, d/b, p/c, 12/52, Latt et al, *Med J Aust* 2002;**176**:530–4) or targetted naltrexone, ie. prior to situations that might have a high risk of heavy drinking (n = 153, RCT, p/c, 8/52, Kranzler et al, *J Clin Psychopharmacol* 2003;**23**:294–304). Cochrane concludes that naltrexone 50 mg/d significantly decreases relapse in the short-term (NNT = 7), but that medium-term treatment gives no benefit. More long-term, combination and low drop-out trials are needed (RCT = 27, Srisurapanont and Jarusuraisin, *Cochrane Database Syst Rev* 2005;**1**:CD001867). A systematic review and meta-analysis concluded that naltrexone is safe and effective, reduces relapse rates, time to relapse and drinking frequency, suggesting a different application for each drug (s = 33, Bouza et al, *Addiction* 2004;**99**:811–28; comment by Feeney, *EBMH* 2005;**8**:14). There are, however, a number of negative trials, eg. 50 mg/d did not reduce alcohol use or relapse (n = 209, RCT, 12/12, Krystal et al, *N Engl J Med* 2001;**345**:1734–9; comment by Chick, *EBMH* 2002;**5**:80; n = 171, RCT, d/b, p/ c, 12/52, Gastpar et al, *J Clin Psychopharmacol* 2002;**22**:592–8) and, although another trial showed reduced relapse to heavy drinking, this was not statistically significant on any other measure of alcohol consumption (n = 202, p/c, 12/52, Guardia et al, Alcohol Clin Exp Res 2002;**26**:1381–7). Since one trial came to the stunning conclusion that, while naltrexone is only moderately effective in reducing alcohol intake, its efficacy is far greater in people who actually take it (n=97, p/c, Volpicelli et al, Arch Gen Psychiatry 1997;**54**:737–42) a long-acting naltrexone injection (Vivitrex®; n=315, RCT, p/c, DASNDSG, Alcohol Clin Exp Res 2004;**28**:1051–9) may help, eg. 380 mg monthly significantly reduced heavy drinking days (n=627 [c=401], RCT, d/b, p/c, 6/12, Garbutt et al, JAMA 2005;**293**:1617–25; comment by Killeen, EBMH 2005;**8**:100).

Reviews: editorial (Prescrire International 1999; **8**:9–11, 12 refs), general (Anton, J Clin Psychiatry 2001;**62**[Suppl 20]:S11–S17).

Ondansetron

Ondansetron, a 5-HT3 antagonist, at 8 mcg/kg/d was superior to placebo in increasing drink-free days, especially for early-onset (pre-25 years) alcoholism (n=271, RCT, Johnson et al, JAMA 2000;**284**:963–71).

Topiramate *

Topiramate up to 300 mg/d was robustly superior to placebo on all measures of alcohol intake, with an accumulating effect (n=150, RCT, d/b, p/c, 12/52, Johnson et al, Lancet 2003;**361**:1677–85; n=150, RCT, p/c, d/b, 12/52, Johnson et al, Arch Gen Psychiatry 2004; **61**:905–12), and it may be useful for curbing alcohol craving in bipolar PTSD sufferers (n=2, Komanduri, J Clin Psychiatry 2003;**64**:612, letter).

Valproate *

Valproate augmentation of TAU decreased heavy drinking in people with bipolar I with comorbid alcohol dependence, an important finding (n=59, RCT, d/b, p/c, 24/52, Salloum et al, Arch Gen Psychiatry 2005;**62**:37–45; enthusiastic review by Le Fauve, EBMH 2005;**8**:79). A pilot study showed some promise in the treatment of acute alcohol withdrawal and may help some symptoms of protracted abstinence (d/b, p/c, 12/52, Brady et al, Drug Alcohol Depend 2002;**67**:323–30). Valproate may also be a suitable alternative to BDZs in withdrawal due to its lack of abuse potential (n=16, RCT, 6/52, Longo et al, J Addict Dis 2002;**21**:55–64).

■ Unlicensed/possible efficacy

Benzodiazepines

Although not recommended in alcoholics for the very real fear of addiction, benzodiazepines have been advocated if they are able to reduce alcohol dependence (as a 'lesser of two evils' strategy). Any use should be well-documented in the patient's notes.

Buspirone

Two trials in anxious alcoholics have shown reduced anxiety, alcohol consumption and drinking days (n=61, 12/52, Kranzer et al, Arch Gen Psychiatry 1994;**51**:720–31), and a significant reduction in alcohol craving and consumption in motivated patients (n=50, d/b, p/c, Bruno, Psychopathology 1989;**22**[Suppl 1]:S49–S59), but no effect on drinking or anxiety has been noted in two other studies (n=66, Alcohol Clin Exp Res 1992;**16**:1007–13; n=156, RCT, Fawcett et al, Alcohol Clin Exp Res 2000;**24**:666–74).

Gabapentin

Gabapentin may be more effective than trazodone for persistent insomnia in alcoholics (n=55, Karam-Hage and Brower, Psych Clin Neurosci 2003;**57**:542–4).

Mirtazapine *

There is a case report of improvement in alcoholism with adjunctive mirtazapine for depression (n=1, Crockford and White, J Clin Psychiatry 2005;**66**:540).

Nalmefene

Nalmefene 20 mg/d reduced relapse to heavy drinking in alcohol dependence, supporting the view that opioid antagonists are effective (n=105, RCT, Mason et al, Arch Gen Psychiatry 1999;**56**:719–24).

Oxcarbazepine *

In a pilot study, oxcarbazepine was as effective as acamprosate in preventing alcohol relapse and as well-tolerated (n=30, RCT, open, 24/52, Croissant et al, Alcohol Clin Exp Res 2006;**30**:630–5; see also case series by Croissant et al, Pharmacopsychiatry 2004;**37**:306–7).

SSRIs (see also fluvoxamine)

Citalopram has produced a modest (16–17%) but significant reduction in alcoholic drink intake and increase in drink-free days in studies of alcoholics (eg. Naranjo et al, Clin Pharmacol Ther 1992;**51**:729–39), possibly by decreasing desire or reducing the reward (see also n = 62, d/b, p/c, Tiihonen et al, Pharmacopsychiatry 1996;**29**:27–9). Fluoxetine 60mg/d reduced alcoholic and total drink intake compared to placebo and to fluoxetine 40mg/d (n = 29, Naranjo et al, Clin Pharmacol Ther 1990;**47**:490–8), as has fluoxetine 20–40mg/d in alcoholics with co-morbid depression (RCT, n = 51, Cornelius et al, Arch Gen Psychiatry 1997;**54**:700–5; review by Haslam, EBMH 1998;**1**:41) but a larger study failed to reproduce these findings (n = 101, RCT, Kranzler et al, Am J Psychiatry 1995;**152**:391–7).

Review: (Naranjo and Knoke, J Clin Psychiatry 2001;**62**[Suppl 20]:S18–S25).

◆ Others

Other drugs tried include imipramine (n = 60, Am J Psychiatry 1993;**150**:963–5), methylphenidate (Clin Neuropharmacol 1986;**9**:65–70), trazodone (open, n = 25, Janiri et al, Alcohol Alcoholism 1998;**33**:362–5) and piracetam (Barnas et al, Psychopharmacology 1990;**100**:361–5).

✳ No efficacy

Amisulpride

Low dose amisulpride 50mg/d is ineffective in preventing relapse in primary alcohol dependence (n = 71, RCT, d/b, p/c, 6/12, Marra et al, Alcohol Clin Exp Res 2002;**26**:1545–52).

Donepezil

While donepezil was ineffective in one study in reversing Wernicke-Korsakoff's disease memory changes (n = 7, s/b, p/c, c/o, 30/7, Sahin et al, Clin Neuropharmacol 2002;**25**:16–20), high dose donepezil has been reported to help the memory deficits from Korsakoff's psychosis (n = 1, Ing et al, Alcohol Alcohol 2001;**36**:553–5; n = 2, Codina et al, Rev Neurol 2002;**35**:341–5).

Fluvoxamine

Fluvoxamine was worse than placebo on measures of abstinence and relapse (n = 493, RCT, d/b, p/c, 12/12, Chick et al, Drug Alcohol Depend 2004;**74**:61–70).

Flupentixol decanoate

After detoxification, flupentixol decanoate 10mg 2/52 actually increased relapses compared to placebo (85% vs 65% for placebo), and so appears to have no role (n = 281, RCT, d/b, 12/12, Weisbeck et al, Alcohol Alcohol 2001;**36**:329–34).

Lithium

Three trials have shown lack of advantage over placebo (eg. n = 22, d/b, 3/12, Olbrich et al, Nervenarzt 1991;**62**:182–6; n = 156, RCT, 6/12, Fawcett et al, Alcohol Clin Exp Res 2000;**24**:666–74).

Olanzapine

Olanzapine was well-tolerated but ineffective in reducing drinking outcomes (n = 60, RCT, b/d, 12/52, Guardia et al, Alcohol Clin Exp Res 2004;**28**:736–45).

1.5 ALCOHOL WITHDRAWAL SYNDROME (AWS)

see also Alcohol dependence and abuse (1.4)

Symptoms

The presentation of AWS includes psychological symptoms (eg. anxiety, insomnia and restlessness), psychotic symptoms (eg. hallucinations), tremor, sweating, tachycardia, gastrointestinal symptoms, GTC seizures, hallucinations and illusions, clouding of consciousness, delirium tremens (DT) and Wernicke's Encephalopathy (WE). WE is the acute phase, lasting for about 48 hours after the last drink, and results from thiamine (B1) deficiency. If untreated it can lead on to the chronic form (Korsakoff psychosis, KP) characterised by severe short-term memory loss. Fits may first occur within 6–8 hours after cessation of alcohol use and peak at 12–24 hours (chronic alcohol consumption causes adaptation and downregulation of GABA receptors and upregulation of NMDA, so sudden withdrawal leads to hyperexcitability and hence seizures). In DT, seizures may occur (either primary or secondary to hypoglycaemia, hypomagnesaemia or hyponatraemia) as may suicidal ideation, gross disorientation, delusions, violence and marked tremor. DT peaks on the 3rd or 4th day, and physical complications are common, eg. pulmonary infection and hepatic encephalopathy. Risk factors for alcohol withdrawal delirium include concurrent infection, tachycardia, symptoms of withdrawal with blood levels above 1 g/L, and a history of epileptic seizures or delirious episodes (n = 334, Palmstierna et al, Psychiatr Serv 2001;**52**:820–3).

Role of drugs

Seizures and psychiatric disturbances are serious problems and treatment of severe AWS is essential. Withdrawal symptoms in hospital may be underestimated and this may lead to undertreatment. A meta-analysis and practice guideline (Chang and Steinberg, Med Clin North Am 2001;**85**:1191–212) concludes that:

- benzodiazepines are suitable agents for alcohol withdrawal
- dosage should be individualised according to withdrawal severity, comorbidity and history of withdrawal seizures
- beta-blockers, clonidine, carbamazepine ameliorate withdrawal severity but evidence of their effect on delirium and seizures is lacking
- phenothiazines ameliorate withdrawal but are less effective than benzodiazepines in reducing delirium or seizures
- thiamine (IM or IV) should be an additional first-line treatment.

Reviews: management of Korsakoff psychosis (Smith and Hillman, Adv Psychiatr Treat 1999;**5**:271–8), management of acute AWS (Kosten and O'Connor, N Engl J Med 2003;**348**:1786–95), anticonvulsants in AWS (Malcolm et al, Am J Addict 2001;**10**[Suppl]:S16–S23), alcohol-related seizures (Ahmed et al, Hosp Med 2000;**61**:793–6) and in the elderly (Kraemer et al, Drugs Aging 1999;**14**:409–25).

BNF listed

Benzodiazepines

Benzodiazepines are the drugs of choice for treating acute alcohol withdrawal (meta-analysis of 11 RCTs, n = 1286, Holbrook et al, Can Med Ass J 1999;**160**:649–55). Chlordiazepoxide (and diazepam) are the established treatments in the UK. Lorazepam (n = 186, p/c, D'Onofrio et

al, N Engl J Med 1999;**340**:915–9; reviewed in EBMH 1999;**2**:107; plus correspondence from Sosis et al, N Engl J Med 1999;**341**:609–10) has also been used, as it has an intermediate half-life and no active metabolites, both particularly useful in the elderly or those with hepatic damage. Doses may also be adjusted in a more refined, symptom-triggered way, with adequate monitoring of symptoms in patients with particular needs (Saitz et al, JAMA 1994;**272**:519–23 plus editorial 557–8; see also symptom-triggered out-patient detoxification with variable dose chlordiazepoxide, n = 108, Wiseman et al, J Clin Psychiatry 1998;**59**:289–93; and oxazepam, n = 117, RCT, Daeppen et al, Arch Intern Med 2002;**162**:1117–21). Withdrawal symptoms may be underestimated and hence undertreated. Beware of an extended metabolism in liver damage (see 3.6), and of respiratory depression.

Reviews: chlordiazepoxide withdrawal regimens (Chick, Adv Psychiatr Treat 1996;**2**:249–57), chlordiazepoxide vs clomethiazole (Duncan and Taylor, Psychiatr Bull 1996;**20**:601–3), general (Peppers, Pharmacotherapy 1996;**16**:49–58).

Clomethiazole (chlormethiazole) *

Regarded as safe and effective treatment of AWS at up to 16 capsules/d, reducing over five to nine days, it has a low addictive potential (Schied et al, Acta Psychiatr Scand 1986;**73**[Suppl 329]:S136-39). Dependence (mainly psychological) can be seen in some patients on longer-term therapy (Br Med J 1987;**294**:592) and clomethiazole may markedly suppress REM sleep in AWS (n = 20, RCT, p/c, d/b, 13/7, Gann et al, Pharmacopsychiatry 2004;**37**:228-35). The dangers of toxicity may have been exaggerated.

Reviews: clomethiazole home detoxification schedules, and counter to the argument that clomethiazole is highly toxic (Sowerby and Hunter, J Substance Misuse 1997;**2**:62–3, 114–7), general (Duncan and Taylor, Psychiatr Bull 1996;**20**:6013).

Vitamin B supplementation *

Classic signs of vitamin deficiency may only occur in extreme depletion and so are easily missed, being interpreted as intoxication. B vitamins act as co-enzymes for essential carbohydrate metabolism. Deficiency of nicotinamide, riboflavine (B_2) and pyridoxine (B_6) can cause neuropathies. Thiamine (B_1) must be primary and priority treatment to reverse the mental confusion secondary to thiamine deficiency (Wernicke's encephalopathy). Oral thiamine has a saturable absorption mechanism which allows only about 4.5 mg of a single dose to be absorbed. Thiamine 100 mg TDS allows about 13.5 mg to be absorbed, adequate only for mild deficiency. In chronic alcohol misusers oral absorption can be reduced by 70%. Large oral doses are thus ineffective and adequate parenteral therapy should be routine, and is essential to treat or prevent KP (review, Thompson, *Alcohol Alcohol* 2000;**35**[Suppl 1]:S2–S7). Indeed, only 16% patients with WE recovered when given low parenteral thiamine doses (50–100 mg/d) and 20% died (see Thompson et al, *Alcohol Alcohol* 2002;**37**:513–21). The parenteral dose necessary is about 500–1000 mg for three to five days. Although anaphylaxis has been reported with 'Parentrovite®' (Link) the incidence is about one report for every 5000000 IM ampoules used. It may be necessary to administer glucose after thiamine when administering thiamine to prevent Wernicke's Encephalopathy (Chataway and Hardman, *Postgrad Med J* 1995;**71**:249–53).

Reviews: * Thompson et al, *Alcohol Alcohol* 2002;**37**:513–21, McIntosh et al, *Psychiatr Bull* 2005; **29**:94–7.

● Unlicensed/some efficacy

Baclofen *

Baclofen (30 mg/d, n = 15) was as effective as diazepam (n = 19) in uncomplicated AWS (n = 37, RCT, 10/7, Addolorato et al, *Am J Med* 2006;**119**:13–8).

Carbamazepine *

An effective and useful treatment, carbamazepine is probably active via an anti-kindling effect. It is non-addictive and its metabolism is generally little affected by liver dysfunction but may be inhibited by higher doses of alcohol. Carbamazepine may be as potent as clomethiazole in AWS (n = 37, RCT, s/b, Seifert et al, *Addict Biol* 2004;**9**:43–51). Higher blood

levels would thus occur in the same person than if abstinent, so beware of enhanced side-effects (Sternebring et al, *Eur J Clin Pharmacol* 1992;**43**:393–7). It has also been used for outpatient detoxifications due to its safety and lack of abuse potential (Ballard et al, *Br J Psychiatry* 1991;**158**:133), supported by a retrospective study (Franz et al, *Eur Arch Psychiatry Clin Neurosci* 2001; **251**:185–92).

Oxcarbazepine *

A pilot study suggested that oxcarbazepine was more effective than carbazepine in AWS, with less craving (n = 29, RCT, s/b, Schik et al, *Addict Biol* 2005;**10**:283–8).

■ Unlicensed/possible efficacy

Alcohol IV

IV alcohol can be used if aggressive therapy is needed (Anon, *Drug Intell Clin Pharm* 1990; **24**:1120–2).

Antipsychotics

Decreased dopamine activity may occur in DT (*Postgrad Med J* 1990;**66**:1005–9) so care is needed with anti-dopaminergic drugs, as this may aggravate symptoms and lower the seizure threshold. NMS may also occur and not be recognised. Temperature regulation and liver function pose further difficulties.

Beta-blockers

Beta-blockers, such as atenolol and propranolol, may be useful in treating some symptoms of mild to moderate AWS, eg. tachycardia and tremor, and to reduce craving, but are generally not recommended (Neff and McQueen, *Drug Intell Clin Pharm* 1991;**25**:31–2). The variable kinetics of propranolol in cirrhosis and portal hypertension must be considered (Cales et al, *Br J Clin Pharmacol* 1989;**27**:763–70; comparison with diazepam, Worner, *Am J Drug Alcohol Abuse* 1994;**20**:115–24).

Gabapentin *

A gabapentin reduction regimen has been used in out-patient detoxifications, with minimal abuse potential and lack of cognitive impairment (Bozikas et al, *Prog Neuropsychopharmacol Biol Psychiatry* 2002;**26**:197–9). Although gabapentin may be a useful alternative as an adjunct (n = 49, open, retrospective, Voris et al, Subst Abuse 2003;**24**:129–32), augmentation of clomethiazole is well-tolerated but ineffective (n = 61, RCT, d/b, 7/7, Bonnet et al, J Clin Psychopharmacol 2003;**23**:514–19), although it may be as effective as phenobarbital (n = 27, RCT, open, Mariani et al, Am J Addict 2006;**15**:76–84).

Lofexidine

Several studies have shown lofexidine (eg. 0.4mg qds for 2–3 days) to be superior to placebo in controlling withdrawal symptoms (eg. n = 23, Cushman and Sowers, Alcohol Clin Exp Res 1989;**13**:361–4), but in a recent RCT lofexidine appeared as an adjunct to chlordiazepoxide, with more withdrawal, hypotension and adverse effects and poorer retention with the combination compared to chlordiazepoxide alone (n = 72, RCT, Keaney et al, Alcohol Alcohol 2001;**36**:426–30).

Mirtazapine

Adjunctive mirtazapine 30–60mg/d reduced anxiety and depressive symptoms during the detox process (n = 68, 4/52, Liappas et al, J Psychopharmacol 2004;**18**:88–93).

Phenobarbital

Phenobarbital is an anticonvulsant and may help reduce withdrawal tremors (Simon, N Engl J Med 1988;**319**:715–6; Rodgers and Crouch, Am J Health-Sys Pharm 1999;**56**:175–8).

Propofol

Benzodiazepine refractory AWS has been successfully treated with propofol infusion (n = 4, McCowan and Marik, Critical Care Med 2000;**28**:1781–4; n = 1, J Clin Psychiatry 2004; **65**:134–5).

Tiapride

A retrospective study concluded that tiapride has potential efficacy (Franz et al, Eur Arch Psychiatry Clin Neurosci 2001;**251**:185–92).

Valproate *

A review has concluded that only two of the six available studies show a significant effect for valproate and that it should not become a standard treatment (Lum et al,

Ann Pharmacother 2006;**40**:441–8), although adjunctive valproate (500mg TDS) may help reduce benzodiazepine doses in AWS, particularly with more severe withdrawal symptoms (n = 36, RCT, 7/7, Reoux et al, Alcohol Clin Exp Res 2001;**25**:1324–9).

◆ Others

Other drugs tried include **buprenorphine** (for abrupt withdrawal; Fudala et al, Clin Pharmacol Ther 1990;**47**:525–34), **clonidine** (for tremor, tachycardia and hypertension; J Stud Alcohol 1987;**48**:356–70), **dexamethasone** (as 4mg injections; n = 110, Arch Int Med 1991;**114**:705–6), **flumazenil** (for AWS; n = 20, RCT, s/b, Gerra et al, Curr Ther Res 1991;**50**:62–6), **hydroxyzine** (100mg IM every six hours; Dilts et al, Am J Psychiatry 1977;**134**:92), **magnesium sulphate** (Ann Pharmacother 1992;**26**:650–2), **nitrous oxide** (rapid relief of AWS; n = 104, Br J Psychiatry 1991; **159**:672–5), and **phenytoin** (in pre-existing epilepsy; N Engl J Med 1988;**319**:715–6).

＊ No efficacy

Fluvoxamine

A trial of fluvoxamine in alcoholic Korsakoff syndrome showed no therapeutic role and included two apparently fluvoxamine-induced episodes of depression (n = 8, O'Carroll et al, Psychopharmacol 1994;**116**:85–8).

ALZHEIMER'S DISEASE
see Dementia (1.13)

ANOREXIA AND BULIMIA NERVOSA
see Eating disorders (1.16)

1.6 ANXIETY DISORDER
(generalised) — Generalised Anxiety disorder (GAD) includes also Panic disorder (1.21) with or without Agoraphobia (1.3), OCD (1.20) and Social phobia (1.27)

Symptoms

There are numerous symptoms of generalised anxiety disorder (although anxiety can in itself be a symptom of many conditions), but they can be classified into two main groups:

- **Psychological symptoms** include fearful apprehension, irritability, poor concentration, restlessness, being easily fatigued, sensitivity to noise, disturbed sleep (lying awake worrying, waking intermittently, unpleasant dreams, but not usually early morning waking) and poor memory (due to poor concentration).
- **Physical symptoms** are mainly due to overactivity of the sympathetic system or increased muscle tension, eg. gastrointestinal (dry mouth, difficulty swallowing, wind, loose motions, etc), CNS (tinnitus, blurred vision, dizziness), respiratory (constricted chest, difficulty inhaling, overbreathing), cardiovascular (palpitations, heart pain, missed beats, neck throbbing), genitourinary (increased micturition, lack of libido and impotence), muscular tension (tension headache, tremor) and panic attacks (sudden episodes of extreme anxiety or apprehension). Anxiety must be differentiated from depression, early schizophrenia, dementia, drugs/alcohol abuse including withdrawal and physical illness, eg. thyroid dysfunction (n = 169, Simon et al, *J Affect Disord* 2002;**69**:209–17).

Role of drugs *

Anxiolytics used as a 'first-line' measure are quite rational, but it is difficult to assess the longer-term effectiveness of these drugs, as anxiety tends to vary for reasons other than pharmacotherapy. The decision for longer-term treatment must be considered on an individual basis, with the risk:benefit analysis varying with the disability caused by the symptoms and the age of the person. The SSRIs and venlafaxine are effective across the range of anxiety disorders and are generally considered first-line. Initial worsening and rare suicidal ideation can occur so specific monitoring is needed early in treatment. BDZs are effective but use is not recommended by NICE and should only be used in the short-term unless anxiety is treatment-resistant. TCAs, antipsychotics and anticonvulsants can be tried in resistant cases but need an individual risk-benefit assessment. Efficacy should be assessed at 12 weeks and, if successful, continued for six months (BAP evidence-based guidelines Baldwin et al, *J Psychopharmacol* 2005;**19**:567–96). Psychological

interventions include explanations, reassurance, support and, in more persistent conditions, cognitive and behavioural therapy (Hoehn-Saric, *CNS Drugs* 1998;**9**:85–98).

Reviews: * evidence-base for drugs, review (Baldwin et al, *J Psychopharmacol* 2005; **19**: 567–96; Baldwin and Polkinghorn, *Int J Neuropsychopharmacol* 2005;**8**:293–302), pharmacotherapy (s = 48, Mitte et al, *J Clin Psychopharmacol* 2005;**25**:141–50; comment by Swinson, *EBMH* 2005;**8**:111), general (Rickels and Rynn, *J Clin Psychiatry* 2002;**63**[Suppl 14]:S9–S16; Hallström, *Hosp Med* 2000;**61**:8–9; Bell and Wilson, *Prescriber* 2000;**11**:46–8), practical advice on diagnosis and treatment (Birtwistle and Baldwin, *Prescriber* 2001;**12**:89–101), use of antidepressants (Scott et al, *Adv Psychiatr Treat* 2001;**7**:275–82), in primary care (Livingstone and Jarvie, *Prescriber* 2002;**13**:17–28) and in children (Coyle, *N Engl J Med* 2001;**344**:1326–7; *N Engl J Med* 2001;**344**:1279–85).

BNF listed

BENZODIAZEPINES

Benzodiazepines may be extremely useful for chronic anxiety and should not be overlooked (rational defence of BDZ prescribing: Williams and McBride, *Br J Psychiatry* 1998;**173**:361–2). Use of benzodiazepines can be restricted to short-term (up to four weeks) or intermittent courses. Prior benzodiazepine exposure does not predispose patients to more severe discontinuation symptoms in subsequent courses (review, Rickels and Freeman, *J Clin Psychiatry* 2000;**61**:409–13). Although the benzodiazepines have a relative lack of toxicity in overdose, there is some difference between different drugs, eg. temazepam (with rapid absorption and

> Benzodiazepines are indicated for short-term relief of severe anxiety. Other treatment methods should then be started, eg. relaxation, psychotherapy, treating any underlying depression, etc. Caution is advised for the use of benzodiazepines, eg. use for short-term use, and avoid in depression and personality disorder.

high sedative effect) and possibly flurazepam have a greater toxicity in overdose than other benzodiazepines, eg. diazepam, clonazepam, and oxazepam (303 overdose study by Buckley et al, Br Med J 1995;**310**:219–21). All are capable of being fatal in overdose (especially combined with alcohol) and should not be prescribed for patients at high risk of overdose. Users of benzodiazepines are also at greater risk of road-traffic accidents, especially if combined with alcohol (involved in accidents, n = 19 386 over three years, Barbone et al, Lancet 1998;**352**:1331–6). A retrospective review of hip fractures indicated that doses of > 3 mg/d diazepam (or equivalent) increased the risk of hip fractures by 50%, especially after initiation and after more than a month of treatment. Shorter half-life drugs did not appear to reduce the risk (n = 1 222 + 4 888, Wang et al, Am J Psychiatry 2001;**158**:892–8). In the UK, the National Institute for Health and Clinical Excellence (NICE) does not recommend the routine use of benzodiazepines or venlafaxine.

Reviews: guidelines for the clinical use of benzodiazepines (Nelson and Chouinard, Can J Clin Pharmacol 1999;**6**:69–83), advantages and disadvantages, mode of action (Lader, Eur Neuropsychopharmacol 1999;**9**[Suppl 6]:S399–S405; Argyropoulos and Nutt, Prescriber 2001; **12**:21–8), CSM warning about driving (Curr Prob Pharmacovig 1999;**25**:17).

Alprazolam *

Alprazolam (review by Verster and Volkerts, CNS Drug Rev 2004;**10**:45–76) was once claimed to have some antidepressant activity, probably due to inadequate trial design (review by Greenblatt and Wright, Clin Pharmacokinetics 1993;**24**:453–71). From 2063 BDZ overdoses, those with alprazolam (n = 131) were more likely to be admitted to ITUs and it appeared more toxic than other BDZs (n = 2063, Isbister et al, Br J Clin Pharmacol 2004;**58**:88–95).

Chlordiazepoxide

Chlordiazepoxide has a slower onset of action and many active metabolites.

Clobazam

Clobazam is licensed for the short-term (two to four weeks) treatment of anxiety. See entry under epilepsy (1.17.1).

Diazepam

Diazepam is the standard longer-acting benzodiazepine, with sedative, anxiolytic and muscle relaxant properties (among others). It has a long half-life and many active metabolites.

Lorazepam

A shorter-acting benzodiazepine with potent receptor-binding properties. Dependence has been a particular problem with this drug, giving it a bad press.

Oxazepam

A shorter-acting benzodiazepine (the ultimate metabolite of diazepam and some other benzodiazepines) with no active metabolites.

There are many other benzodiazepines available commercially in the UK and elsewhere, eg. **bromazepam, clorazepate, quazepam**.

Non-benzodiazepines

Beta-blockers

Propranolol at 20–60 mg/d may be useful for somatic anxiety symptoms such as tachycardia, sweating, tremor, etc and for short-term problems. Studies have shown propranolol to be less effective than diazepam (n = 26, d/b, p/c, c/o, Hallström et al, Br J Psychiatry 1981;**139**:417–21) and more effective than placebo (n = 57, p/c, Hudson, Br J Clin Pract 1988;**42**:419–26). 80–120 mg/d may be too high a dose in many patients and can lead to cardiac symptoms. The best response appears to be in doses sufficient to reduce resting pulse by 7 bpm (Hallström et al, Br J Psychiatry 1981;**139**:417–21), and in patients presenting with autonomic complaints, eg. palpitations, shortness of breath, sweating, rapid ventilation, etc.

Buspirone *

Buspirone is a non-benzodiazepine anxiolytic with negligible sedative, hypnotic, anticonvulsant and muscle relaxant properties. In general, it is considered as effective as the benzodiazepines in GAD, with a lower incidence of dependence, a better side-effect profile and less memory and cognitive impairment (Pecknold, Drug Saf 1997;**16**:118–32), although it has been noted that the efficacy studies were not performed in patients diagnosed with GAD using current criteria (review, Roerig, *J Am Pharm Assoc* 1999;**39**:811–21). It has a slow onset of action and may be underused, as it needs four weeks at 10mg TDS for optimum efficacy. Buspirone possibly acts on 5-HT$_{1A}$ receptors and has no effect on withdrawal in benzodiazepine-dependent persons. Indeed, patients with GAD who have recently discontinued BDZs may suffer more ADRs and respond slower to buspirone than those who have neither had BDZs nor discontinued more than a month before (n=735, DeMartinis et al, *J Clin Psychiatry* 2000;**61**:91–4). Buspirone does not significantly reduce anxiety symptoms in opioid-dependent individuals (n=36, RCT, p/c, McRae et al, *Am J Addict* 2004;**13**:53–63). It has a low 'peak' effect and so the abuse potential is low and abrupt discontinuation has not been shown to produce withdrawal symptoms. Cochrane concludes that buspirone is superior to placebo but less effective than BDZs (s=36, n=5908, Chessick et al, *Cochrane Database Syst Rev* 2006;**3**:CD006115).

Reviews: general (Apter and Allen, *J Clin Psychopharmacol* 1999;**19**:86–93), clinical pharmacology and therapeutic applications (Fulton and Brogden, *CNS Drugs* 1997;**7**:68–88), pharmacokinetics (Mahmood and Sahajwalla, *Clin Pharmacokinet* 1999;**36**:277–87, 48 refs; Salazar et al, *J Clin Pharmacol* 2001;**41**:1351–8).

Escitalopram *

Escitalopram is now licensed for anxiety, with a 10mg/d starting dose and a 20mg/d maximum. There may be significant improvement of GAD symptoms as early as the first week and the majority of patients responded by week eight with a significant improvement in their functioning (n=315, RCT, d/b, p/c, 8/52, Davidson et al, *Depress Anxiety* 2004;**19**:234–40). Several large studies have shown that escitalopram 10mg/d and 20mg/d are equally effective for GAD and superior to paroxetine and placebo (n=681, RCT, d/b, 12/52, Baldwin et al, *Br J Psychiatry* 2006;**189**:264–72; n=121, d/b, 24/52, Bielski et al, *Ann Clin Psychiatry* 2005;**17**:65–9; pooled results analysis; s=3, n=850, RCT, d/b, d/b, 8/52, Goodman et al, *J Affect Disord* 2005;**87**:161–7; s=3, RCT, p/c, Stein et al, *Ann Clin Psychiatry* 2005;**17**:71–5).

Escitalopram also seems effective in the long-term (n=526[c=299], open, 24/52, Davidson et al, *J Clin Psychiatry* 2005;**66**:1441–6).

Hydroxyzine

Hydroxyzine is a poorly studied antihistamine related to the phenothiazines which may be mildly useful in some cases. Data is scarce but hydroxyzine 50mg/d was as effective as bromazepam (but with less drowsiness) and both were more effective than placebo in GAD (n=334, RCT, d/b, 3/52, Llorca et al, *J Clin Psychiatry* 2002;**63**:1020–7; comment by Akhondzadeh, *EBMH* 2003;**6**:91).

Paroxetine *

Paroxetine is licensed in the UK for GAD, and a number of RCTs have shown 20–50mg/d to be rapidly effective (eg. n=324, RCT, p/c, Pollack et al, *J Clin Psychiatry* 2001;**62**:350–7). Paroxetine 20mg/d may be adequate (n=384, RCT, d/b, p/c, Leibowitz et al, *J Clin Psychiatry* 2002;**63**:66–74; n=278, RCT, d/b, p/c, 12/52, Baldwin et al, *Br J Psychiatry* 2006;**189**:264–72) and 40mg/d may be only slightly more effective than 20mg/d (n=566, RCT, d/b, p/c, 8/52, Rickels et al, *Am J Psychiatry* 2003;**160**:749–56). Paroxetine was also effective and well-tolerated for long-term management of GAD and reduces relapse (n=652, d/b, p/c extension, 32/52, Stocchi et al, *J Clin Psychiatry* 2003;**64**:250–8; MS).

Reviews: * overview of studies (s=4, n=1800, RCT, d/b, p/c, Rickels et al, *J Clin Psychiatry* 2006;**67**:41–7), use in anxiety (Snyderman et al, *Expert Opin Pharmacother* 2004;**5**:1799–806).

Pregabalin *

Pregabalin is newly licensed for anxiety and 300mg/d was reasonably well-tolerated, significantly superior to placebo and equivalent to alprazolam in GAD (n=454, RCT, d/b, p/c, 4/52, Rickels et al, *Arch Gen Psychiatry* 2005;**62**:1022–30). Pregabalin 400mg/d is well-tolerated, and equivalent to venlafaxine for anxiety (n=21, RCT, d/b, p/c, 6/52, *J Clin Psychiatry* 2006;**67**:771–82; MS). It may also be a quick-acting anxiolytic with few withdrawal symptoms, when compared to lorazepam (n=276, RCT, p/c, 6/52, Pande et al, *Am J Psychiatry* 2003;**160**:533–40).

Venlafaxine XL *

Venlafaxine (as Efexor® XL, Wyeth) is licensed for GAD and 75 mg/d is considered to be the optimum dose (Melichar et al, J Psychopharmacol 2001;**15**:9–12). For long-term treatment of GAD, 75 mg and 150 mg/d (but not 37.5 mg/d) have both been shown to be superior to placebo, showing a sustained effect (n=541, p/c, d/b, 24/52, Allgulander et al, Br J Psychiatry 2001;**179**:15–22, MS; n=377, RCT, 8/52, Rickels et al, Am J Psychiatry 2000;**157**:968–74; Feighner et al, J Affect Disord 1998;**47**:55–62). It is also effective for depression with anxiety, eg. 75–225 mg/d was slightly more effective than fluoxetine (20–60 mg/d) in 92 patients with co-morbid GAD and MDD (n=368, 12/52, Silverstone and Salinas, J Clin Psychiatry 2001;**62**:523–9; see also n=359, RCT, Silverstone and Ravindran, J Clin Psychiatry 1999;**60**:22–8). Higher doses are not routinely recommended but can be used, eg. venlafaxine up to 225 mg/day was superior to placebo in non-depressed outpatients with generalised anxiety disorder (n=251, RCT, 6/52, Gelenberg et al, JAMA 2000;**283**:3082–8). In a Wyeth pooled analysis of the five RCTs, venlafaxine was found to be as well-tolerated and effective in older adults for anxiety as in younger adults (n=1839, Katz et al, J Am Geriatr Soc 2002;**50**:18–25).

Review: * general (Thase, Expert Rev Neurother 2006;**6**:269–82).

● Unlicensed/some efficacy

Antipsychotics *

Antipsychotics have little proven efficacy and marked side-effects. Some atypicals have been used but the evidence for this currently makes it a costly strategy, eg. olanzapine PRN is an expensive antihistamine. The use of PRN anti-psychotics makes assessment of the underlying causes of agitation more difficult, especially as akathisia can be a side-effect. Antipsychotics should be used carefully and only for infrequent, sustained agitation (review by Druckenbrod et al, Ann Pharmacother 1993;**27**:645–8). Adjunctive low-dose **risperidone** (0.5–1.5 mg/d) was superior (but not statistically) to placebo as add-on to existing anxiolytics (n=40, RCT, d/b, p/c, 5/52, Brawman-Mintzer et al, J Clin

Psychiatry 2005;**66**:1321–5), and up to 3 mg/d may be useful in refractory anxiety disorders (n=30[c=21], open, 8/52, Simon et al, J Clin Psychiatry 2006;**67**:381–5).

Mirtazapine *

Mirtazapine (15–45 mg/d) has been shown to be effective within a week for the symptoms of GAD with comorbid depression (n=10, open, 8/52, Goodnick et al, J Clin Psychiatry 1999;**60**:446–8). Mirtazapine 30 mg produced response in 78% and remission in 36% in a pilot study (n=44, open, 12/52, Gambi et al, J Psychopharmacol 2006;**20**:483–7) and 15 mg/d may be as effective as diazepam 10 mg/d in reducing insomnia and anxiety when given the night before surgery (Sorensen et al, Acta Psychiatr Scand 1985;**71**:339–46; see also an outpatient study: n=40, d/b, p/c, Sitsen and Moors, Drug Invest 1994;**8**:339–44).

SSRIs

(see also paroxetine and escitalopram)

SSRIs have some efficacy in anxiety, with paroxetine and escitalopram licensed. Lower doses may be needed initially, as SSRIs may increase symptoms over the first 1–2 weeks of treatment. **Citalopram** has been shown to be effective in 85% patients with GAD, including some who had failed with other SSRIs (n=13, 12/52, Varia and Rauscher, Int Clin Psychopharmacol 2002;**17**:103–7), and also in children (n=17, open, Prince et al, Psychopharmacol Bull 2002;**36**:100–7). **Fluvoxamine** CR was superior to placebo for anxiety in adults, with few sexual side-effects (n=300, RCT, d/b, p/c, 12/52, Westenberg et al, J Clin Psychopharmacol 2004;**24**:49–55) and it may be mildly effective for anxiety in children and adolescents (n=128, RCT, 8/52, RUPPAS, N Engl J Med 2001:**344**:1279–85; critique by Hazell, EBMH 2001;**4**:116). **Sertraline** 50–150 mg/d was more effective than placebo for GAD (n=370, RCT, d/b, p/c, 12/52, Allgulander et al, Am J Psychiatry 2004;**161**:1642–9), including acute treatment (n=326, RCT, d/b, p/c, 10/52, Brawman-Mintzer et al, J Clin Psychiatry 2006;**67**:874–81) and 50 mg/d may be safe and effective in children and adolescents with GAD (n=22, aged 5–17 years, RCT, d/b, 9/52, Rynn et al, Am J Psychiatry 2001;**158**:2008–14).

Tricyclic antidepressants

Although not recommended by NICE, tricyclics may be useful for persistent or disabling anxiety that is not part of an adjustment/stress reaction. They may take several weeks to act but may be very potent, eg. imipramine may be at least as effective as diazepam and trazodone in generalised anxiety, although the antidepressants had more side-effects, such as akathisia (n = 230, d/b, p/c, 8/52, Rickels et al, Arch Gen Psychiatry 1993;**50**:884–95).

■ Unlicensed/possible efficacy

Duloxetine *

A sub-analysis of four RCTs in depression suggested some potential effects on anxiety subcomponents of the HAMD-17 score (s = 4, RCT sub-analysis, Depress Anxiety 2003;**18**:53–61).

Gabapentin

In patients with a history of alcohol dependency or abuse, gabapentin 100–900mg/d may produce sustained clinical improvement in symptoms of anxiety (n = 4, Pollack et al, Am J Psychiatry 1998,**155**,992–93; review by Norton and Quarles, Hosp Pharm 2001;**36**:843–5, 12 refs). Gabapentin 800mg has reduced public-speaking provoked anxiety (n = 32, d/b, p/c, de-Paris et al, J Psychopharmacol 2003;**17**:184–8).

Kava kava

Kava kava has been reported to be as effective as sub-therapeutic buspirone and a drug I'd never heard of (opipramol), with a 75% response rate for all treatment arms which must say something about the illness severity in the trial (n = 129, RCT, 8/52, d/b, Boerner et al, Phytomedicine 2003;**10**[Suppl 4]:S38–S49).

Passionflower

Passionflower has an anxiolytic effect, with a low incidence of drowsiness compared to oxazepam (n = 36, RCT, d/b, p/c, 4/52, Akhondzadeh et al, J Clin Pharm Ther 2001;**26**:363–7).

Quetiapine *

Quetiapine 150–300mg/d monotherapy may have some efficacy in anxiety (n = 13[c = 10], open, 12/52, Schutters et al, J Clin Psychiatry 2005;**66**:540–2).

Riluzole *

Riluzole 100mg/d was rapidly effective in 80%, producing remission in 53% over 2–3 weeks (n = 18[c = 15], open, 8/52, Mathew et al, Am J Psychiatry 2005;**162**:2379–81).

Testosterone

Undiagnosed hypogonadism presenting as GAD has been treated successfully with testosterone injections (n = 1, Cooper and Ritchie, Am J Psychiatry 2000;**157**:1884).

Tiagabine *

Tiagabine up to 16mg/d (mean 10mg/d) was as effective as paroxetine in GAD (n = 40, open, RCT, 10/52, Rosenthal, J Clin Psychiatry 2003;**64**:1245–9). Response was noted in 76% patients who took tiagabine 8–20mg/d (mean 13mg/d) as adjunctive therapy for anxiety (n = 18[c = 17], open, 8/52, Schwartz et al, Ann Clin Psychiatry 2005;**17**:167–72). However, in the major RCT tiagabine had no significant effect on GAD using LOCF, although one sub-analysis suggested some efficacy in some patients (n = 266, RCT, d/b, p/c, 8/52, Pollack et al, J Clin Psychiatry 2005;**66**:1401–8).

Trazodone

Trazodone has been claimed to be equipotent with some benzodiazepines, eg. a trial showed trazodone to be at least as effective as diazepam and imipramine in generalised anxiety, although the antidepressants had more side-effects (n = 230, d/b, p/c, 8/52, Rickels et al, Arch Gen Psychiatry 1993;**50**:884–95).

Valproate

There has been some speculation that valproate may have anxiolytic actions (Am J Psychiatry 1990;**147**:950–1) via an effect of enhancing GABA.

◆ Others

Other drugs tried include **barbiturates** (such as amylobarbital), **mianserin** (n = 106, d/b, 6/52, Bjertnaes et al, Acta Psychiatr Scand 1982;**66**:199–207; Murphy, Br J Clin Pharmacol 1978;**5**:S81–S85), **nabilone** (n = 8, RCT, Glass et al, J Clin Pharmacol 1981;**21**[Suppl 8–9]:S383–

S96) and **St John's wort** (n = 100, d/b, 2/52, Panijel, *Therapiewoche* 1985;**41**:4659–68).

✳ No efficacy

Caffeine

Caffeine consumption should be calculated in anxiety (*see Caffeinism 1.30*), as higher intakes can cause nervousness, anxiety, restlessness, irritability and palpitations, probably by an abnormal sensitivity to caffeine (Bruce *et al*, *Arch Gen Psychiatry* 1992;**49**:867–9) via antagonism of adenosine receptors (*Arch Gen Psychiatry* 1985;**42**:233–43). One study, however, of chronic schizophrenic in-patients showed no change in anxiety when caffeine was removed from the diet (n = 26, Mayo *et al*, *Br J Psychiatry* 1993;**162**:543–5).
Review: anxiogenic effects of caffeine (Bruce, *Postgrad Med J* 1990;**66**[Suppl 2]:S18–S24).

Homeopathy

Classical homeopathy was no different in one study to placebo, although both groups had high response rates (n = 44, RCT, d/b, p/c, 10/52, Bonne *et al*, *J Clin Psychiatry* 2003;**64**:282–7).

Ondansetron

One study showed 4 mg/d to be no better than placebo, although placebo response was high (n = 97, RCT, Romach *et al*, *J Clin Psychopharmacol* 1998;**18**:121–31).

Yohimbine

Yohimbine increases self-rated anxiety in anxiety-prone children (n = 32, Sallee *et al*, *Am J Psychiatry* 2000;**157**:1236–42).

1.7 ATTENTION DEFICIT HYPER-ACTIVITY DISORDER (ADHD), including HYPERKINETIC DISORDER

Symptoms ✳

Attention deficit hyperactivity disorder (ADHD) is characterised by a developmentally inappropriate degree of gross motor activity, impulsivity, inattention to detail and temper outbursts. Children with ADHD have extreme and persistent restlessness, sustained and prolonged motor activity and difficulty in organising and maintaining attention to work or play. They are impulsive, easily distracted, fidget, careless, reckless, prone to accidents, have learning difficulties (partly due to poor concentration) and often have antisocial behaviour and a fluctuating mood. Onset is before seven years of age. Symptoms usually fade out by puberty but learning and concentration difficulties and antisocial behaviour may persist into adult life and may, but not always, lead to poor achievement. Predisposing factors include obstetric complications and psychosocial adversity. Studies implicate dysregulation of frontal-subcortical-cerebellar catecholamine circuits, including abnormal dopamine transport and impaired neurotransmission (Biederman and Faraone, *Lancet* 2005;**366**:237–48).

Role of drugs ✳

Pharmacotherapy is useful for the treatment of severe hyperkinesis or in those resistant to non-drug measures as part of a treatment package. A robust study of medication and/or behavioural therapy in children (7–10 years) with ADHD indicated strongly that careful medication management was effective in reducing core ADHD symptoms, was superior to behavioural therapy and, with some limited evidence, that the combination was more effective than either alone or some indirect outcome measures (n = 579, NTA-CG, *Arch Gen Psychiatry* 2000;**56**:1073–86; review by Sawyer and Graetz, *EBMH* 2000;**3**:82). The main medicine management strategy is the use of stimulants and a major meta-analysis has shown robust and consistent evidence that stimulants are more effective than placebo for improving overt and covert aggressive behaviours in ADHD (s = 28, n = 683, Connor *et al*, *J Am Acad Child Adolesc Psych* 2002;**41**:253–61; comment by Klein, *EBMH* 2002;**5**:108). Methylphenidate is clearly the first-line stimulant and a meta-analysis of 62 RCTs (n = 2897) shows short-acting methylphenidate is effective in under 18s (but unproven beyond that: Schachter *et al*, *CMAJ* 2001;**165**:1475–88; review by Connor, *EBMH* 2002;**5**:50). Stimulants have an immediate effect compared to a delayed effect from noradrenergic agents, eg. pemoline and antidepressants (Wilens *et al*, *J Atten Disord* 2002;**5**:189–202). Lack of response to one stimulant does not necessarily predict lack of response to a different one (eg. Elia *et* *al, Psychiatry Res* 1991;**36**:141–55). There is a natural reluctance by many prescribers to use stimulants in younger children and so mild symptoms should be treated with environmental changes, but moderate to severe symptoms may require drug therapy. Combining psychosocial treatment with methylphenidate may make no difference to stimulant responsive children with ADHD (n = 103, RCT, 24/12, Abikoff *et al, J Am Acad Child Adolesc Psychiatry* 2004;**43**:802–11; comment by Scahill, *EBMH* 2005;**8**:9).

Reviews: * extensive overviews (meta-analysis, Klassen *et al, Can J Psychiatry* 1999;**44**:1007–16; various, *J Clin Psychiatry* 1998 [Suppl 7], 3–79), general (Olfson, *Am J Manag Care* 2004;**10**(Suppl 4):S117–S24; Williams *et al, Br J Gen Pract* 1999;**49**:563–71, 167 refs; McNicholas and Gringras, *Prescriber* 2000;**5**:19–29), ADHD in adults (Ashton *et al, J Psychopharmacol* 2006; **20**:602–10, Maidment, *J Psychopharmacol* 2003; **17**:332–6; 28 refs; Gadow and Weiss, *Arch Gen Psychiatry* 2001;**58**:784–5), problems in the management of ADHD (Zametkin and Ernst, *N Engl J Med* 1999;**340**:40–7, 39 refs), stimulants vs atomoxetine (s = 5, Gibson *et al,Ann Pharmacother* 2006;**40**:1134–42).

NB: Drug trials need to be interpreted carefully as different diagnostic criteria have been used in different studies.

BNF listed

Atomoxetine *

Atomoxetine is a noradrenaline reuptake inhibitor (NARI) with minimal effects on other transmitters. Efficacy in ADHD has been shown in a number of RCTs (eg. n = 291, two studies, RCT, d/b, p/c, 12/52, Spencer *et al, J Clin Psychiatry* 2002;**63**:1140–7). Atomoxetine takes 3–4 weeks to work, so if switching from a stimulant you may need to keep the stimulant going for a few weeks while the atomoxetine kicks in. Once daily dosing of atomoxetine seems equally effective and as well-tolerated as twice a day (n = 218, RCT, d/b, Adler *et al, Ann Clin Psychiatry* 2006;**18**:107–13; n = 153, RCT, p/c, 7/52, Weiss *et al, J Am Acad Child Adolesc Psychiatry* 2005;**44**:647–55, MS; comment by Barton, *EBMH* 2006;**9**:7) and may be effective throughout the day, including the next morning, unlike methylphenidate (n = 197, RCT, d/b, p/c,

8/52, Kelsey *et al, Pediatrics* 2004;**114**:1–8, MS). In a meta-analysis of long-term follow-up data, atomoxetine had only a minor effect on height, with none on those with the lowest height (n = 412, >2 years, Spencer *et al, Pediatrics* 2005;**116**:74–80). Atomoxetine was superior to placebo in maintaining response over 9/12 for people who responded in an open-label treatment phase (n = 416, RCT, d/b, p/c, 9/12, Michelson *et al, J Am Acad Child Adolesc Psychiatry* 2004;**43**:896–904, MS). Atomoxetine has also been shown to be effective in adults (two RCTs reported together, n = 280 + 256, RCT, d/b, p/c, 10/52, Michelson *et al, Biol Psychiatry* 2003;**53**:112–20, MS; see also n = 384, two years, Adler *et al, J Clin Psychiatry* 2005;**66**:294–9; MS). Atomoxetine does not seem to make tics worse in ADHD with comorbid tic disorders (n = 148, RCT, d/b, p/c, < 18/52, Allen *et al, Neurology* 2005;**65**:1941–9; MS). Atomoxetine is non-stimulant, with minimal abuse potential (comparison with methylphenidate, n = 16, d/b, p/c, Heil *et al, Drug Alcohol Depend* 2002;**67**:149–56) and no discontinuation syndrome (Wernicke *et al,J Clin Psychopharmacol* 2004;**24**:30–5, MS). In 2006, the UK MHRA issued guidance that patients should be monitored for signs of depression, suicidal thoughts or suicidal behaviour and referred for appropriate treatment if necessary, as increased suicidal thoughts or behaviour have been in association with atomoxetine (s = 12, n = 1357), although the incidence was only 0.4% and with no completed suicides.

Reviews: * general (Christman *et al, Pharma-cotherapy* 2004;**24**:1020–36; Barton, *Arch Dis Child* 2005;**90**(Suppl 1);26–9; Corman *et al, Am J Health Syst Pharm* 2004;**61**:2391–9).

Dexamfetamine

Amfetamine is clearly superior to placebo on a variety of key measures, remaining effective over the 15 months in one trial (n = 62, RCT, Gillberg *et al, Arch Gen Psychiatry* 1997;**54**:857–64; review by Hall, *EBMH* 1998;**1**:86). A trial of dexamfetamine in adults with ADHD showed a significant effect in the short-term, with more data needed to justify long-term therapy (n = 68, RCT, Paterson *et al, Aust N Z J Psychiatry* 1999;**33**:494–502). Exacerbation of chronic tic disorder by methylphenidate or dexamfetamine has not been shown over at least one year (n = 19, d/b, p/c, Nolan et al, Pediatrics 1999;103:730–7).

Methylphenidate *

At appropriate doses of methylphenidate (10–80 mg/d), a large proportion of children (and adults: Spencer et al, Arch Gen Psychiatry 1995;52:434–43) with ADHD obtain re-mission of symptoms. Methylphenidate's mode of action may be blockade of central dopamine transporters (Volkow et al, Am J Psychiatry 1998;155:1325–31), and/or may enhance the motivation to complete a task by increasing dopamine (n = 16, Volkow et al, Am J Psychiatry 2004;161:1173–80). Predictors of a positive response include younger age, demonstrable inattention, normal or near normal IQ, low anxiety (Buitelaar et al, J Am Acad Child Adolesc Psychiatry 1995; 34:1025–32), high levels of hyperactivity at school and relatively low age (n = 36, RCT, Zeiner et al, Acta Pediatr 1999;88:298–303). The new SR preparations (eg. Concerta® XL, Janssen-Cilag) have made dosing much easier (n = 321, RCT, d/b, p/c, Greenhill et al, ADHD Study Group, Pediatrics 2002;109:E39; OROS system equivalent to TDS: n = 282, RCT, Wolraich et al [Concerta Study Group], Pediatrics 2001;108:883–92). The response to methylphenidate in ADHD does not appear to be moderated by co-morbid anxiety (n = 91, RCT, 4/12, Diamond et al, J Am Acad Chold Adolesc Psychiatry 1999;38:402–9; reviewed in EBMH 1999;2:108). Methylphenidate (along with psychosocial treatment) may improve daily academic performance, 17% in one study (n = 45, RCT, p/c, 6/52, Evans et al, Exp Clin Psychopharmacol 2001;9:163–75). In adult ADHD, 'robust' dosing (mean 1 mg/kg/d) may be highly effective (response 76% vs 19% placebo) compared to more traditional dosing (n = 146, RCT, d/b, p/c, 6/52, Spencer et al, Biol Psychiatry 2005;57:456–63; n = 45, RCT, d/b, p/c, c/o, Kooij et al, Psychol Med 2004;34:973–82). Although some tics have been reported to worsen with methylphenidate (Gadow et al, Arch Gen Psychiatry 1995;52:444–55), normal doses probably neither cause nor exacerbate tics

(n = 91, p/c, d/b, Law and Schachar, J Am Acad Child Adolesc Psychiatry 1999;38:944–51; reviewed in EBMH 2000;3:31).

Reviews: pharmacokinetics and efficacy (Kimko et al, Clin Pharmacokinet 1999;37:457–70, 75 refs), side-effects (review, Rappaport and Moffitt, Clin Psychol Rev 2002;22:1107–31).

● Unlicensed/some efficacy

Bupropion *

There is a growing body of evidence supporting the use of bupropion in ADHD. Bupropion XL up to 450 mg/d was effective (53% vs 31% for placebo) for ADHD, providing well-tolerated and sustained benefit throughout the day (n = 162, RCT, d/b, p/c, 8/52, Wilens et al, Biol Psychiatry 2005;57:793–801). Bupropion (mean 3.3 mg/kg/d) and methylphenidate (mean 0.7 mg/kg/d) were equipotent in children with ADHD in one trial (n = 15, RCT, 6/52, Barrickman et al, J Am Acad Child Adolesc Psychiatry 1995;34:649–57), and in adolescents with substance misuse disorders (n = 13, open, 5/52, Riggs et al, J Am Acad Child Adolesc Psychiatry 1998;37:1271–8), and thus provides a pharmacological alternative to stimulants in ADHD (review, Popper, Child Adolesc Psychiatr Clin North Am 2000;9:605–46). Use in adult ADHD has also been investigated. Bupropion and methylphenidate were superior (but not statistically) to placebo in adult ADHD (n = 30, RCT, d/b, p/c, 7/52, Kuperman et al, Ann Clin Psychiatry 2001;13:129–34) and bupropion up to 400 mg/d was clinically and significantly superior (76% improved) to placebo (37% improved) and, although the exclusion criteria were unclear, further trials are warranted (n = 40, RCT, 6/52, Wilens et al, Am J Psychiatry 2001;158:282–8; reviewed by Ferre and Nutt, EBMH 2001;4:92).

Clonidine

Clonidine has been widely used for ADHD, especially if resistant to stimulants. A thorough meta-analysis of 11 studies indicates that clonidine 0.1–0.3 mg/d has a moderate effect in reducing core ADHD symptoms (better in those without comorbid disorders), although less effective than stimulants, and associated with many side-effects (although obviously not the stimulant ADRs). Parents' efficacy ratings correlated negatively with the sedation caused by clonidine (n = 150, Connor et al, J Am Acad Child Adolesc Psychiatry 1999;**38**:1551–9; reviewed by Greenhill, EBMH 2000;**3**:74). Clonidine augmentation of psychostimulants can be used to improve conduct, but not hyperactivity, and may reduce stimulant adverse effects (n = 67, RCT, p/c, 6/52, Hazell and Stuart, J Am Acad Child Adolesc Psychiatry 2003;**42**:886–94). Most studies are small and a large RCT is needed to identify its role (review, Chafin et al, J Pediatr Pharm Pract 1999;**4**:308–15, 32 refs).

Modafinil *

Modafinil appears to be promising in ADHD, eg. once-daily modafinil (170–425 mg/d) was effective in children and adolescents on all rating systems, and well-tolerated (n = 246, RCT, d/b, p/c, 9/52, Biederman et al, Pediatrics 2005;**116**:777–84; positive comment by Barr and Clarke, EBMH 2006;**9**:68). Modafinil significantly improves ADHD symptoms at school and home and no withdrawal symptoms were seen on abrupt withdrawal (n = 190, RCT, d/b, p/c, 9/52, Swanson et al, J Clin Psychiatry 2006;**67**:137–47), with once daily dosing better tolerated than divided doses (n = 248 [c = 223], RCT, d/b, p/c, 4/52, Biederman et al, J Clin Psychiatry 2006;**67**:727–35).

Selegiline *

In an active comparison, selegiline and methylphenidate were equally effective for child and adolescent ADHD (n = 40, RCT, 60/7, Mohammadi et al, J Child Adolesc Psychopharmacol 2004;**14**:418–25).

Tricyclics

Tricyclics are considered useful in patients non-responsive or intolerant of stimulants. Imipramine, clomipramine, nortriptyline and desipramine have been used in doses of 10–150 mg/d (mean 80 mg). In a retrospective, naturalistic study, tricyclics were shown to be effective at antidepressant doses (n = 37, Wilens et al, J Nerv Ment Dis 1995;**183**:48–9), although other authors have suggested that lower doses (eg. 25–50 mg/d) are effective (Ratey et al, J Child Adolesc Psychopharmacol 1992;**2**:267–75). They produce drowsiness and

irritability, but are less likely to cause insomnia than stimulants. Sudden death, including cardiac arrest, has been reported with relatively low plasma levels (Riddle et al, J Am Acad Child Adolesc Psychiatry 1991;**30**:104–8) and so close monitoring is warranted.

■ Unlicensed/possible efficacy

Antipsychotics *

Some antipsychotics have been used for uncontrollable and explosive behaviour, but their side-effect profile makes them unsatisfactory and potentially dangerous. This potential for long-term side-effects and worsening cognitive learning function usually outweighs their potential advantages. Risperidone may be at least as effective as methylphenidate for ADHD in children and adolescents with moderate learning disabilities (n = 45, s/b, 4/52, Filho et al, J Am Acad Child Adolesc Psychiatry 2005;**44**:748–55; see also Hardan et al, J Am Acad Child Adolesc Psychiatry 1996;**35**:1551–6).

Buspirone

A pilot study suggested buspirone may help hyperactive behaviour in ADHD (n = 8, Niederhofer, Hum Psychopharmacol 2003; **18**: 489–92).

Fluoxetine

Serotonin function may be abnormal in ADHD (Fargason and Ford, South Med J 1994;**87**:302–9) and fluoxetine 20–60 mg/d may produce some statistical improvements in some rating scales (n = 22, open, Barrickman et al, J Am Acad Child Adolesc Psychiatry 1991;**30**:762–7).

Gabapentin

A number of case reports exist, eg. aggression, temper and violence responded almost completely ('a miracle') to gabapentin 900 mg/d in a 15-year-old boy with ADHD (among other diagnoses) resistant to other therapies (n = 1, Ryback and Ryback, Am J Psychiatry 1995;**152**:1399). There is a report of rapid and marked improvement with 200 mg/d as an adjunct to methylphenidate (n = 1, Hamrin and Bailey, J Child Adolesc Psychopharmacol 2001;**11**:301–9).

Lithium

In adult ADHD, lithium (up to 1200mg/d) was equivalent to methylphenidate (up to 40mg/d) on most outcome measures in one study (RCT, d/b, c/o, 16/52, Dorrego et al, J Neuropsychiatry Clin Neurosci 2002;14:289–95).

MAOIs

MAOIs are not considered as effective as stimulants but may help some non-responders, eg. tranylcypromine has been considered as effective as stimulants but the dietary restrictions proved too difficult to manage.

Nicotine

Daily transdermal nicotine reduced hyperactivity and learning problems in a pilot study, but was poorly tolerated and so other methods of nicotinic receptor modulation may be worth investigating (n = 10, RCT, d/b, p/c, 2/52, Shytle et al, World J Biol Psychiatry 2002;3:150–5).

Reboxetine *

Reboxetine may have some efficacy in stimulant-resistant ADHD (n=31, RCT, open, 6/52, Ratner et al, J Am Acad Child Adolesc Psychiatry 2005;44:428–33).

Venlafaxine

There may be a possible role in child and adult ADHD at 56.25–300mg/d (n = 10, open, Findling et al, J Clin Psychiatry 1996;57:184–9; case reports by Pleak and Gormly, Wilens et al, Am J Psychiatry 1995;152:1099–100).

Zinc *

There is some evidence for zinc's efficacy (review by Arnold and DiSilvestro, J Child Adolesc Psychopharmacol 2005;15:619–27).

◆ Others

Other drugs tried include **levodopa/carbidopa** (Pediatr Ann 1985;14:383–400) and **thyroid** (n = 1, N Engl J Med 1993;328:997–1001).

✳ No efficacy

Barbiturates

These have been tried but excitation and agitation may be counter-productive.

Benzodiazepines

As for barbiturates.

Caffeine

Caffeine is ineffective as a minor stimulant (Dulcan, Pediatr Ann 1985;14:383–400).

Donepezil *

Adjunctive donepezil seems poorly tolerated and ineffective for residual ADHD and cognitive symptoms (n = 13 [c = 7], open, 12/52, Wilens et al, J Child Adolesc Psychopharmacol 2005;15:947–55).

1.8 AUTISTIC DISORDER

Symptoms

Autism is a neurodevelopmental disorder, characterised by an excessive or morbid dislike of others or society, not responding with normal human emotions towards other people, a morbid self-centred attitude and with major impairments or abnormalities in language, communication, reciprocity, social interactions, imagination and behaviour. The main features include 'autistic aloneness', poor speech and language development, an obsessive desire for sameness, bizarre behaviour or mannerisms, a restricted repertoire of activities and interests, rituals and compulsive behaviour. Onset is not later than three years of age, the incidence four in 10000, or up to 20 in 10000 if including associated conditions (Gillberg and Wing, Acta Psychiatr Scand 1999;99:399–406). Up to 25% develop seizures in adolescence, 75% have an IQ in the retarded range, and up to 60% need long-term residential care. There is growing evidence that dietary gluten could be implicated in autism, and that a gluten-free diet may ameliorate symptoms, particularly if implemented at a very early stage (review by Shattock and Whiteley, Pharm J 2001;267:17–19).

Role of drugs

Drugs may be of limited use in treating some of the more severe behavioural symptoms. SIB is common (see 1.25) and may be helped by low dose antipsychotics, to which autistic individuals seem very sensitive and so lower doses may be needed. A therapeutic window may exist, and higher doses may be counter-productive. Family support, education, skills training, behavioural therapy and social support can be significant aspects of the overall management.

Reviews: general (Volkmar et al, J Child Psychol Psychiatry 2004;**45**:135–70; Goldson, Adv Pediatr 2004;**51**:63–109, Drugs Therapy Perspectives 1998;**12**:5–8), drug therapy (Palermo and Curatolo, J Child Neurol 2004;**19**:155–64; Owley, CNS Spectrum 2002;**7**:663–9; Posey and McDougle, Expert Opin Pharmacother 2001; **2**:587–600), genetics (Muhle et al, Pediatrics 2004;**113**:472–86), ADHD in autism (Aman and Langworthy, J Autism Dev Disord 2000;**30**:451–9).

● Unlicensed/some efficacy

Antipsychotics *

Low-dose antipsychotics have a role to play. As adverse reactions can be significant, a 'start low and go slow' routine is recommended. **Risperidone** is now the standard first-line antipsychotic in autism and, although a review concluded risperidone does not effect the core symptoms of autism, it helps behavioural aspects, eg. irritability, aggression, hyperactivity and stereotyping (Chavez et al, Ann Pharmacother 2006;**40**:909–16; n=101, RCT, d/b, p/c, 8/52, McCracken et al, N Engl J Med 2002;**347**:314–21), eg. 0.5–3.5mg/d had significant effects on overall non-specific behavioural symptoms (n=101, RCT, d/b, p/c, 8/52, McDougle et al, Am J Psychiatry 2005;**162**:1142–8; comment by Fombonne, EBMH 2006;**9**:6). Long-term use seems safe and effective, eg. for up to three years (n=35, open, one year, Reyes et al, Eur Child Adolesc Psychiatry 2006;**15**:97–104) and a long-term discontinuation study suggested a significant relapse prevention efficacy, reducing disruptive behaviour in about half the children taking it (n=36, d/b, 24/52, Troost et al, J Am Acad Child Adolesc Psychiatry 2005;**44**:1137–44), although this may disappear rapidly on discontinuation (n=32, 6/12, d/b, Autism Network, Am J Psychiatry 2005;**162**:1361–9). It is well-tolerated (n=101, RCT, d/b, p/c, 8/52, Aman et al, J Child Adolesc Psychopharmacol 2005;**15**:844–5), although raised prolactin and weight gain are risks so monitor carefully (n=20, 24/52, Gagliano et al, J Child Adolesc Psychopharmacol 2004;**14**:39–47). Although risperidone appears to have the best evidence,

other antipsychotics have been used. A review of 19 studies of atypicals concluded that risperidone (n=133, s=13) may be effective in reducing hyperactivity, aggression and repetitive behaviour (with low EPS), **olanzapine** (n=11, s=3; eg. see n=12, RCT, open, 6/52, Malone et al, J Am Acad Child Adolesc Psychiatry 2001;**40**:887–94) and **clozapine** (open, n=3, Zuddas et al, Am J Psychiatry 1996;**153**:738) may also be effective, but there is little evidence that **amisulpride** (RCT, n=9) or **quetiapine** (open, n=6) are useful in this population (Barnard et al, J Psychopharmacol 2002;**16**:93–101). Olanzapine 5–10mg/d (mean 8mg) may be an alternative (n=12, RCT, open, 6/52, Malone et al, J Am Acad Child Adolesc Psychiatry 2001;**40**:887–94). **Haloperidol** has been widely used, with 0.5–3mg/d used to reduce behavioural symptoms (eg. aggression and SIB) and improve learning (n=60, 6/12, Perry et al, J Am Acad Child Adolesc Psychiatry 1989;**28**:87–92; n=45, p/c, d/b, Anderson et al, J Autism Dev Dis 1989;**19**:227–39).

■ Unlicensed/possible efficacy

Antidepressants *

Serotonin reuptake inhibitors may have a role to play, particularly in adults with strong behavioural rigidity. Children and adolescents may be more sensitive to SSRIs and so, once again, 'start low and go slow' is the advice. A review of **SSRIs** in autism concludes that there are significant improvements in global functioning, anxiety and repetitive behaviour and they are well-tolerated, but methodological weaknesses mean the findings are not robust (s=3, RCT; s=10, open; Kolevzon et al, J Clin Psychiatry 2006;**67**:407–14; review by Moore et al, Ann Pharmacother 2004;**38**:1515–9). **Clomipramine** may be superior to placebo and desipramine in autistic symptoms, anger and ritualism (n=12, d/b, c/o, 10/52, Arch Gen Psychiatry 1993;**50**:441–7), reduce compulsions and adventitious movements (n=5, open, Brasic et al, Neurology 1994;**44**:1309–12), and as an alternative to haloperidol for some symptoms (RCT, n=36, p/c, 7/52, Remington et al, J Clin Psychopharmacol 2001;**21**:440–4). **Fluoxetine** liquid (mean 10mg/d) was superior to placebo for repetitive behaviours in autism (n = 45, RCT, d/b, p/c, c/o, 2×8/52, Hollander et al, Neuropsychopharmacology 2005;**30**:582–9) and there are two cases of dramatic response of OCD–like behavioural symptoms in autistic adults (Koshes, Am J Psychiatry 1997; **154**:578). Low dose **venlafaxine** (18.75 mg/d) may help reduce SIB and ADHD-like symptoms in autism (n = 3, Carminati et al, Prog Neuropsychopharmacol Biol Psychiatry 2006; **30**:312–5).

Cicloserin

Cicloserin was well-tolerated and improved CGI and ABC measures of social withdrawal (n = 12, 6/52, Posey et al, Am J Psychiatry 2004;**161**:2115–7).

Cyproheptadine

Cyproheptadine plus haloperidol was superior to haloperidol alone for ABC-C (aberrant behaviour) listed symptoms (RCT, d/b, p/c, 8/52, Akhondzadeh et al, J Clin Pharm Ther 2004;**29**:145–50).

Levetiracetam

Levetiracetam may improve some symptoms (n = 10, open, Rugino and Samsock, J Dev Behav Pediatr 2002;**23**:225–30).

Memantine *

Memantine 10 mg/d has been used successfully for disruptive behaviour in autism (n = 1, Erickson and Chambers, J Clin Psychiatry 2006; **67**:1000).

Methylphenidate

The considerable negative effects on tantrums and moods may sometimes be outweighed by the positive effects on attention and stereotype behaviour. Two studies have shown a significant reduction in hyperactivity in autism from 10–50 mg/d (n = 10, d/b, p/c, c/o, Quintana et al, J Autism Dev Disord 1995;**25**:283–94; n = 13, d/b, p/c, c/o, Handen et al, J Autism Dev Disord 2000;**30**:245–55).

Mirtazapine

Mirtazapine was only modestly effective in treating some autism-related symptoms (n = 26, open, Posey et al, J Child Adolesc Psychopharmacol 2001;**11**:267–77).

Naltrexone

Three controlled studies have shown disappointing results (eg. n = 23, d/b, p/c, c/o, 4/52, Willemsen-Swinkels et al, Biol Psychiatry 1996;**39**:1023–31). Although 1 mg/kg/d may reduce withdrawal, hyperactivity and SIB, with sedation being the only major side-effect (J Am Acad Child Adolesc Psychiatry 1989;**28**:200–6), most other measures do not improve. There may be a therapeutic window, with doses of 10–25 mg/d optimal in some people.

Omega-3 fatty acids

A case of rapid response of anxiety and agitation in autism has been reported (n = 1, Johnson and Hollander, J Clin Psychiatry 2003; **64**:848–9).

Valproate

Two open trials have suggested some improvement in behavioural symptoms associated with autism, eg. 91% who completed one trial showed sustained improvement in autistic spectrum symptoms, eg. aggression and impulsivity, particularly if an EEG abnormality or seizure history was present (n = 14, open pilot, Hollander et al, J Clin Psychiatry 2001;**62**:530–4; see open, Plioplys, Arch Pediatr Adolesc Med 1994;**148**:220–2).

◆ Others

Other drugs tried include **buspirone** (eg. n = 14, open, Ratey et al, J Clin Psychiatry 1989;**50**:382–4; n = 4, Realmuto et al, J Clin Psychopharmacol 1989;**9**:122–5), **carbamazepine** (eg. Gillberg, J Autism Dev Disord 1991;**21**:61–77), **clonidine** (n = 9, d/b, p/c, Fankhauser et al, J Clin Psychiatry 1992;**53**:77–82; n = 8, p/c, d/b, c/o, Jaselskis et al, J Clin Psychopharmacol 1992;**12**:322–7), **lithium** (eg. n = 2, Kerbeshian et al, J Clin Psychopharmacol 1987;**7**:401–5) and high dose **pyridoxine**.

✱ No efficacy

Lamotrigine

Lamotrigine was ineffective on all measures in one study (n = 28, RCT, p/c, 18/52, Belsito et al, J Autism Dev Disord 2001;**31**:175–81).

Secretin

Despite much interest, a complete lack of

significant effect has been demonstrated (eg. n = 95, RCT, Dunn-Geier et al, Dev Med Child Neurol 2000;**42**:796–802; n = 20, RCT, Owley et al, Med Gen Med 1999;**6**:E2; n = 56, open, Chez et al, J Autism Dev Disord 2000;**30**:87–94; Roberts et al, Pediatrics 2001;**107**:E71; reviewed by Levy, EBMH 2002;**5**:22; n = 56, RCT, p/c, 4/52, Owley et al, J Am Acad Child Adolesc Psychiatry 2001;**40**:1293–99; multiple doses showing no symptomatic improvement n = 6, d/b, p/c, c/o, Sponheim et al, Acta Paediatrica 2002;**91**:540–5). It thus remains an almost completely unproven therapy (review by Patel et al, Pharmacotherapy 2002: **22**:905–14).

1.9 BENZODIAZEPINE DEPENDENCE and WITHDRAWAL *

Although short-term benzodiazepine use at standard doses is usually without significant risk of toxicity and dependence, higher dose and longer-term use has potentially significant risks. The SDS (Severity of Dependence Scale) can be used to accurately detect the potential BDZ dependence (de la Cuevas et al, Addiction 2000;**95**:245–50; reviewed by Law, EBMH 2000;**3**:119). In a review of a number of BDZ withdrawal strategies, minimal intervention (leaflet or group meeting) and clinician-led systematic discontinuation are both more effective than TAU (s = 29, Voshaar et al, Br J Psychiatry 2006;**189**:213–20), although psychotherapy during BDZ tapering may actually be detrimental to long-term outcomes (n = 180 [c = 170], RCT, 15/12, Oude Voshaar et al, Br J Psychiatry 2006;**188**:188–9). Lorazepam, alprazolam and diazepam may be more liable to abuse than chlordiazepoxide and oxazepam (Griffiths and Wolf, J Clin Psychopharmacol 1990; **10**:237–43), probably due to the more rapid absorption and higher receptor potency. Pre-treatment with imipramine or buspirone in people with panic disorder withdrawing from BDZs appears ineffective and had no effect on status at 12 weeks (n = 40, p/c, 12/52, Rynn et al, J Clin Psychopharmacol 2003;**23**:505–8).

Reviews: withdrawal syndrome (Petursson, Addiction 1994;**89**:11455–9), general (Ferguson, Prescriber 1999;**10**:118–21; Rickels et al, J Clin Psychopharmacol 1999;**19**[Suppl 2]:S12–S6), techniques and outcomes of BDZ

detoxifications (Ferguson, Prescriber 2005; **16**: 20–7; n = 82, Charney et al, J Clin Psychiatry 2000;**61**:190–5).

BNF listed

Antidepressants
Antidepressants may be useful for treating any concurrent depression and some are anxiolytics in their own right. However, pre-treatment with imipramine or buspirone is no better than placebo in reducing anticipatory BDZ-withdrawal symptoms or anxiety (n = 40, p/c, Rynn et al, J Clin Psychopharmacol 2003; **23**:505–8).

Benzodiazepines
Transferring from the current benzo-diazepine to diazepam (if necessary) is a common strategy, as diazepam is a longer-acting benzodiazepine and possibly easier to withdraw from. Addition of an SSRI seems of limited value (n = 230, d/b, p/c, Zitman and Couvee, Br J Psychiatry 2001;**178**:317–24). If withdrawing chronic BDZs from geriatric in-patients, short-term (one week) substitution with a low-dose BDZ at night to help sleep may be effective (RCT, d/b, p/c, Petrovic et al, Eur J Clin Pharmacol 2002;**57**:759–64).

● Unlicensed/some efficacy

Buspirone
Caution is advised as buspirone has been reported to aggravate withdrawal symptoms

---

Characteristics of benzodiazepine users:

- Elderly maintained symptom-free by low and unchanging doses.
- Chronic physical disorders controlled by BDZs (eg. epilepsy).
- Where quality of life is so improved by BDZs that long-term use, preferably with intermittent/variable doses, is justified (eg. chronic or severe anxiety or insomnia and an inadequate personality, people who relapse to alcohol and other more dangerous substances when BDZ-free).

(1.6). However, buspirone (38 mg/d) and imipramine (180 mg/d) have been used successfully in patients with GAD discontinuing long-term BDZs, introduced before a tapered discontinuation (n = 107, d/b, Rickels et al, Am J Psychiatry 2000;**157**:1973–9), and buspirone 15 mg/d may relieve lorazepam withdrawal symptoms, with no rebound anxiety on withdrawal (n = 44, RCT, Delle Chiaie et al, J Clin Psychopharmacol 1995;**15**:12–9). Buspirone may

be helpful if established before BDZ withdrawal, to manage underlying anxiety.

Carbamazepine

Carbamazepine 600–800 mg/d has been shown to be effective in benzodiazepine withdrawal in several studies (eg. Ries et al,

---

How to minimise the risks of dependence:

- Carefully select patients (eg. avoid especially dependence-prone, lower education, multiple drug users, those with a criminal background).
- Keep the dose low.
- Stop where possible, eg. use shorter courses.
- Use intermittent or variable doses.
- Use antidepressants if depression mixed with anxiety is present.
  (Darke et al, Addiction 1994;**89**:683–90)

Patients where withdrawal should not be attempted:

- *Older medically ill or with spasticity or epilepsy:* Benzodiazepine usually prescribed by a non-psychiatrist. Seldom abused, doses not escalated, effective long-term. Care with subtle cognitive changes can occur.
- *Psychiatric patients with panic or agoraphobic disorders:* Seldom abused, doses not escalated, necessary long-term.
- *Psychiatric patients with recurrent dysphoria:* Long-term indications for use less clear. Abuse of other drugs often occurs.
- *Chronic sleep-disordered problems:* Drug may be active or preventing a rebound syndrome.

Risk factors for poor withdrawal (need to seek specialist advice): *

- Previously severe withdrawal (including history of seizures) or post-withdrawal reaction.
- Elderly or infirm.
- History of abuse of alcohol/other drugs.
- Concomitant severe medical or psychiatric illness (including personality problems).
- High dose/longer-term use (eg. > 30 mg/d diazepam equivalent > 1 year).
- Cluster B personality/Borderline PD (n = 76, Vorma et al, Subst Use Misuse 2005;**40**:499–510).
- High neuroticism, higher behavioural inhibition and low social support (n = 41, 28/52, O'Connor et al, Addict Behav 2004;**29**:583–93).

Withdrawal symptoms in the dependent patient:

- *Psychological:* Tension (to above pre-treatment levels), restlessness, agitation, panic attacks.
- *Physical:* Dry mouth, sweating, tremor, sleep disturbance, lethargy, headache, nausea, palpitations.
- *Mental:* Impaired memory and concentration, confusion.
- *Moderate:* Perceptual changes (ie. hypersensitivity to light/sound), dysphoria, flu-like symptoms, anorexia, sore eyes, depersonalisation, depression, abnormal sensations of movement, rebound insomnia.
- *Severe:* (rare) Convulsions, psychoses (eg. visual hallucinations, paranoia), delusions.

J Psychoactive Drugs 1991;**23**:73–6), including that of high dose (up to 300 mg/d) diazepam (Neppe and Sindorf, J Nerv Ment Dis 1991;**179**:234–5) and in people with panic disorder (Klein et al, Am J Psychiatry 1994; **151**:1760–6). Up to 800 mg/d also reduces the chance of withdrawal convulsions and can minimise withdrawal symptoms (eg. emotional lability), especially if withdrawal is abrupt. It may also reduce the incidence of relapse (n = 40, RCT, 12/52, Schweizer et al, Arch Gen Psychiatry 1991;**48**:448–52).

■ Unlicensed/possible efficacy

Antihistamines
These may be useful as non-benzodiazepine hypnotics where insomnia is a problem.

Clonidine
This may be a helpful adjunct in withdrawal, especially at relatively high dose.

Flumazenil
IV flumazenil has been used to reduce BDZ craving, lower relapse rates and improve outcomes in BDZ withdrawal (n = 50, RCT, p/c, 6/52, Gerra et al, Addict Biol 2002;**7**:385–95). Caution is needed in BDZ dependence.

Melatonin
Controlled-release melatonin has been successfully used to facilitate discontinuation of benzodiazepines (n = 34, d/b, 6/52, Garfinkel et al, Arch Intern Med 1999;**159**:2456–60).

Oxcarbazepine *
Oxcarbazepine has been used successfully (Croissant et al, Pharmacopsychiatry 2005; **38**:222–3).

Topiramate
Successful management of rapid BDZ-withdrawal with topiramate has been reported (n = 1, Cheseaux et al, Hum Psychopharmacol 2003;**18**:375–7).

Valproate
150–1200 mg/d may reduce the intensity of symptoms in protracted withdrawal (eg. n = 4, Apelt and Emrich, Am J Psychiatry

1994;**147**:1990), as well as acting as an anticonvulsant (Apelt and Emrich, Am J Psychiatry 1990;**147**:950–1).

◆ Others

Other drugs tried include **phenobarbital** (J Psychoact Drugs 1983;**15**:85–95, 99–104) and **propranolol** (Postgrad Med J 1988; **64** [Suppl]:40–4).

✱ No efficacy

Antipsychotics
Low dose anxiolytic use may be useful but may make withdrawal symptoms worse (Anon, Lancet 1987;**i**:78–9).

1.10 BIPOLAR MOOD DISORDER

1.10.1 PROPOPHYLAXIS AND MAINTENANCE
1.10.2 MANIA AND HYPOMANIA
1.10.3 BIPOLAR DEPRESSION
1.10.4 RAPID-CYCLING BIPOLAR DISORDER

Introduction
Bipolar mood disorder is a life-long illness with a variety of presentations, phases and sub-divisions. DSM-IV divides the condition into bipolar I (one or more manic or mixed episodes, wide mood swings), bipolar II (the most common form, one or more episodes of depression with at least one hypomanic but no manic episode) and bipolar III (pseudobipolar, often triggered by antidepressants, and which may present as a mixed state). There are many other classifications and sub-categories.

Diagnosis
Bipolar disorder is frequently unrecognised, misdiagnosed and inadequately treated. A survey of members of US bipolar association 'Chapters' showed that over 33% sought professional help within a year of the onset of symptoms. Of these, 69% were misdiagnosed (mostly unipolar depression), there was an average of four physicians seen before getting an accurate diagnosis, and over 33% waited over 10 years before getting a diagnosis (n = 600, Hirschfeld et al, J Clin Psychiatry 2003;**64**:161–74), a finding stunningly similar to a previous

survey (Lish et al, J Affect Disord 1994;**31**:281–94). The **average** time from the onset of symptoms to starting maintenance therapy is 8–10 years (n = 56, Goldberg and Ernst, J Clin Psychiatry 2002;**63**: 985–91; Baldessarini et al, Am J Psychiatry 1999;**156**:811–2), and may be even longer with women (n = 360, Viguera et al, Bipolar Disord 2001;**3**:245–52). Sadly, many suicide attempts are made during this latency period before lithium is started, the only mood stabiliser proven to reduce suicides. A longer delay also results in poorer social functioning over the last year, more annual hospitalisations and a higher likelihood of suicide attempts, regardless of the polarity of the first episode (n = 56, Goldberg and Ernst, J Clin Psychiatry 2002;**63**:985–91). A delay in starting mood stabilisers does not necessarily ultimately adversely influence the prophylactic outcome, but illness severity prior to prophylaxis does predict outcome, although those with a more severe illness were more likely to be treated early, with better outcomes (n = 147, Baethge et al, Acta Psychiatr Scand 2003;**107**:260–7). Excess mortality has been shown in bipolar (n = 15 386) and unipolar (n = 39 182) disorder in Sweden, both in terms of suicides and from natural causes (population study, Osby et al, Arch Gen Psychiatry 2001;**58**:844–50); but suicide rates are significantly reduced by long-term medication with an antidepressant, neuroleptic, or lithium, or combinations thereof (n = 406, 22 years, Angst et al, J Affect Disord 2002;**68**:167–81). Poor outcome is associated with anxiety (n = 124, Feske et al, Am J Psychiatry 2000;**157**:956–62) and concurrent personality disorders (n = 59, Dunayevich et al, J Clin Psychiatry 2000;**61**:134–9).

1.10.1 PROPOPHYLAXIS AND MAINTENANCE

Role of drugs

The optimum outcomes in bipolar occur with the appropriate and consistent prescribing of mood stabilisers, training for the person to cope with stresses and risk factors, and family support. Lithium, valproate, some atypicals and carbamazepine are widely used for the prophylaxis of bipolar disorder, although the evidence for carbamazepine and perhaps valproate is not robust. It is clear that well-being and functioning

are inversely proportional to the number of bipolar episodes, and so strategies to reduce relapse must be rigorously followed, especially minimising difficult-to-treat bipolar depression (n = 64, retrospective, MacQueen et al, Acta Psychiatr Scand 2000;**101**:374–81). Unfortunately, inappropriate use of antidepressants in un-diagnosed bipolar may lead to cycle worsening in many (n = 85, naturalistic, Ghaemi et al, J Clin Psychiatry 2000;**61**:804–8). CBT can significantly help to reduce risk factors for relapse and produce better outcomes in combination with mood stabilisers (review of combination approaches, Rothbaum and Astin, J Clin Psychiatry 2000;**61**[Suppl 9]:68–75). Regular compliance is important but be aware that impaired verbal learning and memory in bipolar could passively limit treatment adherence (n = 40, Cavanagh et al, Br J Psychiatry 2002;**180**:293–5, 320–6). There is an overlap with ADHD, anxiety and personality disorder, eg. labile effect, irritability, mood instability, stress, low mood/dysphoria, and many have warned of over-diagnosing BPD and under-diagnosing bipolar disorder.

Reviews: bipolar disorder (Müller-Oerling-hausen et al, Lancet 2002;**359**:241–7, 75 refs), diagnosis and treatment in children and adolescents (Silva et al, CNS Drugs 1999;**12**:437–50), genetics (Potash and DePaolo, Bipolar Disord 2000;**2**:8–26), suicide and bipolar (Jamison, J Clin Psychiatry 2000;**61**[Suppl 9]:S47–S51), longitudinal course (Suppes et al, J Clin Psychiatry 2000;**61**[Suppl 9]:23–30, 134 refs), BAP guidelines on bipolar disorder (Goodwin et al, J Psychopharmacol 2003;**17**:149–73), suicide reduction with anticonvulsants (Yerevanian et al, J Affect Disord 2003;**73**:223–8).

Comparisons

Active comparisons between mood stabilisers are rare, eg. valproate was superior to placebo and lithium in the only RCT (n = 372, RCT, Bowden et al, Arch Gen Psychiatry 2000;**57**:481–9) and lithium outdid carbamazepine in clinical response in bipolar patients, based on inter-episodic morbidity, drop-out rate, and rehospitalisation, with 2.5 times higher drop-out rate with CBZ (n = 171, 2.5 years, Kleindienst and Greil, Psychol Med 2002;**32**:493–501). In a unique comparison, stable bipolars who had received less than 6/12 treatment with either carbamazepine or lithium, were randomised to receive either lithium or carbamazepine. Relapse with lithium (12/44) was lower than with carbamazepine (21/50) (both as monotherapy). Almost all lithium relapses occurred within the first three months' treatment, whereas carbamazepine carried a constant risk of 40% per year, suggesting lithium was more effective as a mood stabiliser (n = 94, RCT, d/b, two years, Hartong et al, J Clin Psychiatry 2003;**64**:144–51).

BNF listed

Carbamazepine

Long-term therapy in affective disorders is well-established, either as an alternative to lithium or used in combination in treatment-resistant cases, although it is rapidly falling out of favour. Carbamazepine is reported to be better for early onset illness and with an alternating pattern of mood. However, six studies of maintenance carbamazepine in bipolar disorder have shown equivocal results, eg. incomplete protection, and so some uncertainty remains (reviewed by Keck et al, J Clin Psychiatry 1998;**59**[Suppl 6]:S74–S81, 114 refs). Indeed, one study showed that only 18% of carbamazepine-treated bipolars remained stable for 3–4 years, and another showed a 50% relapse rate (n = 24, open, four years, Post et al, J Clin Psychopharmacol 1990;**10**:318–27). A comparison of 10 studies of carbamazepine against lithium shows a roughly similar efficacy (n = 572, table in Davis et al, Acta Psychiatr Scand 1999;**100**:406–17). There has, however, been an increased interest in carbamazepine as a consequence of two studies on an SR preparation for use in mania and in a follow-on study as relapse prevention, and although 69% discontinued early, only 14% of the 77 completers relapsed (n = 92, open, 6/52, Ketter et al, J Clin Psychiatry 2004;**65**:668–73). Trough carbamazepine levels of 7 mg/L or above are strongly associated with therapeutic response in bipolar patients (Taylor and Duncan, Psychiatr Bull 1997;**21**:221–3) and thus may require higher doses (eg. 600 mg/d) than are currently recommended. There is little evidence for a rebound mania on discontinuation (eg. n = 6, Macritchie and Hunt, J Psychopharmacol 2000;**14**:266–8). It has been suggested that the

best thing you can do with carbamazepine in bipolar is to stop it and allow other drugs to reach therapeutic levels.

Lithium

The use of lithium in bipolar was first published by Cade (Med J Aust 1949;**36**:49–52) and it is now widely used for the treatment and prophylaxis of bipolar illnesses and, with care, can be successful and safe. It is effective in bipolar I and II, by reducing relapses and increasing inter-episodic intervals (eg. Tondo et al, Am J Psychiatry 1998;**155**:638–45).

Efficacy: Although the nine major placebo-controlled trials of lithium as prophylaxis of bipolar disorder have methodological flaws (eg. most used an abrupt lithium-withdrawal control group, which has now been shown to increase relapse in its own right), their findings are of great importance. There are some who have doubted lithium's efficacy, despite it having a known dose-response curve, and withdrawal produces relapse (n = 865, s = 19, RCTs, Davis et al, Acta Psychiatr Scand 1999;**100**:406–17). Lithium clearly reduces the risk of relapse in bipolar disorder (61% with placebo, 33% with lithium), particularly for manic episodes (systematic review and meta-analysis, n = 770, Geddes et al, Am J Psychiatry 2004;**161**:217–22; review by Bauer, EBMH 2004;**7**;72). Bauer's review states it to be the first published, methodologically rigorous meta-analysis of RCT, d/b, p/c trials in relapse prevention, and concludes that lithium reduces the risk of relapse in affective relapse, especially manic, but that there is less evidence that it prevents depressive relapses. Response may be a familial trait (n = 146, Grof et al, J Clin Psychiatry 2002;**63**:942–7). Another meta-analysis showed a non-significant trend towards better responses to lithium in recent times (Baldessarini and Tondo, Arch Gen Psychiatry 2000;**57**:187–90), so despite the lack of any commercial promotion of lithium, it still apparently works.

Prophylaxis: Lithium appears highly effective as prophylactic therapy, provided it is taken and monitored regularly, and the dose and therapy reviewed regularly to minimise side-effects, especially those of weight gain and cognitive dulling. Commencing lithium within the first ten years of illness predicts better preventative outcomes than beginning prophylaxis later, both in major depression, recurrent and bipolar patients (n = 270, Franchini et al, Eur Arch Psychiatry Clin Neurosci 1999;**249**:227–30). The prophylactic efficacy is probably maintained for at least ten years (n = 86, mean 8.2 years, Berghofer et al, Acta Psychiatr Scand 1996;**93**:349–54). Data is accumulating that long-term lithium markedly reduces the excess mortality of people with recurrent affective disorders (retrospective study, n = 273, Müller-Oerlinghausen et al, Acta Psychiatr Scand 1996;**94**:344–7), probably at least in part by (see next section) reducing suicide (Gershon and Soares, Arch Gen Psychiatry 1997;**54**:16–20). Lithium maintenance yields striking long-term reductions of depressive as well as manic morbidity in both bipolar disorder subtypes, with greater overall benefits in bipolar II patients and with earlier treatment (n = 317, retrospective, Tondo et al, Am J Psychiatry 1998; **155**:638–45). Regular lithium use over five years has been shown to produce a drastic reduction in time in hospital as 'almost the rule', but irregular use leads to a much poorer outcome (n = 402, Maj et al, Am J Psychiatry 1998;**155**:30–5). Adjunctive CBT may enhance the effectiveness of lithium in long-term bipolar prophylaxis (n = 15, Fava et al, J Clin Psychiatry 2001;**62**:556–9).

The main problems appear to be when therapy is given to carelessly selected patients given insufficient support (see compliance), education and supervision, illustrated by naturalistic studies which show a poorer outcome than controlled trials. Goodwin argues strongly that treatment with lithium should be for at least two years (and more probably three years at the minimum), and that up to two years it may have at best no beneficial effect (premature stopping resulting in premature recurrence of mania).

Suicide reduction: Reduced suicide rates have been strongly suggested by many studies, something unique in bipolar to lithium (Baldessarini and Jamison, J Clin Psychiatry 1999;**60**[Suppl 2]:S117–S22). An analysis of 22 studies on lithium maintenance showed that suicide was 82% less frequent during lithium treatment, not accounted for by discontinuation

(22 studies, meta-analysis, n = 5647, Tondo et al, Acta Psychiatr Scand 2001;**104**:163–72), although this has been disputed in one retrospective study of selected suicides (Coryell et al, Acta Psychiatr Scand 2001;**104**:193–7; editorial comment by Gelenberg, Acta Psychiatr Scand 2001;**104**:161–2; review by Burgess, EBMH 2002;**5**:52) although excess mortality has also been reported with lithium (n = 133, retrospective over 16 years, Brodersen et al, Br J Psychiatry 2000;**176**:429–33). The effect may be further enhanced by psychotherapy (two years, Rucci et al, Am J Psychiatry 2002;**159**:1160–4) and, although suicide protection may be incomplete, suicide is seven-fold lower than in non-lithium treated patients (meta-analysis by Müller-Oerlinghausen, Eur Arch Psychiatry Clin Neurosci 2001;**251**[Suppl 2]:S72–S75), as are suicide attempts or successful suicide (2.7 times higher with valproate than lithium; n = 20 638, Goodwin et al, JAMA 2003;**290**:1467–73).

Mode of action: Lithium may exert its effect via many mechanisms, eg. inositol monophosphatase enzyme inhibition, decreasing inositol concentrations, inhibiting secondary messenger systems, inhibition of Protein Kinase C activity (which may stabilise aberrant neuronal signals in critical areas of the brain, an action shared with valproate and tamoxifen; Manji et al, J Clin Psychiatry 1996;**57**[Suppl 13]:S34–S46), neuroprotection, glycogen synthase kinase 3-beta inhibition (GSK-3b regulates gene expression, and inhibiting it increases expression of neuroprotective agents, such as heat shock protein), increased human brain grey matter (Moore et al, Lancet 2000;**356**:1241–2), up-regulation of Bcl-2 (major neuroprotective protein, with speculated rebound reduction in Bcl-2 production on withdrawal: Manji et al, J Clin Psychiatry 2000;**61**[Suppl 9]:S82–S96), protection from glutamate apoptosis (programmed cell death) and serotonin regulation (although acute tryptophan depletion does not reverse the effect on mood and suicidality in bipolar I: n = 19, RCT, Hughes et al, Br J Psychiatry 2000;**177**:447–51). Some of the long-term benefits of lithium may be mediated by neurotrophic effects.

Review: Mode of action (Shaldubina et al, Prog Neuropsychopharmacol Biol Psychiatry 2001; **25**:855–66).

Dosing: Once-daily lithium reduces side-effects, simplifies dosage requirements and reduces renal damage. Alternate daily lithium is not recommended (n = 50, d/b, Jensen et al, J Affect Disord 1996;**36**:89–93).

Plasma levels: Plasma levels of 0.4–0.8 mmol/L are generally considered safe and effective as prophylaxis, but below 0.4–0.6 mEq/L may be less protective against relapse (eg. n = 94, RCT, d/b, Gelenberg et al, N Engl J Med 1989;**321**:1489–93). There was no difference in the protection against affective disorder relapse between high (0.8–1.0 mmol/L) and low (0.5–0.8 mmol/L) serum lithium levels (naturalistic, n = 91, Vestergaard et al, Acta Psychiatr Scand 1998;**98**:310–5), but only a third completed two years lithium prophylaxis successfully, and alcohol or other medication abuse was associated with poor outcome. In the elderly, a third to half less lithium may be needed due to reduced clearance (n = 9, Hardy et al, J Clin Psychopharmacol 1987;**7**:153–8). Lithium plasma levels may need to be higher in children and adolescents as the brain-to-serum concentration ratio appears to be correlated positively with age (n = 27, Moore et al, Am J Psychiatry 2002;**159**:1240–2).

Monitoring: Plasma monitoring is often poor, with many litigation cases for poor monitoring, eg. a substantial proportion of patients still do not receive adequate TDM (no tests for 12 months in 37% lithium users, n = 718, Marcus et al, Am J Psychiatry 1999;**156**:1014–8). Local databases may be a successful way round this (Holmes and Bazire, Bipolar Disorders 2003;**5**[Suppl 1]:S53).

Compliance or concordance: The main reason for lithium failure is non-compliance (either complete or erratic), and the patient (and any partner or caregiver) should be aware of the long-term commitment needed. Specialised care, eg. via lithium or mood clinics, may improve patient and professional compliance with lithium use (Guscott and Taylor, Br J Psychiatry 1994;**164**:741–6). Future compliance to lithium after discharge from hospital (and hence likelihood of readmission within one year) has been predicted by measuring pre- and post-leave levels, the so-called lithium level-to-dose ratio (LDR) (Terao and Terao, Lithium 1994;**5**:115–16). For a general review

of strategies to improve compliance, see Schou (Acta Psychiatr Scand 1997;**95**:361–3).

Discontinuation: Early (particularly manic) relapse in bipolar illness following lithium discontinuation is now well accepted. Several important studies have shown a significant risk from rapid discontinuation. If stopped in under 14 days, the risk of relapse is much higher (median 50% risk of relapse within four months, 100% over 3.5 years) than with slower (15–30 days) withdrawal, with a significant excess over the first six months (n = 161, Baldessarini et al, J Clin Psychiatry 1996;**57**:441–8; n = 78, Baldessarini et al, Am J Psychiatry 1997;**154**:551–3). At seven-year follow-up, relapse was more common after acute lithium discontinuation, the excess morbidity being attributable to the first episode/relapse after discontinuation (n = 42, seven years, Cavanagh et al, Acta Psychiatr Scand 2004;**109**:91–5). Even controlled lithium discontinuation leads to a high relapse in people who had had a good response for at least five years, so be careful (n = 32, up to nine years, Yazici et al, J Affect Disord 2004;**80**:269–71). Since lithium has been shown to reduce mortality, discontinuation is also likely to be associated with increased mortality (review by MacQueen and Joffe, Acta Psychiatr Scand 2004;**109**:81–2).

Abrupt decrease: Decreasing lithium levels, (either through erratic compliance or major changes in dose) is also a powerful predictor of relapse (n = 94, Perlis et al, Am J Psychiatry 2002;**159**:1155–9). Indeed, the original paper that claims that >0.8 mmol/L is superior to lower levels (n = 94, RCT, d/b, Gelenberg et al, N Engl J Med 1989;**321**:1489–93) notes that many in the lower level group had rapid reductions in levels which may have contributed to relapse.

Lithium refractoriness: Lithium discontinuation in stable patients, despite adequate lithium levels, has been reported to induce a refractory state (eg. Bauer, Am J Psychiatry 1994;**151**:1522). However, two studies of lithium maintenance treatment periods (mean four years) were unable to show this (n = 86, Tondo et al, Am J Psychiatry 1997;**154**:548–50; n = 28, Coryell et al, Am J Psychiatry 1998;**155**:895–8), although the latter study has been criticised as being underpowered (Maj, Am J Psychiatry 1999;**156**:1130; plus reply). In a longitudinal study of clinic-attending bipolars compliant with lithium for at least a year, and without co-morbid substance misuse, retreatment showed a slightly reduced efficacy. There was no tendency for lesser responses later in treatment (n = 360, longitudinal, Tondo et al, Br J Psychiatry 2001;**178**[Suppl 41]:S184–S190). See also discontinuation above for discussion of relapse.

Reviews: * general (Baldessarini et al, Harv Rev Psychiatry 2002;**10**:59–75; Dinan, Br Med J 2002;**324**:989–90), review of good practice (Watson and Young, Curr Opin Psychiatry 2001;**14**:57–63), neurobiology and mode of action (Lenox and Hahn, J Clin Psychiatry 2000;**61**[Suppl 9]:S5–S15, 123 refs), metabolic adverse effects (Livingstone and Rampes, J Psychopharmacol 2006;**20**:347–55), historical perspectives (Soares and Gershon, J Clin Psychiatry 2000;**61**[Suppl 9]:16–22, Nemeroff, J Clin Psychiatry 2000;**61**[Suppl 9]:S3–S4), pharmacokinetics and pharmacodynamics (Kilts, J Clin Psychiatry 2000;**61**[Suppl 9]:41–6), prophylaxis (editorial review, Vestergaard, Acta Psychiatr Scand 2000;**101**:341–2), adverse effects (Geisler and Schou, Adv Drug React Bull 2001;**206**:787–90), long-term treatment (Kleindienst and Greil, Eur Arch Psychiatry Clin Neurosci 2003;**253**:120–5), in combination with other mood stabilisers (Goodwin, J Clin Psychiatry 2003;**64**[Suppl 5]:S18–S24, 58 refs) and recent research (Maj, Bipolar Disorder 2003; **5**:180–8), in renal disease (Smith et al, J Clin Psychiatry 2005;**66**:396–9).

Olanzapine *

Olanzapine is indicated for the prevention of recurrence in patients with bipolar disorder whose manic episode has responded to olanzapine. In people with mania responding to olanzapine in the acute phase, maintenance olanzapine reduced relapse to subsequent mood disorder compared to placebo, although people with an index depressive episode in the open phase were excluded (n = 361, RCT, p/c, 48/52, Tohen et al, Am J Psychiatry 2006;**163**:247–56; MS; comment by Citrome, EBMH 2006;**9**:73). Olanzapine 5–20 mg/d may be more effective than lithium (0.6–1.2 mEd/L) in preventing manic and mixed episode relapse in the specific sub-group

of olanzapine responders, but both were comparable in depressive relapse (n = 431, RCT, d/b, 12/12, Tohen et al, Am J Psychiatry 2005;**162**:1281–90; MS). Adjunctive therapy in resistant bipolar (average dose 8.1 mg/d) shows some promise (n = 23, open, Vieta et al, J Clin Psychopharmacol 2001;**21**:469–73). The time to remission of mania with olanzapine was slower than with valproate, and rates of bipolar relapse were the same for both treatment arms (n = 251, RCT, d/b, 47/52, Tohen et al, Am J Psychiatry 2003;**160**:1263–71; MS). In a longer-term study, however, a sustained mood stabilising effect was evident in only 26% (7/27) of those taking olanzapine as an add-on (n = 125, 15/12, Narendran et al, J Clin Psychiatry 2001;**62**:509–16). In a sponsor's re-analysis, olanzapine and lithium were as effective over one year at reducing relapse, although olanzapine may have short-term advantages (n = 431, RCT, d/b, 12/12, Ketter et al, J Clin Psychiatry 2006;**67**:95–101, MS).

+ Combinations

There has been an increased use of polypharmacy in refractory bipolar disorder over recent decades (n = 178, Frye et al, J Clin Psychiatry 2000; **61**:9–15).

Lithium + antipsychotics

Lithium is frequently used with antipsychotics in maintenance therapy, although the evidence is poor, eg. flupentixol was ineffective as an adjunct to lithium (n = 11, d/b, c/o, Esparon et al, Br J Psychiatry 1986;**148**:723–5). Quetiapine (mean 175 mg/d) was effective in 56% as an adjunct to lithium or valproate (n = 16, retro chart review, 18/12, Prog Neuropsychopharmacol Biol Psychiatry 2003;**27**:863–6). Anecdotal reports indicate an additive effect, eg. with clozapine, risperidone and olanzapine (reviewed by Freeman and Stoll, Am J Psychiatry 1998;**155**:12–21). See also 'some efficacy' section.

Lithium + calcium-channel blockers

Although there are some reports of efficacy, potential drug interactions make this combination hazardous (reviewed by Freeman and Stoll, Am J Psychiatry 1998;**155**:12–21).

Lithium + carbamazepine

This combination has been widely used and can seem safe and effective, especially for rapid-cycling. Some retrospective and prospective studies have shown a well-tolerated and improved prophylactic effect compared to lithium monotherapy (eg. n = 33, Small et al, Psychopharmacol Bull 1995;**31**:265–72). Occasional neurotoxic reactions have been reported, but mostly in patients with pre-existing brain damage (n = 5, Shukla et al, Am J Psychiatry 1984;**141**:1604–6). An additive anti-thyroid effect may occur, lowering T4 and free T4 levels (n = 23, Kramlinger and Post, Am J Psychiatry 1990;**147**:615–20), although the addition of carbamazepine to lithium has also been claimed to help to counteract lithium-induced sub-clinical hypothyroidism, possibly improving efficacy (six years, Bocchetta et al, Acta Psychiatr Scand 1996;**94**:45–8).

Lithium + lamotrigine

Case reports indicate this may be a useful combination (eg. Calabrese et al, Am J Psychiatry 1996;**153**:1236) and since lamotrigine is better at preventing relapse to depression and lithium at preventing relapse of mania, the combination might be ideal, meriting further study.

Valproate + antipsychotics

Many combinations are used, although there is little data to show a proven efficacy. Reports of valproate used effectively with clozapine and risperidone have appeared (reviewed by Freeman and Stoll, Am J Psychiatry 1998;**155**:12–21). See also 'some efficacy'.

Valproate + carbamazepine

There have been several reports of efficacy, eg. when valproate was added to carbamazepine non-responders, 69% responded (n = 29, Schaff et al, J Clin Psychiatry 1993;**54**:380–4).

Valproate + lamotrigine

An open study has indicated some efficacy (reviewed by Freeman and Stoll, Am J Psychiatry 1998;**155**:12–21), although the incidence of rash appears higher and valproate increases lamotrigine levels (see 4.5.4).

● Unlicensed/some efficacy

Antidepressants

See bipolar depression (1.10.3) for use in bipolar disorder, with notes about the risk of inducing a switch to mania in bipolar depression. The one dissenting voice is the study that showed that continuing antidepressants after a depressive episode was **not** associated with an increased risk of manic episodes, but early discontinuation was associated with significantly increased depressive relapse (n = 84, one year, naturalistic, Altshuler et al, Am J Psychiatry 2003; **160**:1252–62).

Antipsychotics (see also olanzapine) *

The main roles of antipsychotics in bipolar disorder are:

1. Adjunctive to mood stabilisers for management of acute mania (see 1.10.2) or psychotic depression.
2. Adjunctive maintenance in treatment-resistance.

There is no compelling evidence that anti-psychotics, as such, are effective as mood stabilisers alone in bipolar disorder, although they may help prevent relapse of mania. Olanzapine is licensed for relapse prevention of olanzapine-responsive mania (see BNF section). Many other antipsychotics are licensed for bipolar mania and might thus have some relapse prevention efficacy. **Risperidone** is licensed for acute mania or mixed episodes in bipolar mania. Cochrane concludes that there is a need to study risperidone in the long-term treatment of bipolar disorder (Rendell and Geddes, Cochrane Database Syst Rev 2006;**4**:CD004999). **Quetiapine** is licensed in the short-term treatment of acute manic episodes and may have some applications as an alternative or adjunct in bipolar or schizoaffective disorders (n = 145, open, Zarate et al, J Clin Psychiatry 2000;**61**:185–9), and a pilot study in bipolar or schizoaffective patients poorly responsive to mood stabilisers, suggested that quetiapine (50–400 mg/d) may have some potential (n = 20, open, 12/52, Sajatovic et al, J Clin Psychiatry 2001;**62**:728–32). Results from a monotherapy relapse prevention study were also encouraging (n = 28, open, 12/12, Altamura et al, J Affect Disord 2003;**76**:267–71).

Clozapine may have some significant mood stabilising effects in treatment-resistant bipolar or schizoaffective patients, eg. as add-on therapy compared to placebo (n = 38, RCT, p/c, Suppes et al, Am J Psychiatry 1999;**156**:1164–9; see also n = 193, Banov et al, J Clin Psychiatry 1994;**55**:295–300; n = 34/91, open, Ciapparelli et al, J Clin Psychiatry 2000;**61**:329–34), and a longer trial showed some efficacy to improve symptoms in bipolar with psychotic features (n = 37, open, two years, Ciapparelli et al, J Clin Psychiatry 2003;**64**:451–8). **Aripiprazole** is licensed for mania relapse prevention in USA supported by several studies, eg. 15–30 mg/d was superior to placebo for reducing relapse in bipolar mania in those responding over 6/52 (n = 161, RCT, d.b, p/c, 6/12, Keck et al, J Clin Psychiatry 2006;**67**:626–37; see also n = 262, RCT, d/b, p/c, 3/52, Keck et al, Am J Psychiatry 2003;**160**:1651–8; observations by Jagadheesan and Muirhead, Am J Psychiatry 2004;**161**:1926–7; review by Lyseng-Williamson and Perry, CNS Drugs 2004;**18**:367–76).
Reviews: atypicals in bipolar and schizoaffective disorders (Ghaemi and Goodwin, J Clin Psychopharmacol 1999;**19**:354–61), olanzapine in bipolar I (Bhana and Perry, CNS Drugs 2001;**15**:871–904, 110 refs).

Lamotrigine *

Lamotrigine is licensed in the US (but not the UK) for the maintenance treatment of bipolar I depression and relapse prevention (See bipolar depression 1.10.3). The mode of action may be inhibiting excess glutamate release but it doesn't down-regulate pkC nor MARCKS so may be different to lithium and valproate (review by Hahn et al, J Clin Psychiatry 2004;**65**:791–804).
Reviews: * use in bipolar (Bhagwagar and Goodwin, Expert Opin Pharmacother 2005; **6**:1401–8).

Valproate

While valproate is now licensed for mania, valproate salts are not yet actually licensed as mood stabilisers (and unlikely ever to be), albeit widely used for this purpose (review, Davis et al, Acta Psychiatr Scand 1999;**100**:406–17). The one-year study comparing divalproex, lithium and placebo (2:1:1) just failed to show

divalproex to be superior to lithium or placebo in the time to any mood episode, but there was a noticeable trend for divalproex (40/52) over placebo (28/52) and lithium (24/52), and it was superior to placebo on nearly all secondary measures (n = 372, RCT, Bowden et al, Arch Gen Psychiatry 2000;**57**:481–9). Case studies and open trials (eg. Calabrese et al, J Clin Psychopharmacol 1992;**12**[Suppl 1]:S53–S56) suggest a therapeutic effect, particularly in prevention of mania or mixed episodes. Valproate may also reduce depressive symptoms compared to lithium (sub-analysis of Bowden study by Gyulai et al, Neuropsychopharmacol 2003;**28**:1374–82). Valproate may be highly effective in some bipolar patients refractory to lithium and carbamazepine (n = 24, Denicoff et al, Am J Psychiatry 1997;**154**:1456–8). There is also some data that valproate may allow reduction in the doses of antipsychotics needed in bipolar disorder with psychosis, or even replace them (Reutens and Castle, Br J Psychiatry 1997;**170**:484–5). See also entry under mania/hypomania (1.10.2).

■ Unlicensed/possible efficacy

Calcium-channel blockers

Verapamil 120–450 mg/d showed some promise as a mood stabiliser. Diltiazem has also been suggested to be effective (n = 8, open, 12/12, Silverstone and Birkett, J Psychiatry Neurosci 2000;**25**:276–80). They may have some role as add-on therapy in resistant cases.

Cannabis *

A review of cannabinoids in bipolar concluded that there were no published studies of efficacy but much anecdotal evidence (Ashton et al, J Psychopharmacol 2005;**19**:293–300).

Gabapentin

See bipolar depression (1.10.3). Despite lacking efficacy in acute states, gabapentin added to a mood stabiliser (lithium, valproate or carbamazepine) appeared to have some prophylactic effects (n = 25, RCT, d/b, p/c, 12/12, Vieta et al, J Clin Psychiatry 2006;**67**:473–7).

Omega-3 fatty acids

In a not very stringent four-month trial, omega-

3 fatty acids produced a significantly longer remission than placebo, as well as scoring higher on most other outcome measures (n = 30, d/b, Stoll et al, Arch Gen Psychiatry 1999;**56**:407–12; general review by Greener, Prog Neurol Psychiatry 1999;**3**:26–7).

Oxcarbazepine

There are case reports of success in bipolar II with co-morbid substance abuse (n = 4, Nasr, Am J Psychiatry 2002;**159**:1793). See also carbamazepine.

Pramipexole

See bipolar depression (1.10.3).

Tamoxifen

There is some interest in tamoxifen as a mood stabiliser, in that it shares some intra-cellular properties with lithium, eg. PKc inhibition (see lithium in this section).

Tiagabine

There are case reports of tiagabine 4 mg/d used successfully as adjunctive therapy in multiple drug-resistant bipolar disorder, continuing to be effective over several months (n = 2, Schaffer and Schaffer, Am J Psychiatry 1999;**156**:2014–15), although it was at best only modestly effective in refractory bipolar, with several significant ADRs in a small trial (n = 13, open, Suppes et al, Bipolar Disord 2002;**4**:283–9).

Topiramate

There is some open evidence accumulating for topiramate, but RCTs are awaited to confirm this. In one study, mild improvement was seen in 47% and marked-to-moderate in 13% bipolars treated with topiramate, (mean 180 mg/d), with a dose-related response and weight loss, as well as significant side-effects (n = 76, open, Ghaemi et al, Ann Clin Psychiatry 2001;**13**:185–9), and there is a report of success in recurrent mania in bipolar I (n = 1, Letmaier et al, Int Clin Psychopharmacol 2001:**16**:295–8). Adjunctive topiramate has been used successfully in mania and depression in treatment-resistant bipolar (n = 19, open, 12/52, Vieta et al, World J Biol Psychiatry 2003;**4**:172–6). Another open, uncontrolled, retrospective study of topiramate as add-on maintenance in bipolar

had low drop-outs and low relapses, an encouraging thought (n = 56, open, one year, Lykouras and Hatzimanolis, Curr Med Res Opin 2004;**20**:843–7).

Vitamins and minerals

A trial of 36 dietary nutrients has produced a 55–66% reduction in bipolar symptoms and a reduction in medication levels, leading to suggestions that bipolar disorder is an inborn error of metabolism, although the mechanism is unknown (n = 11, 6/12, Kaplan et al, J Clin Psychiatry 2001;**62**:936–44).

1.10.2 MANIA AND HYPOMANIA

Symptoms

Hypomania, the more common and milder form of mania, includes an abnormal elation of mood, alternating with irritability, great energy, inability to concentrate, flight of ideas (rapid changing of the subject with some connections) and insomnia. Obsessive preoccupation with some idea, activity or desire may occur. The main presenting symptoms are a euphoric and labile mood (irritable, angry, grandiose), bright or untidy appearance, low sleep requirement, increased drive and energy, reduced insight, pressure of speech, flight of ideas, expansive thought and an overactive and intrusive manner.

Role of drugs *

Hypomania or mania represents a particular phase of a bipolar (or rarely a unipolar) illness. Both usually require specific long-term mood-stabiliser drug treatment for the bipolar component (ie. lithium, valproate, atypicals, carbamazepine, etc), and non-specific shorter-term treatments (eg. antipsychotics, benzodiazepines) for the insomnia, agitation and hyperactivity to calm the patient and prevent exhaustion and harm. A night of sleep deprivation is likely to escalate any manic patient to a higher degree of mania and so hypnotic/sedative use should be considered appropriate (n = 67, Wehr et al, Arch Gen Psychiatry 1982;**39**:559–65). Any co-morbid substance misuse should be tackled at the same time, as recovery from mania is poorer in people with a history of substance abuse (retrospective review, n = 204, Goldberg et al, J Clin Psychiatry 1999;**60**:733–40). After recovery from a manic episode with an antipsychotic and a mood stabiliser, many people receive antipsychotics long-term. This may not always be the best thing to do, as one study showed that those continuing antipsychotics long-term had a quicker onset of depression, were more likely to discontinue, and have more EPS and dysphoria — a good collection of detrimental effects (n = 27, RCT, p/c, d/b, 6/12, Zarate and Tohen, Am J Psychiatry 2004;**161**:169–71). Most response to drugs occurs in the first few weeks and the data on some antipsychotics and valproate is robust. Lithium is an effective antimanic but difficult to use in the short and long-term. Evidence for an antimanic effect for valproate (particularly in mixed states) is better than carbamazepine. Treatment goals for mania should be:

1. Discontinue any agents that may induce symptoms, including antidepressants and substances of misuse (see 5.7 for lists).
2. Stabilise any medical conditions.
3. Start non-specific calming medications, eg. BDZs, antipsychotics.
4. Start specific mood-stabilisers or relapse prevention agents (see 1.10.1) preferably when the patient is able to consent to longer-term therapy.

For very good reasons, in the real world patients presenting with mania are very different to those in clinical trials and inclusions, exclusions and differing assessments of severity (USA tend to rate the same presentation as more severe than UK) may have led to the over-estimating of anti-manic drug efficacy (Storosum et al, Eur Neuropsychopharmacol 2004;**14**:19–23). Indeed, only a small percentage (16%) of acute manic patients presenting in a routine mental hospital would seem to qualify for a standard placebo-controlled RCT (n = 74, Storosum et al, Eur Neuropsychopharmacol 2004;**14**:319–23).

See bipolar mood disorder (1.10.1) for maintenance strategies.

Reviews: * treatment of acute mania and resistant mania (Holtzheimer and Neumaier, CNS Spect 2003;**8**:917–20 and 924–8; Keck and McElroy, Psychopharmacol Bull 2001;**35**:130–48), anticonvulsants in mania (Cookson and Elliott, J Psychopharmacol 2006;**20**[Suppl]:23–30), loading strategies for lithium, valproate and CBZ (Keck et al, Bipolar Disord 2000;**2**:42–6, 37 refs).

BNF listed

Carbamazepine *

There has been a surge of interest in carbamazepine with the launch of an MR preparation in USA. Carbamazepine MR up to 1600 mg/d was effective in 41% (cf 22% for placebo) as monotherapy in acute bipolar mania (n = 204 [c = 96], RCT, d/b, p/c, 3/52, Weisler et al, J Clin Psychiatry 2004;**65**:478–84) and up to 1600 mg/d was superior to placebo in acute mania (n = 239 [c = 144], RCT, d/b, p/c, 3/52, Weisler et al, J Clin Psychiatry 2005;**66**:323–30; pooled results analysis; n = 443 [c = 240], RCT, Weisler et al, CNS Drugs 2006;**20**:219–31). The previous five RCTs of carbamazepine in acute mania show a response rate equivalent to lithium and chlorpromazine (review by Keck et al, J Clin Psychiatry 1998;**59**[Suppl 6]:S74–S81, 114 refs). Doses of up to 1600 mg/d or more have been used in resistant patients (Ballenger, J Clin Psychiatry 1988;**49**[Suppl 1]:S13–S19), but no loading dose strategies have been published in bipolar (see Keck et al, Bipolar Disord 2000;**2**:42–6).

Review: * acute mania (Owen, Drugs Today [Barc] 2006;**42**:283–9).

Lithium *

Lithium may be effective in acute mania/hypomania, although the onset of action may be delayed for five to seven days or longer (unless perhaps if loading doses are used). It is difficult to use in mania due to the need to monitor blood levels, problems with stopping later or prematurely, and the need for two to three years minimum treatment duration. Serum levels of 0.9–1.4 mmol/L may be necessary in the short-term for a therapeutic effect and should be reduced once mood is normalised. Loading with lithium in mania is surprisingly poorly studied but has been tried with rapid success, many responding within 48 hours. The only recent study available showed that in 15 manic in-patients given 20 mg/kg/d for up to 10 days, only five completed the trial (although seven drop-outs improved sufficiently to allow discharge and only two had ADRs). All had levels > 0.6 mmol/L after the first day, which was generally well-tolerated and showed a rapid improvement, although this needs confirming in a full study (n = 15, open, Keck et al, Bipolar Disord 2001;**3**:68–72). At least four previous depressive or 10–12 previous manic episodes are associated with reduced antimanic response to lithium (Swann et al, Acta Psychiatr Scand 2000;**101**:444–51). It may be that patients who have had more than about 10 previous manic episodes may respond less well to lithium than previously (n = 154, Swann et al, Am J Psychiatry 1999;**156**:1264–6; n=40, RCT, d/b, p/c, 4/52, Kafantaris et al, J Am Acad Child Adolesc Psychiatry 2004;**43**:984–93).

Review: efficacy and side-effects in mania (Bowden, J Clin Psychiatry 2000;**61**[Suppl 9]: S35–S40).

Olanzapine *

Olanzapine is licensed in many countries for acute mania. The starting dose is 15 mg/d as monotherapy or 10 mg/d in combination. Two manufacturers' RCTs have shown efficacy as monotherapy in mania, eg. in acute mania, response to olanzapine (49%) was better than placebo (24%) (n = 139, RCT, 3/52, Tohen et al, Am J Psychiatry 1999;**156**:702–9, MS) and olanzapine (mean 17mg/d) produced a significantly greater improvement in mania scores and protocol-defined remission in acute mania than valproate (mean 1400mg/d), with more weight gain, somnolence, dry mouth and increased appetite, but less nausea (n=248, RCT, d/b, 3/52, Tohen et al, Am J Psychiatry 2002;**159**:1011–17, MS). Olanzapine is also useful as an adjunct, eg. it was superior to placebo as an add-on to valproate or lithium in manic and mixed bipolar episodes, although weight gain with olanzapine was significant (n = 344, RCT, d/b, 6/52, Tohen et al, Arch Gen Psychiatry 2002;**59**:62–9, MS; comment by Gardner, EBMH 2002;**5**:89). In a sub-analysis of a larger trial, acute dysphoric mania seems to respond better to lithium or valproate if olanzapine is added (n = 85, RCT, d/b, p/c, 6/52, Baker et al, Br J Psychiatry 2004;**185**:472–8, MS). Cochrane concludes that olanzapine is effective in mania, possibly more so than valproate but with more weight gain and somnolence (n = 1422, s = 6, Rendell et al, Cochrane Database Syst Rev 2003;**3**:CD004040). It has been suggested that some comparative studies didn't use loading doses of valproate (the initial dose

was 750mg/d) which may have postponed the response from valproate, and that somnolence may have helped valproate dosing (Lu, EBMH 2003;**6**:28). Olanzapine 'Velotabs' produce a plasma level profile similar to oral tablets but may be a suitable alternative to injections in some cases by assuring compliance.

Reviews: * short-term management of bipolar I mania (Bhana and Perry, CNS Drugs 2001;**15**:871–904), evidence for relapse prevention following mania (Dando and Tohen, J Psychopharmacol 2006;**20**[Suppl]:31–8).

Quetiapine *

Quetiapine is licensed as monotherapy for the short-term treatment of acute manic episodes associated with bipolar I disorder. Two RCTs have shown efficacy, eg. quetiapine was as effective as haloperidol in acute mania but better tolerated, with a final dose range of 400–800mg/d (n = 302, RCT, d/b, p/c, 12/52, McIntyre et al, Eur Neuropsychopharmacol 2005;**15**:573–85) and up to 800mg/d was as effective as lithium and both were superior to placebo in bipolar mania using YMRS (n = 302, RCT, d/b, p/c, 12/52, Bowden et al, J Clin Psychiatry 2005;**66**:111–21). Quetiapine was at least as effective as valproate in adolescent mania (n = 50, RCT, d/b, 28/7, DelBello et al, J Am Acad Child Adolesc Psychiatry 2006;**45**:305-13; n = 30, RCT, d/b, p/c, 6/52, Delbello et al, J Am Acad Child Adolesc Psychiatry 2002;**41**:1216–23). Rapid dose-titration (200mg, 400mg and 600mg/d on successive days) may be as well-tolerated and as effective as the standard five-day titration, although additional bp monitoring would be prudent (open, 5/7, Pae et al, Int Clin Psychopharmacol 2005;**20**:327–30). Quetiapine is also useful as an adjunct, eg. it was superior to placebo when added to lithium or valproate semisodium, and well-tolerated (n = 191 [c = 105], RCT, 21/7, d/b, p/c, Sachs et al, Bipolar Disord 2004;**6**:213–23) and 500mg/d (range300–700mg/d) was superior to placebo when combined with lithium or divalproex for bipolar mania, and was well-tolerated (n = 402, RCT, d/b, p/c, 6/52, Yatham et al, J Clin Psychopharmacol 2004;**24**:599–606). Results from a monotherapy relapse prevention study were also encouraging (n = 28, open, 12/12, Altamura et al, J Affect Disord 2003;**76**:267–71).

Risperidone *

Risperidone is licensed in UK for monotherapy in bipolar mania. Two RCTs have shown efficacy, eg. risperidone was more effective than placebo (42% vs. 13% remission) in bipolar mania (n = 291, RCT, d/b, p/c, 3/52, Gopal et al, J Clin Psychiatry 2005;**66**:1016–20, MS; comment by Khanna, EBMH 2006;**9**:40; see also n = 259, RCT, p/c, 3/52, Hirschfeld et al, Am J Psychiatry 2004;**161**:1057–65) and in acute mania (YMRS > 20) risperidone 1–6mg/d produced significant improvement in severe mania (n = 290, RCT, d/b, p/c, 3/52, Khanna et al, Br J Psychiatry 2005;**187**:229–34, MS). Although there is much controversy about this second study, the mania was severe and with low drop-outs shows that risperidone also works in very ill patients. It is also useful as an adjunct, eg. risperidone plus mood stabiliser (lithium or valproate) was as effective as haloperidol plus mood stabiliser and more effective than a mood stabiliser alone in acute mania (n = 156, RCT, d/b, p/c, 3/52, Sachs et al, Am J Psychiatry 2002;**159**:1146–54). Onset can be rapidly effective (within a week) as an adjunctive treatment to mood stabilisers in mania, especially if carbamazepine-treated patients are excluded (n = 151, RCT, d/b, p/c, 3/52, Yatham et al, Br J Psychiatry 2003;**182**:141–7; see 4.5.1 for reasons). In a further sub-analysis of this trial, it appears risperidone can be safely combined with valproate or lithium in acute mania (n = 79, 12/52, Yatham et al, Int Clin Psychopharmacol 2004;**19**:103–9). Cochrane concludes that risperidone is effective in mania as both monotherapy and adjunctive treatment (s = 6, n = 1343, Rendell et al, Cochrane Database Syst Rev 2006;**1**:CD004043).

Reviews: * general (Nguyen and Guthrie, Ann Pharmacother 2006;**40**:674–82; Fenton and Scott, CNS Drugs 2005;**19**:429–44).

Valproate semisodium *

Valproate semisodium (aka divalproex) is licensed in the UK as monotherapy for acute mania. Several RCTs have shown efficacy. A robust trial showed valproate to be as effective as lithium in acute mania, independently of a prior responsiveness to lithium (n = 174, RCT, p/c, 21/7, Bowden et al, JAMA 1994;**271**:918–24). Valproate may be more effective than

lithium and as effective as (but better tolerated than) olanzapine (n = 348, s = 3, RCT, d/b, Hirschfeld et al, J Clin Psychiatry 2003;**64**:841–6; MS). A realistic study under realistic conditions, including more severely ill patients, suggests that prompt rapid stabilisation with valproate may allow transition to maintenance without antipsychotics (n = 136, RCT, d/b, p/c, 21/7, Müller-Oerlinghausen et al, J Clin Psychopharmacol 2000;**20**:195–203; review by Swann, EBMH 2000;**3**:113). A comparison of valproate and olanzapine showed an equivalent effect but with fewer side-effects from valproate (n = 120, RCT, d/b, 12/52, Zajecka et al, J Clin Psychiatry 2003;**63**:1148–55). There appears to be a linear relationship between valproate serum concentration and response in acute mania, best response being above 94mcg/ml, presumably as trough levels, although this is unclear in the paper (n = 374, s = 3, RCT, Allen et al, Am J Psychiatry 2006;**163**:272–5). Subsequently, oral loading doses of valproate are probably more rapidly effective in mania, eg. 20mg/kg/d may give a rapid response, often within three days (n = 36, RCT, 6/7, McElroy et al, J Clin Psychiatry 1996;**57**:142–6). Even more aggressive dosing (30mg/kg/d on days one and two, then 20mg/kg/d days 3–10) may produce more rapid therapeutic levels in acute mania, with no adverse effects (n = 59, RCT, Hirschfeld et al, J Clin Psychiatry 1999;**60**:815–18). High-dose IV valproate (20mg/kg) over 30 minutes had no effect in acute mania (n = 7, Phrolov et al, J Clin Psychiatry 2004;**65**:68–70), but IV has been successfully used for adolescent mania (n = 5, Thakur et al, Eur Child Adolesc Psychiatry 2004;**13**:258-61). Valproate infusion (initially 125mg over one hour) has been used and may also be rapidly effective (n = 1, Herbert and Nelson, Am J Psychiatry 2000;**157**:1023–4). Valproate augmentation of TAU decreased heavy drinking in bipolars with co-occurring alcohol dependence (n = 59, RCT, d/b, p/c, 24/52, Salloum et al, Arch Gen Psychiatry 2005;**62**:37–45). Cochrane concludes that there is consistent if limited evidence that valproate is effective in acute mania; it may be less effective than olanzapine but with less sedation and weight gain (s = 10, Macritchie et al, Cochrane Database Syst Rev 2003;**1**:CD004052). While sodium valproate and Depakote® (Sanofi-Synthelabo) are very similar (Fisher and Broderick, *Psychiatr Bull* 2003;**27**:446–8), and while Depakote® may be more tolerable than valproic acid, it may be associated with longer in-patient stays and higher relapse rates (n = 9260, six years, Wassef *et al*, *Am J Psychiatry* 2005;**162**:330–9).

Reviews: general (Bowden, *Bipolar Disord* 2003;**5**:189–202), loading dose strategies (Keck *et al*, *Bipolar Disord* 2000;**2**:42–6).

+ Combinations

In acute mania, combinations are rightfully commonly used. A recent meta-analysis has concluded that adding an antipsychotic to an established mood stabliser is more effective than a mood stabliser alone (s = 8, n = 1124, RCT, Smith *et al*, *Acta Psychiatr Scand* 2007;**115**:12–20).

Review of combinations in mania: Mondimore *et al*, *J Clin Psychiatry* 2003;**64**[Suppl 5]:S25–S31, 73 refs).

Antipsychotics + benzodiazepines
See individual drugs or groups in this section (see also Acute Psychiatric Emergency *1.1*).

Lithium/valproate + antipsychotics
A review of these combinations concluded that the slow onset of action of lithium/valproate means they are more adjuncts to antipsychotics initially, rather than vice versa (Cookson, *Br J Psychiatry* 2001;**178**[Suppl 41]:S148–S56). See also individual antipsychotics in BNF listed section.

Lithium + carbamazepine
Carbamazepine can be used in resistant cases in combination with lithium (review of literature in *Compr Psychiatry* 1990;**31**:261–5). See 4.4 for neurotoxicity warning.

Valproate + lithium
Divalproex may successfully augment lithium in resistant rapid-cycling mania in elderly patients (n = 4, Schneider and Wilcox, *J Affect Disord* 1998;**47**:201–5) and in adults (n = 12, open, Reischies *et al*, *Neuropsychobiol* 2002;**46**[Suppl 1]:S22–S27).

● Unlicensed/some efficacy

Antipsychotics
(see also olanzapine, quetiapine and risperidone in BNF listed section) *

There is some evidence that hypomania has a hyperdopaminergic component and so treatment with dopamine-blocking drugs may be rational, although the majority of even refractory bipolars can be stabilised without long-term antipsychotics (n = 133, Brotman *et al*, *J Clin Psychiatry* 2000; **61**:68–72). A review of 15 RCTs showed that antipsychotics produce a more rapid antimanic effect than lithium (predictably), but lithium is superior at three weeks (Keck *et al*, *J Clin Psychiatry* 1998; **59**[Suppl 6]:S74–S81). **Amisulpride** (about 700mg/d) was effective for mania in a pilot study (n = 20[c = 14], open, 6/52, Vieta *et al*, *J Clin Psychiatry* 2005;**66**:575–8). **Aripiprazole** is licensed for acute mania (and relapse prevention) in USA and supported by several RCTs. Aripiprazole was significantly superior to haloperidol in acute bipolar I mania sustained over 12 weeks and better tolerated (n = 347, RCT, d/b, 12/52, Vieta *et al*, *Br J Psychiatry* 2005; **187**:235–42; comment by Centorrino, *EBMH* 2006;**9**:41, noting that despite the relatively high haloperidol comparative dose and inclusion/exclusion criteria, it is clear aripiprazole is effective and well-tolerated in acute mania). Aripiprazole was also superior to placebo (53% vs 32% responders) and well-tolerated in mania or mixed episodes (n = 272, RCT, d/b, p/c, 3/52, Sachs *et al*, *J Psychopharmacol* 2006;**20**:536–46). **Haloperidol** was superior to placebo at up to 8mg/d (n = 302, RCT, d/b, p/c, 12/52, McIntyre *et al*, *Eur Neuropsychopharmacol* 2005;**15**:573–85) and Cochrane concludes that haloperidol is superior to placebo and equivalent to other antimanic antipsychotics (but possibly inferior to aripiprazole), albeit poorly tolerated (s = 15, n = 2022, Cipriani *et al*, *Cochrane Database Syst Rev* 2006;**3**:CD004362). **Ziprasidone** is licensed in the USA for acute mania and 40–80mg BD produced a rapid (within two days) and sustained improvement in acute bipolar symptoms in one study (n = 210, RCT, p/c, d/b, 3/52, Keck *et al*, *Am J Psychiatry* 2003;**160**:741–8); 80–160mg/d was rapidly effective and well-tolerated for bipolar mania and mixed episodes (n = 202, RCT, d/b, p/c, Potkin et al, J Clin Psychopharmacol 2005; **25**:301–10). Although obviously problematic, **clozapine** (mean 500mg/d) may be effective in 72% treatment-resistant manics or schizo-affectives (n=25, open, Calabrese et al, Am J Psychiatry 1996;**153**:759–64). Another study showed significant improvement relative to TAU in bipolar (n=38, RCT, one year, Suppes et al, Am J Psychiatry 1999;**156**:1164–9), and up to 550mg/d was effective in treatment-refractory psychotic mania (n=22, open, 12/52, Green et al, Am J Psychiatry 2000;**157**:982–6). A pilot study showed **zotepine** (mean 250mg/d) monotherapy is effective in severe mania (n=12[c=10], open, 3/52, Amann et al, Bipolar Disord 2005;**7**:471–6).

Benzodiazepines *

For a group of drugs regularly used in mania, there is remarkably little robust evidence for the efficacy of benzodiazepines, but use is supported by extensive clinical experience. Short-term medium or high doses of benzodiazepines can be used alone or as adjuvants to other therapies in acute phases of hypomania, eg. diazepam by itself, lorazepam (Salzman et al, Psychosomatics 1986;**27**:17–21), or clonazepam at 4–16mg/d (n=12, RCT, d/b, c/o, Chouinard et al, Biol Psychiatry 1983;**18**:451–66). For acute symptoms they have a rapid onset, are highly sedative and are well-tolerated, with no EPSE side-effect risk, but have little or no long-term role. A meta-analysis concluded that the data supported the safe and effective use of clonazepam in mania, although there wasn't exactly a lot to meta-analyse (Curtin and Schulz, J Affect Disord 2004; **78**:201–8).

Phenytoin

Phenytoin augmentation of haloperidol in acute mania was more effective than haloperidol alone, and may indicate that blockade of voltage-activated sodium channels is a common therapeutic mechanism for anticonvulsants in acute mania (n=39, RCT, 5/52, Mishory et al, Am J Psychiatry 2000;**157**:463–5).

■ Unlicensed/possible efficacy

Allopurinol *

YMRS improved when allopurinol (300mg/d)

was added to lithium and haloperidol in acute mania, albeit not quite statistically significant (n=82, RCT, d/b, p/c, Akhondzadeh et al, Bipolar Disord 2006;**8**:485–9).

Levetiracetam *

A pilot trial of adjunctive levetiracetam 500–2000mg/d showed some improvement in most manic patients, but was not wildly encouraging (n=34, open, 8/52, Post et al, J Clin Psychiatry 2005;**66**:370–4). There is a well-documented case of acute mania responding to levetiracetam up to 2500mg/d (n=1, Goldberg and Burdick, Am J Psychiatry 2002;**159**:148), and up to 4g/d appears to have some antimanic effect when used with haloperidol (n=10, open, 28/7, Grunze et al, J Clin Psychiatry 2003;**64**:781–4).

Omega-3 fatty acids

Fish oils may have some application (reviewed by Maidment, Acta Psychiatr Scand 2000;**102**:3–11, 40 refs).

Oxcarbazepine *

Oxcarbazepine has been used successfully in acute mania at 2400mg/d compared with haloperidol 42mg/d, where it had a slower onset of action but fewer side-effects (n=42, Emrich, Int Clin Psychopharmacol 1990;**5**[Suppl 1]:S83–S88). In a comparison with lithium in acute mania, oxcarbazepine was equally effective, but with a slower onset and was less well-tolerated (n=58, d/b, mentioned by Grant and Faulds, Drugs 1992, **43**, 873–88), and as an add-on to lithium was effective in 60%, and may be helpful long-term in some patients (n=17, open, 8/52+12/12, Benedetti et al, J Affect Disord 2004;**79**:273–7). Oxcarbazepine was also not significantly superior to placebo in youths (7–18 years) with bipolar mania (n=116, RCT, d/b, p/c, 7/52, Wagner et al, Am J Psychiatry 2006;**163**:1179–86).

Propofol *

Propofol has been effective as an IV drip in multidrug, severe, life-threatening mania (n=1, Cluver and Hardesty, J Clin Psychiatry 2006; **67**:165–6).

Topiramate *

Data on topiramate as an adjunct is mixed.

Open trials have suggested modest efficacy for topiramate in mania (n = 14, open, 4/52, Bozikas et al, Prog Neuropsychopharmacol Biol Psychiatry 2002;26:1203–6; 50% response, n = 10, open, 28/7, Calabrese et al, J Clin Psychopharmacol 2001;21:340–2), and as an adjunct in resistant bipolar depression and mania (n = 34, open, Vieta et al, J Clin Psychopharmacol 2002;22:431–5). Topiramate (mean 180 mg/d) as an adjunct to mood stabilisers reduced the severity of manic and depressive bipolar symptoms, as well as reducing tremor and weight (n = 109, open, 16/52, McIntyre et al, Can J Psychiatry 2005;50:415–22), although a manufacturer's analysis concluded there was no evidence to support use as monotherapy in mania (s = 4, RCT, Kushner et al, Bipolar Disord 2006; 8:15–27). Two short exposures (with a gap) to topiramate as an add-on to existing mood stabilisers both showed improvement in manic symptoms, indicating that response was linked to the addition of topiramate (n = 11, Grunze et al, J Clin Psychiatry 2001;62:464–8; although the number of authors [nine] almost out-numbered the number of patients). Topiramate and risperidone combined may be useful for short and long-term management of mania (n = 58[c = 41], open, 12/12, Vieta et al, J Clin Psychiatry 2003;64:834–9). Cochrane concluded there was as yet insufficient evidence for use as monotherapy or adjunctive for acute episodes of bipolar disorder (Vasudev et al, Cochrane Database Syst Rev 2006;1:CD003384).

Review: use in mood disorders, (Chengappa et al, Bipolar Disord 2001;3:215–32, 98 refs).

Verapamil

One study showed that up to 320 mg/d was as effective in acute mania as lithium (n = 20, RCT, d/b, 4/52, Garza-Trevino et al, Am J Psychiatry 1992;149:121–2). However, a short random-assignment, parallel-group in-patient trial found no benefit on psychosis for verapamil over placebo (n = 32, RCT, 3/52, Janicak et al, Am J Psychiatry 1998;155:972–3). A naturalistic study in bipolar women suggested that verapamil was effective in mania with a response rate comparable to other mood stabilisers, but an RCT would be needed to confirm this (n = 10437 women, open, Wisner et al, Biol Psychiatry 2002;5:745–52).

Zonisamide *

Adjunctive zonisamide has improved mania and depression in many patients but mood deteriorated in 32% patients and there was a high discontinuation rate, although nearly all lost weight (n = 62, open, 8/52, McElroy et al, J Clin Psychiatry 2005;66:617–24).

◆ Others

Other drugs tried include **dexamfetamine** (Clower, Psychopharmacol Bull 1988;24:168), **clonidine** (in antipsychotic-resistant mania; Jouvent et al, Br J Psychiatry 1988;152:293), **doxepin** 100 mg/d (n = 1, Kaye, Am J Psychiatry 1992;146:802–3), **levothyroxine** (0.3–0.5 mg/d for rapid or 48-hour cycling mania; n = 7, Stancer and Persad, Arch Gen Psychiatry 1982;39:311–2), **methylene blue** (to reduce pathotoxic vanadium ion concentrations; n = 31, d/b, c/o, two years, Naylor et al, Biol Psychiatry 1986;21:915–20; Moody et al, Biol Psychiatry 1989; 26:850–2) and **spironolactone** (n = 1, Gillman and Lichtigfeld, Br Med J 1986;292:661–2).

* No efficacy

Antidepressants

Antidepressants can either precipitate mania by provoking a mood switch or exacerbate existing or developing mania. A retrospective study of patients discharged from hospital with bipolar I depression or mania showed a relatively high use of antidepressants in bipolar mania (either alone or in combination) and, although this included some trazodone for insomnia, the rest was not for insomnia, a worrying finding (n = 1864, Lim et al, Bipolar Disord 2001;3:165–73).

Caffeine

A high caffeine intake will risk disturbing sleep patterns and exacerbating mania.

Fosphenytoin

IV fosphenytoin appears ineffective in acute mania (n = 7, open, 1 hour; Applebaum et al, J Clin Psychiatry 2003;64:408–9).

Gabapentin

The only two double-blind placebo-controlled studies failed to show any advantage as an adjunct over placebo in mania (eg. n = 117, Pande, gabapentin study group, *Bipolar Disord* 1999;1[Suppl 1]:S17; Pande *et al, J Clin Psychopharmacol* 1999;**19**:341–8), and the trend was towards a negative effect. However, a number of case reports (eg. Stanton *et al, Am J Psychiatry* 1997;**154**:287) and open studies (n = 25, up to 1440mg/d, Cabras *et al, J Clin Psychiatry* 1999;**60**:245–8) had suggested a potential effect in mania in some people, a good advert for evidence-based approaches to treatment.

Lamotrigine *

Lamotrigine is not considered effective in mania. It has no efficacy in acute mania and only delays time to manic relapse in pooled data. It may be more effective in male bipolar patients with fewer prior medication trials (n = 45, Obrocea *et al, Biol Psychiatry* 2002;**51**:253–60).

Tiagabine

Tiagabine has no detectable anti-manic activity as monotherapy or adjunctive therapy compared to standard treatments (n = 8, open, 14/7, Grunze *et al, J Clin Psychiatry* 1999; **60**:759–62).

1.10.3 BIPOLAR DEPRESSION

Bipolar depression is longer-lasting than unipolar depression (up to 50% may still be depressed at one year, Hlastala *et al, Depress Anxiety* 1997;**5**:73–83), frequently misdiagnosed (a substantial proportion of antidepressant–refractory depression is probably undiagnosed bipolar; n = 26, Inoue *et al, J Affect Disord* 2006;**95**:61–7) and is often characterised by psychomotor-retarded melancholic symptoms, atypical features and psychosis (n = 39 + 39, Mitchell *et al, J Clin Psychiatry* 2001;**62**:212–6). It is clear that well-being and functioning are inversely proportional to the number of bipolar episodes and so strategies to reduce relapse must be rigorously followed, especially minimising difficult-to-treat bipolar depression (n = 64, retrospective, MacQueen *et al, Acta Psychiatr Scand* 2000;**101**:374–81). It can be potentiated by substance and alcohol misuse and is much more difficult to treat.

The general principles of management include:
1. **Avoid inducing mixed affective states** with antidepressants, particularly in bipolar III, where the risk of self-harm is high.
2. **Avoid sudden dose changes** or switches.
3. **Optimise antidepressants** (eg. n = 2032, Moller *et al, J Affect Disord* 2001;**67**:141–6) with care, starting with lowest switch risk drugs, eg. SSRIs, mirtazapine, bupropion or moclobemide, but avoiding tricyclics, MAOIs and venlafaxine if possible. Addition of an antidepressant to a mood stabiliser is probably more effective than adding a second mood stabiliser (paroxetine vs lithium or valproate; n = 27, RCT, d/b, 6/52, Young *et al, Am J Psychiatry* 2000;**157**:124–6), particularly in people unable to tolerate higher lithium doses (n = 117, d/b, p/c, 10/52, Nemeroff *et al, Am J Psychiatry* 2001;**158**:906–12). Lamotrigine has a growing reputation as a specific measure for bipolar depression, although most robust data supports prevention of relapse rather than as an acute treatment.
4. **Avoid switching to mania with antidepressants** — in bipolar depression this varies from 31–70%. It usually occurs within the first 12 weeks, is lower if antidepressants used with a mood stabiliser. If depression develops, the best plan is to reduce the antidepressant dose immediately and allow the mood to settle for a month or so. It occurs more often in bipolar II than bipolar I (n = 184, 10/52, Altshuler *et al, Am J Psychiatry* 2006;**163**:313–5). A systematic review of antidepressants in bipolar depression concludes that they do not induce switching to mania, although the switching rate is higher with tricyclics. Use SSRIs first line, although the available data is of short duration and complicated by polytherapy (s = 12, n = 1088, RCTs, Gijsman *et al, Am J Psychiatry* 2004;**161**:1537–47; comment by Masand and Mago, *EBMH* 2005;**8**:35). The switch rates in trials have been reported to be:
   - placebo 7%
   - sertraline 2%
   - bupropion 4%.
   - fluoxetine 0–16%
   - venlafaxine 9%
   - imipramine 9.5–28%
   - tranylcypromine 24%.

References: n=89, d/b, Cohn et al, Int Clin Psychopharmacol 1989;**4**:313–22; n=56, RCT, Himmelhoch et al, Am J Psychiatry 1991; **148**:910–6; n=174, RCT, 10/52, Post et al, Br J Psychiatry 2006;**189**:124–31; n=34, RCT, p/c, d/b, 8/52, Amsterdam and Shults, J Affect Disord 2005;**87**:121–30.

5. **Use mood stabilisers** in the initial acute stage, eg. lithium and valproate.

6. **Minimise antidepressant exposure** by attempting gradual taper after a continuation phase, provided the patient is genuinely euthymic. Consider, however, that premature discontinuing antidepressants within the first 3–6/12 of an episode (n=25) has an up to three times higher relapse rate than those continuing for at least 8/12 (n=19), with no increase in mania in the latter group (n=44, retrospective, one year, Altshuler et al, J Clin Psychiatry 2001;**62**:612–6).

7. **Offer ECT** for patients at immediate risk of self-harm or unable to tolerate antidepressants. ECT may be better in older people.

8. **Check thyroid function** — poor response in bipolar depression may be related to low FTI and high TSH levels, even if in the alleged therapeutic range (n=65, Cole et al, Am J Psychiatry 2002;**159**:116–21).

Reviews: general (Haddad and Dursun, Acta Psychiatr Scand 2002;**105**:401–3; Ghaemi et al, J Clin Psychiatry 2001;**62**:565–9), WFSBP Guidelines (Grunze et al, World J Biol Psychiatry 2002;**3**:115–24).

+ Combinations

Lithium + lamotrigine *

In treatment-resistant bipolars, a retrospective chart review suggested that combining lamotrigine and lithium was effective for acute bipolar depression in 48% patients but that acute manic (14%) and long-term efficacy (29%) appeared less robust (n=21, one year, Ghaemi et al, J Psychiatr Pract 2006;**12**:300–5).

Olanzapine + fluoxetine (OFC) *

The olanzapine-fluoxetine combination (OFC) is marketed as 'Symbyax' and licensed for bipolar depression in the US. The efficacy of Symbyax for the treatment of depressive

episodes associated with bipolar disorder has been established utilising flexible dosing as the following: Symbyax (6/25, 6/50, or 12/50mg/day), olanzapine (5–20mg/day), and placebo (n=833, RCT, d/b, 8/52, Tohen et al, Arch Gen Psychiatry 2003;**60**:1079–88, MS; secondary analysis, n=833, RCT, d/b, p/c, Shi et al, Clin Ther 2004;**26**:125–34, MS). The study included patients with or without psychotic symptoms and with or without a rapid cycling course, although had no fluoxetine arm and so the combination's efficacy might be predominantly from fluoxetine. OFC was modestly superior to lamotrigine for bipolar depressive or manic symptoms (n=410, RCT, d/b, 7/52, Brown et al, J Clin Psychiatry 2006;**67**:1025–33: MS), and there may be some efficacy in relapse prevention (n=560, open, 76/52, Corya et al, J Clin Psychiatry 2003;**64**:1349–56; MS).

Reviews: general (Shelton, Expert Opin Pharmacother 2003;**4**:1175–83; Owen, Drugs Today [Barc] 2006;**42**:185–92).

Lithium + fluoxetine

Fluoxetine-augmentation of lithium in bipolar mood disorder can help prevent breakthrough depression (n=26, open, three-year, Tondo et al, Int J Psychiatry Clin Pract 1997;**1**:203–6).

• Unlicensed/some efficacy

Antidepressants *

Antidepressants can be highly effective in treating bipolar depression, but once mood has lifted there is the risk of inducing a switch to mania or induce rapid-cycling. In adults with bipolar depression, venlafaxine, bupropion and sertraline all produce similar acute responses (49–53%) and remission (34–41%) but the risk of switching to mania or hypomania is variable (see general principles, point 4). **Fluoxetine** may have a low switch rate in bipolar I and II (n=34, RCT, p/c, d/b, 8/52, Amsterdam and Shults, J Affect Disord 2005;**87**:121–30). **Bupropion** has been used as an adjunct in resistant, bipolar depression (n=13, open, Erfurth et al, Neuropsychobiology 2001;**45**[Suppl 1]:S33–S36). **Citalopram** has been shown to be highly effective in bipolar I and II depression, with a robust and sustained response rate and low ADRs (n=45, open, 8/52, Kupfer et *al, Clin Psych* 2001;**62**:985–90). Citalopram and lamotrigine may be useful adjunctives in bipolar depression, with reponse rates rising considerably past the first six weeks (n = 20, RCT, d/b, 12/52, Schaffer *et al, J Affect Disord* 2006;**96**:95–9). **Escitalopram** may have some efficacy in bipolar depression (n = 20, open, 12/52, Fonseca *et al, J Clin Psychiatry* 2006;**67**:81–6). **Moclobemide** 450–750mg/d may be as effective as imipramine (150–250mg/d) in bipolar depression, with less side-effects and less switches to mania (2 vs 6) indicating a useful potential role (n = 156, RCT, 8/52, Silverstone *et al, Acta Psychiatr Scand* 2001;**104**:104–9), although 50% patients were on lithium and 31% were on 750mg moclobemide so there may be an augmentation component in its efficacy. In bipolars developing a new-onset depressive episode, there is no evidence that antidepressants were associated with new-onset suicidality, even in already high-risk populations (n = 425, STEP-BD, Bauer *et al, J Clin Psychiatry* 2006;**67**:48–55). People who had more than six months of antidepressants were less likely to relapse into depression at follow-up of one year (n = 59, open, onw year retrospective, Joffe *et al, Acta Psychiatr Scand* 2005;**112**:105–9), which slightly confuses the picture. One study showed that continuing antidepressants after a depressive episode was **not** associated with an increased risk of manic episodes, but early discontinuation was associated with significantly increased depressive relapse (n = 84, one year, naturalistic, Altshuler *et al, Am J Psychiatry* 2003;**160**:1252–62). **Tricyclics** should be avoided unless covered with mood stabilisers (n = 136, Mundo *et al, J Affect Disord* 2006;**92**:227–30).

Antipsychotics

The main roles of antipsychotics in bipolar depression are as adjunctives to mood stabilisers and as adjunctive maintenance in treatment-resistance.

Reviews: atypicals in bipolar and schizoaffective disorders (Ghaemi and Goodwin, *J Clin Psychopharmacol* 1999;**19**:354–61).

Ethyl-EPA (ethyl-eicopentaenoic acid) *

This omega-3 fatty acid was effective in bipolar depression, with 1–2g/d superior to placebo

(n = 75, RCT, d/b, p/c, 12/52, Frangou *et al, Br J Psychiatry* 2006;**188**:46–50).

Lamotrigine *

Lamotrigine is licensed in the US (but not the UK) for the maintenance treatment of bipolar I depression and relapse prevention. Although there are some unpublished negative studies, lamotrigine appears to significantly delay the time to depressive relapse in bipolar depression, eg. lamotrigine and lithium were superior to placebo for prevention of mood episodes in bipolar I depression, with lamotrigine predominantly and robustly effective against relapse to depression and lithium robustly effective against relapse to mania (n = 463, RCT, p/c, 18/12, Calabrese *et al, J Clin Psychiatry* 2003;**64**:1013–24; comment by Soldani and Ghaemi, *EBMH* 2004;**7**:48, noting high drop-out rate and lithium at high plasma levels; see also n = 1315, RCT, p/c, d/b, 18/12, Goodwin *et al, J Clin Psychiatry* 2004;**65**:432–41). Lamotrigine 50–200mg/d monotherapy is significantly more effective than placebo in bipolar I depression, the effect being seen as early as the third week (n = 195, RCT, Calabrese *et al, J Clin Psychiatry* 1999;**60**:79–88). After an open-label acute mania/hypomania episode treatment trial, both lamotrigine and lithium were superior to placebo for reducing relapse or recurrence of mood disorders in bipolar I, with lamotrigine better for preventing depressive and lithium better for preventing manic episodes (n = 175, RCT, d/b, p/c, ≤18/12, Bowden *et al, Arch Gen Psychiatry* 2003;**60**:392–400). Lamotrigine improves cognitive functioning especially in bipolar depression when used as monotherapy or adjunctive treatment (n = 349 + 966, Khan *et al, J Clin Psychiatry* 2004;**65**:1483–90). In patients with bipolar depression unresponsive to a mood stabiliser and at least one antidepressant, response to lamotrigine was 24% (cf. inositol 17% and risperidone 5%; n = 66, RCT, 16/52, open, Nierenberg *et al, Am J Psychiatry* 2006; **163**:210–6). The mode of action may be inhibition of sodium and calcium channels in presynaptic neurons, and subsequent neuronal membrane stabilisation. Increasing the dose slowly over 6/52 to 200mg/d minimises the incidence of rash.

Reviews: general (Goldsmith *et al, Drugs* 2003;

63:2029–50; Zerjav-Lacombe and Tabarsi, *Can J Psychiatry* 2001;**46**:328–33; Engle and Heck, *Ann Pharmacother* 2000;**34**:258–62, 28 refs), mode of action in mood disorders (Ketter *et al*, *J Clin Psychopharmacol* 2003;**23**:484–95).

Quetiapine *

Two robust RCTs (BOLDER 1 and 2) have shown quetiapine monotherapy to have a significant efficacy in bipolar depression. The first showed response rates in bipolar 1 depression of 58.2% (600 mg/d) and 57.6% (300 mg/d), compared with 36% for placebo (remission was 52.9% vs 28.4%). Treatment emergent mania was 3–4% for both groups (n = 542, RCT, d/b, p/c, 8/52, Calabrese *et al*, *Am J Psychiatry* 2005;**162**:1351–60). In the second study, quetiapine, 300 mg and 600 mg/d monotherapy were equally effective in bipolar I and II depression, with a 53% response rate (n = 542, RCT, 8/52, p/c, Hirschfeld *et al*, *J Clin Psychiatry* 2006;**67**:355–62). A UK licence is due in 2007–8.

■ Unlicensed/possible efficacy

Gabapentin

While gabapentin has no antimanic activity (see *1.10.2*), it may be useful as an adjunct in refractory and co-morbid bipolar patients (review, s = 40, Carta *et al*, *J Affect Disord* 2003;**75**:83–91). Gabapentin was considered moderately to markedly effective in 30% of patients with bipolar or unipolar depression mood disorders (n = 50, retrospective, open, Ghaemi *et al*, *J Clin Psychiatry* 1998;**59**:426–9). Gabapentin augmentation was effective and well-tolerated in mild to moderate bipolar depression (n = 22, open pilot, 12/52, Wang *et al*, *Bipolar Disord* 2002;**4**:296–301). In a trial against lamotrigine, gabapentin was no better than placebo (n = 45, RCT, p/c, d/b, c/o, 6/52, Obrocea *et al*, *Biol Psychiatry* 2002;**51**:253–60). **Reviews:** Letterman and Markowitz, *Pharmacotherapy* 1999;**19**:565–72; Maidment, *Ann Pharmacother* 2001;**35**:1264–9.

Inositol *

Inositol may be useful in bipolar (as well as unipolar), depression as shown in a trial where 50% responded to 12 g/d inositol (cf 30%

on placebo) (n = 24, RCT, 6/52, Chengappa *et al*, *Bipolar Disord* 2000;**2**:47–55). In a second trial, patients with bipolar depression unresponsive to a mood stabiliser and at least one antidepressant, response to inositol was 17% (cf lamotrigine 24% and risperidone 5%; n = 66, RCT, 16/52, open, Nierenberg *et al*, *Am J Psychiatry* 2006;**163**:210–6).

Ketoconazole

Ketoconazole, 400 mg/d has been used as add-on therapy in resistant bipolar depression, with no increase in manic symptoms (n = 6, open, Brown *et al*, *Bipolar Disord* 2001;**3**:23–9).

Levetiracetam *

A pilot trial of adjunctive levetiracetam 500–2000 mg/d showed a modest improvement in some depressed patients, but was not wildly encouraging (n = 34, open, 8/52, Post *et al*, *J Clin Psychiatry* 2005;**66**:370–4).

Methylphenidate

In one study, methylphenidate was effective and tolerable in 78% depressed bipolars, although use of a stimulant such as methylphenidate would in theory risk switching to mania (n = 14, open, 12/52, El-Mallakh, *Bipolar Disord* 2000; **2**:56–9).

Modafinil *

In remitted bipolar depression with hypersomnia, modafinil may be effective as an adjunct to mood stabilisers and antidepressants (n = 2, Fernandes and Petty, *Ann Pharmacother* 2003;**37**:1807–9).

Oxcarbazepine *

Oxcarbazepine as add-on to lithium in bipolar depression was effective in 60% and may be successful in most over the longer-term (n = 17, open, 8/52+12/12, Benedetti *et al*, *J Affect Disord* 2004;**79**:273–7).

Pramipexole

Pramipexole is a dopamine agonist and was clearly superior (60% response) to placebo (9%) in bipolar depression, when used as an adjunct to either lithium or valproate (n = 21, RCT, d/b, p/c, 6/52, Zarate *et al*, *Biol Psychiatry* 2004;**56**:54–60) and a mean 1.7 mg/d added to existing mood stabilisers produced a 67% response (cf 20% with placebo) in bipolar depression (n = 22, RCT, o/p, p/c, 6/52, Goldberg et al, Am J Psychiatry 2004;**161**:564–6).

Review: Whiskey and Taylor, *Psychiatr Bull* 2004;**28**:438–40).

Valproate *

Valproate may reduce depressive symptoms compared to lithium (sub-analysis of Bowden study by Gyulai et al, *Neuropsychopharmacol* 2003;**28**:1374–82).

Zonisamide *

Adjunctive zonisamide (mean 236 mg/d) may have some potential in bipolar depression in some patients (n = 12, retrospective chart analysis, Baldassano et al, *Bipolar Disord* 2004;**6**:432–4).

1.10.4 RAPID-CYCLING BIPOLAR DISORDER

Introduction *

Rapid-cycling bipolar disorder is a variant of bipolar mood disorder, where four or more mood episodes occur in one year. Although it is relatively uncommon (eg. one in six presenting with bipolar have a rapid-cycling pattern) and often a transient condition (about 80% will resolve in a year), the clinical significance of the sub-group is that it accounts for up to 80% of lithium non-responders, that antidepressant therapy of depressive phases can induce or worsen cycling (eg. Wehr and Goodwin, *Am J Psychiatry* 1987;**176**:633–6) and that rapid-cycling is a risk factor for suicide. Rapid-cyclers suffer substantial depressive morbidity and are at higher risk of suicide attempts (n = 345, mean 13 years, Coryell et al, *Arch Gen Psychiatry* 2003;**60**:914–20). Rapid-cycling is slightly more common in women.

Role of drugs *

There will probably always be a lack of robust data on the pharmacotherapy of rapid-cycling, as research is complicated by the unpredictable and spontaneously remitting nature of the condition. The initial actions must be:

1. Reduce or stop any cycle-promoters (eg. antidepressants).

2. Add or optimise mood stabilisers (start with lithium for treatment-naïve patients).
3. Add other drugs, eg. lithium, atypicals, lamotrigine, perhaps valproate.
4. Minimise ADRs.
5. Recognise that full benefits may not be apparent for several months so do not abandon treatment too early.

References: n = 500, STEP-BD, Schneck et al, *J Clin Psychiatry* 2006;**67**[Suppl 11]:22–7; Coryell, *CNS Drugs* 2005;**19**:557–69; s = 20, Kupka et al, *J Clin Psychiatry* 2003;**64**:1483–94).

If ineffective, drugs may be used in combination. Levothyroxine and nimodipine may be effective in some patients not responsive to first-line drugs and may be worth a therapeutic trial.

Reviews: * definitions (Maj et al, *Am J Psychiatry* 1999;**156**:1421–4), general (Mercer, *Curr Psychiatr Rep* 2007;**9**:53–62; Goodnick et al, *Expert Opin Pharmacother* 2001;**2**:1963–73), use of novel anticonvulsants (Calabrese et al, *J Clin Psychiatry* 2002;**63**[Suppl 3]:S5–S9).

BNF listed

Carbamazepine

Several studies (eg. n = 18, open, 6/12, Joyce, *Int Clin Psychopharmacol* 1988;**3**:123–9) have shown a long-term response rate ranging from 20–70%. The original carbamazepine study (n = 32, Kishimoto et al, *Br J Psychiatry* 1983;**143**:327–31) showed a particular effect in rapid-cycling. Doubt has, however, been raised about long-term efficacy as many people seem to lose the therapeutic response over several years (n = 24, open, four years, Post et al, *J Clin Psychopharmacol* 1990;**10**:318–27).

Lithium

Although around 80% of rapid-cyclers are lithium non-responsive (as opposed to 41% of non-rapid cyclers), that still leaves 20% who do respond and lithium undoubtedly has some effect, probably by reducing the intensity of relapses rather than the actual number. Lithium response may be better if the sequence of relapse is mania, depression and then remission rather than depression, then mania and remission (Grof et al, *Prog Neuropsychopharmacol Biol Psychiatry* 1987;**11**:199–203). Poor compliance with lithium, particularly if intermittent (eg.

frequent abrupt stopping), may complicate treatment by inducing relapse. The STEP-BD study is beginning to provide some much-needed information.

+ Combinations

Carbamazepine + valproate

Synergy has been reported (n=1 and review: Ketter et al, J Clin Psychopharmacol 1992;12:276–81).

Lithium + carbamazepine

The combination can be useful in rapid-cyclers non-responsive to the individual drugs (eg. n=16, retrospective, Di Costanzo and Schifano, Acta Psychiatr Scand 1991;83:456–9). See interactions for cautions on the use of this combination (4.5.1).

Lithium + levothyroxine

Low dose levothyroxine added to lithium in one rapid-cycler produced complete euthymia within seven days (n=1, Bernstein, J Clin Psychopharmacol 1992;12:443–4).

Lithium + valproate

Open studies have included this combination in rapid-cyclers, and reported an additive or potentiating effect, sometimes within a matter of days (mentioned by Sharma and Persad, Lithium 1994;5:117–25).

Thyroid + tricyclic

Sub-therapeutic doses of T_3 tri-iodothyronine 25–50mcg/d (n=1, Cooke, Am J Psychiatry 1990, 147, 255) or T_4 levothyroxine up to 0.1mg/d have been used as augmentation to tricyclics and phenelzine (although care is needed with any use of antidepressants in rapid-cycling). This may be effective particularly in rapid-cycling disorder (n=11, open, Bauer and Whybrow, Arch Gen Psychiatry 1990;47:435–40) rather than equally in all depressions. See also levothyroxine/liothyronine.

Topiramate + clozapine *

There is one case of topiramate augmentation of clozapine retaining effectiveness for three years with no significant ADRs (n=1, Chen et al, Clin Neuropharmacol 2005;28:136–8).

● Unlicensed/some efficacy

Lamotrigine

In the largest and only prospective placebo-controlled study in rapid-cycling disorder, lamotrigine was well-tolerated, and appeared useful in some rapid-cyclers (n=324, open + n=182, d/b maintenance phase, Calabrese et al, J Clin Psychiatry 2000;61:841–50) with survival rates favouring lamotrigine (significantly so in bipolar II patients), with 41% stable without relapse at 6/12 (cf 26% placebo). Lamotrigine may be effective compared to lithium in a trial in refractory rapid-cycling (n=14, RCT, open, one year, Walden et al, Bipolar Disorder 2000;2:336–9; n=6, open, Jusumakar and Yatham, Am J Psychiatry 1997;154:1171–12). The optimum dose appears to be 50–200mg/d, although doses as high as 600mg/d have been used.

Levothyroxine/thyroxine/liothyronine

Levothyroxine has potential efficacy at 0.3–0.5mg/d (or liothyronine 140–400mcg/d) for rapid or 48-hour cycling mania. In one open study, 91% showed clear-cut improvement of rapid-cycling on levothyroxine, supranormal free levothyroxine levels being necessary for clinical response, with minimal side-effects (n=11, open, Bauer and Whybrow, Arch Gen Psychiatry 1990;47:435–40). Significant response was seen in a two-year study with high-dose levothyroxine (n=6, open, Afflelou et al, Encephale 1997;23:209–17) and 0.25–0.3mg/d, creating a slightly hyperthyroid state, was shown to be effective (via an unplanned dose reduction) in a lady with long-standing resistant rapid-cycling (n=1, Extein, Am J Psychiatry 2000;157:1704–5).

Valproate *

Valproate seems as effective as lithium in preventing relapse in recently stabilised rapid-cyclers (n=60 [n=254 in stabilisation phase], RCT, d/b, 20/12, Calabrese et al, Am J Psychiatry 2005;162:2152–61).

■ Unlicensed/possible efficacy

Calcium-channel blockers

There have been reports of response to nimodipine (highly lipophilic, allowing adequate

CNS concentrations and minimal peripheral effects) in rapid-cycling with a very marked response in some patients (n = 12[c=9], RCT, d/b, p/c, Pazzaglia et al, Psychiatry Res 1993;**49**:257–72; Goodnick, J Clin Psychiatry 1995;**56**:330), with 90–180 mg/d optimal. Verapamil is poorly lipophilic with a low central effect.

Clonazepam

Cases exist of clonazepam being useful as an adjunct to lithium in lithium-refractory bipolars (n = 5, open, Aronson et al, Am J Psychiatry 1989;**146**:77–80).

Clozapine

A number of case reports indicate clozapine may be effective in treatment-resistant rapid cycling (n = 2, Calabrese et al, J Clin Psychopharmacol 1991;**11**:396–7; n = 3, Suppes et al, Biol Psychiatry 1994;**36**:338–40).

Gabapentin

Some of the studies of gabapentin in mania included some rapid-cycling patients and moderate efficacy was reported (but see mania) by Shelton and Calabrese (Curr Psychiatry Reports 2000;**2**:310–15).

Levetiracetam *

There are cases of adjunctive treatment improving depression, interrupting rapid cycling (n = 2, Braünig and Krüger, J Psychopharmacol 2003;**17**:239–41) and in multiple drug-resistant rapid-cycling (n = 1, Kaufman, Epilepsy Behav 2004;**5**:1017–20).

Olanzapine

Ten rapid-cyclers were classified as responding to olanzapine during dysphoric mania (n = 13, open, 4/52, Gonzalez-Pinto et al, J Clin Psychopharmacol 2002;**22**:450–4).

Quetiapine *

Successful use with co-morbid anxiety and social phobia has been reported (n = 1, Valerius et al, Pharmacopsychiatry 2005;**38**:225–6).

✱ No efficacy

Antidepressants

Antidepressants may induce rapid-cycling,

especially in women prior to the first episode (but not in men, Yildiz and Sachs, J Clin Psychiatry 2003;**64**:814–18) and since up to 50% of cases may be antidepressant-induced, discontinuation has to be first-line treatment (n = 51, open, Wehr et al, Am J Psychiatry 1988;**145**:179–84; see also Coryell et al, Arch Gen Psychiatry 1992;**49**:126–31). Antidepressants should only be used in rapid-cyclers in low dose and only in acute severe depression.

1.11 BORDERLINE PERSONALITY DISORDER

see also Aggression (1.2)

There are a large number of personality disorders, of which borderline personality disorder is but one. Treating personality disorders (and hence personality itself) is obviously somewhat controversial. Patients with BPD present for treatment more often than schizoid, paranoid and avoidant personality types. Research is now often directed towards treating symptom clusters rather than the underlying personality disorder, eg. anxiety, aggression and impulsiveness.

Symptoms

The main symptoms of BPD are of a deeply ingrained maladaptive pattern of behaviour, recognisable from adolescence and continuing through most of adult life. Such people show continued boredom, anger, unstable relationships, impulsive self-harmful behaviour (eg. gambling, stealing, binge-eating or drinking), variable moods, recurrent suicide threats or behaviour, and uncertainty about their personal identity.

Role of drugs *

BPD may account for up to 7.5% of psychiatric admissions, with a raised incidence of psychiatric morbidity and mortality, and are users of a wide range of medication and services (n = 664, Bender et al, Am J Psychiatry 2001;**158**:295–302). Pharmacotherapy will not alter ingrained character traits or the effects of abuse, but they may produce modest benefits with the occasional striking result, and be more effective if combined with psychotherapy. Drug therapy, however, is fraught with problems. Side-effects may be grossly exaggerated to avoid treatment and patients may be actively antimedication.

Cochrane concludes that current data for pharmacological interventions in BPD is poor, but that there may be a positive effect from antidepressants (Binks et al, Cochrane Database Syst Rev 2006;1:CD005653).Therapeutic alliances (eg. giving a drug a 'trial'), and not abandoning the patient if the drugs work, may help.

Reviews: general (Various, Am J Psychiatry 2001;**158** (Oct Suppl):S25–S43; Soloff, Psychiatr Clin North Am 2000;**23**:169–92), classification, epidemiology, diagnosis and assessment, intervention and management (Marlowe and Sugarman, Br Med J 1997;**315**:176–9).

• Unlicensed/some efficacy

Antipsychotics *

It has been generally accepted that patients with DSM-IV borderline or schizotypical personality disorders may gain significant benefit from psychotherapy and small doses of antipsychotics. Low dose **risperidone** may be effective and well-tolerated, eg. risperidone (mean 3.27 mg/d) helped as an add-on to existing therapies to improve BPD symptomatology, especially aggression and overall functioning (n=15, open, 8/52, Rocca et al, J Clin Psychiatry 2002;**63**:241–4). **Olanzapine** may be effective against a range of psychopathological symptoms in females with BPD (weight gain being the only significant side-effect; n=28, d/b, p/c, 6/12, Zanarini and Frankenburg, J Clin Psychiatry 2001;**62**:849–54), with 5–10 mg/d significantly superior to placebo for a mixed sample of BPD individuals (n=40, d/b, p/c, 12/52, Bogenschutz and Nurnberg, J Clin Psychiatry 2004;**65**:104–9, MS). Two small open trials of **clozapine** (25–100 mg/d) in severe BPD produced a general improvement in symptoms in one study (n=12, Benedetti et al, J Clin Psychiatry 1998;**59**:13–107) and significantly reduced SIB, aggression, seclusion and violence in the other (n=7, Chengappa et al, J Clin Psychiatry 1999;**60**:477–84). **Quetiapine** (mean 250 mg/d, range 175–400 mg/d) may be well-tolerated and significantly improve impulsivity and other symptoms in severe BPD (n=23, open, 12/52, Villeneuve and Lemelin, J Clin Psychiatry 2005;**66**:1298–303; see also n=14[c=11], open, 12/52, Bellion et al, J Clin Psychiatry 2006;**67**:1042–6). **Aripiprazole**

15 mg/d may improve many measures of BPD (n=52, RCT, d/b, p/c, 8/52, Nickel et al, Am J Psychiatry 2006;**163**:833–8) and a low starting dose may facilitate response (n=3, Mobascher et al, Pharmacopsychiatry 2006;**39**:111–2). **Haloperidol** and **trifluoperazine** may improve anger, hostility and behavioural symptoms, but have been largely superseded, especially as two studies showed haloperidol to be no better than placebo (Soloff et al, Arch Gen Psychiatry 1993;**150**:377–85) and with poor tolerability (n=54, 16/52, Cornelius et al, Am J Psychiatry 1993;**150**:1843–8).

SSRIs *

Some studies suggest that SSRIs may have a role, eg. irritability and aggression improved in the 44% completers in a trial of 50–200 mg/d **sertraline** (n=16, 8/52, Kavoussi et al, J Clin Psychiatry 1994;**55**:137–41). Another study showed that 20–60 mg/d **fluoxetine** significantly reduced anger and distress, with a significant placebo effect also being detectable (n=22, p/c, Selzman et al, J Clin Psychopharmacol 1995;**15**:23–9). Fluoxetine was partially effective in reduced impulsive aggressive behaviour in another study, but with high drop-out rates (n=40, RCT, Coccaro and Kavoussi, Arch Gen Psychiatry 1997;**54**:1081–8; review by Hawton, EBMH 1998;**1**:79) and combining with IPT may improve outcomes (n=39[c=32], 6/12, Bellino et al, Can J Psychiatry 2006;**51**:453-60). **Fluvoxamine** may significantly improve rapid mood shifts in female BPDs, but not impulsivity and aggression (n=38, RCT, d/b, p/c, c/o, 24/52 total, Rinne et al, Am J Psychiatry 2002;**159**:2048–54). Careful dose titration is needed to minimise agitation.

Topiramate *

Two RCTs have shown topiramate to help to reduce anger in men (n=42, RCT, d/b, p/c, 8/52, Nickel et al, Biol Psychiatry 2005;**57**:495–9) and women (n=29, RCT, d/b, p/c, 8/52, Nickel et al, J Clin Psychiatry 2004;**65**:1515–9; IS), and in both studies participants lost weight. In another study, topiramate (up to 200 mg/d) reduced stress and some other symptoms, although SIB was not an outcome measure and the exclusion criteria included anyone suicidal or abusing drugs or alcohol, so the cohort was pretty limited (n=56, RCT, d/b, 10/52, Loew et al, J Clin Psychopharmacol 2006;**26**:61–6; comment by Killaspy, EBMH 2006;**9**:74).

Valproate

Valproate significantly reduced irritability and anger, impulsiveness and relationship tempestuousness in women with co-morbid bipolar II and BPD and was well-tolerated (n=20, RCT, p/c, d/b, 6/12, Frankenburg and Zanarini, J Clin Psychiatry 2002;**63**:442–6), supporting a previous study in impulsive aggression in SSRIs non-responders (n=10, open, Kavoussi and Coccaro, J Clin Psychiatry 1998;**59**:676–80).

■ Unlicensed/possible efficacy

Antidepressants

Some symptoms of BPD are shared with depression, eg. self-condemnation, emptiness, hopelessness, boredom and somatic complaints (Rogers et al, Am J Psychiatry 1995;**152**:268–70), and so the use of anti-depressants may have some logic. See tricyclics and SSRIs in this section.

Carbamazepine

Carbamazepine may be useful for aggression and episodic dyscontrol and, although the latter is not epileptic, there are some common precipitating factors (eg. prodromal symptoms, severe disturbance and post-episode relief of tension). Carbamazepine has been suggested as superior to placebo for behaviour control (n=16, d/b, p/c, c/o, 6/52, Cowdry and Gardner, Arch Gen Psychiatry 1988;**45**:111–9; n=14, Gardner and Cowdry, Am J Psychiatry 1986;**143**:519–22) but an RCT failed to show any effects (n=20, RCT, 30/7, de la Fuente and Lotstra, Eur Neuropsychopharmacol 1994; **4**:479–86).

Lamotrigine *

Lamotrigine was relatively well-tolerated and highly significantly effective for anger in women with BPD (n=27, RCT, d/b, p/c, 8/52, Tritt et al, J Psychopharmacol 2005;**9**:287–91).

Lithium

Lithium has been reported to be useful

for episodic dyscontrol and aggression, affective disorder in BPD, emotionally unstable adolescents and in alcoholics with a PD. Anecdotally, it produced a state of 'reflective delay', although the consequences of erratic compliance would be a significant disadvantage.

Methylphenidate

There is one case where methylphenidate was thought to have been effective in a patient with both ADHD and BPD (n=1, Van Reekum and Links, Can J Psychiatry 1994;**39**:186–7), although this is open to debate (see amfetamines in this section).

Oxcarbazepine *

Oxcarbazepine 1.2–1.5g BD may have a potential role (n=17, open, Bellino et al, J Clin Psychiatry 2005;**66**:1111–5).

Tricyclics

Generally tricyclics are considered ineffective (or even detrimental) in depression associated with BPD, although they may help, particularly in females and those with a history of depression and hypersomnia. Unstable or drug-abusing males may be more likely to be non-responders (review: Akiskal et al, Arch Gen Psychiatry 1980;**37**:777–83).

* No efficacy

Amfetamines

Dexamfetamine has been used but, with the exception of the occasional patient, has proved ineffective. It may be possible to test for amfetamine responsiveness (reviewed by Stein in Br J Psychiatry 1992;**161**:167–84).

Benzodiazepines

Benzodiazepines are considered to be contra-indicated in BPD due to their potential to disinhibit and induce rage reactions and dependence, eg. **alprazolam** was shown to be significantly worse than placebo for behavioural control (n=16, d/b, p/c, c/o, 6/52, Cowdry and Gardner, Arch Gen Psychiatry 1988;**45**:111–9), and the only major study showed **alprazolam** to be no better than placebo in children with anxious or avoidant disorders (n=30, d/b, p/c,

Simeon et al, J Am Acad Child Adolesc Psychiatry 1993;**31**:29–33). The occasional use of rapidly absorbed short-acting drugs (eg. **lorazepam**) may have some limited use in patients with intermittent explosive disorders.

MAOIs

Although there was some evidence that MAOIs are effective in depression associated with BPD, two studies have shown phenelzine 60 mg/d to be no better than placebo except for a minor effect on hostility and anger (eg. n = 108, RCT, d/b, p/c, 5/52, Soloff et al, Arch Gen Psychiatry 1993;**150**:377–85), and a 90 mg/d follow-up study of those phenelzine responders found it to be poorly tolerated and having only a mild effect on irritability and depressive symptoms (n = 54, d/b, p/c, 21/52, Cornelius et al, Am J Psychiatry 1993;**150**:1843–8).

Phenytoin

Two ancient studies showed an often negative effect (eg. Rosenblatt et al, Curr Ther Res 1976;**19**:332–6).

Reboxetine *

There is a case of worsening symptoms with reboxetine (n = 1, Anghelescu et al, J Neuropsychiatry Clin Neurosci 2005;**17**:559–60).

1.12: CATATONIA
see also Schizophrenia (1.23)

Symptoms

Catatonia is usually a rare and potentially lethal type of schizophrenia, dominated by psychosis, catalepsy, stupor, extreme negativism, resistant rigidity, hyperpyrexia, excitement (purposeless motor activity not influenced by external stimulii), echopraxia, grimacing or posturing. It has been linked with neuroleptic malignant syndrome (eg. Fink, Biol Psychiatry 1996;**39**:1–4) and may be associated with mixed (rather than pure) manic episodes in bipolars, and so may be misdiagnosed (n = 27, Krüger et al, J Affect Disord 2003;**74**:279–85).

Role of drugs

ECT is generally considered the treatment of choice for various forms of catatonia, eg. organic, lethal and schizophrenic. Organic catatonia often responds to treatment of the underlying cause, eg. withdrawal of the offending drug. Antipsychotic-induced catatonia is also potentially fatal and must be treated symptomatically. A careful history may elicit a drug-symptom association and the potentially offending drug(s) stopped. Antipsychotics are generally unhelpful.

Reviews: general (Singerman and Raheja, Ann Clin Psychiatry 1994;**6**:259–66), drug-induced (Duggal and Singh, Drugs Today [Barc] 2005;**41**:599-607), clinical features, diagnosis, management and prognosis (Taylor and Fink, Am J Psychiatry 2003;**160**:1233–41).

+ Combinations

Lorazepam + dexamfetamine
See separate drugs/groups.

Lorazepam + ECT
Concurrent or sequential use may be successful (n = 5, Petrides et al, Biol Psychiatry 1997;**42**, 375–81).

Thyroid hormone + reserpine
There is a case report of the combination successfully abolishing periodic catatonia (n = 1, Komori et al, Acta Psychiatr Scand 1997;**96**:155–6).

● Unlicensed/some efficacy

Benzodiazepines *
There are many reports of successful benzodiazepine use in catatonia, eg. 1.5–2 mg IV **lorazepam** has improved antipsychotic-induced catatonia (n = 4, Fricchione et al, J Clin Psychopharmacol 1983;**3**:338–42) and lorazepam IM (or diazepam IV if lorazepam failed) showed a 100% success rate over 24 hours (n = 14, Huang, Psychiatry Clin Neurosci 2005;**59**:52–5). Low-dose lorazepam has treated excited catatonia, where higher doses worsened the condition (n = 1, Pruett and Rizvi, J Child Adolesc Psychopharmacol 2005;**15**:1005-10), and in an open study comparing lorazepam and ECT, 76% responded to lorazepam (IV and/or oral) within five days, most who failed responded promptly to ECT and a positive response to initial parenteral challenge with lorazepam predicted a positive outcome

(n = 28, open, Bush et al, Acta Psychiatr Scand 1996;**93**:137–43). In another open study, short-term benzodiazepine administration (oral lorazepam 2 mg or **diazepam** 10 mg IM followed, if needed, by 2–18 mg oral lorazepam over 48 hours) was successful in 88% showing catatonic symptoms (n = 18, open, Ungvari et al, Acta Psychiatr Scand 1994;**89**:285–8), although the effect may only be short-term (n = 18, RCT, Ungvari et al, Psychopharmacology [Berl] 1999; **142**:393–8). **Clonazepam** at 2.5 mg/d orally or 1 mg IV (n = 3, Am J Psychiatry 1989;**146**:1230; n = 1, Kumar, Aust N Z J Psychiatry 2001;**35**:391) and **midazolam** (mentioned in Am J Psychiatry 1991;**148**:809) have also been used.

Zolpidem

There have been a number of reports of dramatic improvement in catatonia with zolpidem (eg. Mastain et al, Rev Neurol 1995; **151**:52–6), to the extent that it has been used as a diagnostic tool for catatonia, eg. by inducing resolution in people thought to have schizophrenia and allowing interviews to take place (eg. Thomas et al, Lancet 1997;**349**:702; Zaw and Bates, Lancet 1997;**349**:1914).

■ Unlicensed/possible efficacy

Antipsychotics *

These have been used (referred to in Am J Psychiatry 1992;**149**:144–5) but are generally considered unhelpful (see also below). There are cases of catatonic schizophrenia responsive to **amisulpride** (n = 1, French and Eastwood, Can J Psychiatry 2003;**48**:570), **clozapine** (n = 2, Dursun et al, J Psychopharmacol 2005;**19**:432–3) and **risperidone** (n = 2, Valevski et al, Clin Neuropharmacol 2001;**24**:228–31; n = 1, Cook et al, Arch Gen Psychiatry 1996;**53**:82–3) including periodic catatonia (Duggal and Gandotra, Can J Psychiatry 2005;**50**:241–2) has been reported. High dose **olanzapine** 30 mg/d has been used to successfully treat lethal catatonia (n = 1, Cassidy et al, J Psychopharmacol 2001;**15**:302–4).

Carbamazepine

Carbamazepine may be a useful alternative in lorazepam-resistant patients (n = 9, Kritzinger and Jordaan, Int J Neuropsychopharmacol 2001; **4**:251–7).

Memantine *

There are case reports of rapid, significant response of catatonic schizophrenia to memantine 10 mg/d (n = 1, Carpenter et al, Ann Pharmacother 2006;**40**:344–6) and 20 mg/d (n = 1, Thomas, Am J Psychiatry 2005;**162**:626; Carroll et al, Ann Clin Psychiatry 2006; **18**:133–4).

Valproate *

Valproate has been reported to have a prophylactic effect in catatonia (n = 1, Yoshida et al, J Clin Psychopharmacol 2005;**25**:504–5).

Vitamin B12 deficiency

There is a case of complete remission of catatonia with B12 replacement (n = 1, Berry et al, Acta Psychiatr Scand 2003;**108**:156–9).

◆ Others

Other drugs tried include **barbiturates** (thiopental and amobarbital; referred to by Masiar, Am J Psychiatry 1992;**149**:144–5), **bromocriptine** (n = 1, Mahmood, Br J Psychiatry 1991;**158**:437–8), IV **dantrolene** (n = 2, Pennati, Am J Psychiatry 1991; **148**:268), **dexamfetamine** (n = 1, Smith and Lebegue, Am J Psychiatry 1991;**148**:1265), and **lithium** (n = 1, Pheterson et al, J Am Acad Child Adolesc Psychiatry 1985;**24**:235–7).

1.13 DEMENTIA including behavioural and psychological symptoms of dementia (BPSD), Alzheimer's disease, Lewy body dementia, etc

Symptoms

Dementia is an acquired progressive and irreversible reduction in the level of previously attained intellectual, memory and personality/emotional functioning. The main clinical features include disturbed behaviour (disorganised, inappropriate, distracted, restless, antisocial), lack of insight, impaired thinking (slow, impoverished, incoherent, rigid), poverty of speech, low mood, poor cognitive function (forgetfulness, poor attention, disorientation in time and later place), and impaired memory. Some dementias can be treated, eg. if caused by vitamin depletion (eg. B_{12}, folic acid, thiamine), infections (encephalitis, neurosyphilis) or drug toxicity.

Alzheimer's disease is a form of dementia

characterised by amyloid plaques and neuro-fibrillary tangles, with reduced levels of acetylcholine and other transmitters in the brain. The degree of dementia is clearly associated more with the degree of neurofibrillary pathology than with the amyloid plaque burden. It usually presents as a steady deterioration. The main features of its insidious onset are forgetfulness, lack of spontaneity, disorientation, depressed mood, decline in self-care, poor sleep (waking disorientated and perplexed) and intellectual impairment (dysphasia, dyspraxia, language decline).

Lewy body dementia is a variant of Alzheimer's disease and is more common in men. The key features include early onset, persistent and well-formed visual hallucinations, and motor features of Parkinsonism. Patients may be extremely sensitive to antipsychotics, which may result in a sudden onset of EPSEs, profound confusion and deterioration, and can lead to death (McKeith et al, Br Med J 1992;**305**:673–8; CSM warning in Curr Problems 1994;**20**:6).

Role of drugs *

An extensive review (Schmitt et al, CNS Drugs 2004;**18**:827–44) concluded that there are six classes of agents for dementia (management and prevention or delay):

- cholinesterase inhibitors
- NMDA receptor blockers (eg. memantine)
- antioxidants (including gingko biloba)
- anti-inflammatory agents
- neurotrophic factors (including HRT)
- antiamyloid agents (inc cholesterol lowering drugs).

The use of cholinesterase inhibitors (ChEIs) remains massively controversial. In the UK, NICE has advised against their use (based on cost-effectiveness). However, they clearly help many people, but the problem seems to be in identifying which ones. Drug trials have many exclusions and extrapolation of the results to the general population is open to question, but even delaying admission to a nursing home by one month would pay for a year's drug. Unfortunately, the only extended trial failed to show an effect on time to institutionalisation or any other measure (n = 565, RCT, d/b, three years, Courtney et al, Lancet 2004;**363**:2105–15), concluding that donepezil was not cost-effective (although the trial has shortcomings, see correspondence in Lancet).

However, several independent reviews have concluded that the ChEIs are effective. A major systematic review and meta-analysis showed cholinesterase inhibitors to have a modest effect on neuropsychiatric and functional outcomes in Alzheimer's, but long-term outcomes, such as quality of life and caregiver burden, are unclear (s = 29, Trinh et al, JAMA 2003;**280**:210–16; comment by Lahiri and Farlow, EBMH 2003;**6**:94). Another review suggested the ChEIs result in a modest but significant therapeutic improvement, with an NNT of 7, and an NNH of 12 (s = 16, n = 5159 + 2795 controls, Lanctôt et al, CMAJ 2003;**169**:557–64).

Reviews: * general (Evans et al, Int J Neuro-psychopharmacol 2004;**1**:1–19; Lanctôt et al, CMAJ 2003;**169**:557–64), anticholinesterases (Holden and Kelly, Adv Psychiatr Treat 2002;**8**:89–96), newer drug treatments (Reichman, Ann Gen Hosp Psychiatry 2003;**29**:1; Gauthier, Can Med Assoc J 2002;**166**:616–23, 36 refs; Bullock, Br J Psychiatry 2002;**180**:135–9), Lewy body dementia (Zesiewicz et al, Curr Treat Options Neurol 2001;**3**:507–18; McKeith, Br J Psychiatry 2002;**180**:144–7; Swanberg and Cummings, Drug Saf 2002;**25**:511–23, 112 refs), use of mood stabilisers (Tariot et al, Adv Drug Deliv Rev 2002;**54**:1567–77), ChIEs and memantine in Alzheimer's in adults with Down's syndrome (Prasher, Int J Geriatr Psychiatry 2004;**19**:509–15), long-term treatment (Johannsen, CNS Drugs 2004;**18**:757–68).

1.13.1 MANAGEMENT OF DEMENTIA AND BPSD

BNF listed

CHOLINESTERASE INHIBITORS (ChEIs) *

Although there is little to clinically separate the three currently available ChEIs, there are slight differences between them. Donepezil inhibits AChE, rivastigmine inhibits AChE and BuChE (which gives more side-effects initially but may have advantages in later illness), and galantamine both inhibits AChE and enhances ACh's action on nicotinic receptors (review by

Stahl, *J Clin Psychiatry* 2000;**10**:710–11). ChEIs may offer continued benefit for up to two years in moderately-severe AD (n=994[c=575], RCT, d/b, two years, Bullock et al, *Curr Med Res Opin* 2005;**21**:1317–27) and in more severe AD (n=145, RCT, p/c, 24/52, Feldman et al, *Int J Geriatr Psychiatry* 2005;**20**:559–69). Cochrane concludes that all three are effective, there is no evidence that they are **not** cost-effective, and that donepezil may be slightly better tolerated, although careful titration of galantamine and rivastigmine might overcome this (s=13, RCT, d/b, p/c, Birks, *Cochrane Database Syst Rev* 2006;**1**:CD005593). However, another systematic review concluded that the available studies are flawed and show small clinical effects, and questions the rationale for using them at all (s=22, RCT, d/b, Kaduszkiewicz et al, *Br Med J* 2005;**331**:321–7).
Reviews: Comparison (Bullock, *Br J Psychiatry* 2002;**180**:135–9), cost-effectiveness (Clegg et al, *Int J Technol Assess Health Care* 2002;**18**:497–507), kinetics and dynamics (Jann et al, *Clin Pharmacokinet* 2002;**41**:719–39).

Donepezil *

Donepezil is a piperidine-based reversible selective acetylcholinesterase inhibitor licensed for the symptomatic treatment of mild or moderate Alzheimer's disease. The dose is 5mg/d for the first month, increasing to 10mg/d as tolerated. CYP2D6 ultrarapid metabolisers may have lower steady-state plasma levels that normals, and show no improvement as a consequence, a possible explanation of interindividual variation (n=42, Varsaldi et al, *Eur J Clin Pharmacol* 2006;**62**:721–6). Withdrawal effects are rare (n=2, Singh and Dudley, *Int J Geriatr Psychiatry* 2003;**18**:282–4), probably as its half-life is 70 hours. In the early stages of Alzheimer's, donepezil 10mg/d may improve daily cognitive functioning (n=153, RCT, d/b, p/c, 24/52, Seltzer et al, *Arch Neurol* 2004;**61**:1852–6) and may be effective in more advanced stages (MMSE 5–17) of Alzheimer's disease (n=290, RCT, p/c, d/b, 24/52, Feldman et al, *Neurology* 2001, **57**, 613–20). Donepezil may be easier to use and improve cognition and functions in mild to moderate Alzheimer's compared to galantamine (n=120, RCT, s/b, 12/52, Jones et al, *Int J Geriatr Psychiatry*

2004;**19**:58–67, MS; review by Warner, *EBMH* 2004;**7**:77). In moderate Alzheimer's, a systematic review and meta-analysis concluded donepezil was effective for cognitive and global function in AD for up to six months (s=10, Whitehead et al, *Int J Geriatr Psychiatry* 2004;**19**:624–33; comment by Lanctôt, *EBMH* 2005;**8**:15, noting AD2000 was published too late to be included in the analysis). Donepezil slows the decline in moderate to severe Alzheimer's and reduces caregiver burden (n=290, RCT, d/b, p/c, Feldman et al, *J Am Ger Soc* 2003;**51**:737–44; comment by Hancock and Charlesworth, *EBMH* 2004;**7**:20). Donepezil maintains its effectiveness over one year while remaining well-tolerated (n=286, RCT, p/c, one year, Winblad et al, *Neurology* 2001;**57**:489–95; n=431, p/c, Mohs et al, *Neurology* 2001;**57**:481–8; n=25, open, 12/12, Rocca et al, *Prog Neuropsychopharmacol Biol Psychiatry* 2002;**26**:369–73; n=423, Doody et al, *Dement Geriatr Cogn Disord* 2001, **12**, 295–300), and even over two years in open-labelled extensions, although even after this time the benefits are lost within six weeks of stopping (n=763, open, two years, Doody et al, *Arch Neurol* 2001, **58**, 427–33). In a follow-on study in severe Alzheimer's (MMSE 1–10), donepezil improved cognition and preserved function over an extended period (n=248[c=194], RCT, d/b, p/c, 6/12, Winblad et al, *Lancet* 2006;**367**:1057–65). Donepezil may also help emotional and behavioural symptoms in AD (n=25, open, Weiner et al, *J Clin Psychiatry* 2000, **61**, 487–92; n=28, open, Paleacu et al, *Clin Neuropharmacol* 2002;**25**:313–7). The AD-2000 trial concludes that donepezil does not delay the time to institutionalisation or progression of disability in Alzheimer's, but this may be because of a number of design and practical reasons (n=565, RCT, d/b, p/c, 60/52, AD2000 CG, *Lancet* 2004;**363**:2105–15; review by Standridge, *EBMH* 2004;**7**:112). Donepezil may be used in Lewy body dementia, but abrupt withdrawal can lead to acute cognitive and behavioural decline (n=19, 20+6/52, Minett et al, *Int J Geriatr Psychiatry* 2003;**18**:988–93). In mild cognitive impairment, donepezil 10mg/d (cf. placebo) may slow the progression to Alzheimer's over the first year but not over three years (n=769, three years,

RCT, p/c, d/b, Petersen et al, N Engl J Med 2005;352:2379–88). It might have some non-significant efficacy in mild cognitive impairment (n=270, RCT, d/b, p/c, 24/52, Salloway et al, Neurology 2004;63:651–7) but it has no effect as a cognitive enhancer in healthy elderly volunteers (n=26, RCT, 2/52, p/c, Beglinger et al, J Clin Psychopharmacol 2005;25:159–65). In vascular dementia donepezil may help (n=603, RCT, p/c, 24/52, Black et al, Stroke 2003, 34, 2320–30; see also s=2, n=1219, 24/52, Malouf and Birks, Cochrane Database Syst Rev 2004;1:CD004395). Cochrane concludes that donepezil produces modest improvements in cognitive function, ADL, and behaviour over one year (Birks et al, Cochrane Database Syst Rev 2006;1:CD001190).

Reviews: * general (Shigeta and Homma, CNS Drug Rev 2001;7:353–68; Drugs Ther Perspect 2001;17:1–6), tolerability (Jackson et al, Br J Clin Pharmacol 2004;58[Suppl 1]:1–8).

Galantamine *

Galantamine is a reversible competitive acetyl-cholinesterase inhibitor, but also stimulates pre- and post-synaptic nicotinic receptors and is indicated for mild to moderate Alzheimer's disease. Doses of the plain tablets should be twice a day, starting at 4mg BD for 4/52, then 8mg BD for 4/52, increasing to 12mg BD if appropriate, and with meals. The availability of sustained release capsules (Galantamine XL) has allowed once a day dosing. High dose galantamine (24mg/d) is associated with a significant reduction in caregiver burden (n=978, p/c, 21/52, Cummings et al, Am J Psychiatry 2004;161:532–8). There appears to be no rebound from abrupt discontinuation.

A range of studies have shown effectiveness. Galantamine 16–24mg/d was significantly superior to placebo (n=978, RCT, 5/12, Tariot et al, Neurology 2000;54:2269–76), with the benefit sustained over 12 months with the 24mg/d dose (n=636, RCT, 6/12 plus 6/12 extension, Raskind et al, Neurology 2000; 54:2261–8) and 24–32mg/d was superior to placebo on basic and ADL scores, but not behaviour, with an 82% completion rate at the higher dose (n=386, RCT, d/b, p/c, 3/12, Rockwood et al, J Neurol Neurosurg Psychiatry 2001;71:589–95). Galantamine may also be

effective in advanced moderate Alzheimer's disease (sub-analysis, 12/12, Blesa et al, Dement Geriatr Cogn Disord 2003;15:79–87). Over the long term, galantamine 24mg/d and donepezil 10mg/d are both effective over one year, with galantamine producing a better response on cognition than donepezil (n=182, RCT, s/b, 12/12, Wilcock et al, Drugs Aging 2003;20:777–89). Cognitive benefits appear to be sustained for at least 36 months (n=194, 119 completers, RCT, d/b, p/c, 36/52, Raskind et al, Arch Neurol 2004;61:252–6). Galantamine may also be effective for patients with vascular dementia or Alzheimer's disease combined with cerebrovascular disease (n=396+196 controls, 6/12, Erkinjuntti et al, Lancet 2002;359:1283–90; MS). Two extension studies have shown efficacy over two years (24mg/d was safe and effective; Pirttila et al, Eur J Neurol 2004;11;734–41) and 18 months (n=288, RCT, open, Lyketsos et al, Am J Geriatr Psychiatry 2004;12:473–82). A pooled analysis also suggested galantamine might improve behavioural symptoms as well (s=3, n=2033, RCT, d/b, p/c, 3-6/12, Herrmann et al, Am J Geriatr Psychiatry 2005;13:527–34). Cochrane concludes that it is effective at doses of 16–32mg/d, with a consistent effect at 3–6 months (s=10, Loy and Schneider, Cochrane Database Syst Rev 2006;1:CD001747).

Reviews: general (Lilienfeld, CNS Drug Rev 2002;8:159–76; Denzig and Kershaw, CNS Spectr 2004;9:377–92), kinetics (Farlow, Clin Pharmacokinet 2003, 42, 1383–92), use in vascular dementia (Erkinjuntti, J Neurol Sci 2002; 15:125–130).

Rivastigmine *

Rivastigmine is a carbamate-derived 'pseudo-irreversible' acetylcholinesterase (preferentially the G1 sub-type) and butylcholinesterase inhibitor licensed for the treatment of mild to moderately severe Alzheimer's disease and for mild to moderate dementia in patients with idiopathic Parkinson's disease. The dose must be titrated at a minimum of weekly intervals to reduce side-effects. A number of trials have shown some efficacy. Rivastigmine 6–12mg/d may also have a sustained effect in advanced moderate Alzheimer's disease (n=44, RCT, p/c, 12/12, Karaman et al, Dement Geriatr Cogn

Disord 2005;**19**:51–6; see also s = 3, n = 117, RCTs, p/c, d/b, 6/12, Burns et al, Int J Geriatr Psychiatry 2004;**19**:243–9). Rivastigmine may be useful in people with rapidly progressing AD (s = 4, n = 517, 26/52, Farlow et al, Dement Geriatr Cogn Disord 2005;**20**:192–7). A sub-group analysis suggested that rivastigmine may be more effective and better tolerated than donepezil in Lewy body dementia (n = 49, RCT, d/b, Touchon et al, Curr Med Res Opin 2006;**22**:49–59). Rivastigmine may also improve dementia in Parkinson's disease but increases nausea, vomiting and tremor (n = 541 [c = 410], RCT, d/b, 24/52, Emre et al, N Engl J Med 2004;**351**:2509–18; comment by Chow, EBMH 2005;**8**:41). Rivastigmine may have some use in Lewy body dementia, with a return to pre-treatment levels of function 3/52 after discontinuation (n = 92 completers, RCT, d/b, p/c, 23/52, Wesnes et al, Dement Geriatr Cogn Disord 2002;**13**:183–92; n = 8, open, Maclean et al, Int Psychogeriatr 2001, **13**, 277–88; 98/52, Grace et al, Int Psychogeriatr 2001;**13**:199–205). Cochrane concludes from seven trials that rivastigmine was beneficial at 6–12mg/d in mild to moderate Alzheimer's (n = 3370, Birks et al, Cochrane Database Syst Rev 2000;**4**:CD001191; review in EBMH 2000; **3**:10).

Reviews: general (Williams et al, Clin Ther 2003; **25**:1634–53), pharmacoeconomics (Lamb and Goa, Pharmacoeconomics 2001;**19**:303–18), kinetics (Gobburu et al, J Clin Pharmacol 2001; **41**:1082–90).

NON-ANTICHOLINESTERASES

Memantine *

Memantine is licensed in the UK and some European countries for moderate to severe dementia (not just mild to moderately severe) Alzheimer's disease, a unique indication. Memantine is a NMDA antagonist. It replaces the magnesium ion that blocks NMDA receptors, so acts as a voltage-dependent, non-competitive NMDA-antagonist, blocking the effect of excess glutamate release, thought to be responsible for many symptoms and for disease progression. It appears to have a neuroprotective action (review, Jann, Expert Opin Investig Drugs 2000;**9**:1397–406). The

dose is 5mg/d for the first week, adding 5mg/d each week up to a maximum of 20mg/d as divided doses. Side-effects seem low compared to placebo but include hallucinations, confusion, dizziness, headache and tiredness. For NNTs are 3–6 for global outcomes, 7 for cognitive improvement and 3–6 for ADL improvements (s = 2, Livingston and Katona, Int J Geriatr Psychiatry 2004;**19**:19–25). Memantine has also, uniquely, been shown to reduce deterioration in moderate to severe Alzheimer's disease (MMSE 3–14, mean 7.9) compared to placebo, based on CIBIC-plus and ADCS-ADLsev, and with low drop-outs (n = 252, RCT, p/c, 28/52, Reisberg et al, N Engl J Med 2003;**348**:1333–41). In a sub-analysis, memantine seemed to enhance autonomy in moderate to severe Alzheimer's disease, possibly lengthening independency (n = 252, RCT, 28/52, Rive et al, Int J Geriatr Psychiatry 2004;**19**:458–64). An open extension study showed a sustained effect in moderate to severe Alzheimer's disease (n = 175 [c = 136], open, 24/52, Reis-berg et al, Arch Neurol 2006;**63**:49–54). A chart-review showed memantine helped some Lewy body dementia patients (n = 7) although some (n = 4) worsened (n = 11, Sabbagh et al, J Alzheimer's Dis 2005;**7**:285–9). Memantine may be used for mild, moderate (n = 531, Ruther et al, Pharmacopsychiatry 2000;**33**:103–8), and severe dementia (n = 166, RCT, Winblad and Poritis, Int J Geriatr Psychiatry 1999;**14**:135–46). In mild to moderate vascular dementia memantine improved cognition and was well-tolerated (n = 579, RCT, d/b, p/c, 28/52, Wilcock et al, Int Clin Psychopharmacol 2002;**17**:297–305). Adjunctive memantine may allow a reduction in antipsychotic doses in severe AD with aggression (n = 1, Sleeper, Ann Pharmacother 2005;**39**:1573–6). Cochrane concludes that there is a small beneficial effect at six months in moderate to severe Alzheimer's disease, but no detectable effect in vascular or mild to moderate Alzheimer's disease (Areosa et al, Cochrane Database Syst Rev 2005;**2**:CD003154).

Reviews: * general (Rossom et al, Am J Geriatr Pharmacother 2004;**2**:303–12; Molinuevo et al, Am J Alz Dis Other Dement 2004;**19**:10–8; Mobius et al, Drugs Today [Barc] 2004;**40**:685–95; Robinson and Keating, Drugs 2006;**66**:1515–

34), in vascular dementia (Mobius and Stoffler, *Int Psychogeriatr* 2003;**15**[Suppl 1]:207–13).

+ Combinations

Donepezil + gabapentin
Behavioural control from gabapentin may augment the cognitive improvement from donepezil (n=2, Dallocchio *et al*, *J Clin Psychiatry* 2000;**61**:64).

Memantine + ChEI *
In patients stable on donepezil, addition of memantine may significantly improve physical and mental health in moderate to severe Alzheimer's (n=404[c=322], RCT, d/b, p/c, Tariot *et al*,*JAMA* 2004;**291**:317–24; review by McShane, *EBMH* 2004;**7**:76) and significantly lowered NPI scores and reduce agitation-related stress (d/b, p/c, 24/52, Cummings *et al*, *Neurology* 2006;**67**:57–63). Memantine has been added to rivastigmine when deterioration continues despite treatment (n=202, open, 12/52, Dantoine *et al*, *Int J Clin Pract* 2006;**60**:110–8). A survey of patients taking memantine with AChIs suggested that the combination was safe and well-tolerated (n=158, open, mean 4/52, Hartmann and Mobius, *Int Clin Psychopharmacol* 2003;**18**:81–5).
Reviews: * memantine and galantamine (Grossberg *et al*, *J Clin Pharmacol* 2006;**46**[7 Suppl 1]:17S–26S), memantine and donepezil (Xiong and Doraiswamy, *Geriatrics* 2005;**60**:13–4).

● Unlicensed/some efficacy

Antipsychotics *
Antipsychotics are widely used as symptomatic treatments of aggressive, agitated behaviour and as sedatives. With the availability of newer agents, the use of traditional agents such as phenothiazines may be unnecessary clinically, although not without some financial implications. Antipsychotics should not be used as substitutes for poor standards of care, but must be adjuncts to other interventions, and be monitored and reviewed regularly.
Stroke: While we know that risperidone and olanzapine have potential problems, there is a good evidence that they are effective in BPSD (Lee *et al*, *Br Med J* 2004;**329**:75–8) and the

alternative agents are without proven efficacy (Tariot, *EBMH* 2005;**8**:16). Early in 2004, data suggesting an increased risk of cerebrovascular adverse events (eg. stroke, TIAs), including fatalities, were reported in trials of risperidone in elderly patients with dementia-related psychosis. As a consequence, the UK CSM recommended that risperidone and olanzapine not be used for behavioural problems in elderly people with dementia. Sadly, the options left are other atypicals (with no proof of safety data) or older typicals (from which we thought we had moved on). Cochrane concludes that risperidone and olanzapine reduce aggression in dementia, but the risk of severe CVA and EPSE means that they should not be used routinely unless there is marked distress (s=16, RCT, p/c, Ballard and Waite, *Cochrane Database Syst Rev* 2006;**1**:CD003476). A meta-analysis of published and unpublished data concluded that atypicals are associated with a small increase in risk of death compared to placebo in dementia, although this should be considered along with the efficacy and safety of alternatives (s=15, RCT, Schneider *et al*, *JAMA* 2005;**294**:1934–43). A comparison of quetiapine, risperidone and olanzapine prescribed in the elderly for dementia or other indications showed no significant differences in CVA/TIA events, although dementia appeared to be an important risk factor (n=18236, 26/52, Layton *et al*, *J Psychopharmacol* 2006;**20**:473–82). Another review concluded that antipsychotics are not particularly effective, there is most evidence for risperidone and olanzapine, but the effect is modest and increases the risk of stroke (s=29, Sink *et al*, *JAMA* 2005;**293**:596–608). Finally, an enormous Medicaid analysis was unable to show that atypicals (including risperidone) were more likely to cause CVEs than haloperidol or benzodiazepines (n=8 million, Finkel *et al*, *Int Psychogeriatr* 2005;**17**:617–29) but, overall, ADRs from the atypicals may be the limiting factor (n=421, RCT, d/b, p/c, Schneider *et al*, *N Engl J Med* 2006;**355**:1525–38).

Lack of adverse safety data on strokes for **quetiapine** has led to increased use in elderly demented patients with behavioural problems. Quetiapine 25–150mg/d has become standard therapy in dementia and may reduce aggression and behaviour in Alzheimer's (eg. open, 12/52,

Scharre and Chang, *Alz Dis Assoc Disord* 2002;**16**:128–30). Neither rivastigmine nor quetiapine were effective for institutionalised, agitated, demented patients, but quetiapine was associated with significantly greater cognitive decline (n=80[c=71], RCT, p/c, d/b, 26/52, Ballard et al, *Br Med J* 2005;**330**:874).

Regardless of the problems, **risperidone** seems effective at an optimum dose of 1 mg/d, eg. for aggression and behavioural disturbances (n=344, d/b,13/52, De Deyn et al, *Neurology* 1999;**53**:946–55), and in 82% patients with behavioural and psychological symptoms associated with dementia, without impairing cognitive performance (n=34, open, 8/52, Rainer et al, *J Clin Psychiatry* 2001;**62**:894–900). Maximum benefit may occur after 7–10 days with minimal sedation (n=5, Jeanblanc and Davis, *Am J Psychiatry* 1995;**152**:1239). Starting at very low doses (eg. 0.25 mg/d) using the syrup formulation improves tolerability. Risperidone (mean 0.95 mg/d) may significantly improve aggression, agitation and psychosis in dementia (n=337, RCT, p/c, 12/52, Brodaty et al, *J Clin Psychiatry* 2003;**64**:134–43). Additional care is needed in Lewy body dementia as, although psychotic and behavioural symptoms may respond well to low dose, severe EPSEs (especially rigidity) have occurred at 1 mg/d. Olanzapine and risperidone appear equally effective for dementia-related behaviour disturbances (n=19, s/b, Ellingrod et al, *Pharmacother* 2002;**22**:1–5; n=39, d/b, 14/7, Fontaine et al, *J Clin Psychiatry* 2003;**64**:726–30). Risperidone also seems helpful for BPSD and sleep disturbance (n=338[c=321], 12/52, open, Duran et al, *Int Psychogeriatr* 2005;**17**:591–604). Risperidone was superior to haloperidol for BPSD, eg. agitation, wandering and diurnal variations (n=114, RCT, d/b, c/o, 18/52, Suh et al, *Int J Geriatr Psychiatry* 2006;**21**:654–60). Low-dose **olanzapine**, eg. 5–10 mg/d (but not 15 mg/d) has been shown to be superior to placebo in treating agitation, aggression and psychosis in patients with Alzheimer's disease (n=206, RCT, d/b, p/c, 6/52, Street et al, *Arch Gen Psychiatry* 2000;**57**:968–76). Olanzapine 7.5 mg/d reduced symptoms of psychosis, with 1 mg/d ineffective and 2.5 mg/d a reasonable starting dose (n=652, RCT, 10/52, d/b, p/c, De Deyn et al, *Int J Geriatr Psychiatry* 2004;**19**:115–

26). In a sub-group analysis, olanzapine had some effect in reducing the emergence of psychosis in people with Alzheimer's disease who didn't have psychosis when they started treatment, if that makes sense (n=165, RCT, Clark et al, *J Clin Psychiatry* 2001;**62**:34–40, MS). It has also been used in Lewy body dementia, eg. decreased psychotic symptoms but no exacerbation of EPS (n=29, RCT, Cummings et al, *Dement Geriatr Cogn Disord* 2002;**13**:67–73, sub-analysis), although only two tolerated 2.5–7.5 mg/d with clear improvement, and five could not tolerate it or gained no benefit (n=8, open, Walker et al, *Int J Geriatr Psychiatry* 1999; **14**:459–66). **Zotepine** 12.5–150 mg/d was well-tolerated and effective on two measures of behavioural and psychological symptoms of dementia, but not most other measures (n=24, 8/52, open, Rainer et al, *CNS Drugs* 2004;**18**:49–55).

Review: general plus algorithm (Defilippi and Crismon, *Pharmacotherapy* 2000;**20**:23–33, 43 refs).

Ginkgo biloba *

Ginkgo biloba (GB) 120 mg/d stabilised and in some cases improved cognitive function for 6–12 months in patients with mild to moderate Alzheimer's and multi-infarct dementia (n=155) compared to placebo (n=54), (RCT, Le Bars et al, *JAMA* 1997;**278**:1327–32). It must be given for 1–3 months before the full therapeutic effect is seen (review in *Medical Letter* 1998;**40**:63–64). In a trial of mild to severe Alzheimer's, the placebo group showed a significant decline in all measures (ADAS-cog, GERRI and CGI), while the GB group were considered to have at least slightly improved on some scales (n=309, d/b, p/c, 26/52, Le Bars et al, *Dement Geriatr Cogn Disord* 2000;**11**:230–7). GB (special extract EGb 761) has been shown to be equivalent to donepezil and superior to placebo on MMSE (RCT, d/b, p/c, 24/52, Mazza et al, *Eur J Neurol* 2006;**13**:981–5). A rigorous meta-analysis by Oken et al (*Arch Neurol* 1998; **55**:1409–15; reviewed by Bernabei, *EBMH* 1999;**2**:82), concluded that GB was effective in mild to moderate Alzheimer's, and only slightly inferior to donepezil and rivastigmine. However, it fails to boost memory in healthy older adults (n=230, p/c, 6/52, Solomon et al, *JAMA* 2002;**288**:835–40).

Reviews: Barnes, *Pharm J* 2002;**269**:160–2; Maidment, *Psychiatr Bull* 2001;**25**:353–6.

SSRIs (see also no efficacy)

Some studies have shown a potential effect with **citalopram**, eg. improved confusion, mood, restlessness and irritability in Alzheimer's, but not vascular dementia (n=98, RCT, d/b, 4/52, Nyth and Gottfries, *Br J Psychiatry* 1990;**157**:894–901), improved cognition and emotional functioning (eg. Nyth *et al*, *Acta Psychiatr Scand* 1992;**86**:138–45; review by Pollock *et al*, *Consultant Pharm* 1999;**14**:1251–8), and superiority over placebo (favourably with perphenazine) for behavioural disturbances associated with dementia (n=85, RCT, d/b, 17/7, Pollock *et al*, *Am J Psychiatry* 2002;**159**:460–5). A trial showed slight improvement in confusion/ anxiety with **fluvoxamine**, but not cognition or behaviour (n=46, RCT, d/b, p/c, Olafsson *et al*, *Acta Psychiatr Scand* 1992;**85**:453–6), and fluvoxamine augmentation of perphenazine may be effective in reducing psychosis in Alzheimer's patients (n=20, d/b, p/c, Levkovitz *et al*, *J Nerv Ment Dis* 2001;**189**:126–9).

■ Unlicensed/possible efficacy

Aromatherapy

Melissa, an essential balm oil, may reduce agitation in severe dementia (n=71, d/b, p/c, Ballard *et al*, *J Clin Psychiatry* 2002;**63**, 553–8) and lavender oil (two hours a day) produced a modest but significant reduction in agitation in dementia in a cunningly placebo-controlled trial (n=15, p/c, *Int J Geriatr Psychiatry* 2002; **17**:305–8).
Review: Holmes and Ballard, *Adv Psychiatr Treat* 2004;**10**:296–300.

Buspirone

There have been reports of vocal grunts, rocking, difficult behaviour and choreoathetoid movements improving with buspirone (eg. n=1, Hamner *et al*, *J Clin Psychopharmacol* 1996;**16**:261–2).

Carbamazepine

Carbamazepine proved useful in one trial for hostility and aggression in demented patients who had not responded to antipsychotics

(n=21, RCT, 6/52, Olin *et al*, *Am J Geriatr Psychiatry* 2001;**9**:400–5), and in another for nursing home patients with agitation and dementia, where it showed significant short-term efficacy with generally good safety and tolerability (6/52, 51 sites, RCT, Tariot *et al*, *Am J Psychiatry* 1998;**155**:54–61).

Cicloserin

Cicloserin 5–50mg/d (a partial agonist acting at the NMDA glycine receptor complex) has been shown to enhance implicit memory in Alzheimer's patients, supporting the development of NMDA receptor-mediated glutamatergic interventions for the treatment of Alzheimer-related memory disorders (n= 108, p/c, d/b, 10/52, Schwartz *et al*, *Neurology* 1996;**46**:420–4). Cicloserin 100mg/d produced a significant improvement in cognitive scores in one short trial (n=17, RCT, Tsai *et al*, *Am J Psychiatry* 1999;**156**:467–9).

Cyproterone *

Cyproterone was effective for aggression and impulsive behaviour but not aberrant motor behaviour in Alzheimer's or vascular dementia (n=19, open, Caparros-Lefebvre and Dewailly, *Rev Neurol* [Paris] 2005;**161**:1071–8).

Gabapentin

Gabapentin has been used for behavioural agitation in Alzheimer's, sexual disinhibition in dementia (n=3, Alkhalil *et al*, *Am J Ther* 2004;**11**:231–5), and in aggressive and agitated demented elderly patients, where 70% were much or greatly improved (n=24, case series, Hawkins *et al*, *Am J Geriatr Psychiatry* 2000;**8**:221–5; review by Miller, *Ann Pharmacother* 2001;**35**:427–31, 28 refs).

Insulin

Elevating insulin levels (with or without hyperglycaemia) improves memory in people with Alzheimer's (n=23 + 14 controls, Craft *et al*, *Arch Gen Psychiatry* 1999;**56**:1135–40).

Lamotrigine

A case of frontal lobe dementia responded well to lamotrigine up to 100mg/d, but not to other treatments (n=1, 6/12, Devarajan *et al*, *Am J Psychiatry* 2000;**157**:1178, letter).

Levodopa *

In people with dementia with Lewy bodies, levodopa produced 36% 'responders' for motor symptoms (n = 14 [c=10], Molloy et al, J Neurol Neurosurg Psychiatry 2005; **76**:1200–3).

Lithium *

There is some evidence that lithium could have some preventative role in Alzheimer's disease, possibly by blocking accumulation of amyloid-beta peptides (n = 1423, Terao et al, Prog Neuropsychopharmacol Biol Psychiatry 2006; **30**:1125–8), but a case-control study failed to show that lithium protects against the onset of dementia (Dunn et al, Alzheimer Dis Assoc Disord 2005; **19**:20–2).

Methylphenidate

Methylphenidate 10mg/d has been used successfully for chronic apathy in dementia (n = 2, RCT, d/b, c/o, Jansen et al, J Am Geriatr Soc 2001; **49**:474–6).

Naftidrofuryl

This is a cerebral vasodilator with some limited effect on cognitive and global functioning (eg. n = 84, RCT, Emeriau et al, Clin Ther 2000; **22**:834–44; Goldline, Clin Ther 2000; **22**:1251–2).

Piracetam

Piracetam stimulates ACh release. Mild effects may occur when used alone or with an ACh precursor, although Cochrane concludes that the evidence is not robust enough to prove an effect (Flicker et al, Cochrane Database Syst Rev 2001; **2**:1011).

Testosterone *

Men with Alzheimer's disease receiving weekly testosterone enanthante 100mg performed clinically significant better in spatial and memory tests, but with no change in aggression or unwanted behaviour (n = 32, RCT, p/c, 6/52, Cherrier et al, Neurology 2005; **64**:2063–8).

Trazodone

Modest reductions of agitation in AD, with fewer side-effects than placebo have been shown (comparisons with haloperidol: n = 28, RCT, Sulzer et al, Am J Geriatr Psychiatry 1997;

5:60–9; n = 149, RCT, 16/52, Teri et al, Neurology 2000; **55**:1247–8).

Valproate *

Valproate has been used to help behavioural symptoms of Alzheimer's disease, but tolerated doses were less than 1000mg/d (n = 20, RCT, d/b, p/c, Profenno et al, Curr Alzheimer Res 2005; **2**:553–8). A recent trial showed no benefit of valproate in agitation at 800mg/d (n = 153 [c=110], RCT, d/b, p/c, 6/52, Tariot et al, Am J Geriatr Psychiatry 2005; **13**:942–9), and an earlier RCT was unable to show an advantage for valproate over placebo in aggressive behaviour in people with dementia (n = 42, RCT, d/b, p/c, c/o, 3/52 per arm, Sival et al, Int J Geriatr Psychiatry 2002; **17**:579–85). Other studies have, however, suggested an effect in some people, eg. in patients (68–95 years) unresponsive to other pharmacotherapies; divalproex 750–2500mg/d for 5–34 weeks was generally well-tolerated and was moderately effective in decreasing physical agitation and aggression (n = 16, open, Herrmann, Can J Psychiatry 1998; **43**:69–72) with 86% response rates reported (n = 46, open, 6/52, Porteinsson et al, Am J Geriatr Psychiatry 2003; **11**:434–40). Low-dose use may help reduce a broad range of disturbed behaviour in aggressive demented patients (n = 39, open, 12/52, Sival et al, Int J Geriatr Psychiatry 2004; **19**:305–12).

Zolpidem

This has been used for dementia-related insomnia and night-time wandering (Shelton and Hocking, Ann Pharmacother 1997; **31**:319–22).

◆ Others

Other drugs tried include **amantadine** (n = 33, Jibiki et al, Acta Therapeutica 1993; **19**:389–96) and **naltrexone** and **naloxone** (review in Ann Pharmacother 1993; **27**:447–80).

* No efficacy

Combination hormone therapy

Contrary to popular belief, estrogen-based combination hormone replacement therapy (HRT) does not appear to protect against cognitive decline, and may actually double the risk of dementia in postmenopausal women over 70 (n = 4000, RCT, d/b, p/c, Shumaker et al, JAMA 2003;**289**:2651–62, 2663–72; comment by Sherwin and McGill, EBMH 2003;**6**:111). See also some efficacy section in prophylaxis.

Melatonin *

There is no evidence that melatonin helps cognitive and non-cognitive symptoms of dementia (Jansen et al, Cochrane Database Syst Rev 2006;**1**:CD003802).

Nicotine

Studies have shown reduced nicotinic cholinergic receptors in the frontal cortex. Nicotine may stimulate the release of acetylcholine in this area. Nicotine is known to improve attention, memory, vigilance and information processing in (so far) healthy humans, but transdermal nicotine (up to 21 mg/d) had no significant effect on cognitive functions in patients with Alzheimer's disease (n = 18, p/c, d/b, c/o, Snaedal et al, Dementia 1996;**7**:47–52). Cochrane concludes that there is no reliable evidence for a beneficial effect (Lopez-Arrieta et al, Cochrane Database Syst Rev 2000;**2**:CD000149).

Prednisone

Prednisone 10–20 mg/d has been shown to be ineffective (n = 138, RCT, 56/52, Aisen et al, Neurology 2000;**54**:588–93), despite initial enthusiasm from a pilot study, where 20 mg/d showed some short-term effect in suppressing acute phase proteins, which have a role in plaque formation (n = 20, open, Aisen et al, Dementia 1996;**7**:201–6).

Selegiline

Selegiline may improve MMSE scores, but with no apparent effect on brain lesions or degenerative changes in brain tissue (n = 17, Alafuzoff et al, Eur J Clin Pharmacol 2000;**55**:815–9), although one trial (with questionable methodology) of 10 mg/d indicated some slowing of the disease (n = 341, RCT, Sano et al, N Engl J Med 1997;**336**:1216–22). Cochrane concludes that the evidence is lacking, and that there was no justification for use or any need for further studies (Birks and Flicker, Cochrane Database Syst Rev 2003;**1**:CD000442).

Another review of available studies (n = 1073) indicated only small short-term improvement in cognition and ADL in Alzheimer's, which disappeared after 4–6 weeks (Wilcock et al, Int J Geriatr Psychiatry 2002;**17**:175–83).

Sertraline

Sertraline augmentation of donepezil for BPSD in Alzheimer's is ineffective, although, as they say, 'there may be a sub-group who respond' (n = 24 + 120, RCT, d/b, p/c, 12/52, Finkel et al, Int J Geriatr Psychiatry 2004;**19**:9–18).

1.13.2 PROPHYLAXIS AND PREVENTION OF DEMENTIA

This section may be useful in helping advise patients, carers, friends and relatives about possible strategies for reducing the risk of dementia, especially where a family history exists.

● Unlicensed/some efficacy

NSAIDs

A recent systematic review indicates that regular NSAIDs protect against Alzheimer's disease, with the duration of use being an important predictor of this protective effect, reducing the risk by an average of 28%, but with aspirin having a less significant impact (n = 13211, s = 9, Etminan et al, Br Med J 2003;**327**:128–30). Two huge studies have shown that the risk of Alzheimer's disease (but not vascular dementia) is reduced by 55% (NSAIDs at any time and aspirin; n = 3227, Breitner et al, Neurology 2002;**59**:880–6) or by 80%, with a greater effect with more NSAID-taking years (minimum two years), and provided the NSAID was started before the early signs of the disease are apparent (n = 6989, prospective, mean seven-year follow-up, Stricker et al, N Engl J Med 2001;**345**:1515–21). Not all the data, however, is positive. A trial of diclofenac/misoprostol in Alzheimer's disease showed no significant differences, but with a trend towards the NSAID having some positive effects (n = 41, RCT, 25/52, Scharf et al, Neurology 1999;**53**:197–201). A five-year case-control study of post-mortem brain tissue showed no significant differences in the amount of inflammatory glia, plaques, or tangles in either diagnostic group, and so, while long-term NSAIDs in people with Alzheimer's disease may enhance cognitive performance, they may not alleviate the progression of the pathological changes (n = 22, Halliday et al, Arch Neurol 2000;**57**:831–6; see also postmortem study, Mackenzie, Neurology 2000;**54**:732–5). Rofecoxib and naproxen do not slow cognitive decline in people actually with mild to moderate Alzheimer's (n = 351, RCT, d/b, p/c, one year, Aisen et al, JAMA 2003;**289**:2819–26; comment by Jacoby, EBMH 2003;**6**:110) so any effect must be prophylactic.

Reviews: general (Br Med J 2003;**327**:128; Neurology 2003;**60**:1591–7; Flynn and Theesen, Ann Pharmacother 1999;**33**:840–9).

■ Unlicensed/possible efficacy

Antihypertensives

Cognition appears preserved in elderly patients taking long-term antihypertensives (55% reduction in risk of dementia cf placebo, Forette et al, Arch Intern Med 2002;**162**:2046–52; n = 1900, Murray et al, Arch Intern Med 2002;**162**:2090–6).

Estrogen (oestrogen)

Estrogen is a potent chemical factor that prevents vascular disease and improves blood flow in diseased vessels, including blood flow in regions of the brain affected by Alzheimer's disease. Estrogen also has direct effects on neuronal function that may play an important role, not only in the preservation of neurons, but in the repair of neurons damaged by disease processes. Endogenous estrogen levels may decline in post-menopausal women in whom Alzheimer's disease develops (n = 143, Manly et al, Neurology 2000;**54**:833–8). A number of trials have shown a potential effect in reducing the risk of developing dementia in postmenopausal women (meta-analysis by Yaffe et al, JAMA 1998;**279**:688–95; review by Whalley, EBMH 1998;**1**:119). Long-term HRT may slow mental decline in older women, especially those over 85 (n = 2000, Carlson et al, Neurology 2001;**57**:2210–16), and high-dose transdermal 17-beta-estradiol improved cognition in women with Alzheimer's disease (n = 20, RCT, p/c, 8/52, Asthana et al, Neurology

2001;**57**:605–12). Estrogen HRT (oral or transdermal) enhanced verbal memory and performance in non-demented cognitively intact older women (n = 184, Maki et al, Am J Psychiatry 2001;**158**:227–33). However, some recent trials have failed to show a protective effect from, eg. conjugated estrogens (n = 120, RCT, 12/12, Mulnard et al, JAMA 2000;**283**:1007–15; Shaywitz and Shaywitz, JAMA 2000;**283**:1055–6; editorial, review by Hogervorst and McShane, EBMH 2000;**3**:83; n = 50, d/b, 12/52, Wang et al, Neurology 2000;**54**:2061–6) and from short-term estrogens (n = 42 women, RCT, 16/52, Henderson et al, Neurology 2000;**54**:295–302). Estrogen replacement therapy (ERT) did not appear to slow the decline in cognitive functioning in postmenopausal women (n = 2859, Alves de Moraes et al, Am J Epidemiol 2001;**154**:733–9) or reduce the risk of developing Alzheimer's disease (n = 112481 + 108925, case-control, Seshadri et al, Arch Neurol 2001;**58**:435–40). Indeed, short-term estrogen may increase disturbed and aggressive behaviour in dementia in the elderly (n = 16, RCT, d/b, p/c, 4/52, Kyomen et al, Am J Psychiatry 2002;**159**:1225–7).

Reviews: general (Monk and Brodaty, Dement Geriatr Cogn Disord 2000;**11**:1–10; Shepherd, J Am Pharm Assoc 2001;**41**:221–8).

Fish and n-3 fatty acids

People who eat fish at least once a week have 60% lower risk of developing Alzheimer's disease compared with people who never, or seldom, eat fish (n = 815, Morris et al, Arch Neurol 2003;**60**:940–6).

Raloxifene *

Raloxifene, a selective estrogen receptor modulator for osteoporosis, at 120mg/d (but not 60mg/d) may produce a 33% reduced risk of cognitive impairment in postmenopausal women (n = 5386, three years, Yaffe et al, Am J Psychiatry 2005;**62**:683–90).

Statins *

The use of statins (lovastatin and pravastatin but not simvastatin) has been reported to substantially lower the risk of developing dementias (n = 1364, Jick et al, Lancet 2000;

356:1627–31; n = 60,000, Josefson, *Br Med J* 2000;**321**:1040). Atorvastatin 80 mg/d showed significant improvements in MMSE over 12/12 (n = 67[c = 63], RCT, p/c, 3/12, Sparks *et al, Arch Neurol* 2005;**62**:753–7). However, a cross-sectional study showed statin use over 4–5 years had no association with a lower incidence of dementia (n = 355 from n = 4895, Zandi *et al, Arch Gen Psychiatry* 2005;**62**:217–24), a cohort study failed to show reduced risk of dementia in people taking statins (n = 2798, Rea *et al, Arch Neurol* 2005;**62**:1047–51) and Cochrane concludes that there is no good evidence for the use of statins to delay Alzheimer's disease (Scott and Laake, *Cochrane Database Syst Rev* 2001;**4**: CD003160).

Vitamins *

Alzheimer's disease has been linked to low levels of B12 or folate, with twice the risk of developing the disease if deficient (n = 370, *Neurology* 2001;**56**:1188). A study in Hawaii suggested that vitamin E and C supplements may protect against vascular dementia and may improve cognitive function in later life in men (n = 3385, Masaki *et al, Neurology* 2000;**54**:1265–72). Two large studies have shown that high dietary intake of vitamin C and vitamin E may lower the risk of Alzheimer's disease (n = 5395, six years, Engelhart *et al, JAMA* 2002;**287**:3223–9), and that vitamin E from food (but not other antioxidants or supplements) may lower the risk of Alzheimer's (n = 815, Morris *et al, JAMA* 2002;**287**:3230–7). Also, patients taking combined vitamin E (1000 u/d) and donepezil 5 mg/d declined at a slower rate than expected and a prospective study might be revealing (n = 130, retrospective, one year, Klatte *et al, Alz Dis Assoc Disord* 2003;**17**:113–16). Vitamin E in mild cognitive impairment does not reduce the progression to Alzheimer's (n = 769, RCT, p/c, Petersen *et al, N Engl J Med* 2005;**352**:2379–88; comment by Blacker, *EBMH* 2006;**9**:20). In patients with mild cognitive impairment, Vitamin E 2000 IU (cf placebo) had no effect on impairment and did not slow the progression to Alzheimer's (n = 769, three years, RCT, p/c, d/b, Petersen *et al, N Engl J Med* 2005;**352**:2379–88).

1.14 DEPRESSION
see also Bipolar mood disorder (*1.10*), Dysthymia (*1.15*), Rapid-cycling bipolar disorder (*1.10.4*) and Mania and hypomania (*1.10.2*)

Depression is a common illness, affecting up to 3% of the population per year, but remains under-diagnosed, under-treated (especially in men and in those under 30) and antidepressants appear under-represented in suicides (n = 5281 suicides, Isacsson *et al, Br J Psychiatry* 1999;**174**:259–65). Detection in primary care may be better than perceived by some (n = 18414, Thompson *et al, Br J Psychiatry* 2001;**179**:317–23), although treatment is adequate in fewer than 50% patients (n = 9090, Kessler *et al, JAMA* 2003;**289**:3095–105). The overall cost of depression (eg. work, family, other illnesses) is high for this eminently treatable condition.

Symptoms
Depression presents with a mixture of biological symptoms (insomnia or hypersomnia, diurnal variation in mood, low appetite, fatigue or loss of energy, constipation, loss of libido, weight loss or gain) and psychiatric symptoms (depressed mood, loss of interest or pleasure, poor memory, psychomotor agitation or retardation, recurrent thoughts of death or suicide, anxiety, feelings of worthlessness or guilt, including delusions, etc). Depression does not include the normal reaction to the death of a loved one. Atypical depression includes the symptoms of depression, plus two from hypersomnia, hyperphagia, rejection sensitivity and severe lethargy (n = 579, Posternak and Zimmerman, *Arch Gen Psychiatry* 2002;**59**:70–6).

Causes
Precipitating factors can include prescribed or OTC drugs and substance misuse, physical illness and stress, eg. bereavement, loss of job, birth of child, break-up of relationship, work stress, poor social background and the time of year.

Role of drugs
Although most depressions will resolve with time, antidepressants have a major role in hastening this recovery and reducing suffering. Antidepressants are effective, not addictive, and do not generally

lose efficacy with prolonged use. Adequate doses are needed for clinical effect, and continuation for an appropriate period will minimise relapse. A viable option is combining medicines with long-term maintenance CBT (Blackburn and Moore, *Br J Psychiatry* 1997;**171**:328–34) or IPT (n = 187, RCT, elderly, Reynolds *et al*, *JAMA* 1999;**281**:39–45), where a combination is generally more effective than either individually (meta-analysis, DeRubeis *et al*, *Am J Psychiatry* 1999;**156**:1007–13; disputed by Taylor *et al*, *Am J Psychiatry* 2000;**157**:1025–6). In patients either randomised to counselling or antidepressants, or who were allowed to choose for themselves between drugs and counselling, no differences were found either in the initial characteristics or in the outcomes, and both were equally effective at eight weeks, so expressing a preference had no apparent effect or benefit on outcomes (n = 323, Bedi *et al*, *Br J Psychiatry* 2000;**177**:312–8). Studies of antidepressants in children are not very robust and tend to exaggerate the positive outcomes and underestimate side-effects (*Br Med J* 2004; **328**:879; see also *Lancet* 2004;**363**:1341–5).

Treatment of depression *

The general principles of treatment of depression (with antidepressants) can be summed up by the six Ds:

- Diagnosis
- Drug-related
- Drug
- Dose
- Duration
- Discontinuation

1. **Diagnosis:** Making, or being able to make, a diagnosis helps. An obvious statement, but diagnosis does start with D.

2. **Drug-related causes eliminated:** This might include excessive caffeine intake, other drugs liable to cause depression (see 5.5), and physical (eg. low folate levels) and environmental causes.

3. **Drug:** All the main antidepressants appear to have broadly similar efficacy as first-line treatments in depression and so antidepressant choice will be based upon the features of depression, suicide risk, concomitant therapy, concurrent illness, side-effect tolerability, time to reach therapeutic dose, cost and special considerations, eg. cognitive impairment and driving. As non-compliance or inadequate dosage are the main causes of drug failure, the choice of drug should consider these factors. Deaths from overdose are mostly from TCAs (predominantly dosulepin and amitriptyline) and most often in deprived areas (Shah *et al*, *Psychol Med* 2001;**31**:1203–10). Nearly all antidepressants can be given once a day.

Onset of action: * Although commonly thought that antidepressants take four weeks to work, it is more accurate to say that or 'time to substantial remission' (full statistical separation from placebo) may take four weeks in clinical trials (partly because trials are not powered to detect an earlier onset). The onset of action may actually be much quicker, shown by two meta-analyses. One showed that 23% of all drug-placebo differences occur within the first week and 57% were apparent by week 2 (s = 47, n = 8500, d/b, p/c, Pasternak and Zimmerman, *J Clin Psychiatry* 2005;**66**:148–58), with separation by day 5 reported (review by Mitchell, *Br J Psychiatry* 2006;**188**:105–6) and the second showed symptomatic improvement in depression by the end of the first week, continuing at a reduced rate for at least six weeks (s = 28, n = 5872, RCT, Taylor *et al*, *Arch Gen Psychiatry* 2006;**63**:1217–23). A systematic review with meta-analysis of available studies concludes that antidepressants increase sustained response rate at two weeks compared to placebo, with less residual long-term symptoms (s = 8, n = 7121, RCT, d/b, p/c, Papakostas *et al*, *J Clin Psychopharmacol* 2006;**26**:56–60; comment by Artigas, *EBMH* 2006;**9**:78). Perhaps it might be more realistic to say that in 90% cases, substantial improvement occurs within the first two weeks but that the benefit continues to build over several weeks. There is some data that mirtazapine (and perhaps venlafaxine) may act slightly quicker than some SSRIs, especially if more aggressive dosing strategies are used.

4. **Dose:** The therapeutic range of the newer antidepressants has been established through dose-finding studies but is less clear for the tricyclics (see TCAs for discussion). Once-daily dosing is as effective as multiple daily doses, regardless of drug half-life (meta-analysis of 22 studies by the Scrabble players favourite Yyldyz, and Sachs, *J Affect Disord* 2001;**66**:199–206; review by Barbui, *EBMH* 2002;**5**:57). A 20-year study has shown that recovery from MDD is significantly more likely with higher levels of antidepressant

doses, whereas recovery was no more likely with lower doses than placebo (n = 285, Leon et al, Am J Psychiatry 2003;**160**:727–33). See tricyclics and other antidepressants for advice on dosing, eg. the need for tricyclic doses of 125–150mg/d in 95% adults.

5. Duration:

5a. Acute therapy — antidepressants must be increased to therapeutic doses, with SSRIs the standard first-line therapy. The patient must be monitored for akathisia, anxiety, agitation and suicidal ideation early in treatment. If depression remains completely unchanged at four weeks of therapeutic dosing, an alternate drug should be tried. Minimal improvement within the first four weeks should indicate a further two-week trial, then change to an alternate drug if there is no further response (n = 593, Quitkin et al, Arch Gen Psychiatry 1996;**53**:785–92). If there is no response by eight weeks, the trial should 'be declared a failure' (n = 840, 12/52, open, Quitkin et al, Am J Psychiatry 2003;**160**:734–40). These times should probably be doubled in the elderly and in chronic depression (Gelenberg and Chesen, J Clin Psychiatry 2000;**61**:712–21).

5b. Continuation therapy — proper treatment of depression requires relief not just of acute symptoms but continued treatment while the person remains vulnerable. Inadequate or no treatment for six months post-response in controlled trials has resulted in relapse rates as high as 50% (cf 20% with adequate treatment, although compliance was not certain in these cases). If a first episode of depression remits in 12 weeks, continued treatment for six months minimises the risk of relapse, but longer therapy confers little additional benefit, except in people with additional relapse risk factors (n = 395, RCT, 52/52, Reimherr et al, Am J Psychiatry 1998;**155**:1247–53). A systematic review and meta-analysis concludes that continuing antidepressants for longer, eg. 12 months after acute treatment reduces the relapse rate by 70% in people with recurrent depression (n = 4410, s = 31, Geddes et al, Lancet 2003;**361**:653–61; comment by Donoghue, EBMH 2003;**6**:84). People who continue with their initial antidepressant (rather than need to switch or just discontinue) also have lower relapse/recurrence rates over two years (retrospective study, n = 4052, Melfi et al, Arch Gen Psychiatry 1998;**55**:1128–32). Continuation doses should be the **same or close**

to the therapeutic dose (RCT, three years, Frank et al, J Affect Disord 1993;**27**:139–45). In the elderly, therapy for up to two years after recovery may be needed (Int J Geriatr Psychiatry 1992;**7**:617–9; Anon, Br J Psychiatry 1993;**162**:175–82). Patients should also be advised that antidepressants are not 'addictive' as such. If stopped prematurely (less than 13 weeks), antidepressants are still likely to be effective if reintroduced on relapse (n = 501, Fava et al, Psychother Psychosom 2002;**71**:195–9).

5c. Relapse prevention and prophylactic therapy — longer-term relapse prevention has been shown for a number of antidepressants, eg. imipramine over 3–5 years (n = 128, RCT, d/b, p/c, three years, Frank et al, Arch Gen Psychiatry 1990;**47**:1093–9; Kupfer et al, Arch Gen Psychiatry 1992;**49**:769–73), paroxetine in old age (n = 116, RCT, d/b, p/c, two years, Reynolds et al, N Engl J Med 2006;**354**:1130–8) and venlafaxine (PREVENT, two years, in press, 2007) but not sertraline (RCT, d/b, p/c, two years, Wilson et al, Br J Psychiatry 2003;**182**:492–7). Long-term antidepressant treatment in recovered depressed people is, however, often 'strikingly inadequate', even in previous suicide attempters (Oquendo et al, Am J Psychiatry 2002;**159**:1746–51). Long-term management benefits depressed patients by increasing long-term compliance and, hence, prolonging remission (n = 211, RCT, Rost et al, Br Med J 2002;**325**:934–7), since 75% have a further episode, usually within 2–3 years, if untreated. Those likely to benefit from maintenance (Kasper and Eder in Winkler et al, Curr Opin Psychiatry 2002;**15**:63–8) include those with chronic depression, three episodes, or two episodes with risk factors (late or early onset, short interval between episodes, rapid onset, dysthymia, positive family history, co-morbidity, incomplete response and low work adjustment). In a 10-year prospective study of multiple recurrences of major depression, the risk of recurrence increased by 16% with each successive episode, but the risk of recurrence progressively decreased as duration of recovery increased (n = 318, Solomon et al, Am J Psychiatry 2000;**157**:229–33), so keeping people well pays dividends.

General minimum treatment duration recommendations:

- First episode — six months post-recovery (see 3 above).
- Second episode — 2–3 years.
- Third episode — five years or longer.

- Fourth episode — you should need a very good reason to stop.

Review: Maintenance (WFSBP Guidelines, Bauer et al, World J Biol Psychiatry 2002;**3**:69–86).

6. Discontinuation: When discontinuing therapy is considered appropriate, slowly reduce doses over a minimum of four weeks. Discontinuation syndromes have been reported for nearly all antidepressants, but particularly paroxetine and venlafaxine. Discontinuation symptoms usually appear within 1–3 days of stopping treatment and they can improve within a week (although can last much longer), while recurrence of depression begins after three weeks and continues to worsen. See switching antidepressants in 2.2.2 for a further review, eg. symptoms and management.

Treatment-resistant depression *
True 'treatment-resistant' depression often needs a systematic approach to solve. Remember also that resistant depression may be undiagnosed bipolar (see 1.13.3).

1. Escalate antidepressant doses for an adequate duration: An appropriate action for drugs with a dose-response curve, eg. up to 300 mg/d or more of a tricyclic or other drug (eg. venlafaxine), or to tolerance (monitoring plasma levels carefully), remembering that a few people have multiple copies of, eg. CYP2D6 and may rapidly metabolise tricyclics. Treatment for up to 9–17 weeks may also be needed (review; Greenhouse et al, J Affect Disord 1987;**13**:259–66). SSRIs tend to have a flat dose response curve, so switching is probably the best ploy (review; Corruble and Guelfi, Acta Psychiatr Scand 2000;**101**:343–8).

2. Check blood levels: Levels of 300–400 mcg/L of tricyclics have been used by some in true refractory cases (see Hodgkiss et al, Hum Psychopharmacol 1995;**10**:407–15). This also detects possible ultrarapid 2D6 metabolisers. Dosulepin, amitriptyline and clomipramine have been the tricyclics preferred for high dose therapy.

3. Switch drugs: Ensure all drug classes have been tried optimally, eg. SSRIs, tricyclics, SNRIs, NASSAs, RIMAs (eg. moclobemide at much higher doses than are currently recommended, eg. over 600 mg/d) and MAOIs (see Chapter 2.2.5 for advice on switching antidepressants).

4. Augment or combine: Use logical combinations of antidepressants, (see later in this section), eg. mirtazapine, lithium, carbamazepine

(but not with tricyclics, where it reduces plasma levels, see 4.5.1), valproate, or lithium/SSRI/tryptophan. SSRIs should not routinely be used with tricyclics, unless with regular blood level testing, or at all with MAOIs or tryptophan (see 4.3.4).

5. Assure compliance: For example, taking plasma levels. Around 42% people stop antidepressants within the first 30 days (mostly from ADRs), 30% in the next 60 days (mostly due to lack of efficacy) and only 28% carry on beyond three months (n = 829, Olfson et al, Am J Psychiatry 2006;**163**:101–8).

6. Check folate levels: See adjunctive therapy.

7. Consider individual CBT: This should be considered in combination with antidepressants and may be effective but requires a high level of expertise (n = 240, RCT, p/c, 16/52, DeRubeis et al, Arch Gen Psychiatry 2005;**62**:409–16).

Review: drug treatments (O'Reardon et al, Curr Opin Psychiatry 2000;**13**:93–8).

Bipolar depression
See separate section (1.10.3).

Loss of antidepressant efficacy (tachyphylaxis)
Loss of antidepressant efficacy (also termed 'operational tolerance', or more graphically as 'poop-out') has been reported during long-term maintenance treatment in 4–33% patients with antidepressants and may be significantly less common with venlafaxine (4%) and tricyclics than with SSRIs (14%) (n = 237, Posternak and Zimmerman, J Clin Psychiatry 2005;**66**:705–7). There is, however, no sound data to support the view that antidepressants may actually worsen the course of depression (except perhaps bipolar depression). Possible mechanisms might include non-compliance, loss of initial placebo response, loss of true drug effect, pharmacological tolerance, accumulation of detrimental metabolites, change in illness pathology, unrecognised rapid cycling, switching and cycle acceleration in bipolars, antidepressant-inducing paradoxical effects and a genuine lack of prophylactic efficacy (review by Fava, J Clin Psychiatry 2003;**64**:123–33). Strategies to overcome loss of efficacy include:

1. Increase the dose (logical, and works with, eg. fluoxetine, ie. n = 41, RCT, d/b, p/c, Fava et al, Am J Psychiatry 1994;**151**:1372–4).

2. Decrease the dose (this may work if the

dose has exceeded any 'therapeutic window', but is poorly supported by published data).

3. **Addition** of dopamine antagonists, eg. bromocriptine.
4. **Augment** with mood stabilisers, anti-convulsants, thyroid, another antidepressant, etc.
5. **Drug holiday** (although this is poorly supported by the literature).
6. **Switch** to a different drug or class.
7. **Ensure compliance**.

Reviews: study and review (Byrne and Rothschild, J Clin Psychiatry 1998;**59**:279–88).

Suicidality *

The role of antidepressants in reducing or causing suicide or suicidal ideation has been controversial. However, of the 14 studies published to August 2006, 12 support the hypothesis that increased antidepressant use reduces suicide and two don't (one is inconclusive, one disagrees). The main issues are as follows:

• **Depression is a risk factor for suicide:** Suicide practically does not occur without the presence of mental health problems, most commonly depression, then alcoholism. Depressed individuals who have committed suicide have seldom been treated with antidepressants.

• **Antidepressants reduce the incidence of suicides:** The absolute risk of suicide during acute antidepressant treatment is about 1 in 3000, and of serious suicide attempt is 1 in 1000, with no evidence of a statistically significant increase in suicide or ideation in the month after starting treatment with newer antidepressants (n=65103, Simon et al, Am J Psychiatry 2006; **163**:41–7). In Denmark, the suicide rate (1995–1999) had dropped in all groups, but particularly in people treated with SSRIs or older antidepressants (n=438625) compared to those not treated with antidepressants (n=1199057) (four years, Søndergård et al, Acta Psychiatr Scand 2006;**114**:168–76). In Sweden, an annual on-going educational programme (interactive seminars, 1995–2002) for GPs, has led to antidepressant use increased from 25% below national average to the same level, while suicide decreased to the national average (Henriksson and Isacsson, Acta Psychiatr Scand 2006;**114**:159–67).

• **Antidepressants do not cause suicides but might cause a short-term increase in suicidal ideation:** Antidepressants have been associated with the emergence of suicidal tendencies but an analysis of all FDA antidepressant trials was unable to find any link with increased suicide with any antidepressants compared to placebo (n=49277, Khan et al, Am J Psychiatry 2003;**160**:790–2). In a comparison of UK patients taking amitriptyline, fluoxetine, paroxetine and dosulepin, suicidal behaviour was slightly increased in the first month of starting antidepressants (especially days 1–9) probably due to akathisia, but no difference between the drugs or in people aged 10–19 years (n=159810, Jick et al, JAMA 2004;**292**:338–43). Another systematic review showed that suicide attempt risk in people taking an SSRI is 2.3 times higher than placebo and 1.9 times higher than other interventions, but slightly less than TCAs (s=702, n=87650, Fergusson et al, Br Med J 2005;**330**:396). To put this into perspective, and add some balance, a thorough review of death/suicide and dependence concluded that while SSRIs have problems, they are less than depression itself and the tricyclics (Nutt, J Psychopharmacol 2003;**17**:355–64), and a chart analysis showed that there was a five-fold increase in suicidal behaviour after discontinuation of antidepressants (TCAs and SSRIs), suggesting a possible protective effect (n=521, Yerevanian et al, Acta Psychiatr Scand 2004;**110**:452–8). A meta-analysis of SSRI:placebo RCTs showed no increased risk of suicide in adults on SSRIs (s=477, n=>40000, RCTs, Gunnell et al, Br Med J 2005;**330**:385), in a nested case-control study there was no evidence of increased risk of suicide compared to TCAs (n=146095, Martinez et al, Br Med J 2005;**330**:389–93), and a case control study in people taking antidepressants, SSRI use was no more common in people who committed suicide than those who died of natural causes or an accident (n=4949, Isacsson et al, Acta Psychiatr Scand 2005;**111**:286–90; comment by Cipriani, EBMH 2005;**8**:113).

• **Antidepressants need to be treated with respect:** SSRIs and other newer agents have low toxicity in overdose but the tricyclics and some older antidepressants can be toxic in overdose.

Reviews: * extensive (Mann, N Engl J Med 2005;**353**:1819–34), evidence-based guidelines for pharmacotherapy (BAP Guidelines; Anderson et al, J Psychopharmacol 2000;**14**:3–20), depression in old age (Anderson, Age Ageing 2001;**30**:13–7), atypicals in treatment-resistance (Thase, J Clin Psychiatry 2002;**63**:95–103), atypical depression (n=591, Angst et al, J Affect Disord 2002;**72**:125–38), genetics of this familial disorder (Sullivan et al, Am J Psychiatry 2000;**157**:1552–62), rapid-onset strategies (Blier, J Clin Psychiatry 2001;**62**[Suppl 15]:S12–S17).

Types of antidepressants *

There are many classifications of antidepressants, based on a simple putative mode of action. It is important to remember that reuptake inhibition by antidepressants is just the start of a cascade of events involving changes in the sensitivities of receptors at (somatodendritic) sites, eg. $5HT_{1A}$ receptors, at pre- and post-synaptic sites, as well as changes in neuronal signal transduction beyond the receptor and gene expression. All neurotransmitter systems seem inter-dependent. On a transmitter mechanism basis, the following may, however, be useful:

1. Norepinephrine and serotonin reuptake inhibition, eg. tricyclics, venlafaxine (150mg/d and above), duloxetine.
2. Serotonin reuptake inhibition, eg. SSRIs, venlafaxine (lower dose).
3. Norepinephrine reuptake inhibition, eg. reboxetine.
4. $5-HT_2$ blockade plus serotonin reuptake inhibition, eg. trazodone.
5. Monoamine oxidase inhibition, eg. moclobemide, MAOIs.
6. Pre-synaptic alpha-2-autoreceptor and heteroceptor blockade, eg. mirtazapine.
7. Serotonin precursor, eg. tryptophan.
8. Dopamine reuptake blockers, eg. bupropion (also used for smoking cessation).
9. Melatonin M1 and M2 agonists, eg. agomelatine.

BNF listed

SELECTIVE SEROTONIN REUPTAKE INHIBITORS (SSRIs)

The SSRIs are now first choice drugs in depression in most patients due to their safety in overdose and heart disease and better side-effect profile (eg. lacking anticholinergic, sedation and weight gain effects). The increase in prescribing of SSRIs has coincided with a fall in the suicide rate in many countries, implying that SSRIs are not a major cause of suicide. Although chemically distinct from each other, the SSRIs are essentially more similar than different and are all effective antidepressants, but their ADR profiles and potential for interactions may show clinical differences.

Reviews: general (Vaswani et al, Prog Neuropsychopharmacol Biol Psychiatry 2003; **27**: 85–102), differences in their pharmacological and clinical profiles (Anderson and Edwards, Adv Psychiatr Treat 2001;**7**:170–80).

Citalopram

Citalopram has been shown to be effective and well-tolerated in studies against standard antidepressants. A review of 30 RCTs showed citalopram to be superior to placebo, of comparable efficacy to other antidepressants and well-tolerated from 20–60mg/d, with linear pharmacokinetics and minimal drug interactions (Keller, J Clin Psychiatry 2000;**61**:896–908, 81 refs; reviewed by Silva de Lima, EBMH 2001;**4**:80), with a particularly robust effect in melancholic depression seen at 40–60mg/d (n=650, RCT, Feighner and Overø, J Clin Psychiatry 1999;**60**:824–30). Relapse prevention has been shown over 15 months in adults (n=427, RCT, 44–77/52, Hochstrasser et al, Br J Psychiatry 2001;**178**:304–10) and in the elderly (n=121, RCT, 48/52, Klysner et al, Br J Psychiatry 2002; **181**:29–35; review by Appelberg, EBMH 2003;**6**:24). In patients who had responded to citalopram 40mg/d for four months, halving the dose to 20mg/d for a maintenance phase (two years) resulted in a 50% relapse rate, reinforcing the view that full-dose maintenance therapy is required (n=50, Franchini et al, J Clin Psychiatry 1999;**60**:861–5, comment by Somawalla, J Clin Psychiatry 2001;**62**:993). Citalopram may be well-tolerated and superior to placebo in children (7–11 years) and adolescents (12–17 years) for MDD (n=174, RCT, d/b, p/c, 8/52, Wagner et al, Am J Psychiatry 2004;**161**:1079–83), although not recommended in the UK. It has a very low incidence of drug interactions (4.3.2.1).

Reviews: general (Joubert et al, Hum Psychopharmacol 2000;**15**:439–510) and safety (Nemeroff, Psychopharmacol Bull 2003;**37**: 96–121).

TABLE 1.1: THE RATIONALE AND RISKS FOR COMBINATIONS OF ANTIDEPRESSANTS

	Citalopram/escitalopram	Fluoxetine	Fluvoxamine	Paroxetine	Sertraline	Tricyclics	MAOIs	Venlafaxine	Mirtazapine	Reboxetine	Trazodone	Duloxetine	Moclobemide	Flupentixol
Fluoxetine	SS LR-HH													
Fluvoxamine	SS LR-HH	SS LR-HR												
Paroxetine	SSU LR-HH	SS LR-HH	SS LR-HR											
Sertraline	SS LR-HH	SS-C4/5/5 LR-HH	SS LR-HH	SS LR-HH										
Tricyclics	SS-C4/5 LR-HH-CI	SS-C4/5 LR-HH-CI SM-LDT	SS-C4/5 LR-HH-CI SM-LDT	SS-C4/5 LR-HH-CI SM-LDT	SS-C4/5 LR-HH-CI									
MAOIs	(SS)-C4/5 SR-HH	(SS)-C4/5 SR-HH	(SS)-C4/5 SR-HH	(SS)-C4/5 SR-HH	(SS)-C4/5 SR-HH	(SS) SR-HH-CI								
Venlafaxine	SS LR-HH	SS-C4/5 LR-HH	SS LR-HH	SS MR-HH-CI	SS-C4/5 LR-HH	SS LR-HH	SS-C4/5 SR-HH							
Mirtazapine	SSU LR-UH	(SS) LR-UH	SSU LR-UH	SSU C4/5 LR/LH	SSU C4/5 LR-LH	SSU C4/5 LR-MH	SSU C4/5 SR-MH	SSU HR-LH						
Reboxetine	SSU SR-UH VM	SSU SR-UH VM	SSU SR-UH VM	SSU SR-UH VM	SSU SR-UH VM	SSU C4/5 LR-MH	SSU C4/5 LR-HH	SSU LR-UH	SSU MR-UH					
Trazodone	SS LR-HH	SS LR-HH	SS LR-UH	SS LR-UH	SS LR-UH	(SS) SR-MH	(SS)-C4/5 SR-HH	SS LR-HH	SSU SR-UH	SSU SR-UH VM				
Duloxetine	(SS)-C4/5 SR-MH	(SS)-C4/5 SR-LH	(SS)-C4/5 SR-MH	(SS) LR-HH	(SS) LR-HH	(SS)-C4 SR-LH	(SS)-C4 SR-HH	(SS)-C4/5 SR-HH	SSU SR-UH	SSU SR-UH VM	(SS) SR-UH			
Moclobemide	(SS)-C4/5 SR-MH	(SS)-C4/5 SR-LH	(SS)-C4/5 SR-MH	(SS) LR-HH	(SS) LR-HH	(SS) SR-MH	(SS)-C4/5 SR-HH	(SS)-C4/5 SR-HH	SSU SR-UH	SSU SR-UH	(SS) SR-UH	(SS) SR-UH		
Flupentixol	SSU LR-UH	SSU LR-UH	SSU LR-UH	SSU LR-UH	SSU LR-UH	SSU LR-UH	SSU LR-UH	SSU LR-UH	SSU LR-UH	SSU LR-UH	SSU LR-UH	SSU LR-UR	SSU LR-UH	
Tryptophan	(SS)-C4/5 UR-MH	(SS)-C4/5 UR-MH	(SS)-C4/5 UR-MH	(SS)-C4/5 UR-MH	(SS)-C4/5 UR-MH	(SS)-C4/5 UR-MH	(SS)-C4/5 UR-MH	(SS) UR-MH	SSU UR-LH	SSU UR-LH	(SS) UR-MH	(SS) UR-MH	SSU UR-MH	SSU UR-LH

SS	serotonin syndrome very possible
(SS)	serotonin syndrome possible or rarely reported
SSU	serotonin syndrome unlikely
LR	low rationale
SR	some rationale
HR	high rationale
UR	unknown rationale
LH	relatively low hazard or risk
MH	medium hazard or risk either known or predicted
HH	high hazard or risk of problems known or predicted so specialist monitoring required
UH	unknown or undocumented hazard specialist monitoring required and limit dose of tricyclic
VM	consider venlafaxine (>200mg/d) or mirtazapine instead for combined 5-HT and NA/NE reuptake blockade
CI	see Chapter 1 for data on positive use of combination
C4/5	see Chapters 4 or 5 for data on risk of interaction or adverse consequences

Escitalopram *

Escitalopram (the most serotonin transporter-selective compound tested; Owens et al, Biol Psychiatry 2001;**50**:345–50) is the pharmacologically active enantiomer of citalopram (a mix of R- and S-citalopram) and at least twice as potent on a mg for mg basis (eg, n = 380, RCT, d/b, 8/52, Wade et al, Int Clin Psychopharmacol 2002;**17**:95–102). There is accumulating evidence that R-citalopram antagonises escitalopram at serotonin recep-tors (eg. Storustovu et al, Br J Pharmacol 2004;**142**:172–80); ecitalopram binds to the primary binding site **and** the allosteric site; whereas R-citalopram blocks the allosteric site in a dose-dependent manner, reducing the antidepressant effect on the primary site. R-citalopram has a greater affinity for the serotonin transporter than escitalopram (Sanchez, Basic Clin Pharmacol Toxicol 2006; **99**:91–5) and may also have a longer half-life (R-citalopram is metabolised slower than escitalopram), which might lead to an accumulating negative effect. The recommended dose for depression is 10 mg/d increasing to a maximum 20 mg/d. Escitalopram has now been shown to be superior to citalopram in a large number of settings. In severely depressed out-patients with MADRS scores above 30 (n = 290 [c = 269], RCT, d/b, 8/52, Moore et al, Int Clin Psychopharmacol 2005;**20**:131–7), in depressed out-patients, where escitalopram 10 mg/d was at least as effective as citalopram 40 mg/d with few other differences (n = 491, RCT, d/b, p/c, 8/52, Burke et al, J Clin Psychiatry 2002;**63**:331–6), more effective than citalopram and placebo (n = 469, 8/52, d/b, Lepola et al, Int Clin Psychopharmacol 2003;**18**:211–17) and with a long-term relapse prevention efficacy (n = 590 [c = 437], open, 12/12, Wade et al, Ann Clin Psychiatry 2006;**18**:83–9). An active comparison showed escitalopram at least as good as citalopram (n = 357, RCT, d/b, 24/52, Colonna et al, Curr Med Res Opin 2005;**21**:1659–68) and in a direct comparison, escitalopram 20 mg/d had a superior effect to citalopram 40 mg/d (76% vs 61% responders, 56% vs 43% adjusted remitters) (n = 280 [c = 259], RCT, d/b, 8/52, Moore et al, Int Clin Psychopharmacol 2005;**20**:131–7). A robust meta-analysis concluded that escitalopram was superior to citalopram at weeks one and eight, with greater efficacy in very severely depressed patients (n = 1262, s = 4, 8/52, RCTs, Auquier et al, Int J Psych Clin Pract 2003;**7**:259–68; see also a pooled analysis; Kper et al, Int Clin Psychopharmacol 2006;**21**:105–10). An analysis of two RCTs suggested escitalopram was superior to citalopram at one week and was superior on all efficacy parameters (Lepola et al, Int Clin Psychopharmacol 2004;**19**:149–55). A meta-analysis suggested escitalopram was superior in efficacy to all comparator antidepressants with fewer ADR-related drop-outs (s = 10, n = 2687, RCT, d/b, Kennedy et al, J Psychiatr Neurosci 2006;**31**:122–31). When rapidly titrated to maximum dose, escitalopram 20 mg/d appears at least as effective as venlafaxine XL 225 mg/d and is significantly better tolerated (n = 195, RCT, d/b, 8/52, Bielski et al, J Clin Psychiatry 2004;**65**:1190–6) and in a two-study reanalysis, escitalopram appeared more effective than venlafaxine for severe depression (s = 2, c = 483, 8/52, Montgomery and Andersen, Int Clin Psychopharmacol 2006;**21**:297–309).

Reviews: * general (Murdoch and Keam, Drugs 2005;**65**:2379–404; Waugh and Goa, CNS Drugs 2003;**17**:343–62), extensive (Dhillon et al, CNS Drugs 2006;**20**:763–90), pharmacoeconomics (Croom and Plosker, CNS Drugs 2004;**18**:469–73), comparison with citalopram (Sanchez et al, Psychopharmacol [Berl] 2004;**174**:163–76).

Fluoxetine *

Fluoxetine is licensed across the world for depression, with or without anxiety. Although 20 mg/d is the standard dose (UK maximum 80 mg/d), some resistant depressions may respond to 60–80 mg/d. It has been shown to be clearly superior to placebo and slightly superior to tricyclics with significantly fewer drop-outs (rigorous meta-analysis, 30 trials, n = 4120, Bech et al, Br J Psychiatry 2000;**176**:421–8), with 20 mg as the most effective dose (n = 417, meta-analysis by Beasley et al, J Clin Psychiatry 2000;**61**:722–8) and evidence of relapse prevention (n = 140, RCT, 48/52, Gilaberte et al, J Clin Psychopharmacol 2001;**21**:417–24, MS). There is an interesting independent review suggesting inferior efficacy to other antidepressants (s = 131, Cipriani et al, J Clin Psychiatry 2006;**67**:850–64). Claims of suicidal

ideation (n = 6, Teicher et al, Am J Psychiatry 1990;**147**:207–10) have been disproven (n = 10614, Tollefson et al, Ann Clin Psychiatry 1993;**5**:209–24), as fluoxetine shows a slight reduction in suicidal behaviour, rather than an increase (n = 185, Leon et al, Am J Psychiatry 1999;**156**:195–201). A long half-life may prove a problem in the elderly, although missed doses become less important in continuation and prophylactic therapy and discontinuation symptoms are rare. Twice-weekly dosing (Megna and Devitt, Ann Pharmacother 2001; **35**:45–7), and a weekly tablet (see 7.2) have been used. Cochrane calls for better trials with fluoxetine, a somewhat futile hope unless used as a comparator (Cipriani et al, Cochrane Database Syst Rev 2005;**19**:4185).
Reviews: * safety and side-effects (Wernicke, Expert Opin Drug Saf 2004;**3**:495–504, MS).

Fluvoxamine

Fluvoxamine is licensed in UK for depression. The starting dose should be 100–150 mg/d and lack of response at 6/52 accurately predicts non-response (n = 72, open, Morishita and Arita, Psychiatry Clin Neurosci 2003;**57**:177–81). It has been compared with and shown to be as effective as many standard tricyclics, eg. clomipramine (n = 86, RCT, d/b, 8/52, Zohar et al, Hum Psychopharmacol 2003;**18**:113–19), although imipramine was more effective in depressed in-patients (n = 141, RCT, d/b, 4/52, Van Den Broek et al, Psychopharmacol (Berl) 2004;**175**:481–6). It may have a higher incidence of nausea and vomiting than other SSRIs.

Paroxetine *

Paroxetine is licensed for depression, including that accompanied by anxiety. It has a flat dose-response curve, with 20 mg/d optimum and no significant advantage for escalating dosage to 40 mg/d (n = 544, RCT, Benkert et al, Acta Psychiatr Scand 1997;**95**:288–96). Several short-term trials comparing it with standard tricyclics have been published. Relapse prevention has been shown with paroxetine in old age (n = 116, RCT, d/b, p/c, two years, Reynolds et al, N Engl J Med 2006;**354**:1130–8). Paroxetine's half-life increases from 10 to 21 hours on chronic dosing, but reduces when this is stopped, which may in part explain the many

reports of discontinuation effects (see 2.2.2), which have received much media attention in recent years. In 2006, the UK CHM warned that young adults (18–29 years of age) are at a higher risk of suicidal behaviour than older adults, so careful and frequent monitoring is important, especially if a patient experiences worsening of symptoms or if new symptoms arise after starting treatment.
Reviews: general (Wagstaff et al, Drugs 2002; **62**:655–703; Bourin et al, CNS Drug Rev 2001;**7**:25–47).

> ### Switching or discontinuing antidepressants
>
> For a table on switching antidepressants and the gaps needed, or advice on the problems of discontinuing, see Chapter 2.2.5.

Sertraline

The pharmacological profile of sertraline is similar to fluoxetine, but with a shorter half-life. The standard dose is 50 mg/d, although 100 mg/d is routinely used. Response to the higher dose may be quicker than 50 mg/d (n = 44, 10/52, Suri et al, J Clin Psychiatry 2000;**61**:942–6). Efficacy in chronic major depression has been shown (eg. n = 635, RCT, Keller et al, J Clin Psychiatry 1998;**59**:598–607), as has relapse prevention (n = 161, RCT, 4/12, Keller et al, JAMA 1998;**280**:1665–72; see also Baldessarini et al, JAMA 1999;**282**:323–4). In recurrent depression (three or more episodes of MDD in four years) both sertraline 50 mg/d and 100 mg/d were superior to placebo in preventing recurrences in people switched to sertraline for the continuation phase of the study (n = 371, RCT, p/c, d/b, 18/12, Lépine et al, Am J Psychiatry 2004;**161**:836–42) but not in the elderly (RCT, d/b, p/c, two years, Wilson et al, Br J Psychiatry 2003;**182**:492–7). Sertraline may be effective also in delusional depression (comparison vs paroxetine, n = 46, d/b, Zanardi et al, Am J Psychiatry 1996;**153**:1631–3) and in the elderly (n = 210, over 60 years, RCT, 12/52, Bondareff et al, Am J Psychiatry 2000;**157**:729–36). Patients in a community nursing home-stabilised on sertraline once-daily for 12 or more weeks, have been successfully changed to equivalent doses of sertraline three times a week (n=44, Karki et al, J Pharm Technol 2000;**16**:43–6). Sertraline has a favourable drug interaction profile (4.3.2.5).

Reviews: pharmacokinetic profile (DeVane et al, Clin Pharmacokinet 2002;**41**:1247–66).

TRICYCLICS

Doses of 125–150mg/d of tricyclics are effective in depression and clearly superior to placebo. A controversial systematic review and meta-analysis concluded that low-dose tricyclics (≤100mg/d) are effective in some patients with depression with fewer ADR drop-outs, although the optimum dose was not studied and poor CYP2D6 metabolisers will account for some low-dose responders (Furukawa et al, Br Med J 2002; **325**:991–1000; constructively critical comment by Ruhé, EBMH 2003;**6**:46). The meta-analysis by Bollini et al (Br J Psychiatry 1999;**174**:297–303), concluding that 'sub-therapeutic' antidepressant doses are effective is only justified if considering fluoxetine 30mg/d as sub-therapeutic, which it isn't (for a good review of the use of sub-therapeutic doses of TCAs, see Donoghue (Acta Psychiatr Scand 1998;**98**:429–31). If using tricyclics, a therapeutic dose must be used before assessing the response, because as they say, 'Half a whole is nothing', and half a dose only gives you side-effects.

In England and Wales, deaths (1993–1997) from overdose have risen, with 20% antidepressant-related, 95% from TCAs (predominantly dosulepin and amitriptyline) and most often in deprived areas (n=2503, Shah et al, Psychol Med 2001;**31**:1203–10). Patients taking tricyclics are five times more likely to have road traffic accidents than untreated controls (Edwards, editorial in Br Med J 1995;**311**:887–8).

In the UK, NICE recommends performing an ECG before prescribing tricyclics in depressed people at significant risk of cardiovascular disease, and that SSRIs should be first-line rather than a (cheaper) tricyclic.

Reviews: * toxicity (Nutt, J Psychopharmacol 2005;**19**:123–4, pointing out the relative toxicity and sub-therapeutic dosing), cardiovascular toxicity from tricyclic poisoning (Thanacoody and Thomas, Toxicol Rev 2005;**24**:205–14).

Amitriptyline

A widely-used tricyclic with potent anticholinergic, sedative, weight-gaining properties and a long half-life (meta-analysis of amitriptyline vs the rest: Barbui and Hotopf, Br J Psychiatry 2001;**178**:129–44; reply by Thompson, Br J Psychiatry 2001;**178**:99–100). Cochrane concludes that amitriptyline is at least as effective as other antidepressants, but with a higher side-effect burden (Guaiana et al, Cochrane Database Syst Rev 2003; **2**:CD004186).

Amoxapine

Amoxapine is structurally similar to maprotiline. It has a high incidence of seizures (up to 36% in overdose), as well as renal failure, endocrine and EPS. It has been discontinued in the UK.

Clomipramine

Clomipramine is a potent tricyclic with an active metabolite, with a possible added advantage in treating depression with an obsessional component. On one measure, clomipramine has been shown to have superior efficacy to imipramine and citalopram (two trial comparison by Fuglum et al, Acta Psychiatr Scand 1996;**94**:18–25). Clomipramine doses of 25, 50, 75, 125 and 200mg/d all show improvement, with 125 and 200mg/d showing the greatest improvement, although there was no placebo control group (n=151, d/b, 6/52, DUAG, Clin Pharmacol Ther 1999;**66**:152–65). Once daily dosage can be appropriate.

Dosulepin (dothiepin)

Dosulepin is an established tricyclic in the UK, although in the UK NICE recommends that it is only initiated by specialist mental health professionals (including GPs with a special interest in mental health). It has significant sedative effects and impairment of concentration and memory and has been shown to be more toxic than other tricyclics, particularly due to its proconvulsive and cardiac arrhythmic effects (Buckley et al, Lancet 1994;**343**:159–62), so should not be used in someone actively suicidal. It is frequently prescribed in the community at sub-therapeutic antidepressant doses (eg. 75mg/d) which must be a major cause of treatment failure. Although often prescribed to aid sleep, both dosulepin and fluoxetine disrupt REM sleep and no sleep-promoting effects were seen from dosulepin (n = 12, RCT, 5/52, d/b, p/c, Wilson et al, J Psychopharmacol 2002;**16**:321–31).

Doxepin

Doxepin is a standard tricyclic with moderate sedation, which may have fewer anticholinergic and cardiac effects than older tricyclics. It has an active metabolite and is suitable for once or twice daily dosing. It is not to be discontinued in the UK, despite rumours to the contrary.

Imipramine

Imipramine is an established standard tricyclic suitable for once daily administration. NICE states that women tolerate imipramine more poorly than men. Psychotic depression shows high response rate to imipramine (n = 52, Bruijn et al, J Affect Disord 2001;**66**:165–74). Stimulant side-effects may be troublesome as may the anticholinergic effects, especially in the elderly, and it may provoke fragmentation of motor activity during sleep (n = 52, Volkers et al, Eur Neuropsychopharm 2002;**12**:273–8).

Lofepramine

Lofepramine is an established UK tricyclic and NICE's tricyclic of choice. It may have relatively fewer side-effects than other tricyclics, eg. it has minimal sedative effects and impairment of concentration and memory compared with dosulepin (Allen et al, J Psychopharmacol 1993;**7**:33–8). It is surprisingly safe in overdose, with lofepramine seeming to block the cardiotoxic effects of the main metabolite, desipramine (full review by Lancaster and Gonzalez, Drugs 1989;**37**:123–40).

Maprotiline

Maprotiline has cardiac effects similar to the older tricyclics and the greatest incidence of seizures in overdose (and even at standard doses), compounded by its unusually long half-life. Use should be restricted to patients where these risks are absolutely minimal.

Nortriptyline

Nortriptyline is a mildly sedative tricyclic with low cardiotoxic side-effects and suitable

for once daily administration. In treatment-resistant depression (failing 1–5 adequate trials) 40% may respond (12% remission) to nortriptyline, although 35% may not tolerate the treatment (n = 92, open, 6/52, Nierenberg et al, J Clin Psychiatry 2003;**64**:35–9). In a study of melancholic depression in elderly patients, it was shown to be significantly more effective than fluoxetine (n = 22, Roose et al, Am J Psychiatry 1994;**151**:1735–9). It is as effective as paroxetine but less well-tolerated (n = 116, RCT, 12/52, Mulsant et al, Am J Geriatr Psychiatry 2001;**9**:406–14; n = 59, RCT, 18/12, Bump et al, Depress Anxiety 2001;**13**:38–44), but avoidant personality disorder predicts a poor response (n = 92, open, 6/52, Papakostas et al, J Clin Psychiatry 2003;**64**:1357–61, IS).

Switching or discontinuing antidepressants

For a table on switching antidepressants and the gaps needed, or advice on the problems of discontinuing, see Chapter 2.2.5.

Trimipramine *

Structurally related to levomepromazine, trimipramine has significant sedative properties, which can be useful for hypnotic and anxiolytic purposes. High-dose trimipramine (300–400 mg/d, plasma levels higher than 160 ng/ml) has been shown to significantly improve delusional depression (n = 15, open, 4/52, Frieboes et al, Pharmacopsychiatry 2003; **36**:12–7).

OTHER ANTIDEPRESSANTS

Duloxetine *

Duloxetine is an SNRI that also weakly inhibits dopamine reuptake, but has no histamine, dopamine, cholinergic or adrenergic receptor affinity. The standard dose is 60 mg/d and although is no published evidence that 120 mg/d is more effective some believe that to be the case. Efficacy has been shown in two major studies (n = 267, RCT, d/b, p/c, 9/52, Detke et al,

J Psychiatry Res 2002;**36**:383–90; n = 245, RCT, d/b, p/c, 9/52, Detke et al, J Clin Psychiatry 2002; **63**:308–15). Duloxetine 40–80 mg/d was at least as effective as paroxetine 20 mg/d for the emotional and physical symptoms of depression (RCT, d/b, p/c, Goldstein et al, J Clin Psychopharmacol 2004;**24**:389–99; MS). A follow-on study showed some relapse prevention efficacy (n = 278, RCT, p/c, d/b, 26/52, Perahia et al, Br J Psychiatry 2006;**188**:346–53; MS).

Reviews: * use in depression (Kirwin and Goren, Pharmacother 2005;**25**:396–410).

Mianserin

Mianserin is a tetracyclic with prominent $5HT_{2A}$ and $5HT_{2C}$ antagonist properties, a good safety profile in overdose, low cardiotoxicity and marked sedative properties. Mianserin has been shown to be effective at 20–60 mg/d in prophylaxis of recurrent depression (n = 22, 18/12, Kishimoto et al, Acta Psychiatr Scand 1994;**89**:46–51).

Mirtazapine *

Mirtazapine blocks presynaptic alpha-2 adreno-receptors (increasing norepinephrine transmission) and indirectly enhances serotoninergic transmission, with additional $5\text{-}HT_2$ and $5\text{-}HT_3$ receptor blockade minimising the incidence of serotoninergic side-effects, eg. nausea, headache and sexual dysfunction. The dose range is 15–45 mg/d and the optimum starting dose of 30 mg/d is well-tolerated. In a number of double-blind trials, mirtazapine has been shown to be as effective over six weeks as reference antidepressants and as well-tolerated as fluoxetine but significantly more effective at three and four weeks of therapy (n = 135, RCT, Wheatley et al, J Clin Psychiatry 1998;**59**:306–12). Mirtazapine has been shown to be as effective as fluoxetine in severe depression (n = 297[c=292], RCT, d/b, 8/52, Versiani et al, CNS Drugs 2005;**19**:137–46; n = 36[c = 31], RCT, d/b, 6/52, Amini et al, J Clin Pharm Ther 2005;**30**:133–8). In a comparison with venlafaxine, mirtazapine was as effective (62% vs 52% response) for melancholic depression, evident from week four and with lower drop-outs in the mirtazapine group (n = 157, RCT, 8/52, Guelfi et al, J Clin Psychopharmacol 2001;**21**:425–31). Mirtazapine

may also be well-tolerated and very effective as an adjunctive in antidepressant-resistant persistent MDD (n = 26, RCT, d/b, p/c, 4/52, Carpenter et al, Biol Psychiatry 2002;**51**:183–8). A meta-analysis of all three completed comparative studies of mirtazapine versus SSRIs (fluoxetine, paroxetine and citalopram) showed a similar AD profile, but hinted at superior efficacy and a robust faster onset of action, statistically significant in all three studies in the first few weeks (reviewed by Thompson, J Clin Psychiatry 1999, **60**[Suppl 17], 18–22; discussion 46–8; n = 298 + 285 from three studies, Quitkin et al, J Clin Psychiatry 2001, **62**, 358–61; further studies with similar results include n = 212, RCT, d/b, 6/52, Szegedi et al, J Clin Psychiatry 2003;**64**:413–20 and n = 197, RCT, 24/52, Wade et al, Int Clin Psychopharmacol 2003;**18**:133–41). An earlier onset of action is related to better overall outcomes. Relapse prevention is significantly superior to placebo (n = 156, RCT, d/b, 40/52, Thase et al, J Clin Psychiatry 2001;**62**:782–8). Mirtazapine started immediately after stroke may reduce the incidence of post-stroke depression (n = 70, RCT, open, one year, Niedermaier et al, J Clin Psychiatry 2005;**5**:1619–23; critical comment by Ween, EBMH 2005;**8**:74). Orodispersable 'SolTabs' are available worldwide, and have been compared with sertraline (n = 345, RCT, d/b, 8/52, Behnke et al, J Clin Psychopharmacol 2003;**23**:358–64).

Reviews: general (Nutt, Hum Psychopharmacol 2002;**17**[Suppl 1]:S37–S41), kinetics (Timmer et al, Clin Pharmacokinet 2000;**38**:461–74, 56 refs), in the elderly (case reports, Raji and Brady, Ann Pharmacother 2001;**35**:1024–7).

Moclobemide

Moclobemide (a reversible inhibitor of monoamine oxidase-A) inhibits only MAO-A and not MAO-B, so an excess of tyramine in the body will displace moclobemide from MAO-A, allowing tyramine metabolism to occur, MAO-B remaining free. This results in a 'cheese-reaction', usually only at amounts above 100–150 mg of tyramine (see 4.3.4), unlikely under normal conditions. A meta-analysis of 38 double-blind and two single-blind trials with moclobemide (n = 2416) showed it to be about equipotent with imipramine or sedative tricyclic antidepressants in agitated-anxious depressive patients, and all were clearly superior to placebo (Delini-Stula et al, J Affect Disord 1995;**35**:21–30). Another review of studies indicates that moclobemide may be useful in typical severe depression with melancholia (Paykel, Acta Psychiatr Scand 1995;**91**[Suppl 386]:S22–S27). A review of moclobemide overdose toxicity concludes that overdose is benign even with massive ingestions (only one death reported), but overdose in combination with other serotonergic agents can cause severe serotonin toxicity (n = 106, Isbister et al, Br J Clin Pharmacol 2003;**56**:441–50).

Review: Bonnet, CNS Drug Rev 2003;**9**:97–140.

Reboxetine

Reboxetine is a selective norepinephrine reuptake inhibitor with no dopamine, histamine, adrenergic nor serotonin effects at 8 mg/d, but a weak anticholinergic action. Analysis of four RCTs indicates reboxetine to be significantly more effective than placebo in severe depression (s = 4, RCT, d/b, p/c, 8/52, Montgomery et al, J Clin Psychopharmacol 2003;**23**:45–50). A higher level of social functioning has been shown with reboxetine, using a validated scale (SASS), although comparison of nortriptyline and fluoxetine failed to show any difference in SASS scores, suggesting that noradrenergic drive enhancement was not essential for improved social functioning (n = 188, open, 13/52, Luty et al, J Psychopharmacol 2001;**15**:257–64). Relapse prevention has been shown against placebo (n = 283, d/b, p/c, 46/52, Versiani et al, J Clin Psychiatry 1999;**60**:400–6), with reboxetine being well-tolerated. Reboxetine may improve cognitive processing in depressed adults compared to paroxetine and placebo (n = 74, Ferguson et al, Int Clin Psychopharmacol 2003;**18**:9–14). Reboxetine has also been used successfully to treat multi-drug resistant depression in Parkinson's disease (n = 1, Lemke, J Clin Psychiatry 2000;**61**:872; n = 16, open, 4/52, Lemke et al, J Clin Psychiatry 2002;**63**:300–4). There is no effect on reaction time (Hindmarsh, Eur Neuropsychopharmacol 1997;[Suppl 1]:S17–S21). Interest in use as an SSRI adjunct must be tempered by the lack of safety data.

Reviews: general (Hajos et al, CNS Drug Rev 2004;**10**:23–44, Page, CNS Drug Rev 2003;**9**:327–42).

Trazodone

Trazodone increases NE and 5-HT turnover with low cardiotoxicity and anti-cholinergic side-effects, but a higher incidence of drowsiness and nausea, so it makes a good hypnotic as well. It is best taken with food to reduce peak blood levels.

Venlafaxine *

Venlafaxine is an SNRI (combined 5-HT and NE reuptake blocker), with minimal effects on other transmitters (except dopamine, where it has a not insignificant effect at higher doses). It is an effective antidepressant and there is evidence for a dose-response relationship (eg. n = 147, RCT, Mehtonen et al, J Clin Psychiatry 2000;**61**:95–100), with 5-HT reuptake inhibition across the dosage range, NE reuptake inhibition becoming significant from 150 mg/d (n = 32, Harvey et al, Arch Gen Psychiatry 2000;**57**:503–9) and dopamine reuptake inhibition above 225 mg/d. Three systematic reviews and meta-analyses have provided some indication that venlafaxine may be more effective at higher doses than certain SSRIs, with comparable tolerability (s = 32, Smith et al, Br J Psychiatry 2002;**180**:396–404; Stahl et al, Biol Psychiatry 2002;**52**:1166–74), but both show only a weak advantage over other drugs, and a meta-analysis of eight comparable d/b studies in MDD indicated that remission (as opposed to response) rates with venlafaxine were significantly (10%) higher and earlier than with an SSRI (fluoxetine), with doses of > 150 mg/d necessary for remission (Thase et al, Br J Psychiatry 2001;**178**:234–41, MS), although these have been criticised as insufficiently objective.

The UK MHRA have seen some sense and reduced their previous restrictions (comment by Taylor and Scott, J Psychopharmacol 2006; **20**:597–601) on venlafaxine:

- Still to be reserved as second-line treatment.
- Shared care is only required for initiation in severely depressed people or in hospitalised patients who require doses of 300 mg daily, or above.

- Is only contraindicated in patients with an identified high risk of a serious cardiac ventricular arrhythmia or with uncontrolled hypertension. No baseline ECG is needed, but regular bp is recommended.

Although studies suggest a higher overdose toxicity with venlafaxine compared to SSRIs this may be due to increased use in patients at higher risk factors for suicide (including severity of depression), eg. venlafaxine (n = 27096) patients were 4–6 times more likely to have been previously hospitalised for depression than fluoxetine (n = 134996) and citalopram (n = 52035) which might also explain the higher reported suicide rate with venlafaxine (n = 214127, Mines et al, Pharmacoepidemiol Drug Saf 2005;14:367–72, MS). There is a moderate relationship between dose and plasma venlafaxine levels, but a higher correlation between plasma levels and MADRS improvement (n = 89, Charlier et al, J Psychopharmacol 2002;16:369–72). Higher-dose venlafaxine (range 375–600 mg/d) may be more effective in severe depression but has more side-effects (except weight gain) than standard dose (75–300 mg/d), but is not associated with higher drop-outs (n = 70, open, Harrison et al, J Psychopharmacol 2004;18:200–4). It seems to have a relatively high fatal toxicity index (Buckley and McManus, Br Med J 2002;325:1332–3) and discontinuation effects may be significant (see 2.2.5). The sustained release preparation (Efexor XL®, Wyeth) probably gives a reduced incidence of initial nausea and has a once a day dosage. Although the UK SPCs for XL and plain tablets have different maximum doses, this was just a licensing issue not a difference in absorption or safety. Venlafaxine is not recommended in children and adolescents under 18 years, due to lack of efficacy and an increase in the rate of harmful outcomes, including hostility, suicidal ideation and self-harm.

Review: general (Kienke and Rosenbaum, Depress Anxiety 2000;12[Suppl 1]:50–4).

MONO-AMINE OXIDASE INHIBITORS (MAOIs) *

Isocarboxazid

Isocarboxazid is a hydrazine derivative that irreversibly blocks the MAO enzyme

(editorial by Shader and Greenblatt, J Clin Psychopharmacol 1999;19:105).

Phenelzine *

Phenelzine is a hydrazine derivative that irreversibly blocks the MAO enzyme, and is NICE's MAOI of choice, although they recommend that it is only initiated by specialist mental health professionals (including GPs with a special interest in mental health). Patients with chronic atypical depression are at high risk of relapse if phenelzine is withdrawn six months after the initial response (n = 60, RCT, p/c, Stewart et al, Am J Psychiatry 1997;154:31–6). A comparison of tranylcypromine and phenelzine showed no significant difference between them, with a 52% response rate in severely depressed treatment-resistant patients (n = 77[c = 67], d/b, 5/52, Birkenhäger et al, J Clin Psychiatry 2004;65:1505–10). Phenelzine is as effective as CBT in atypical depression (n = 108, RCT, 10/52, Jarrett et al, Arch Gen Psychiatry 1999;56:431–7).

Tranylcypromine *

Tranylcypromine is a non-hydrazine amfetamine-related MAOI with stimulant effects and a greater incidence of adverse drug interactions. It has been shown to be effective in tricyclic-resistant and anergic bipolar depression in one study (n = 16, RCT, d/b, c/o, Thase et al, Am J Psychiatry 1992;149:195–8). Tranylcypromine (mean 37 mg/d) has significant effect on REM latency and disrupts sleep architecture (n = 23, Jindal et al, Psychopharmacol Bull 2003;37:118–26). The use of concomitant amlodipine can attenuate hypertensive episodes with tranylcypromine, making MAOIs' therapy feasible in some resistant depressions (n = 3, Taylor et al, J Clin Psychiatry 2005;6:657–8).

OTHER ANTIDEPRESSANTS

Lithium (see also combinations)

Use of lithium as monotherapy in the treatment and prophylaxis of unipolar (as well as bipolar) depression has been well-established, and associated with lower mortality (n = 827, mean 81/12, Müller-Oerlinghausen et al, Acta Psychiatr Scand 1992;86:218–22). However, lithium is most effective as an adjunct to antidepressants, where it may show a rapid effect over 1–2 weeks (eg. in the elderly with unipolar MDD, a major protective effect: n=50, two years, Wilkinson et al, Int J Geriatr Psychiatry 2002;**17**:619–22, see also combinations later), although it may be of limited use in people resistant to multiple antidepressants (n=92, RCT, p/c, 12/52, Nierenberg et al, J Clin Psychopharmacol 2003;**23**:92–5). A meta-analysis of placebo-controlled studies has shown that lithium augmentation (600–800mg/d) increases response in depression refractory to tricyclics (eight studies) or SSRIs (one study) (n=234, s=9, RCT, Bauer and Dopfmer, J Clin Psychopharmacol 1999;**19**:427–34; review by Lam, EBMH 2000;**3**:44; Bandolier 2000;**7**:4–5). Much antidepressant response to lithium is probably mood stabilisation in undiagnosed bipolar depression and so sudden withdrawal of lithium would be outright dangerous (Faedda et al, Am J Psychiatry 2001;**158**:1337–9). However, a recent long-term open study has suggested that lithium may be useful in prophylaxis of unipolar depression (n=55, mean 6.7 years, Baethge et al, J Psych Neurol 2003;**28**:355–61). **Reviews:** lithium augmentation in refractory depression (Heit and Nemeroff, J Clin Psychiatry 1998;**59**[Suppl 6]:S28–S33, 36 refs), general review (Rouillon and Gorwood, J Clin Psychiatry 1998;**59**[Suppl 5]:S32–S41; Bauer and Dopfmer, J Clin Psychopharmacol 1999;**19**:427–34). See main entry under bipolar mood disorder (1.10) and bipolar depression (1.10.3).

Tryptophan *

A naturally occurring amino acid and precursor to serotonin, tryptophan is usually used in combination with tricyclic or other antidepressants. Tryptophan deficiency results in a rapid lowering of mood (review by Bell et al, Br J Psychiatry 2001;**178**:399–405) and tryptophan depletion reverses antidepressant-induced remission, so tryptophan might help if low tryptophan levels have occurred. Cochrane concludes that the trial data is limited and unreliable but suggests tryptophan may be superior to placebo (Shaw et al, Cochrane Database Syst Rev 2002;**1**:CD003198), and a further review agrees that the evidence is inadequate (Shaw et al, Aust N Z J Psychiatry 2002;**36**:488–91). Due to a previous

association with eosinophilia-myalgia syndrome (EMS), it is now only licensed in the UK for resistant depression, by hospital specialists, in patients with severe depression continuously for more than two years, after adequate trials of standard drug treatments and as an adjunct to other treatments. These remain harsh restrictions for the low risk involved and possible antidepressant benefits.

AUGMENTATION STRATEGIES
(drugs with no intrinsic antidepressant activity)

Reviews: * general (Drugs Ther Perspect 2001; **17**:6–9; DeBattista, J Psychopharmacol 2006; **20**[Suppl]:11–8).

Atomoxetine *

Atomoxetine 40mg/d added to antidepressants produced a positive response in 60%, worthy of further investigation, although atomoxetine is itself a failed antidepressant monotherapy (n=15[c=11], open, 8/52, Carpenter et al, J Clin Psychiatry 2005;**66**:1234–8; see also n=1, Pilhatsch et al, Pharmacopsychiatry 2006;**39**:79–80).

Folate *

Folate 15mg/d has significantly improved clinical response and recovery from acute psychiatric disorders (review by Reynolds, Br Med J 2002;**324**:1512–5, 32 refs), as low folate levels have been associated with melancholic depression and non-response to antidepressants, eg. fluoxetine (n=127, RCT, p/c, 10/52, Coppen and Bailey, J Affect Disord 2000;**60**:121–30; comment by Goodwin, EBMH 2001;**4**:41). Routine folate levels should be included in the assessment of treatment-resistant depressives (McLaughlin and McMahon, Br J Psychiatry 1993;**162**:572) and oral supplementation with folic acid 800mcg/d improves treatment outcomes (extensive review by Coppen and Bolander-Gouaille, J Psychopharmacol 2005;**19**:59–65, 63 refs, systematic review and meta-analysis by Taylor et al, J Psychopharmacol 2004;**18**:251–6). SAMe (S-Adenosyl-Methionine) is a closely related active form that has been used to enhance the onset of TCAs (n=40, RCT, p/c, 2/52, Berlanga et al, J Psychiatr Res 1992;**44**:257–62).

Leucovorin (metabolised to methylfolate) has a modest effect in SSRI non-response (n = 22, 8/52, Alpert et al, Ann Clin Psychiatry 2002; **14**:33–8).

Levothyroxine (thyroxine)

Subclinical hypothyroidism may predispose to depression (n = 31, life-long histories, Haggerty et al, Am J Psychiatry 1993;**150**:508–10). In a small open study, augmentation with high-dose 150–300mg/d levothyroxine had an antidepressant effect in more than 50% of the previously treatment-resistant patients with chronic depression and/or dysthymia (n = 9, open, 8/52, Rudas et al, Biol Psychiatry 1999;**15**:45, 229–33; review by Joffe, J Clin Psychiatry 1998;**59**[Suppl 5]:S26–S31). Thyroid supplementation may accelerate the onset of tricyclic response in non-refractory depression (5/6 studies found T3 significantly superior to placebo, especially in women: meta-analysis, Altshuler et al, Am J Psychiatry 2001;**158**:1617–22).

Liothyronine (triiodothyronine) *

A meta-analysis of the eight controlled studies showed liothyronine augmentation to produce twice as many responses in refractory depression compared to controls, with moderately large improvements, although one RCT showed negative results (n = 292, s = 8, Aronson et al, Arch Gen Psychiatry 1996; **53**:842–8), and addition of liothyronine to paroxetine did not improve response (speed or total effect) and, in fact, more adverse reactions were seen (n = 106, RCT, d/b, p/c, 8/52, Appelhof et al, J Clin Endocrinol Metab 2004;**89**:6271–6). T3 50mcg/d was effective in 35% treatment-resistant depressives, especially for melancholic MDD (n = 20, open, 4/52, Losifescu et al, J Clin Psychiatry 2005;**66**:1038–42). Sub-therapeutic doses of T$_3$ liothyronine 25–50mcg/d (Cooke, Am J Psychiatry 1990; **147**:255) or T$_4$ levothyroxine up to 0.1 mg/d have been used as augmentation to tricyclics, etc (n = 50, RCT, d/b, p/c, 2/52, Joffe et al, Arch Gen Psychiatry 1993;**50**:387–93). This may be effective, particularly in rapid-cycling bipolar disorder (1.10.4).

Metyrapone *

Metyrapone 1g/d accelerated the response to 'standard' antidepressants (nefazodone or fluvoxamine!) in major depression, possibly by counteracting stress hormones' inhibiting effect on 5HT release in the forebrain (n = 63, RCT, p/c, 5/52, Jahn et al, Arch Gen Psychiatry 2004;**61**:1235–44; comment by Young, EBMH 2005;**8**:72).

Modafinil *

Adjunctive modafinil to SSRIs at the start of treatment may enhance the onset of action in people with MDD and fatigue (n = 29, open, 6/52, Ninan et al, J Clin Psychiatry 2004;**65**:414–20, MS). Adjunctive modafinil may help in patients with fatigue and sleepiness in MDD over the short-term, but the effect wears off 6/52 (n = 136 [c = 118], RCT, d/b, p/c, 6/52, DeBattista et al, J Clin Psychiatry 2003;**64**:1057–64; n = 245 [c = 194], open, p/c, 12/52, Thase et al, CNS Spectr 2006;**11**:93–102).

Nimodipine *

Nimodipine augmentation of fluoxetine seemed to be successful for 'vascular depression' (n = 101, RCT, d/b, p/c, 8/52, Taragano et al, Int Psychogeriatr 2005;**17**:487–98).

Pindolol

Antidepressants, eg. SSRIs may act by inhibiting the 5-HT reuptake pump, increasing 5-HT but this also includes enhancing 5-HT at 5-HT$_{1A}$ receptors situated on the cell body which operate a feedback loop, thus cancelling each other out. Over a period of weeks, however, the pre-synaptic 5-HT$_{1A}$ receptors become desensitised but pindolol selectively blocks 5-HT$_{1A}$ receptors, and inhibits this initial feedback loop to increase the speed of onset of action (although not everyone agrees with this: Cremers et al, Biol Psychiatry 2001;**50**:13–21).

A recent systematic review and meta-analysis concludes that pindolol increases the response to SSRIs in the first two weeks of therapy, but not beyond 2–3 weeks (s = 5, Ballesteros et al, J Affect Disord 2004;**79**:137–47; review Isaac, EBMH 2004;**7**:107). Some positive trials exist (eg. Tome et al, J Affect Disord 1997;**44**:101–9; n = 11, RCT, Perez et al, Lancet 1997;**349**:1594–7; n = 3485, three years, Rasanen et al, J Clin Psychopharmacol 1999;**19**:297–302), but others are negative (eg. Perez et al, Arch Gen Psychiatry 1999;**56**:375–9;

n = 42[c = 38], RCT, d/b, p/c, 6/52, Perry et al, J Clin Psychiatry 2004;**65**:238–43). The explanations possibly including too low doses (eg. 15 mg/d probably needed: n = 8, Rabiner et al, Am J Psychiatry 2001;**158**:2080–2) or use of a racaemic mix (Isaac and Tome, Am J Psychiatry 1997;**154**:1790–1).

Reviews: McAskill et al, Br J Psychiatry 1998; **173**:203–8, discussion by McAllister-Williams and Young, Br J Psychiatry 1998;**173**:536–9.

Vitamin B12 (cyanocobalamin) *

Oral B12 1 mg/d supplementation has been recommended in treatment-resistant depression (Tiemeier et al, Am J Psychiatry 2002;**159**:2099–101; review by Coppen and Bolander-Gouaille, J Psychopharmacol 2005; **19**:59–65).

+ Combinations I: combined antidepressants

There is some evidence that combined NE and 5-HT reuptake blocking drugs can produce a quicker antidepressant effect, although it could be that combined drug use produces higher success rates by treating different depressive subgroups. It is better to combine mechanisms of action rather than simply adding drugs, aiming for synergy (de la Gándara et al, Acta Psychiatr Scand 2005;**112**[Suppl 428]:11–3).

Review: * Strategies for combination and augmentation for depression (DeBattista, J Psychopharmacol 2006;**20**[Suppl]:11–8).

Bupropion + tranylcypromine

The cautious use of this combination has been successful in resolving multi-drug resistant depression (n = 1, Pierre and Gitlin, J Clin Psychiatry 2000;**61**:450–1).

Bupropion + venlafaxine/SSRIs/duloxetine *

Bupropion 200–300 mg/d may be useful, eg. 56% of venlafaxine/SSRI-resistant depressed patients responded when bupropion was added (n = 25, Spier et al, Depress Anxiety 1998; **7**:73–5), and in multi-drug resistant depression, bupropion 300 mg/d successfully augmented venlafaxine 450 mg/d (n = 1, Fatemi et al, Ann Pharmacother 1999;**33**:701–3). It may also counteract SSRI/venlafaxine-induced sexual dysfunction (n = 18, open, 8/52, Kennedy et al, J Clin Psychiatry 2002;**63**:181–6). **Duloxetine** (mean 60 mg/d) and bupropion (mean 175 mg/d) was successful (remission 30%, response 60%) in non-responders to initial monotherapy with either drug (n = 10, open, Papakostas et al, Depress Anxiety 2006;**23**:178–81).

Reviews: * reduced side-effects (Zisook et al, Biol Psychiatry 2005;**59**:203–10).

Buspirone + SSRIs

Buspirone shares some pharmacodynamic properties with pindolol and augmentation of SSRIs may produce marked improvement in resistant depressed patients (n = 30, 5/52, Dimitriou and Dimitriou, J Clin Psychopharmacol 1998;**18**:465–9), eg. addition of 20–60 mg/d buspirone to SSRI non-responders produced significant reductions in MADRS scores at the end of week one compared to placebo, but both groups were equivalent at six weeks (n = 102, RCT, p/c, d/b, 6/52, Appelberg et al, J Clin Psychiatry 2001;**62**:448–52). However, another RCT failed to show any advantage of adding buspirone to an SSRI in treatment-resistant depression (n = 119, Landen et al, J Clin Psychiatry 1998;**59**:664–8), although both the placebo (47%) and buspirone (51%) response rates were high, and an open label extension produced a higher (70%) response rate. In another trial, buspirone appeared actually to slow the onset of action of fluoxetine (n = 120, RCT, open, 12/52, Onder and Tural, J Affect Disord 2003;**76**:223–7), so great care is needed.

Lithium + tryptophan + antidepressants (eg. clomipramine, SSRI or phenelzine)

Variously known as Triple Therapy or the MRC, Newcastle or London Cocktail, there have been reports of 55% remission rates in severe depression, eg. from:

- clomipramine (to 150 mg/d or to tolerance eg. 300–400 mg/d) plus
- tryptophan (2–4 g/d) plus
- lithium (standard levels).

Alternatives to clomipramine include phenelzine and the SSRIs (n = 20, RCT, Barker et al, Int Clin Psychopharmacol 1987;**2**:261–72). Tryptophan enhances the action of clomipramine on 5-HT sites and improves 5-HT absorption. Lithium also affects 5-HT and is an antidepressant in its own right.

Mirtazapine + venlafaxine/SSRIs

In persistent MDD, addition of mirtazapine 30 mg to existing therapy produced a response rate of 64% cf 20% with placebo (n = 26, RCT, d/b, p/c, 4/52, Carpenter et al, Biol Psychiatry 2002;**51**:183–88; short review in Fava, J Clin Psychiatry 2001;**62**[Suppl 18]:S4–S11). Mirtazapine has also been used with high-dose venlafaxine, the rationale being to use mirtazapine to block 5HT2 and 5HT3 receptors, reducing sexual and anxiety side-effects from venlafaxine, and allowing higher doses to be tolerated.

Reboxetine + SSRIs *

This logical combination has been used successfully with, eg. citalopram in resistant depression (Devarajan and Dursun, Can J Psychiatry 2000;**45**:489–90). Reboxetine added to SSRI/mirtazapine/venlafaxine partial or non-responders produced a well-tolerated improvement (n = 61, open, 6/52, Rubio et al, J Affect Disord 2004;**81**:67–72) and combined escitalopram and reboxetine may provide a rapid response (n = 3, Camarasa et al, Prog Neuropsychopharmacol Biol Psychiatry 2005; **29**:165–8).

SSRIs + SSRIs

Although there are anecdotal reports (eg. Bondolfi et al, Psychopharmacol [Berl] 1996;**128**:421–5), the combination cannot be recommended and risks serotonin syndrome.

Tricyclics + MAOIs

Although extreme caution is advised, this combination is known to be effective in some resistant depressions, eg. combining isocarboxazid and amitriptyline in treatment-resistant depression showed a 50% response, and most remained in remission for up to three years (n = 25, open, Berlanga and Ortega-Soto, J Affect Disord 1995;**34**:187–92). Tranylcypromine plus clomipramine is known to be dangerous (at least two deaths) but other combinations can be used with care in an in-patient setting. Most problems occur when a tricyclic is added to an MAOI. Fewer adverse events have been reported with the reverse. The main adverse events include hyperthermia, delirium, seizures and agitation,

rather than hypertension. It is best to take great care, eg. separate the doses (eg. MAOI in the morning, tricyclic in the evening), add one to the other in low dose and build up slowly or stop all antidepressants, wait a week, and then start both together at low dose and build up again. The last mentioned seems to be the most widely favoured strategy.

Tricyclics + SSRIs

A number of studies have tried to show that combining tricyclics and SSRIs is more effective than monotherapy (eg. n = 30, open, Weilberg et al, J Clin Psychiatry 1989;**50**:447–9), but the evidence is poor, eg. one report (n = 8, open, Seth et al, Br J Psychiatry 1992;**161**:562–5) was so remarkable its findings were contested (Cowen and Power, Br J Psychiatry 1993;**162**:266–7). However, the only double-blind prospective study on the subject showed that high dose fluoxetine (60 mg/d) was, in fact, more effective in partial or non-responders to 20 mg/d than a fluoxetine/desipramine combination (n = 41, RCT, d/b, 4/52, Fava et al, Am J Psychiatry 1994;**151**:1372–4). The improved outcome with the combination in people who did not respond to either alone is, in most people, likely to be due to raised TCA levels (n = 13, Levitt et al, J Clin Psychiatry 1999;**60**:613; critical review of the therapeutic combination by Taylor, Br J Psychiatry 1995;**167**:575–80). The combination should generally be avoided due to the high risk of an adverse interaction (4.3.2). While SSRI overdose is rare, 93% of those reported in England and Wales (1998–2000) occurred in combination with other drugs, especially TCAs (Cheeta et al, Br J Psychiatry 2004;**184**:41–7), so care is needed when prescribing the combination in potentially suicidal patients.

Venlafaxine + SSRIs

SSRIs have been used successfully to augment venlafaxine (n = 4, Gonul et al, Prog Neuropsychopharmacol Biol Psychiatry 2003;**27**:889–91), but the combination is not recommended.

+ Combinations 2: others

Antipsychotics + antidepressants *

Evidence is accumulating that antipsychotics

(especially 'atypicals') may have some role in augmentation of antidepressants, perhaps via 5HT$_{2A/2C}$ antagonism (review by Thase, *J Clin Psychiatry* 2002;**63**:95–103), as well as anxiolytic and anti-irritability effects. There is some evidence for adjunctive **aripiprazole**. A pilot study showed 55% of the completers responding to aripiprazole augmentation of SSRIs in treatment-resistant depression (n = 12[c = 9], open, 8/52, Papakotas *et al*, *J Clin Psychiatry* 2005;**66**:1326–30), aripiprazole (starting at 2.5–10mg/d) augmentation of partially effective antidepressants appeared useful (n = 15[c = 8], open, 8/52, Simon and Nemeroff, *J Clin Psychiatry* 2005;**66**:1216–20) and augmentation produced a response in 14 (47%) of antidepressant non-responders who had failed augmentation with another atypical, although six of these subsequently relapsed (n = 30, retrospective, Barbee *et al*, *Ann Clin Psychiatry* 2004;**16**:189–94). Finally, a pilot study showed that adjunctive aripiprazole (mean 13mg/d) produced response in 70% and remission in 30% treatment-resistant depressives (n = 10, open, 6/52, Patkar *et al*, *Prim Care Companion J Clin Psychiatry* 2006; **8**:82–7). **Olanzapine** plus fluoxetine was no more effective than either drug alone or nortriptyline alone in one trial (n = 500, RCT, d/b, 8/52, Shelton *et al*, *J Clin Psychiatry* 2005;**66**:1289–97, MS; comment by Dodd and Berk, *EBMH* 2006;**9**:42), but in another (n = 28, d/b, 8/52, Shelton *et al*, *Am J Psychiatry* 2001;**158**:131–4) olanzapine and fluoxetine were effective in people resistant to two antidepressants, although two subsequent trials failed to show the effect (although the control groups showed good responses, suggesting they were not resistant; Shelton, *Expert Opin Pharmacother* 2003;**4**:1175–83). A second (open) trial showed a rapid improvement in depressive symptoms in MDD, including TRD (n = 560, open, 76/52, Corya *et al*, *J Clin Psychiatry* 2003;**64**:1349–56, MS). The combination may be more effective than olanzapine alone or placebo for bipolar I depression, with similar low switching to mania in any group, although there was no fluoxetine monotherapy comparison group (n = 833, RCT, d/b, 8/52, Tohen *et al*, *Arch Gen Psychiatry* 2003;**60**:1079–88; MS). Olanzapine may improve sleep in SSRI-treated

patients (n = 12, open, 3/52, Sharpley *et al*, *J Clin Psychiatry* 2005;**66**:450–4). Although **quetiapine** (n = 554, mean dose 318mg/d) and risperidone (n = 175, mean dose 4.4mg/d) produced improvements in HAM-D scores in psychotic depression, quetiapine was superior to risperidone and better tolerated (n = 729, open randomised, 4/12, Sajatovic *et al*, *J Clin Psychiatry* 2002;**63**:1156–63). Quetiapine 50–750mg/d, mean 300mg/d) may be useful with citalopram (n = 25, open, 6/52, Konstantinidis *et al*, *Prog Neuropsychopharmacol Biol Psychiatry* 2006;**32**:242–7). Addition of low dose **risperidone** (0.5–2mg/d) to existing SSRI therapy may produce rapid responses in some SSRI-resistant patients (n = 8, open, Ostroff and Nelson, *J Clin Psychiatry* 1999;**60**:256–9), and in psychotic depression unresponsive to antidepressants responded to risperidone 4mg/d (n = 1, Land and Chang, *J Clin Psychiatry* 1998;**59**: 624). Addition of low-dose risperidone to fluvoxamine from the start of treatment has enhanced onset (n = 36, open, 6/52, Hirose and Ashby, *J Clin Psychiatry* 2002;**63**:733–6). In another study, the addition of a moderate dose of **perphenazine** to a tricyclic did not improve efficacy in late-life psychotic depression (n = 36, RCT, d/b, 4/52, Mulsant *et al*, *J Clin Psychiatry* 2001;**62**:597–604), although I personally now object to late-life being defined as people aged 50 or older. Adjunctive **sulpiride** 100mg/d may accelerate the antidepressant effect of paroxetine 10–40mg/d (n = 41 [c = 33], RCT, open, 12/52, Uchida *et al*, *J Clin Psychopharmacol* 2005;**25**:545–51). With **ziprasidone** augmentation in SSRI-resistance, a 65% completer response suggests a role for ziprasidone (n = 20 [c = 13], open, 6/52, Papakostas *et al*, *J Clin Psychiatry* 2004; **65**:217–21).

Benzodiazepines + SSRIs

Cochrane concludes that the nine studies (n = 679) indicate that BDZ augmentation (eg. clonazepam, n = 80, RCT, 3/52, Smith *et al*, *Am J Psychiatry* 1998;**155**:1339–45) of antidepressants leads to fewer drop-outs and less depression severity at 1–4 weeks, but the effect disappears at 6–8 weeks. This indicates that short-term use may be successful, possibly by minimising initial SSRI side-effects (eg.

anxiety), improving sleep or a direct action (comment by Gijsman, *EBMH* 2001;**4**:45).

Carbamazepine + SSRIs

Carbamazepine augmentation may be useful in SSRI non-responders (n = 6, Steinacher *et al*, *Eur Neuropsychopharmacol* 2002;**12**:255–60), although beware of potential interactions.

Lithium + antidepressants

There are many double-blind controlled trials of augmentation by lithium of tricyclics, sertraline, citalopram, venlafaxine, and other antidepressants, with 10 studies reporting response rates averaging 52% (review by Fava, *J Clin Psychiatry* 2001;**62**[Suppl 18]:S4–S11). For SSRI augmentation, there is evidence of a substantial effect after 1–6 weeks, mostly within 1–2 weeks (review by Zullino and Baumann, *Pharmacopsychiatry* 2001;**34**:119–27), maintained for 6/12 (n = 30, RCT, d/b, p/c, 6/52, open 4/12 extension, Bauer *et al*, *Am J Psychiatry* 2000;**157**:1429–35). Adequate lithium levels (0.4 mmol/L or more) seem necessary. There is a view that all resistant depressions are part of unrecognised bipolar disorder and, hence, the use of lithium is logical (see also BNF section).
Review: * lithium augmentation in refractory MDD (Bschor and Bauer, *Curr Pharm Des* 2006; **12**:2985–92).

Lithium + valproate

A study of refractory depression indicated that sodium valproate (750–1500 mg/d) augmentation of lithium (900–1500 mg/d) was effective in the eight patients who did not respond to lithium alone (n = 10, Sharma *et al*, *Lithium* 1994;**5**:99–103).

MAOIs + stimulants *

There is a review of combining MAOIs (including selegiline and moclobemide) and stimulants (including amfetamines, methylphenidate, atomoxetine and bupropion) which concludes it isn't as dangerous as people think, provided you take care (Feinberg, *J Clin Psychiatry* 2004;**65**:1520–4; 44 refs).

Methylphenidate + SSRIs *

Methylphenidate may be effective as augmentation where incomplete response has occurred with antidepressants, and in the elderly where apathy and withdrawal (but not hopelessness) are prominent features (mentioned by Salzman, *Curr Affective Illness* 1995;**14**:5–13) and, as such, may help where depression is preventing rehabilitation processes. Augmentation of citalopram in elderly depressed patients may be rapidly successful and well-tolerated (n = 16, RCT, d/b, p/c, 10/52, Lavretsky *et al*, *Am J Geriatr Psychiatry* 2006;**14**:181–5; see also n = 10, open, Lavretsky and Kumar, *Am J Geriatr Psychiatry* 2001;**9**:298–303; n = 5, open, Stoll *et al*, *J Clin Psychiatry* 1996;**57**:72–6), and a follow-on study suggested methylphenidate may help accelerate citalopram's onset of action in the elderly (n = 9, open, 10/52, Lavretsky *et al*, *J Clin Psychiatry* 2003;**64**:1410–14; IS). However, the findings from the first nine patients in a discontinued RCT showed there to be no advantage in adding methylphenidate to sertraline, in terms of quicker or better response (Postolache *et al*, *J Clin Psychiatry* 1999;**60**:123–4).

● Unlicensed/some efficacy (see also augmentation)

Antipsychotics (see also adjunctive)

When used as adjuncts for psychotic depression antipsychotics can be effective, but the majority of people do not need them for more than four months (n = 40, open, 15/12, Rothschild and Duval, *J Clin Psychiatry* 2003;**64**:390–6). Many unipolar depressives receive antipsychotics long-term, but discontinuation can result in clear benefits, and so any reluctance to discontinue may be misplaced (n = 55, case note review, Mortimer *et al*, *J Clin Psychiatry* 2003;**64**:668–72). Amisulpride 50 mg/d has been shown to have an antidepressant activity comparable with fluoxetine 20 mg/d, with a similar incidence of side-effects (n = 281, d/b, Smeraldi, *J Affect Disord* 1998;**48**:47–56), and not inferior to paroxetine 20 mg/d for MDD (n = 272, RCT, d/b, 56/7, Cassano *et al*, *Int Clin Psychopharmacol* 2002;**17**:27–32). One case has been reported where **aripiprazole** 30 mg/d replaced a cocktail of drugs and produced a good response (n = 1, Errico and Yates, *Am J Psychiatry* 2005;**162**:626–7). **Risperidone** may improve sleep architecture in a similar way to conventional antidepressants (n = 8, open, 2/52, Sharpley et al, J Clin Psychiatry 2003;**64**:192–6). **Sulpiride** (mean dose 181 mg/d) may be effective and well-tolerated in mild to moderate depression (n = 177, RCT, 6/52, Ruther et al, Pharmacopsychiatry 1999;**32**:127–35). Use of **clozapine** in refractory psychotic depression has been reported (n = 1, Dassa et al, Br J Psychiatry 1993;**163**:822–4). A retrospective study indicated **olanzapine** 10 mg/d may have efficacy, as monotherapy (n = 30, open, Rothschild, J Clin Psychiatry 1999;**60**:116–18). However, in a combined analysis of two RCTs in depression with psychotic features, olanzapine monotherapy showed no advantage over placebo, although the combination showed improvement in one of the less than convincing trials (n = 249, 2 x RCT, 8/52, d/b, Rothschild et al, J Clin Psychopharmacol 2004;**24**:365–73).

Bupropion *

Bupropion (which inhibits presynaptic dopamine and noradrenaline reuptake) is licensed in the USA and other countries for the treatment of depression, as well as smoking cessation. A meta-analysis of original data from seven studies comparing bupropion (n = 732) with SSRIs (n = 731) showed equivalent efficacy and tolerability, except bupropion caused no more sexual dysfunction than placebo (s = 7, RCT, d/b, Thase et al, J Clin Psychiatry 2005;**66**:974–81), less nausea, diarrhoea and somnolence (Nieuwstraten and Dolovich, Ann Pharmacother 2001;**35**:1608–13), and higher cardiovascular, proconvulsive (at doses up to 450 mg/d: Pesola and Avasarala, J Emerg Med 2002;**22**:235–9, especially in patients who have lower body weights) and overdose toxicity. Bupropion 300–450 mg/d helps MDD with decreased energy, pleasure, interest (n = 274, RCT, d/b, p/c, 8/52, Jefferson et al, J Clin Psychiatry 2006;**67**:865–73), sleepiness and fatigue in MDD more than SSRIs (s = 6, n = 1317, RCT, d/b, Papakostas et al, Biol Psychiatry 2006; **60**(12):1350–5). A relapse prevention effect has been shown (n = 423, RCT, d/b, p/c, 44/52, Weihs et al, Biol Psychiatry 2002;**51**:753–61) and in the elderly (although 12 weeks may be needed for optimum response: n = 31, open, 12/52, Steffens et al, Int J Geriatr Psychiatry 2001;**16**:862–5). If switching from fluoxetine to bupropion, there has been a report of a 35% response, 60% part or full response in fluoxetine-resistant depression (n = 29, 8/52, open, Fava et al, Ann Clin Psychiatry 2003;**15**:17–22). The maximum dosage of 450 mg/d should be adhered to since the risk of seizures is dose related (see 3.4).

Reviews: * General (Koley et al, Expert Rev Neurol 2006;**6**:1249–65; Fava et al, Prim Care Companion J Clin Psychiatry 2005;**7**:106–13), what clinicians think of bupropion (Zimmerman et al, J Clin Psychiatry 2005;**66**:603–10).

Carbamazepine

Evidence for use as a pure antidepressant is poor but use with lithium or as a prophylaxis in bipolar disorder is better established (Psychological Med 1989;**19**:591–604). In one study, 44% of patients with resistant depression showed moderate or marked improvement with carbamazepine (n = 16, open, Cullen et al, J Clin Psychiatry 1991;**52**:472–6). See main entry under bipolar mood disorder (1.10.1).

Estradiol/estrogen *

Estrogen receptors occur in the CNS and loss of estrogen has been shown to reduce serotonergic and other functioning (Stahl, J Clin Psychiatry 2001;**62**:317–18; Stahl, Arch Gen Psychiatry 2001;**58**:537–8) and so there has been some interest as augmentation or monotherapy. Estradiol skin patches as monotherapy showed a striking improvement in two trials in severe postnatal depression (PND); the first showed significant effects at one month and three months (n = 37, d/b, p/c, Henderson et al, Lancet 1991;**338**:816–7), and the second showed a sustained improvement over five months with 200 mcg/d transdermal estrogen (n = 61, d/b, p/c, Gregoire et al, Lancet 1996;**347**:930; further support by Lopez-Jaramillo et al, Lancet 1996;**348**:135–6). The sublingual form (n = 2, Ahokas et al, Lancet 1998; **351**:10; 12/52, Soares et al, Arch Gen Psychiatry 2001;**58**:529–34) can be used. Estrogen supplementation of SSRIs may enhance their effectiveness (n = 5, Westlund et al, J Affect Disord 2003;**77**:87–92) in, eg. postnatal depression (where sublingual estradiol produced clinical recovery in 83% at two weeks: n = 23, open, Ahokas et al, J Clin Psychiatry 2001;**62**:332–6) and the menopause (n = 145, Miller et al, *J Am Geriatr Soc* 2002;**50**:1826–30). Low-dose estrogen 0.625 mg/d as augmentation to partially effective SSRIs in perimenopausal depression significantly improved mood, but not memory (n = 17, RCT, d/b, p/c, 6/52, Morgan et al, *J Clin Psychiatry* 2005;**66**:774–80). Although reduced estrogen and progesterone levels are associated with the development of postpartum mood disorders (n = 8, Bloch et al, *Am J Psychiatry* 2000;**157**:924–30), progestogens do not seem to help PND, and may even be detrimental (Lawrie et al, *Cochrane Database Syst Rev* 2000;**2**:CD001690; reviewed in *EBMH* 2000;**3**:19).

Reviews: general (Stahl, *J Clin Psychiatry* 2001; **62**:404–5; Schmidt et al, *Am J Obstet Gynecol* 2000;**183**:414–20).

Lamotrigine
Although its primary action is on voltage-sensitive sodium channels, where it inhibits pathological release of glutamate, lamotrigine may also have an antidepressant effect, particularly as relapse prevention in bipolar depression (see *1.10.3*). Lamotrigine may also be useful as an adjunct for refractory major depression (n = 2, Maltese, *Am J Psychiatry* 1999;**156**:1833; n = 37, retrospective, Barbee and Jamhour, *J Clin Psychiatry* 2002;**63**:737–41), and at 200 mg/d, enhanced the onset of paroxetine in unipolar depression, but not HAM-D scores at the study end-point (n = 40, p/c, d/b, 9/52, Normann et al, *J Clin Psychiatry* 2002;**63**:337–44). In resistant depression, lamotrigine 100 mg/d was not quite statistically superior to placebo as an adjunct to fluoxetine in major depression and bipolar II (n = 23, RCT, d/b, p/c, 6/52, Barbosa et al, *J Clin Psychiatry* 2003;**64**:403–7). Remember that even missing two days' doses means retitrating.

Levothyroxine (thyroxine)
See augmentation.

Liothyronine (triiodothyronine)
See augmentation.

Methylphenidate
Methylphenidate can be used in acute depression (Klein and Wender, *Arch Gen Psychiatry* 1995;**52**:429–33), as it has the major advantage of a rapid action (often within 48 hours) although the effect tends to be transient and it may worsen anxiety and insomnia. The stimulant action of methylphenidate in the elderly may be grossly attenuated and so may not be appropriate in the elderly reporting age-related cognitive decline (n = 60, RCT, p/c, d/b, Turner et al, *Psychopharmacol* [Berl] 2003;**168**:455–64).

Modafinil
Modafinil has been used initially with SSRIs to enhance the onset of action and symptom relief of depression (n = 29, open, 6/52, Ninan et al, *J Clin Psychiatry* 2004;**65**:414–20). Modafinil has also been used successfully to augment phenelzine for residual fatigue in dysthymia (n = 1, Ashton, *Am J Psychiatry* 2004; **161**:1716–7).

Selegiline *
Transdermal selegiline (20 mg/d) was surprisingly effective and well-tolerated in one trial in MDD, as the transdermal route allows higher doses than possible orally, with no need for dietary restrictions (n = 177, RCT, p/c, 6/52, Bodkin and Amsterdam, *Am J Psychiatry* 2002;**159**:1869–75; comment by Benedictis, *EBMH* 2003;**6**:44; see also n = 289, d/b, p/c, 8/52, Amsterdam, *J Clin Psychiatry* 2003;**64**:208–14). One remarkable response in multi-drug resistant depression from selegiline 7.5 mg/d has been reported (n = 1, Higuchi et al, *Clin Neuropharmacol* 2005; **28**:191–2).

St John's wort (SJW)
SJW is available over-the-counter in most European countries in a variety of preparations. The mode of action is not certain but might include serotonin and/or norepinephrine reuptake inhibition (Neary and Bu, *Brain Res* 1999;**816**:358–63), MAO-A and B inhibition and sigma receptor activity (neuropharmacology reviewed by Bennett et al, *Ann Pharmacother* 1998;**32**:1201–8; Butterweck, *CNS Drugs* 2003;**17**:539–62). From the available studies (of variable quality), it would appear that SJW may be useful for mild to moderate depression but perhaps

not for moderate to severe depression. A systematic review and meta-analysis concluded SJW has only minor effects in major depression but older smaller trials in a variety of depressions have shown a marked effect (s = 35, RCT, d/b, Linde et al, Br J Psychiatry 2005;**186**:99–107). Cochrane concludes that the evidence is inconsistent and confusing and study results are probably only applicable to the particular products tested in the studies (s = 37, Linde et al, Cochrane Database Syst Rev 2005;**2**:CD000448). Some of the positive studies include equivalent efficacy to paroxetine (n = 251, RCT, 6/52, Szegedi et al, Br Med J 2005;**330**:503; comment by Ernst, EBMH 2005;**8**:107) and fluoxetine. Other studies suggest it is either more effective than fluoxetine (n = 135, RCT, d/b, p/c, 12/52, Fava et al, J Clin Psychopharmacol 2005;**25**:441–7), equivalent to fluoxetine (n = 70, RCT, d/b, Behnke et al, Adv Ther 2002, **19**, 43–52; n = 149, RCT, 6/52, Harrer et al, Arzneimittelforschung 1999;**49**:289–96) or inferior to fluoxetine (n = 72, RCT, d/b, p/c, Moreno et al, Rev Bras Psiquiatr 2006;**28**:29–32). However, a major rigorous trial failed to show a significant antidepressant or anxiolytic effect in major depression (n = 200, RCT, p/c, 8/52, Shelton et al, JAMA 2001;**285**:1978–86; review by Hawley and Dale, EBMH 2002;**5**:24) and, in a second trial, neither sertraline nor SJW (generously dosed) were effective in moderately-severe depression (n = 340, RCT, d/b, p/c, 8/52, Davidson et al, JAMA 2002;**287**:1807–14; review by Swann, EBMH 2002;**5**:111; vigorous discussion by Jonas et al, JAMA 2002;**288**:446–9), meaning that endorsement of SJW must be tempered with caution. Most studies are short-term (up to 6/52), and many have high (up to 50%) drop-out rates, indicating that transient mild depression may be common in studies. Care is needed in adjunctive therapy (particularly if purchased OTC — see 4.3.3.9).

Reviews: * general (Kelly, Hosp Med 2001; **62**:274–6; Josey and Tackett, Int J Clin Pharmacol Ther 1999;**37**:111–9; Maidment, Psychiatr Bull 2000;**24**:232–4), in the elderly (Vorbach et al, Drugs Aging 2000;**16**:189–97), and ADRs (s = 35, Knüppel and Linde, J Clin Psychiatry 2004;**5**:1470–9).

■ Unlicensed/possible efficacy

Botox injections *

One study showed that people with depression improved two months after botox injections (n = 10, Dermatologic Surg 2006; **32**:645–50).

Buspirone (see also combinations)

An old meta-analysis of studies showed a minor but statistically significant effect at up to 90 mg/d in depressed patients (review in J Psychopharmacol 1993;**7**:283–9). A more recent study showed buspirone to be more effective than placebo but less effective than imipramine in major depression in elderly patients (n = 177, RCT, Schweizer et al, J Clin Psychiatry 1998;**59**:175–83).

Chromium

Chromium picolinate may be an option in atypical depression, with a potential effect within two weeks (n = 15, 8/52, p/c, Davidson et al, Biol Psychiatry 2003;**53**:261–4).

Dexamethasone

A number of studies have shown a rapid and marked improvement, eg. within a week when given 3–8 mg IV (n = 5, 7/7, Arana, Am J Psychiatry 1991;**148**:1401–2; n = 37, 4/7, Arana et al, Am J Psychiatry 1995;**152**:265–7), 8 mg IV twice, four days apart (n = 7, Beale and Arana, Am J Psychiatry 1995;**152**:959–60), and up to 3 mg/d for four days (n = 10, Dinan et al, Acta Psychiatr Scand 1997;**95**:58–61), although other reports indicate that only a minority of patients respond (letter by Wolkowitz et al, Am J Psychiatry 1996;**153**:1112–3). This interesting effect may be via upregulation of glucocorticoid receptors, an effect shared with the SSRIs.

Dexamfetamine

Dexamfetamine may be rapidly effective for depression and fatigue, with one successful trial in men with HIV (n = 23, RCT, 2/52, Wagner and Rabkin, J Clin Psychiatry 2000;**61**:436–40).

Dehydroepiandrosterone (DHEA)

DHEA up to 90 mg/d was successful in 45% treatment-resistant depressives with no placebo response (n = 22, RCT, d/b, p/c, 6/52, Wolkowitz et al, Am J Psychiatry 1999; **156**:646–9) and so larger-scale trials may be warranted.

Donepezil
Donepezil may reduce REM latency in depressed patients (n = 16, c/o, Perlis et al, Biol Psychiatry 2002;**51**:457–62).

Folate
Low RBC folate levels have been linked to depression, persistent depressive symptoms and a poor response to antidepressant medication, an easily rectified problem (eg. n = 2948, Morris et al, Psychother Psychosom 2003;**72**:80–7).

Hydrocortisone
IV hydrocortisone produced a significantly greater and robust improvement in HAM-D scores than ovine CRH or placebo (n = 22, RCT, d/b, p/c, 2/7, DeBattista et al, Am J Psychiatry 2000;**157**:1334–7; comment by Watson and Young, Am J Psychiatry 2001;**158**:1536–7).

Inositol
Inositol is a precursor of an intracellular secondary messenger system for numerous neurotransmitters. The major trial showed no significant effect in SSRI augmentation (n = 27, RCT, p/c, Levine et al, Biol Psychiatry 1999;**45**:270–3) and 12 g/d had no effect in SSRI failures (RCT, d/b, Nemets et al, J Neural Transm 1999;**106**:795–8). Previous work had led to some enthusiasm (eg. n = 28, p/c, Levine et al, Am J Psychiatry 1995; **152**:792–4; Levine et al, Isr J Psychiatry Relat Sci 1995;**32**:14–21).

Ketamine *
There is a case of remarkable antidepressant response to inadvertent ketamine induction 'monotherapy' after seizure-free and hence failed ECT sessions (n = 1, Ostroff et al, Am J Psychiatry 2005;**162**:1385–6).

Ketoconazole
Ketoconazole inhibits cortisol secretion, lowering cortisol levels. It may have a slow-onset antidepressant effect (n = 17, 8/52, Murphy et al, Can J Psychiatry 1998;**43**:279–86), particularly

in hypercortisolemic (but not normal) patients (n = 20, RCT, Wolkowitz et al, Biol Psychiatry 1999;**45**:1070–74). However, limited efficacy in treatment refractory major depression has been noted (n = 16, RCT, Malison et al, J Clin Psychopharmacol 1999;**19**:466–70).

Mifepristone *
Mifepristone 600–1200 mg/d (a glucocorticosteroid receptor antagonist) may be an option for psychotic major depression (PMD), the theory being that 'the psychosis in PMD is caused by excessive activation of the hypothalamic-pituitary-adrenal axis' (n = 30, open, 7/7, Belanoff et al, Biol Psychiatry 2002; **52**:386–92). A longer-term study showed that six days mifepristone led to significant improvement in PMD even in the first week, maintained for four weeks, but probably not to eight weeks (n = 20, open, 8/52, Simpson et al, J Clin Psychiatry 2005;**66**:598–602).

Omega-3 fatty acids (PUFAs)
There is some evidence for an association between PUFAs (polyunsaturated fatty acids) and depression, and studies so far have seen some beneficial effect from ethyl-EPA (review by Peet, Adv Psychiatr Treat 2002;**8**:223–9), eg. rapid response to adjunctive use with paroxetine (n = 1, Puri et al, Arch Gen Psychiatry 2002;**59**:91–2), with maintenance antidepressants (n = 20, d/b, 4/52, Nemets et al, Am J Psychiatry 2002;**159**:477–9), and 1 g/d added to current medication appeared effective in treatment-resistant depression (n = 70, RCT, d/b, p/c, 12/52, Peet and Horrobin, Arch Gen Psychiatry 2002;**59**:913–19). However, DHA (Docosahexaenoic acid, an omega-3 fatty acid) was ineffective as monotherapy in major depression (n = 35, p/c, 6/52, Marangell et al, Am J Psychiatry 2003;**160**:996–8) and a Finnish study showed low dietary intake of omega-3 fatty acids is **not** associated with low mood (n = 29 133, Hakkarainen et al, Am J Psychiatry 2004;**161**:567–9).

Opiates
Some anecdotal cases suggest that oxycodone or oxymorphone may produce a sustained effect in refractory and chronic depression, as well as reducing psychogenic pain and

distress (n = 3, Stoll and Reuter, *Am J Psychiatry* 1999;**156**:2017). Some efficacy has been shown from buprenorphine in refractory, unipolar depression, with a striking response in four (n = 10, open, 6/52, Bodkin *et al*, *J Clin Psychopharmacol* 1995;**15**:49–57; see also Callaway, *Biol Psychiatry* 1996;**39**: 989–90). The potential for abuse limits their use.

Pergolide

Pergolide (a dopamine agonist) has been tried with moderate success as an adjunct, eg. 55% showed improvement within seven days, with doses of 0.5–1 mg/d (n = 20, open, Bouckoms and Mangini, *Psychopharmacol Bull* 1993;**29**:207–11) and if added to tricyclics (n = 20, open, Izumi *et al*, *J Affect Disord* 2000; **61**:127–32).

Phenytoin *

Phenytoin (up to 400 mg/d) was as effective as fluoxetine (up to 21 mg/d) for MDD (n = 33 [c = 28], RCT, d/b, Nemets *et al*, *J Clin Psychiatry* 2005;**66**:586–90).

Pramipexole *

Pramipexole is a dopamine D2/D3 agonist licensed for Parkinson's disease and has been used with some success (n = 22, case series, Ostow, *Am J Psychiatry* 2002;**159**:320–1; n = 174, RCT, p/c, 8/52, Corrigan *et al*, *Depress Anxiety* 2000;**11**:58–65).

Riluzole

In a pilot study in resistant depression, riluzole (mean 170 mg/d) appeared effective for MADRS-rated symptoms as monotherapy (n = 19, open, 6/52, Zarate *et al*, *Am J Psychiatry* 2004;**161**:171–4) and as an adjunct (n = 1, Sanacora *et al*, *Am J Psychiatry* 2004;**161**:2132).

Testosterone

Weekly testosterone cypionate 100–200 mg/d may be effective in some men with late-onset depression, but not earlier-onset depression (n = 15, RCT, 6/52, Perry *et al*, *J Clin Psychiatry* 2002;**63**:1096–101). Testosterone gel may be a non-parenteral route capable of producing an antidepressant effect in men with refractory depression and low testosterone (n = 22, RCT, p/c, 8/52, Pope *et al*, *Am J Psychiatry* 2003;**160**:105–111). However, the antidepressant effects of IM testosterone in hypogonadal men with major depression were equivalent to placebo (n = 30, RCT, d/b, p/c, 6/52, Seidmen *et al*, *J Clin Psychiatry* 2001;**62**:406–12).

Tetracycline antibiotics

Minocycline and demeclocycline have been reported in case studies to have a detectable antidepressant effect (Levine *et al*, *Am J Psychiatry* 1996;**153**:582).

Thyrotropin-releasing hormone (TRH)

Five of eight depressed patients given 500 mcg of protirelin intrathecally responded robustly and rapidly (mood and suicidality), but the effect was shortlived (Marangell *et al*, *Arch Gen Psychiatry* 1997;**54**:214–22). TRH may thus be involved in mood regulation.

Topiramate

Adjunctive topiramate may be beneficial for some obese depressed females (n = 16, open, Carpenter *et al*, *J Affect Disord* 2002;**69**:251–5).

Tramadol

Response of refractory MDD to tramadol (structurally similar to venlafaxine) 300–400 mg/d prescribed for pain has been reported (n = 1, Shapira *et al*, *J Clin Psychiatry* 2001;**62**:205–6).

Valproate *

Valproate can be used to augment tricyclics but is probably only of minimum to moderate potency (n = 55, open, 7/12, Calabrese and Delucchi, *Am J Psychiatry* 1990;**47**:431–4), although response in resistant unipolar depression or dysthymia has been reported (n = 1, Kemp, *Br J Psychiatry* 1992; **160**:121–3) and it may help reduce depressive agitation (n = 12 [c = 9], open, 4/52, DeBattista *et al*, *J Clin Psychopharmacol* 2005;**25**:476–9).

◆ Others

Other drugs tried include **ascorbic acid, captopril** 50–100 mg/d (n = 9, open, *J Clin Psychopharmacol* 1991;**9211**:395–6), **bromocriptine** 10–60 mg/d (McGrath *et al*, *J Clin Psychopharmacol* 1995; **15**: 289–91), **cyproheptadine** (n = 6, RCT, Greenway *et al*, *Pharmacotherapy* 1995;**15**:357–60), **levodopa**

(*J Psychopharmacol* 1990;**4**:152–67), **primidone** (n = 1, Brown *et al*, *Lancet* 1993; **342**:925) and **zotepine** (n = 2, Konig and Wolfersdorf, *Tw Neurol Psychiatry* 1994; **8**:460–3).

* No efficacy

Benzodiazepines

There have been some suggestions that **alprazolam** (n = 30, RCT, d/b, 6/52, Hubain *et al*, *J Affect Disord* 1990; **18**:67–73) and **diazepam** (RCT, d/b, 8/52, Tiller *et al*, *Br J Psychiatry* 1989; **155**:483–9) have some antidepressant activity, but since some depression rating scales include measures of anxiety this probably explains the alleged effect. The BNF states that they should not be used to treat depression. Discontinuing drugs such as clonazepam prescribed for panic/anxiety control can often lead to improvement of depression (see 5.5). Short-term adjunctive use may have some role.

Caffeine

Some depressed people may have increased sensitivity to caffeine (Lee *et al*, *Am J Psychiatry* 1988; **145**:632–5).

Memantine *

Memantine 5–20 mg/d was ineffective for MDD (n = 32, RCT, d/b, p/c, Zarate *et al*, *Am J Psychiatry* 2006; **163**:153–5).

Pyridoxine (vitamin B6) *

Low B6 levels have been associated with depression and supplementary B6 might be useful (n = 140, Hvas *et al*, *Psychother Psychosom* 2004; **73**:340–3), but a review (s = 10 including five RCTs) showed no apparent effect in men although perhaps some minor effect in pre-menopausal women (*Family Pract* 2005; **2**:532–7).

1.15 DYSTHYMIA
see also Depression (*1.14*)

Symptoms:

Dysthymia (literally 'ill-humored') is a low-grade chronic melancholic depression (often with anxiety) of insidious onset, chronic course (lasting at least two years with permanent or intermittent symptoms) and a high risk of relapse. It has few of the physical symptoms of depression and is compatible with stable social functioning. Almost all sufferers eventually develop super-imposed major depression (n = 86, three-year follow-up, Klein *et al*, *Am J Psychiatry* 2000; **157**:931–9). The life-time prevalence rate may be around 3–6%, and higher in the elderly. Dysthymia has been associated with low testosterone levels in men and hence a link made with HPG axis dysfunction (n = 220, open, Seidman *et al*, *Am J Psychiatry* 2002; **159**:456–9). It has been considered by some to be similar to depressive personality disorder or anxiety and, by others, as a way of medicalising (and hence ignoring) social problems or as a way of giving someone a medical diagnosis to allow insurance claims.

Role of drugs

It is clear that antidepressants are effective in dysthymia, with no proven significant differences between classes but they should form part of an overall treatment strategy including, eg. IPT, CBT and other talking therapies. A greater sensitivity to side-effects has been noted in dysthymics, with tricyclics the biggest culprits. SSRIs and moclobemide appear favoured. If one class does not work, switching to another may convey a 40–60% chance of response (Thase, *Curr Opin Psychiatry* 1998; **11**:77–83, 35 refs). Treatment for several months may be necessary for full response (s = 15, Lima and Moncrieff, *Cochrane Database Syst Rev* 2000; **4**:CD001130; review by Thase, *EBMH* 1998; **1**:111). A low (10–20%) placebo response is seen (Frances *et al*, *Int Clin Psychopharmacol* 1993; **7**:197–200).

Reviews: diagnosis and treatment (Rihmer, *Curr Opin Psychiatry* 1999; **12**:69–75, 48 refs), in the elderly (Bellino *et al*, *Drugs Aging* 2000; **16**:107–21).

● Unlicensed/some efficacy

ALCAR (acetyl-l-carnitine) *

ALCAR may be as effective and tolerable as amisulpride (n = 204, RCT, d/b, 12/52, Zanardi and Smeraldi, *Eur Neuropsychopharmacol* 2006; 16:281–7).

Amisulpride *

A number of studies have shown amisulpride to have some efficacy in dysthymia, eg. 50 mg/d was as effective as sertraline 50–100 mg/d, with a significantly faster onset of action (n = 313, RCT, d/b, 12/52, Amore et al, Int Clin Psychopharmacol 2001;**16**:317–24), and as effective as ALCAR (n = 204, RCT, d/b, 12/52, Zanardi and Smeraldi, Eur Neuropsychopharmacol 2006;**16**:281–7). It may also be effective for short-term treatment (n = 100, RCT, open, 8/52, Rocca et al, J Affect Disord 2002;**70**:313–17), and 50mg/d was more effective than increasing the paroxetine dose to 40mg/d in SSRI-resistant dysthymia (n = 60, open, 3/12, Rocca et al, J Psychiatr Res 2002;**112**:145–52). Some dopaminergic side-effects are seen with amisulpride.

Review: substituted benzamides in dysthymia (Pani and Gessa, Mol Psychiatry 2002;**7**:247–53).

Bupropion

Bupropion SR up to 400mg/d was effective in 71% patients in one trial, with those having a history of substance misuse less likely to respond (n = 21, open, 8/52, Hellerstein et al, J Clin Psychopharmacol 2001;**21**:325–9).

MAOIs

Phenelzine at 50–75mg/d and tranylcypromine have both been shown to be as effective as tricyclics, the latter over a two-year period (Br J Psychiatry 1995;**166**:174–83).

Moclobemide

Moclobemide (mean 675mg/d) has been shown to be significantly more effective for dysthymia than imipramine (mean 220mg/d) and placebo, with fewer side-effects (n = 315, RCT, Versiani et al, Int Clin Psychopharmacol 1997;**12**:183–93), confirming previous studies (review by Petursson, Acta Psychiatr Scand 1995;**91**[Suppl 386]:S36–S39).

SSRIs *

Citalopram (mean dose 39mg/d) appeared effective in 73% of 'pure' dysthymics in one study (n = 21, open, 12/52, Hellerstein et al, Int Clin Psychopharmacol 2004;**19**:143–8). Fluoxetine may produce a significant improvement in dysthymic symptoms (n = 35, RCT, p/c, 8/52, Hellerstein et al, Am J Psychiatry 1993;**150**:1169–75), 20mg/d may be more effective than placebo, with 50% of the non-responders at three months improving with a dose increase to 40mg/d (n = 140, RCT, Vanelle

et al, Br J Psychiatry 1997;**170**:345–50), but may have limited efficacy in elderly patients (n = 90 [c = 71], RCT, d/b, p/c, 12/52, Devanand et al, Am J Geriatr Psychiatry 2005;**13**:59–68). **Paroxetine** was superior to psychotherapy and placebo in older dysthymics (n = 415, RCT, 11/52, Williams et al, JAMA 2000;**284**:1519–26). In dysthymia without major depression, **sertraline** up to 200mg/d may be more effective than placebo over a wide range of efficacy and quality of life measures (n = 310, RCT, 12/52, Ravindran et al, J Clin Psychiatry 2000;**61**:821–7), and may improve behaviour and personality in dysthymia (n = 410, RCT, d/b, p/c, Hellerstein et al, Am J Psychiatry 2000;**157**:1436–44). It has also been effective in out-patients, eg. as effective as imipramine (50–30mg/d), but better tolerated (n = 416, RCT, 12/52, Kocsis et al, Am J Psychiatry 1997; **154**:390; n = 310, d/b, 12/52, Ravindran et al, J Clin Psychiatry 2000;**61**:821–7).

Tricyclics

Amitriptyline and desipramine (n = 42, open, 8/52, Marin et al, Am J Psychiatry 1994; **151**:1079–80) have both been studied over 6–12 weeks and found at doses of 150–300mg/d to be 2–3 times more effective than placebo. 50–300mg/d imipramine has been shown to be as effective (but with more drop-outs) as sertraline in long-standing dysthymia, and both were significantly better than placebo (n = 416, RCT, 12/52, Kocsis et al, Am J Psychiatry 1997;**154**:390).

■ Unlicensed/possible efficacy

Chromium

Chromium (as the picolinate) provided a dramatic and complete resolution of dysthymia in a small trial (n = 5, s/b, McLeod et al, J Clin Psychiatry 1999;**60**:237).

Fluvoxamine

Fluvoxamine may be well-tolerated and effective in dysthymic adolescents (n = 21, open, Rabe-Jablonska, J Child Adolesc Psychopharmacol 2000;**10**:9–18).

Mirtazapine

Mirtazapine 15–45mg/d was effective in 73%

of patients with dysthymia, four discontinuing because of sedation (n=15, open, 10/52, Depress Anxiety 1999;**10**:68–72).

Venlafaxine *

Several open studies suggest some efficacy, eg. up to 225mg/d was effective in 71% of the 14 patients who completed a nine-week trial (seven responded quickly to low dose, three only to high dose, n=17, Dunner et al, J Clin Psychiatry 1997;**58**:528–31), and up to 300mg/d may be reasonably effective and generally well-tolerated for elderly patients (n=23[c=28], open, 12/52, Devanand et al, J Geriatr Psychiatr Neurol 2004;**17**:219–24).

◆ Others

Other drugs tried include lithium (eg. Akiskal et al, Arch Gen Psychiatry 1980;**37**:777–83) and valproate (n=1, Kemp, Br J Psychiatry 1992; **160**:121–3).

* No efficacy

St John's wort *

People with dysthymia seem unresponsive to SJW, with placebo-level response, although non-dysthymics may improve (n=150, RCT, d/b, p/c, 6/52, Randlov et al, Phytomedicine 2006;**13**:215–21).

1.16 EATING DISORDERS *

DSM-IV includes three eating disorders; anorexia nervosa (AN), bulimia nervosa (BN) and eating disorders not otherwise specified (EDNOS), the latter including binge-eating disorder. Remission is more likely in BN than AN. Although sociocultural explanations are important and relevant, anorexia, bulimia and obesity may be heterogeneous disorders with complex aetiology, including genes and the environment (review by Collier and Treasure, Br J Psychiatry 2004;**185**:363–5).

Reviews: general (Cooke and Sawyer, Aust Fam Physician 2004;**33**:27–31; Rome, Obstet Gyn Clin North Am 2003;**30**:353–77; Walsh and Klein, Int Rev Psychiatry 2003;**15**:205–16; Hoek and van Hoeken, Int J Eat Disord 2003;**34**:383–96); pharmacotherapy (Pederson et al, Expert Opin Pharmacother 2003;**4**:1659–78; Mitchell et al, Curr Drug Targets CNS Neurol Disord 2003;**2**:17–29), drug treatment of adolescent eating disorders (Ebling et al, Ann Med 2003;**35**:488–501; Sigman, Pediatr Clin North Am 2003;**50**:1139–77; Pederson et al, Expert Opin Pharmacother 2003;**4**:1659–78), general and primary care (Pederson et al, Expert Opin Pharmacother 2003;**4**:1659–78; Mehler, Ann Int Med 2001;**134**,:1048–59; Cooper, Prescriber 2001;46–8; Kaye et al, Ann Rev Med 2000; **51**: 299–313).

1.16.1 ANOREXIA NERVOSA

Symptoms:

The main diagnostic symptoms of anorexia nervosa are:

1. Amenorrhoea in females (absence of three consecutive menstrual cycles).
2. Refusal to maintain body weight over the minimum normal for age and height.
3. Intense fear of gaining weight or becoming fat.
4. Disturbance in body perception, eg. feeling fat even when emaciated.

Anorexia usually starts in the late teens, with distorted body image and relentless dieting. Patients may avoid carbohydrates, induce vomiting, abuse laxatives, take excess exercise, binge eat and suffer depression and social withdrawal. It may occur in up to 2% of schoolgirls and up to four in 100000 of the general population. Psychotherapy may be useful but with only a few small trials is unproven (s=6, Hay et al, Cochrane Database Syst Rev 2003;**4**:CD003909).

Role of drugs

Drug therapy is generally most useful as a supportive measure to treat any concurrent conditions. In severely emaciated patients, enteral feeding or even TPN may be necessary.

Reviews: overall management (Dalle Grave et al, Eat Weight Disord 2001;**6**:81–9; Kruger and Kennedy, J Psych Neurosci 2000;**25**:497–508), use of SSRIs (Vaswani and Kalra, Expert Opin Invest Drugs 2004;**13**:349–57), in teenagers (Serpell and Treasure, Prescriber 1996;**7**:19–25), SSRIs in anorexia (Ferguson et al, Int J Eat Disord 1999;**25**:11–7) and general (Pike, Clin Psychol Rev 1998;**18**:447–75; Marcus and Levine, Curr Opin Psychiatry 1998;**11**:159–63).

+ Combinations

Olanzapine + mirtazapine *

There is a case report of successful use of olanzapine 10mg/d and mirtazapine 30mg/d over six months (n = 1, Wang et al, Prog Neuropsychopharmacol Biol Psychiatry 2006; 30:306–9).

• Unlicensed/some efficacy

Nutritional feeding

TPN may be necessary in severely anorexic patients (review by Jeejeebhoy, Semin Gastrointest Dis 1998;9:183–8) where a life-threatening weight loss has occurred, particularly if accompanied by low potassium levels and where conventional therapies have failed. Weight gain can be significant in a relatively short period and TPN can help avert permanent damage or death. Great care is needed where patients are likely to interfere with the IV line with the possibility of infection in a compromised patient and of embolism. Supervised oral feeding with nutritional supplements can also be an effective acute treatment.

Treatment of any PMS

This may help any premenstrual exacerbations.

Tricyclic antidepressants

The main role of the tricyclics may be in maintenance therapy. Doses of 150mg/d or more for 4–6 weeks may be needed.

■ Unlicensed/possible efficacy

Antipsychotics *

OCD and anorexia have responded to olanzapine 5mg/d, with reduced fixed body perceptions, no weight loss and improved insight (eg. n = 3, Jensen and Mejlhede, Br J Psychiatry 2000;177:87), and a pilot study suggested weight gain was likely in anorexia (but 20% lost weight), although changes in psychopathology were not assessed (n = 20, open, 10/52, Powers et al, Int J Eat Disord 2002;32:146–54). Another small pilot study also suggested that olanzapine may be useful (n=17, open, 6/52, Barbarich et

al, J Clin Psychiatry 2004;65:1480–82), although this has been strongly disputed (Menaster, J Clin Psychiatry 2005;66:654–6). Risperidone has been used (Newman-Toker, J Am Acad Child Adolesc Psychiatry 2000;39:941–2). Low-dose haloperidol has been suggested as an adjunct in severe AN (n = 13, open, 6/12, Cassano et al, Int J Eat Disord 2003;33:172–7).

Citalopram

Citalopram 20mg/d has been used successfully (n = 6, Calandra et al, Eat Weight Disord 1999; 4:207–10). One pilot study suggested some symptom improvement (n = 52, RCT, Fassino et al, Eur Neuropsychopharmacol 2002; 12:453–9), and a 47% satisfactory response rate was seen in another pilot study (n = 32, open, 6/12, Pallanti et al, Eat Weight Disord 1997;2:216–21).

Sertraline

A case has been reported of complete response to sertraline at 50mg/d in a woman only partly responsive to fluoxetine (Roberts and Lydiard, Am J Psychiatry 1993;150:1753).

Tramadol

Tramadol, which has significant MAOI activity and mu-opioid receptor antagonism, has been successful at 225mg/d (n = 1, Mendelson, Am J Psychiatry 2001;158:963–94).

Zinc

Zinc has virtually no side-effects. A four-week trial may help some people (eg. Acta Psychiatr Scand 1990;82:14–7), and 100mg/d produced an increase in BMI twice that of placebo (n = 35, RCT, Birmingham et al, Int J Eat Disord 1994;15:251–5).

◆ Others

Other drugs tried include cyproheptadine (n = 72, RCT, Halmi et al, Arch Gen Psychiatry 1986;43:177–81) and lithium (n = 16, d/b, 16/52, Gross, J Clin Psychopharmacol 1981;1:376–81; Stein et al, Br J Psychiatry 1982;140:526–8).

✳ No efficacy

Fluoxetine *

In an important trial, fluoxetine had no

advantage over placebo in anorexia following weight restoration (n=93, RCT, d/b, p/c, < I year, Walsh et al, JAMA 2006;**295**:2605–12), supporting a previous in-patient trial (n=31, RCT, Attia et al, Am J Psychiatry 1998; **155**:548–51).

Topiramate

Topiramate caused relapse of anorexia in a patient when used for epilepsy (n = 1, Rosenow et al, Am J Psychiatry 2002;**159**:2112–3).

1.16.2 BULIMIA NERVOSA

Symptoms *

The main diagnostic symptoms of bulimia nervosa are:
1. Recurrent binge eating, including lack of control.
2. An urge to overeat (including lack of control of eating during binges).
3. Regular self-induced vomiting, laxative abuse, strict dieting or fasting.
4. Persistent over-concern with body shape and weight.

There must be a minimum of two binge episodes per week for at least three months. Weight and menses are normal. The prevalence rates are about 1% for young women and 0.1% for young men. Mu-opioid receptor binding in bulimic women (n=8) is lower than in healthy women (n=8) in the left insular cortex, the area involved in processing taste, as well as the anticipation and reward of eating (n = 16, Bencherif et al, J Nucl Med 2005;**46**:1349–51).

Role of drugs

A meta-analysis of antidepressants vs placebo in bulimia showed that short-term remission was more likely with antidepressants, with equivalent drop-outs, but with no drug class better than any other (s=16, RCTs, n = 1300, Bacaltchuk et al, Aust N Z J Psychiatry 2000;**34**:310–7). Cochrane concludes that all antidepressants appear equally effective compared to placebo, but with a high drop-out rate (Bacaltchuk and Hay, Cochrane Database Syst Rev 2003;**4**:CD003391; review by Morgan, EBMH 2002;**5**:75–6) and do not work as antidepressants. Adequate doses are needed, eg. at least 150 mg/d equivalent of a tricyclic for adequate duration, eg. at least four

weeks. Side-effects (especially anticholinergic) can be severe and result in non-compliance. Drugs should be part of an individualised programme with nutrition and CBT the most effective interventions. Psychotherapy may be of some use but the evidence is sparce (Hay et al, Cochrane Database Syst Rev 2003;1:CD000562).

Reviews: general (Mehler, N Engl J Med 2003; **28**:875–81; Brambilla, CNS Drugs 2001;**15**:119–36, 99 refs; Kruger and Kennedy, J Psych Neurosci 2000;**25**:497–508), systematic review (Bacaltchuk et al, Aust N Z J Psychiatry 2000;**34**:310–7), and binge-eating disorder (Dingemans et al, Int J Obes 2002;**26**:299–307).

BNF listed

Fluoxetine

Fluoxetine 60 mg/d has a significant effect on binge-eating and purging, eating attitudes, behaviour and food craving and recent trials have confirmed this effect where psychological treatments have been inadequate, eg. it was superior to placebo as maintenance therapy, albeit with a high drop-out rate (n=150, RCT, 16 centres, 12/12, Romano et al, Am J Psychiatry 2002;**159**:96–102; review by Palmer, EBMH 2002;**120**:120; see also n=22, RCT, 8/52, Walsh et al, Am J Psychiatry 2000;**157**:1332–4). Fluoxetine may also be effective in adolescent (12–18) bulimia (n = 10, open, 8/52, Kotler et al, J Child Adolesc Psychopharmacol 2003;**13**:329–35). Fluoxetine has no benefit over a year once weight has been restored (n=93, RCT, d/b, p/c, 12/12, Walsh et al, JAMA 2006;**295**:2605–12). It does not work purely as an antidepressant as the improvement is independent of depression scores and uses higher doses, although any depression may also improve. Its long half-life may help with missed doses.

+ Combinations

Naltrexone + fluoxetine

After a partial response to 60 mg/d fluoxetine, addition of 100 mg/d naltrexone has produced a 'robust' reduction in binge frequency and amount (n = 1, Neumeister et al, Am J Psychiatry 1999;**156**:797).

● Unlicensed/some efficacy

MAOIs

MAOIs can be successful drugs if the dietary restrictions can be overcome.

PMS treatments

Pyridoxine and progesterones, in particular, may help to minimise the effects of premenstrual relapses.

SSRIs (see also fluoxetine above) *

Citalopram may be useful for depressed patients for bulimia, and may be as effective (n = 37, RCT, s/b, Leombruni et al, Adv Ther 2006;23:481–94) or less effective than fluoxetine (n = 37, RCT, s/b, Leombruni et al, Adv Ther 2006;23:481–94). Fluvoxamine 200 mg/d may reduce binge-eating and purging and may be well-tolerated (n = 12, RCT, p/c, 12/52, Milano et al, Adv Ther 2005;22:178–83; see also n = 85, RCT, 9/52, Hudson et al, Am J Psychiatry 1998;155:1756–62). Paroxetine has been reputed to have no beneficial effect in an unpublished study. Sertraline was significantly superior to placebo in most measures in two short studies (n = 34, RCT, d/b, 6/52, McElroy et al, Am J Psychiatry 2000;157:1004–6; n = 18, open, 8/52, Sloan et al, Int J Eat Dis 2004;36:48–54).

Topiramate *

There is growing interest in topiramate in bulimia. Two RCTs have shown that topiramate (median 100 mg/d, range 25–400) may significantly improve binge and purge symptoms of BN (n = 64, RCT, p/c, Hoopes et al, J Clin Psychiatry 2003;64:1335–41, ibid 1449–54; MS), now confirmed by a later RCT (n = 60, RCT, d/b, p/c, 10/52, Nickel et al, Int J Eat Disord 2005;38:295–300). Earlier studies suggested a total response in 50% and marked improvement in 25% in obese-binge eaters (n = 8, open, 16/52, Appolinario et al, Can J Psychiatry 2002;47:271–3). There have also been several published cases of dramatic response (eg. drug-resistant bulimia, topiramate 150 mg/d, n = 1, Knable, Am J Psychiatry 2001; 158:322–3; n = 1, Appolinario et al, Am J Psychiatry 2001;158:967–8; n = 1, Felstrom and Blackshaw, Am J Psychiatry 2002;159:1246–7), and a case series, where topiramate was almost completely successful in stopping binging and purging in three patients with co-morbid mood disorders, but was ineffective in two (n = 5, Barbee, Int J Eat Disord 2003;33:469–72).

■ Unlicensed/possible efficacy

Buspirone *

Buspirone may have similar efficacy to fluoxetine in short-term management of bulimic symptoms (n = 57, open, 12/52, Rajewski and Rybakowski, Psychiatr Pol 2006;40:75–82).

Duloxetine *

There is a case of treatment refractory bulimia responding to duloxetine 120 mg/d, effective over 2/52 and continuing over the next four months (n = 1, Hazen and Fava, J Psycho-pharmacol 2006;20:723–4).

Flutamide

The testosterone receptor antagonist flutamide (250–500 mg/d) produced a rapid and marked improvement in bulimic behaviour in two women (Bergman and Eriksson, Acta Psychiatr Scand 1996;94:137–9).

Ondansetron

Ondansetron was reported to be effective in three small, short-term trials by one group of investigators, and may be an option after failure of conventional therapies (reviews by Fung and Ferrill, Ann Pharmacother 2001; 35:1270–3; Generali and Cada, Hosp Pharm 2001;36:547–52; 572). Decreased binge-eating and vomiting has been shown with ondansetron 24 mg/d, possibly due to pharmacological decrease in vagal neuro-transmission (n = 28, RCT, Faris et al, Lancet 2000;355:792–7; editorial by Kiss, Lancet 2000;355:769–70).

Reboxetine *

In a pilot study, reboxetine 4 mg/d produced a rapid response (50% decrease in bulimic behaviour) in 60% patients (n = 28, RCT, 3/12, Fassino et al, J Psychopharmacol 2004;18:423–8; see also n = 7, open, El-Giamal et al, Int Clin Psychopharmacol 2000;15:351–6).

Stimulants *

In women with comorbid ADHD and

bulimia, complete response in binge eating has been reported with psychostimulants (n = 6, Dukarm, *J Women's Health* (Larchmt) 2005;**14**:345–50).

Tricyclics

Many tricyclics, eg. amitriptyline (*J Clin Psychopharmacol* 1984;**4**:186–93) have been used but are of arguable potency. Poor relapse rates suggest serious limitations with long-term efficacy (RCT, d/b, p/c, 6/12, Walsh et al, *Am J Psychiatry* 1991;**148**:1206–12).

◆ Others

Other drugs tried include **naltrexone** (n = 19, RCT, Marrazzi et al, *Int Clin Psychopharmacol* 1995;**10**:163–72), **trazodone** (n = 42, RCT, Pope et al, *J Clin Psychopharmacol* 1989;**9**:254–9), **valproate** (Tachibana et al, *Jpn J Psychiatry Neurol* 1989;**43**:77–84) and **zinc** (*Arch Intern Med* 1984; **100**:317–8).

* No efficacy

Carbamazepine

No effect on bulimia was seen in one study (n = 6, Safai-Kutti and Kutti, *Am J Psychiatry* 1983;**140**:1225–6).

Clozapine

There is a single case of bulimia acutely worsening on clozapine 350 mg/d (Brewerton and Shannon, *Am J Psychiatry* 1992;**149**:1408).

Cyproheptadine

Although potentially useful in anorexia, it appears to be detrimental in bulimia (n = 72, RCT, d/b, Halmi et al, *Arch Gen Psychiatry* 1986; **43**:177–81).

Lithium

Despite early enthusiasm, lithium is no more effective than placebo (n = 91, Hsu et al, *J Nerv Mental Dis* 1991;**179**:351–5).

Mianserin

No effect was seen at 60 mg/d (n = 50, 8/52, Sabine et al, *Br J Clin Pharmacol* 1983;**15**:S195–S202).

1.16.3 BINGE-EATING DISORDER

Symptoms *

Binge-eating disorder (BED) is characterised by binge-eating of large amounts of food in discrete time periods, which is not then followed by compensatory behaviours such as purging or vomiting. Many (but not all) patients are obese and may seek treatment for this. CBT is effective for behavioural and psychological features of BED but not obesity (n = 108 [c = 86], RCT, 16/52, d/b, p/c, Grilo et al, *Biol Psychiatry* 2005;**57**:301–9). Higher than expected rates of co-morbid psychiatric conditions, especially depression, are seen. There is some controversy about its status and it is not mentioned in DSM-IV (Wilfley et al, *Int J Eat Disord* 2003;**34**[Suppl]:S96–S106).

Role of drugs

Studies on desipramine, fluvoxamine, fluoxetine, sertraline, citalopram, dexfenfluramine, sibutramine and topiramate have shown some efficacy. An open trial of venlafaxine suggested a role.

Reviews: Carter et al, *Int J Eat Disord* 2003; **34**[Suppl]:S74–S88; Appolinario and McElroy, *Curr Drug Targets* 2004, **5**, 301–7; Latzer and Tzchisinki, *Harefuah* 2003;**142**:544–9.

● Unlicensed/some efficacy

Citalopram

Citalopram may be effective in reducing binge-eating frequency, weight and severity (n = 38, RCT, d/b, p/c, 6/52, McElroy et al, *J Clin Psychiatry* 2003;**64**:807–13).

Fluoxetine

Fluoxetine (mean dose 71 mg/d) was well-tolerated and effective in reducing binge-eating frequency, weight and illness severity (n = 60, RCT, d/b, 6/52, Arnold et al, *J Clin Psychiatry* 2002;**63**:1028–33).

Lithium *

In comorbid bipolar and BED, lithium may have a role in augmenting topiramate (n = 12, open, Kotwal et al, *Hum Psychopharmacol* 2006;**21**:425–31).

Memantine *

Memantine has been reported to decrease

appetite and completely suppress BED within 24 hours, and may block the leptin response (n = 5, Hermanussen and Tresguerres, *Econ Hum Biol* 2005;**3**:329–37).

Reboxetine *

A pilot study with reboxetine 8 mg/d produced a remarkable reduction in binge days per week, decreased BMI and improved other measures (n = 9 [c = 5], open, 12/52, Silveira *et al*, *Eat Weight Disorder* 2005;**10**;93–6).

Sibutramine

A full RCT showed sibutramine 15 mg/d to reduce binge episodes, weight and mental state (n = 60, RCT, d/b, p/c, 12/52, Appolinario *et al*, *Arch Gen Psychiatry* 2003;**60**:1109–16), supporting a pilot, where sibutramine 15 mg/d was seen to be markedly effective and well-tolerated for obese patients with binge-eating disorder, seven showing a complete resolution of symptoms (n = 10, open, 12/52, Appolinario *et al*, *J Clin Psychiatry* 2002;**63**:28–30).

Topiramate *

Topiramate at up to 600 mg/d produced an enduring improvement in some patients with BED but was poorly tolerated with a high drop-out rate (n = 61, 14 + 42/52, RCT, d/b, p/c, McElroy *et al*, *J Clin Psychiatry* 2004;**65**:1463–9); see also n = 61, RCT, d/b, p/c, 14/52, McElroy *et al*, *Am J Psychiatry* 2003;**160**:255–61).

Zonisamide

Zonisamide 100–600 mg/d highly significantly reduced binge-eating frequency and other measures and controlled trials are now awaited (n = 15 [c = 8], open, 12/52, McElroy *et al*, *J Clin Psychiatry* 2004;**65**:50–6).

* No efficacy

Fluvoxamine

Fluvoxamine was no better than placebo in BED (n = 20, RCT, d/b, p/c, Pearlstein *et al*, *Arch Women Ment Health* 2003;**6**:1471–51).

1.17 EPILEPSY
see also Status epilepticus (*1.17.1*)

The annual incidence of epilepsy is 50–70 cases per 100 000 (excluding febrile seizure), with a point prevalence of 5–10 per 1000. The lifetime prevalence is 2–5% of the population.

Role of drugs

Drug therapy is probably the single most important aspect in managing seizures. Treatment after a first seizure probably halves the recurrence rate in the next 1–2 years but with no long-term remission in individuals with single or infrequent seizures (n = 1443, RCT, five years, Marson *et al*, *Lancet* 2005;**365**:2007–13). In a systematic review, the NNTs for new anticonvulsants as add-on therapy for refractory epilepsy were topiramate (1000 mg/d = 2.9, 600 mg/d = 3.0), vigabatrin (300 mg/d = 3.3), tiagabine (32 mg/d = 6.5), lamotrigine (500 mg/d = 7.2) and gabapentin (1200 mg/d = 7.4) (Marson *et al*, *Epilepsia* 1997;**38**:859–80; comment in *Bandolier* 1998; **5**:4–5).

Plasma level monitoring for anticonvulsants has been over-used and should be restricted to:

1. Patients on phenytoin or polytherapy where dosage adjustment is necessary due to poor control or dose-related toxicity.
2. People with learning disabilities, where assessing toxicity is difficult.
3. Patients with renal or hepatic disease.
4. Pregnant women.
5. Where poor compliance is suspected.

Discontinuing anticonvulsants

Since all anticonvulsants have side-effects, especially when taken for long periods and even when optimum ranges are adhered to, they should be discontinued when no longer needed. Adults are not always given advice on anticonvulsant discontinuation, with many stopping on their own initiative. A concentration of seizures during or in the first few months after withdrawal suggest that at least some are provoked by drug withdrawal. Other withdrawal effects such as anxiety, agitation and insomnia are a problem, but only occur with the barbiturates and benzodiazepines. Although around 30% children will have a seizure after anticonvulsant withdrawal, the prognosis is still good if a further course of anticonvulsants is taken (n = 40, 12-year follow-up, Bouma *et al*, *J Neurol Neurosurg Psychiatry* 2002;**72**:507–10).

A prognostic index for recurrence of seizures, either on continued treatment or discontinuation, has been advised by the MRC Antiepileptic Drug Withdrawal Study Group (Chadwick et al, Br Med J 1993;**306**:1374–8), based on a four-year study of 1021 patients from six European countries, testing the potential for 26 possible risk factors. This is the only major study of withdrawal in patients in remission:

Starting score (all patients)	-175
Age 16 years or older	+45
Taking > 1 anticonvulsant	+50
Seizures after starting anticonvulsants	+35
History of 1° or 2° GTC seizures	+35
History of myoclonic seizures	+50
EEG in past year	
– not available	+15
– abnormal	+20
Period free from seizures (in years)	+200/t
Total scores =	=T
Then divide the total score by 100 and expontiate (e^x):	$z = e^{t/100}$
Thus, the probability of recurrence of seizures is:	
Continued by treatment	
– by one year	$1 - 0.89^z$
– by two years	$1 - 0.79^z$
Slow withdrawal:	
– by one year	$1 - 0.69^z$
– by two years	$1 - 0.60^z$

This important and accessible paper should be consulted in order to use this predictive model to its optimum. It should prove useful in counselling patients in the community who wish to withdraw from anticonvulsants.

Reviews: * withdrawing anticonvulsants (Chadwick, Epilepsia 2006;**47**[Suppl 1]:58–61; Lhatoo and Sander, Curr Pharm Des 2000;**6**:861–3; Buna, Pharmacotherapy 1998;**18**:235–41), comparative study (n=1013, Chadwick, Brain 1999; **122**:441–8).

Risk factors for relapse on discontinuing anticonvulsants:

- Polytherapy (four or more anticonvulsants).

- Active epilepsy.
- Age (50 years or older).
- Five weeks or less between reductions.
- Longer duration of treatment or illness (more than 30 months is a higher risk).
- Number of seizures before controlled (higher risk of relapse if more than 100 seizures occur before control).
- Interval seizure less than one month at onset of illness.
- Type of seizure: Complex partial seizures, tonic-clonic or combinations of seizures are more likely to relapse than simple partial seizures.
- Number of drugs required before seizure control (ie. time taken to control seizures).
- Abnormal EEG .
- Adult/late onset seizures (after 10–12 years of age).
- Underlying cerebral disorder.
- Withdrawal in less than six months.

Reviews: * general (n=161, RCT, Peters et al, Neurology 1998;**50**:724–30; n=226, Caviedes and Herranz, Seizure 1998;**7**:107–14; n=409, RCT, Chadwick et al, Epilepsia 1996;**37**:1043–50), practical (Crawford, Prescriber 2005;**16**:43–7).

Favourable factors for discontinuing anticonvulsants:

- Primary generalised seizures.
- Childhood onset (after the age of one, better 5–12 years).
- Short duration of epilepsy.
- No cerebral disorder.
- Normal IQ.
- Normal EEG (or no gross abnormalities, underlying neurological disorder or learning disability), before and after discontinuation
- Few seizures documented, especially juvenile myoclonic epilepsy.
- History of non-compliance/concordance without relapse (in which case withdrawal should be encouraged).
- Medication below quoted therapeuticlevels at time of discontinuation.
- More than two years since last seizure, especially in children.

Reviews: * refractory epilepsy (French et al, Epilepsia 2004;**45**:410–23), efficacy and toler-

TABLE 1.2: THERAPEUTIC DRUG MONITORING

Drug	Plasma levels 'Optimum'	'Toxic'	Half-life	Time to steady state	Peak plasma concs	Sample	Sample frequency	Other checks	Comments
Phenytoin TDM essential	40–80 micol/L (10–20mg/l) upper end for partial seizures; <20mmol unlikely to work	>80 micol/L	20–40 hours (up to 140 at higher levels, dose dependent	5 days minimum, 1–5 weeks possibly (variable)	3–12 hours dependent on total daily dose	Aim for trough unless confirmation of toxicity required	Every 3–12 months for well-stabilised patients	Folate, calcium (both with phenytoin)	Non-linear kinetics, so missed doses, changes in absorption, tablet or capsule brand can markedly affect plasma levels
Phenobarbital TDM useful	60–80 micromol/L (10–30mg/l) dependent upon response	>180micromol/L ↑ chance of stupor	50–160 hours, with age	Adults: 10–25 days Children: 8–15 days	2–6 hours	Long t½, so time not vital. Best to be consistent each time	every 6/12 for well-stabilised patients	Folate 6/12	Blood levels can also be useful as a measure of long-term compliance
Carbamazepine TDM fairly useful	20–50micromol/L (4–12mb/l) 20–40 for GTC + polytherapy 30–50 for monotherapy))	>50micromol/L	5–38 hours	1–4 weeks (enzyme induction). Changes stabilise in about a week	2.5–24 hours (mean 6 hours) — less if taken with food	Aim for trough level unless side-effects suspected	Every 6 months for well-stabilised patients	FBC in initial stages of treatment. thyroid? serum sodium	Plasma levels only of real use for anticonvulsant action. Are of limited use (eg. toxicity) in affective disorders
Sodium valproate/ valproic acid TDM unproven	300–700mmol/L (50–100mg/L proposed) Care in the elderly	>700mmol/L but few side-effects or correlation proved	6–20 hours longer in liver disease + polytherapy	30–85 hours	E/C tabs 2–4 hours Sol tabs + syrup: 1–3 hours	Short t½ so need great care interpreting. Only serial levels are accurate	On request	LFT for 6/12 + plasma amylase if in abdominal pain	Levels may be useful where control is poor, or if toxicity suspected. Hepatotoxicity may be dose related

ability (French et al, Neurology 2004;**62**:1252-60), new-onset epilepsy (French et al, Epilepsia 2004;**45**:401–9), managing severe epilepsy in the community (Motterhead, Prescriber 2002;**13**:67–88), TDM of AEDs (Nelson and Gray, Psychiatr Bull 2001;**25**:356–8), modes of action (Stahl, J Clin Psychiatry 2004;**65**:149–50), Lennox-Gastaut Syndrome (Schmidt and Bourgeois, Drug Saf 2000;**22**:467–77, 51 refs), managing epilepsy in teenagers (McLellan and Cross, Prescriber 2002;**13**:24–37), catamenial epilepsy (Foldvary-Schaefer and Falcone, Neurology 2003;**61**[Suppl 2]:S2–S15), absence epilepsy (Manning et al, Trends Pharmacol Sci 2003;**24**:542–9) and the elderly (Stephen and Brodie, Lancet 2000; **355**:1441–6, 50 refs).

BNF listed

FIRST-LINE/MONOTHERAPY DRUGS

A number of reviews have concluded that carbamazepine, phenobarbital and phenytoin are equipotent (Tudur et al, Cochrane Database Syst Rev 2002;**2**:CD001911; Tudur et al, Cochrane Database Syst Rev 2002;**2**:CD001904), but carbamazepine is better tolerated and there may be some sub-types that respond preferentially to one drug. Carbamazepine may be preferable to valproate for partial-onset seizures (Marson et al, Epilepsia 2002;**43**: 505–13).

Carbamazepine

Carbamazepine is a broad spectrum anti-convulsant, licensed for adjunctive or first-line therapy in tonic-clonic and partial seizures (excluding absences and myoclonic seizures). It has been compared with valproate in complex partial and secondary GTC in a large adult study, where they were considered of similar efficacy but with carbamazepine better for complex partial seizures (n = 480, d/b, ≤5 years, Mattson et al, N Engl J Med 1992;**327**:765–71; comments in N Engl J Med 1993;**328**:207–9) and for partial-onset seizures (n = 1265, 5 studies, Marson et al, Epilepsia 2002;**43**:505–13), with fewer long-term side-effects. The sustained release tablets can be used as a once-a-day dosage, with careful monitoring if seizures continue, although lower trough concentrations mean some patients may need twice daily dosing.

Sudden withdrawal may increase cardiac sympathetic activity in sleep which could lead to seizure-induced hypoxia, and predispose to sudden unexpected death in epilepsy (n = 12, Hennessy et al, Neurology 2001;**57**:1650–4). Cochrane concludes carbamazepine and phenobarbital are equally effective, with phenobarbital possibly slightly better for partial onset seizures and carbamazepine for GTC seizures (Tudur Smith et al, Cochrane Database Syst Rev 2003;**1**:CD001904).

Reviews: pharmacokinetics (Graves et al, Pharmacotherapy 1998;**18**:273–81), mode of action (Ambrosio et al, Neurochem Res 2002; **27**:121–30).

Lamotrigine *

Lamotrigine is indicated for adjunctive or monotherapy in partial or generalised epilepsy, Lennox-Gastaut and juvenile myoclonic epilepsy. It is thought to stabilise pre-synaptic neuronal membranes by blockade of voltage-dependent sodium channels, with this secondarily inhibiting the release of excessive excitatory glutamate and aspartate. It is well-tolerated as monotherapy in adults with newly diagnosed epilepsy, at up to 500 mg/d as monotherapy in adults with partial seizures (n = 156, d/b, Gilliam et al, Neurology 1998;**51**:1018–25), as an adjunctive in primary GTC seizures (n = 121 [c = 117], RCT, d/b, p/c, Biton et al, Neurology 2005;**65**:1737–43), in focal and generalised epilepsy (and as effective as, eg. carbamazepine; n = 239, RCT, open, Steinhoff et al, Seizure 2005;**14**:597–605) and in the elderly (n = 208, s = 13, Giorgi et al, Drugs Aging 2001;**18**:621–30). A continuation study has shown a long-term efficacy in epilepsy without serious ADRs over six years (n = 508, open, six year, Faught et al, Epilepsy Behav 2004;**5**:31–6). It may produce significantly fewer untoward cognitive and behavioural effects than carbamazepine (n = 25, RCT, d/b, c/o, 10+10/52, Meador et al, Neurology 2001;**56**:1177–82). Lamotrigine has a good pharmacokinetic profile, eg. long half-life, low protein-binding and few interactions. The 2–5% risk of rashes can be reduced in adults with a starting dose of 25 mg/d for two weeks, then 50 mg/d for two weeks, then increasing every 1–2 weeks, halved if added to valproate (where rash is also more likely to occur,

Gilman, *Ann Pharmacother* 1995;**29**:144–51) or allergic to trimethoprim, and doubled if combined with concurrent enzyme inducing drugs, eg. phenytoin, carbamazepine, etc. The incidence of serious rash and Stevens-Johnson syndrome is relatively rare (higher if a history of previous AED-related rash; n = 988, Hirsch et al, *Epilepsia* 2006;**47**:318–22) but can be life-threatening and must be considered carefully (s = 2, n = 1955, Calabrese et al, *J Clin Psychiatry* 2002;**63**:1012–19). Cochrane concludes that while lamotrigine is much better tolerated than carbamazepine, the latter may be superior for seizure control (s = 5, n = 1384, Gamble et al, *Cochrane Database Syst Rev* 2006;**1**: CD001031), but that it may be effective in drug-resistant partial epilepsy (n = 1243, s = 11, Ramaratnam et al, *Cochrane Database Syst Rev* 2001;**3**:CD001909).

Reviews: general (Arzimanoglou et al, *Rev Neurol* [Paris] 2001;**157**:525–36), safety review of 68 trials, with particular emphasis on rash (Messenheimer et al, *Drug Saf* 1998;**18**:281–96, 28 refs), use in children (Messenheimer et al, *Drug Saf* 2000;**22**:303–12, 35 refs), saliva and serum monitoring (Tsiropoulos et al, *Ther Drug Monit* 2000;**22**:517–21).

Levetiracetam *

Levetiracetam is licensed as monotherapy for partial seizures, with or without secondary generalisation, in people aged 16 or over with newly diagnosed epilepsy. Although structurally related to piracetam, it has a distinct pharmacological profile (Genton and Van Vleymen, *Epileptic Disord* 2000;**2**:99–105) and the mode of action is unclear. The dose is 250mg BD, increasing to a maximum of 1500mg/d. It has been investigated at 1–3g/d for resistant partial seizures, where it has been effective and well-tolerated (n = 294, RCT, Cereghino et al, *Neurology* 2000;**55**:236–42; n = 286, d/b, p/c, Ben-Menachem and Falter, *Epilepsia* 2000;**41**:1276–83; n = 324, RCT, Boon et al, *Epilepsy Res* 2002;**48**:77–89), at 1–2g BD as add-on in refractory epilepsy (n = 119, RCT, 24/52, Betts et al, *Seizure* 2000;**9**:80–7), and in children with partial seizures (n = 24, open, Glauser et al, *Epilepsia* 2002;**43**:518–24). 31% of patients had a greater than 50% reduction in seizures when used as add-on therapy in

another study in refractory partial seizures (n = 324, RCT, 12/52, Shorvon et al, *Epilepsia* 2000;**41**:1179–86). Levetiracetam seems to have long-term efficacy for partial seizures (n = 280, <4 years, open follow-up, Abou-Khalil and Schaich, *Seizure* 2005;**14**:577–85). The upper limit of efficacy may be 4g/d in many patients (n = 29, p/c, Grant and Shorvon, *Epilepsy Res* 2000;**42**:89–95). It is well-tolerated long-term (n = 1422, up to five years, Krakow et al, *Neurology* 2001;**56**:1772–4), the main side-effect being somnolence, which can be minimised by starting at a lower dose. Cochrane concludes that levetiractam is effective as an add-on in localised partial epilepsy (n = 1023, s = 4, 24/52, Chaisewikul et al, *Cochrane Database Syst Rev* 2001;**1**:CD001901) but that more data is needed. It has good bioavailability, rapidly achieves steady-state concentrations, has linear kinetics, minimal protein binding, and minimal metabolism, ie. ideal pharmacokinetic properties although a BD dosage is needed due to its short half-life (review: Perucca and Johannessen, *Epileptic Disord* 2003;**5**[Suppl 1]:S17–S26).

Reviews: * pharmacokinetic profile (Patsalos, *Pharmacol Ther* 2000;**85**:77–85), general (Leach, *Hosp Med* 2004;**65**:740–4; Dooley and Plosker, *Drugs* 2000;**60**:871–93; Betts, *Prescriber* 2001;**12**:39–44).

Oxcarbazepine *

Oxcarbazepine is indicated for partial seizures with or without secondary generalised tonic-clonic seizures (eg. n = 79, RCT, Beydoun et al, *Neurology* 2000;**54**:2245–51). Oxcarbazepine's mode of action mainly involves blocking sodium and calcium channels, but this may differ subtly from carbamazepine (review by Schmidt and Elger, *Epilepsy Behav* 2004;**5**:627–35). A consensus view suggested starting at 150mg/d, and increasing by 150mg/d on alternate days to 900–1200mg/d (Schmidt et al, *Acta Neurol Scand* 2001;**104**:167–70). Oxcarbazepine exerts its action primarily through its metabolite (the monohydroxy derivative, MHD). It can be used as monotherapy (where 2400mg/d is well-tolerated and efficacious: n = 96, RCT, d/b, Sachdeo et al, *Neurology* 2001;**57**:864–71), or adjunctive therapy in adults and children, with an average maintenance dose of 2400 mg/day. About 25–30% of patients who have experienced hypersensitivity to carbamazepine may experience such reactions with oxcarbazepine, in which case oxcarbazepine should be immediately withdrawn. Hyponatraemia can occur, and so regular sodium levels are advisable. If necessary, an abrupt switch from CBZ to oxcarbazepine on a 1:1.5 basis (or 1:1 for doses of CBZ >800 mg/d followed by titration to tolerance if necessary), may be effective and well-tolerated (n=51, retrospective, Homberg et al, Nervenarzt 2001;72:918–23; n=286, RCT, Albani et al, Seizure 2004;13:254–63). It is less likely to induce enzymes than carbamazepine, and probably has minimal autoinduction. Cochrane concludes that oxcarbazepine is better tolerated than phenytoin but that relative efficacy is unproven (Muller et al, Cochrane Database Syst Rev 2006;2:CD003615).

Reviews: general (Bang and Goa, CNS Drugs 2004;18:57–61; Glauser, Pharmacother 2001;21:904–19, 105 refs; Wellington and Goa, CNS Drugs 2001;15:137–63), TDM (Chong and Dupuis, Ann Pharmacother 2002;36:917–20), clinical pharmacokinetics (May et al, Clin Pharmacokinet 2003;42:1023–42), side-effects (Wellington and Goa, CNS Drugs 2001;15:137–63), safety and efficacy (Beydoun, Pharmacotherapy 2000;20:S152–S158), use in affective and schizoaffective disorders (Dietrich et al, Pharmacopsychiatry 2001;34:242–50).

Phenytoin

Phenytoin is a broad spectrum anticonvulsant licensed for adjunctive or first-line therapy in partial or generalised epilepsy (excluding absence and myoclonus) and status epilepticus, and is believed to stabilise the seizure threshold. Phenytoin is not now routinely recommended for use in children as it can cause permanent learning difficulties. A wide range of side-effects and non-linear kinetics make it a difficult drug to use (review of optimising phenytoin by Valodia et al, J Clin Pharm Therap 1999;24:381). Phenytoin has no effect on the prevention of early post-traumatic seizures in children with moderate to severe blunt head injuries (n=102, RCT, p/c, 30/7, Young et al, Ann Emerg Med 2004;43:435–6). A study of 45 patients aimed at establishing dosing rules to minimise toxic effects with phenytoin concluded the following:

1. Increase the dose by 100 mg/d if the steady state plasma level is less than 7 mcg/ml.
2. Increase the dose by 50 mg/d if the steady state plasma level is ≥7 mcg/ml but less than 12 mcg/ml.
3. Increase the dose by 30 mg/d when initial plasma levels are 12 mcg/ml or more. NB the 'optimal' range is only a guide and higher plasma levels may be needed (eg. n=1, Kozer et al, Ther Drug Monit 2002;24:386–9), as interpatient and intrapatient variability in phenytoin protein binding mean serum concentration monitoring is unreliable (n=48,163 samples, Linh Banh et al, Ther Drug Monit 2002;24:379–85).

Topiramate

Topiramate is licensed as monotherapy for partial and generalised tonic-clonic seizures, with or without secondary generalisation. Topiramate is also licensed as adjunctive therapy in Lennox-Gastaut syndrome, (n=98, RCT, p/c, 11/52, Sachdeo et al, Neurology 1999;52:1882–8; n=97, open extension to RCT, Glauser et al, Epilepsia 2000;41[Suppl 1]:S86–S90) and partial seizures. There is a multiple mode of action, including sodium channel blockade, GABA enhancement, glutamate inhibition and weak carbonic anhydrase inhibition, which may explain its effect in resistant epilepsy and severity of side-effects, eg. ataxia, dizziness and somnolence. The optimum dose now appears to be 100 mg/d (as effective as 200 mg/d but with less side-effects). In children, the dose should be 3–6 mg/kg/day (monotherapy) or 5–9 mg/kg/day for adjunctive therapy (n=613, RCT, d/b, 6/12, Privitera et al, Acta Neurol Scand 2003;107:165–75). Twice daily dosing is appropriate and the recommended starting dose is now 25 mg/d for the first week, increased by 25–50 mg/d every one to two weeks to 200–400 mg/d. Slow dose titration is important to minimise side-effects, which are the main reason for drop-outs (n=470, Bootsma et al, Epilepsy Behav 2004;5:380–7). In a pooled analysis of topiramate as add-on therapy, seizures were reduced by more than

50% in 43% of topiramate-treated, and 12% of placebo-treated patients (n=743, s=6, d/b, p/c, Reife et al, *Epilepsia* 2000;**41**[Suppl 1]:S66–S71). A manufacturer's meta-analysis concludes 200mg/d is a good target dose for add-on therapy in patients with partial epilepsy (Peeters et al, *Acta Neurol Scand* 2003;**108**:9–15). Topiramate may have a role in other seizures, with 600mg/d as effective as 800mg/d as add-on therapy in refractory partial epilepsy (n=190, RCT, Privitera et al, *Neurology* 1996;**46**:1678–83), in West Syndrome (n=11, Glauser et al, *Epilepsia* 2000;**41**[Suppl 1]:S91–S94), and in children (n=51, Mohamed, *Seizure* 2000;**9**:137–41). Although plasma level monitoring is not required, plasma concentrations correlate with CSF levels (n=14, Christensen et al, *Ther Drug Monit* 2001;**23**:529–35) and may be of use in older people or those taking interacting drugs (n=344, May et al, *Ther Drug Monit* 2002;**24**:366–74) as levels may be two-fold lower with valproate or lamotrigine (n=116, Contin et al, *Ther Drug Monit* 2002;**4**:332–7). Cochrane concludes that topiramate has efficacy as add-on therapy in partial epilepsy, but long-term and monotherapy were unproven (n=1049, RCT, s=9, Jette et al, *Cochrane Database Syst Rev* 2002;**3**:CD001417) and longer trials are needed.

Reviews: general (Biton et al, *Ann Pharmacother* 2001;**35**:173–9; Kellett et al, *J Neurol Neurosurg Psychiatry* 1999;**66**:759–63), in children (Ormrod and McClellan, *Paediatr Drugs* 2001; **3**:293–319, 95 refs), monotherapy in newly diagnosed epilepsy (Waugh and Goa, *CNS Drugs* 2003;**17**:985–92), pharmacology (Shank et al, *Epilepsia* 2000;**41**[Suppl 1]:S3–S9).

Valproate

This established drug is licensed for first-line or adjunctive therapy in partial, generalised or other epilepsies (excluding absence and myoclonus), including Lennox-Gastaut syndrome and juvenile myoclonic epilepsy idiopathic epilepsy (Nicolson et al, *J Neurol Neurosurg Psychiatry* 2004;**75**:75–9). Valproate should not be used in women of child-bearing potential without a fully informed and documented discussion. The sustained release preparations overcome the short plasma half-life. There is little correlation between blood levels and therapeutic effect and so routine blood level monitoring is of limited use, although saturation protein-binding may occur above 100mg/L, requiring great care. Serious toxicity is rare and careful supervision initially will guard against major problems, eg. liver toxicity.

Reviews: mode of action in epilepsy (Johannsessen and Johannessen, *CNS Drug Rev* 2003;**9**:199–216), pharmacology (Owens and Nemeroff, *Psychopharmacol Bull* 2003; **37**[Suppl 2]:S17–S24) and kinetics (DeVane, *Psychopharmacol Bull* 2003;**37**[Suppl 2]:S25–S42).

BENZODIAZEPINES

Benzodiazepines are excellent anticonvulsant drugs in the short-term, but tolerance limits their long-term use. They may be useful for 'rescue' or special events, eg. holidays and family events, (review by Henriksen, *Epilepsia* 1998;**39**[Suppl 1]:S2–S6).

Clobazam *

Clobazam is licensed as adjunctive therapy in partial or generalised epilepsy and as intermittent therapy. Tolerance can develop and low doses (eg. 10–20mg/d) and intermittent administration can help to minimise this. Sustained response is more likely in patients with a shorter duration of epilepsy, a known etiology and higher clobazam (but not n-desmethylclobazam) plasma levels (n=173, Singh et al, *Epilepsia* 1995;**36**:798–803). It may be effective for stimulus-provoked attacks, catamenial epilepsy (if given for one week in four), in intractable childhood epilepsy (n=63, Sheth et al, *J Child Neurol* 1995;**10**:205–8; n=31, Jan and Shaabat, *Saudi Med J* 2000;**21**:622–4), as add-on in refractory epilepsy (n=97, open, Montenegro et al, *Epilepsia* 2001;**42**:539–42) and as add-on for TLE with hippocampal sclerosis (n=78, retrospective, Montenegro et al, *Can J Neurol Sci* 2005;**32**:93–6).

Reviews: Shorvon, *Epilepsia* 1998;**39**[Suppl 1]:S15–S23; Fisher and Blum, *Epilepsia* 1995; **36**[Suppl 2]:S105–S14.

Clonazepam

Clonazepam is licensed for adjunctive therapy

in partial or generalised epilepsy (including absence and myoclonus), infantile spasms, status and Lennox-Gastaut syndrome. It has marked anticonvulsant properties but its usefulness is limited by tolerance (which may possibly be reversed with flumazenil 1.5 mg IV) and sedation (general review by Tassinari et al, Epilepsia 1998; **39**[Suppl 1]:S7–S14).

Diazepam

Diazepam is occasionally useful orally as an adjunct and in short-term therapy, although studies on it are limited. Use in status epilepticus is well-established. Review by Tassinari et al, Epilepsia 1998;**39**[Suppl 1]:S7–S14.

BARBITURATES

Phenobarbital *

Phenobarbital is licensed as adjunctive or monotherapy therapy in partial or generalised epilepsy (excluding absence and myoclonus). Concerns about cognitive and psychomotor impairment and dependence have rightly limited its use (Cochrane review: Taylor et al, Cochrane Database Syst Rev 2001;**4**:CD002217). Cochrane concludes that carbamazepine and phenobarbital are equally effective, with phenobarbital possibly slightly better for partial onset seizures, and carbamazepine for GTC seizures (Tudur Smith et al, Cochrane Database Syst Rev 2003;**1**:CD001904).

Reviews: * (Kale and Perucca, Br Med J 2004; **329**:1199–200; Kwan and Brodie, Epilepsia 2004;**45**:1141–9).

Primidone

This obsolescent barbiturate is metabolised mainly to phenobarbital but also to phenyl-ethylmalonamide.

ADD-ON OR ADJUNCT THERAPY/OTHERS

Acetazolamide

Although this carbonic anhydrase inhibitor is a potent anticonvulsant, and is occasionally useful for absence and other seizures, rapid tolerance and long-term side-effects render it of limited use (review by Reiss and Oles, Ann Pharmacother 1996;**30**:512–19, 68 refs). It has been used at 10–20 mg/kg as an adjunct in refractory localised epilepsies (n = 37, open, Katayama et al, Brain Dev 2002;**24**:150–4), and in catamenial epilepsy (n = 20, survey, Lim et al, Epilepsia 2001:**42**:746–9).

Ethosuximide

Ethosuximide is primarily useful in absence seizures, but also as adjunctive therapy in GTC and other epilepsies. It is poorly studied and due to its side-effects, eg. gastric upset, has largely now been replaced by valproate.

Gabapentin

Gabapentin is licensed as adjunctive therapy in refractory partial and secondary generalised epilepsy (with a reduction of 50% or more in partial seizures in 25–33% patients, although few become seizure-free). There is a strong dose:response relationship, with much interpatient variability (requiring individual optimisation). A review concludes that gabapentin can be initiated at 900 mg/d and titrated (rapidly) to up to 3600 mg/d, with children treated with 23–78 mg/kg/d (McLean and Gidal, Clin Ther 2003;**25**:1382–406). A TDS dosage is recommended, with no more than 12 hours between doses. The mode of action is not established (review by Kelly, Neuropsychobiology 1998;**38**:139–44). However, 1200 mg/d is probably the minimum effective maintenance dose, although 600, 1200 and 2400 mg/d have been shown to be equipotent in refractory complex partial or secondary generalised seizures (n = 275, RCT, 6/12, Beydoun et al, Neurology 1997;**49**:746–52). Gabapentin may be effective as add-on therapy in children with refractory partial seizures (n = 247, RCT, 12/52, Appleton et al, Epilepsia 1999;**40**:1147–54, and as effective as lamotrigine in newly-diagnosed epilepsy (n = 309, RCT, d/b, 30/52, Brodie et al, Epilepsia 2002;**43**:993–1000). It has a low order of toxicity, uncomplicated kinetics, no clinically important interactions, and plasma levels are not necessary. A rapid discontinuation withdrawal syndrome has been reported (n = 3, Norton, Clin Neuropharmacol 2001; **24**:245–6). Cochrane concludes that gabapentin has efficacy as an add-on in drug-resistant epilepsy, but trials are short-term, with long-term efficacy and monotherapy unproven

(Marson et al, Cochrane Database Syst Rev 2000;**3**:CD001415).

Reviews: general (n = 3100, PMSS, Wilton and Shakir, Epilepsia 2002;**43**:983–92; Prescrire Int 2000;**9**:40–2; Morris, Epilepsia 1999;**40**[Suppl 5]:S63–S70), as monotherapy (Beydoun, Epilepsia 1999;**40**[Suppl 6]:S13–S16).

Piracetam

Piracetam is a GABA derivative, licensed in the UK for cortical myoclonus, in conjunction with other anti-myoclonic therapies (Brown et al, Mov Disorder 1993;**8**:63–8; n = 20, RCT, Koskiniemi et al, J Neurol Neurosurg Psychiatry 1998;**64**:344–8) and up to 70% of patients may become seizure-free if they can swallow enough of it.

Pregabalin *

Pregabalin is a newly licensed adjunctive therapy for adults with partial seizures, with or without secondary generalisation. It is a GABA analog that reduces excitatory neurotransmitter release by binding to alpha(2)-delta protein, modulating voltage-gated calcium channels (Warner and Figgitt, CNS Drugs 2005;**19**:265–72). The target dose is 600 mg/d in divided doses, starting at 150 mg/d, increasing to 300 mg/d after a week, and to a maximum of 600 mg/d after another week. A careful study showed 150, 300 and 600 mg/d to be well-tolerated and equally effective as add-on therapy in refractory partial seizures (n = 453, RCT, d/b, p/c, 12/52, French et al, Neurology 2003;**27**:1631–7; see also n = 287, RCT, d/b, p/c, 12/52, Arroyo et al, Epilepsia 2004;**45**:20–7). Absorption is slightly reduced by food, and plasma level monitoring is unnecessary.

Tiagabine

Tiagabine is licensed in the UK as adjunctive therapy for partial seizures, with or without secondary generalisation. It is a potent GABA reuptake inhibitor in neuronal and glial cells, increasing GABA-mediated inhibition of the CNS. Several studies have shown an effect in refractory partial seizures (14% achieving a 50% or greater increase in seizure-free days, n = 154, d/b, p/c, Kalviainen et al, Epilepsy Res 1998;**30**:31–40) and refractory complex partial seizures (up to 29% had a >50%

reduction in seizures, n = 297, RCT, Uthman et al, Arch Neurol 1998;**55**:56–62). Data on monotherapy is limited. Tiagabine has linear kinetics, a short half-life (requiring BD to QDS dosage), an inducible metabolism and a number of drug interactions (see 4.5.11). Cochrane concludes that tiagabine is effective as adjunctive therapy but is associated with many ADRs (Pereira et al, Cochrane Database Syst Rev 2002;**3**:CD001908).

Reviews: general (Schachter, Expert Opin Pharmacother 2001;**2**:179–87; Drug Ther Bull 2000;**38**:47–8, 17 refs).

Vigabatrin

Vigabatrin is licensed as adjunctive therapy in refractory partial and secondary generalised epilepsy and as monotherapy for West's syndrome. Use is now limited by ocular changes (eg. impaired contrast sensitivity and usually irreversible loss of field) in up to 50% patients (n = 24, Gross-Tsur et al, Ann Neurol 2000;**48**:60–4). It may retain a role in childhood epilepsy (n = 73, survey, Prasad et al, Epilepsia 2001;**42**:54–61). Total vigabatrin exposure is the most significant factor in predicting visual field loss (n = 92, Hardus et al, Epilepsia 2001;**42**:262–7). It should only be used when there is no alternative, accompanied by a baseline and six-monthly peripheral field examination (Hardus et al, Epilepsia 2001;**42**:262–7; n = 17, Paul et al, Epilepsia 2001;**42**:525–30).

Reviews: general (Gidal et al, Ann Pharmacother 1999;**33**:1277–86, 115 refs), use in children (Br Med J 2000;**320**:1404), ocular problems (Newman et al, Eye 2002;**16**:567–71; Spence and Sankar, Drug Saf 2001;**24**:385–404, 33 refs).

Zonisamide *

Zonisamide is licensed for adjunctive therapy for adults with partial seizures, with or without secondary generalisation. Zonisamide may block voltage sensitive calcium channels and enhance the inhibitory effects, eg. GABA. Its half-life is 60 hours, steady state is reached in 13 days, and accumulation occurs. The dose is 25 mg BD for a week, increasing by up to 100 mg a week to a maximum of 300–500 mg/ d, with a dose-dependent effect. Efficacy has been shown in four main trials (eg. n = 351, RCT, d/b, p/c, 24/52, Brodie et al, Epilepsia 2005;**46**:31–41; n = 203, RCT, d/b, p/c, 12/52, Faught et al, Neurology 2001;**57**:1774–9; RCT, d/b, p/c, 12/52, Sackellares et al, Epilepsia 2004;**45**:610–7). Zonisamide has a sulphonamide group and so caution is necessary with unexplained rashes. Cochrane concludes that zonisamide is effective as an add-on in drug-resistant partial epilepsy, but that the therapeutic dose is unclear and long-term studies are needed (s = 4, n = 850, RCT, p/c, Chadwick and Marson, Cochrane Database Syst Rev 2005;**4**:CD001416).

Reviews: * Biton, Expert Rev Neurother 2004; **4**:935–43; Frampton and Scott, CNS Drugs 2005;**19**:347–67.

+ Combinations

Numerous combinations are used but few have been, or can be, assessed systematically.

Valproate + lamotrigine

The combination of valproate and lamotrigine may have some advantage over the drugs individually in refractory complex partial seizures, as well as being well-tolerated if used with care (n = 20, open, c/o, Pisani et al, Epilepsia 1999;**40**:1141–6; Morris et al, Ther Drug Monit 2000;**22**:656–60). See also lamotrigine.

● Unlicensed/some efficacy

Calcium-channel blockers

Cochrane concludes that flunarizine (in refractory childhood seizures: n = 14, open, Hoppu et al, Pediatr Neurol 1995;**13**:143–7; n = 93, RCT, Pledger et al, Neurology 1994;**44**:1830–6) is difficult to use and may have a weak effect but the evidence for nifedipine and nimodipine is not convincing (s = 11, Chaisewikul et al, Cochrane Database Syst Rev 2001;**4**:CD002750).

Carnitine

Intractable epilepsy in a child, who was found to have carnitine deficiency, was treated successfully with L-carnitine 100mg TDS and valproate (n = 1, Shuper et al, Lancet 1999; **353**:1238).

Fluoxetine

In patients with complex partial seizures, addition of fluoxetine resulted in disappearance of seizures in six, and a 30% reduction occurred in the other 11 (n = 17, open, Favale et al, Neurology 1995;**45**:1926–7).

Goserelin

A reduction in the number of attacks in catamenial epilepsy has been shown, although long-term treatment would have problems (Reid and Gangar, Lancet 1992;**339**:253).

Melatonin *

Adjunctive melatonin 6–9mg/d may be neuroprotective in children with epilepsy taking valproate (n = 31 [c = 29], RCT, d/b, p/c, Gupta et al, Br J Clin Pharmacol 2004;**58**:542–7).

Midazolam

Acute childhood seizures have been managed with intranasal midazolam (n = 20, Lancet 1998;**352**:620; reviews by Smith and Carley, Emerg Med J 2005;**22**:436–7; Body and Ijaz, Emerg Med J 2005;**22**:364–5).

Nitrazepam

Nitrazepam has been used successfully (60% had a > 50% reduction in seizures) in Lennox-Gestaut syndrome (n = 14, open, 12/12, Hosain et al, Pediatr Neurol 2003;**28**:16–9).

◆ Others

Other drugs used include **aromatherapy** (ylang ylang, chamomile and lavender: Anon, Pharm J 1993;**251**:798), **buspirone** (in progressive myoclonus epilepsy: Pranzatelli et al, J Neurol Neurosurg Psychiatry 1993;**56**:114–5), **clomiphene** (n = 1, Herzog, Arch Neurol 1988;**45**:209–10), **magnesium** (Walker et al, Anesthesia 1995;**50**:130–5; discussion in Anesthesia 1995; **50**:824–5), **medroxyprogesterone** (in women: Epilepsia 1985;**26**:S40–S51), **progesterone** (especially in women with catamenial exacerbations: n = 25, open, Herzog, Neurology 1995;**45**:1660–2), **propranolol** (synergistic with carbamazepine: n = 1, Renshaw et al, Am J Psychiatry 1990; **147**: 1687–8), and **vitamin E** (300mg/d as add-on: n = 10, Wiehl and Hart, DICP Ann Pharmacother 1991;**25**:362–3).

1.17.1 STATUS EPILEPTICUS

Status epilepticus is a state where multiple seizures occur without complete recovery between seizures. There are a number of different definitions of status epilepticus, but it usually refers to seizures longer than five minutes or two consecutive seizures without regaining consciousness. Mortality can be high, but a rapid and aggressive treatment reduces this risk and any permanent neuronal damage.

Role of drugs *
To prevent permanent brain damage, first-line therapy must be to support with oxygen and a glucose drip if possible. First-line drugs, eg. benzodiazepines are usually successful to abort status epilepticus. Refractory seizures are frequently caused by acute neurological problems, eg. encephalitis, CVA or trauma. Transfer to an ITU may be appropriate. The EFNS guidelines (Meierkord et al, Eur J Neurol 2006;**13**:445–50) recommend lorazepam 4mg IV or diazepam 10mg IV followed by 15–18mg/kg phenytoin (or fosphenytoin equivalents). If still fitting after 10 minutes, repeat lorazepam or diazepam. If refractory, use anaesthetic doses of midazolam, propofol or barbiturates with appropriate EEG monitoring. Cochrane concludes that lorazepam is superior to diazepam or phenytoin for cessation of seizures and carries a lower risk of continuation of status (Prasad et al, Cochrane Database Syst Rev 2005;**4**:CD003723). Isoflurane and desflurane adequately suppress refractory status epilepticus, albeit with complications (n=7, Mirsattari et al, Arch Neurol 2004;**61**:1254–9).

Reviews: general (Riviello and Holmes, Semin Pediatr Neurol 2004;**11**:129–38; Marik and Varon, Chest 2004;**126**:582–91; Sirven and Waterhouse, Am Fam Physician 2003;**68**:469–76; Misra and Singh, J Indian Med Assoc 2002;**100**:299–303; Hirsch and Claassen, Curr Neurol Neurosci Rep 2002;**2**:345–56; Rosenow et al, Epileptic Disord 2002;**4**[Suppl 2]:S41–S51; Silver and Cockerell, Prescriber 2002;**13**:17–25; Fountain, Epilepsia 2000;**41**[Suppl 2]:S23–S30), benzodiazepine routes (Rey et al, Clin Pharmacokin 1999;**36**:409–24, 98 refs) and in the elderly (Waterhouse and DeLorenzo, Drugs Aging 2001;**18**:133–42, 94 refs).

Amylobarbital (sodium)
See the SPC for injection details, which are important for this potentially toxic drug.

Clonazepam
Clonazepam 0.5–1.5mg by slow IV injection (possibly followed by an infusion) may be useful in refractory cases not responsive to diazepam. A prolonged effect may be seen. It is comparable with lorazepam and probably has the lowest respiratory depressant effect of the benzodiazepines (Pharmacy World Sci 1993;**15**:17–28).

Diazepam
Diazepam 0.15–0.25mg/kg (ie. around 10–30mg) given as a slow IV injection over five minutes or rectally (eg. rectal tubes) is first choice treatment in the UK. Rates above 5mg/min IV are associated with respiratory depression. A diazepam infusion at 3mg/kg in 24 hours can be tried for maintenance (n=1, Bertz and Howrie, Ann Pharmacother 1993;**27**:298–301). The speed of rectal absorption is second only to IV absorption (Int J Pharmaceutics 1980;**5**:127). It is also safe and effective when administered by paramedics in out-of-hospital situations (n=205, RCT, p/c, Alldredge et al, N Engl J Med 2001;**345**:631–7).

Fosphenytoin
Fosphenytoin is a water soluble phosphate ester pro-drug converted to phenytoin. It is rapidly absorbed (therapeutic levels in 5–20 minutes) and is licensed for status and as a substitute for oral phenytoin. It is well-tolerated at injection sites (open, Pryor et al, Epilepsia 2001;**42**:245–50) and has complete IM absorption. It can be given up to three times more rapidly IV than phenytoin and can be given IM, where cardiac monitoring is not necessary. Conversion to phenytoin takes about 7–15 minutes, with peak levels at about 30 minutes, and so fosphenytoin is less appropriate for the sole initial treatment of status epilepticus. Although more expensive, fosphenytoin may be cost-neutral due to reduced side-effects (Armstrong et al, Pharmacotherapy 1999;**19**:844–53, 39 refs),

although this has been disputed (editorial by Labiner, *Arch Int Med* 1999;**159**:2631–2, 12 refs; review by DeToledo and Ramsay, *Drug Saf* 2000;**22**:459–66, 58 refs).

Reviews: general (Browne, *Clin Neuropharmacol* 1997;**20**:1–12), kinetics, (Ogutu et al, *Br J Clin Pharmacol* 2003;**56**:112–9).

Lorazepam *

Lorazepam may be preferable to diazepam, due to a longer duration of action (about two hours), shorter elimination half-life, no active metabolites and possibly less respiratory depression. Lorazepam appears more effective than phenytoin, and easier to use than phenobarbital or diazepam plus phenytoin (n = 384, RCT, Treiman et al, *N Engl J Med* 1998;**339**:792–8). In convulsive status epilepticus, lorazepam 4 mg IV was equivalent to diazepam 10 mg IV, but superior in terms of fewer recurrences (Cock and Schapira, *QJM* 2002;**95**:225–31). It is also safe and effective when administered by paramedics in out-of-hospital situations (n = 205, RCT, p/c, Alldredge et al, *N Engl J Med* 2001;**345**:631–7). Intranasal lorazepam is safe and effective in protracted convulsions in children and less invasive than IM paraldehyde (n = 160, RCT, open, Ahmad et al, *Lancet* 2006;**367**:1591–7).

Paraldehyde

Given by IM injection (up to 5 ml per muscle site, glass syringe needed) or rectally (50/50 mixture with arachis oil, 2:1 in oil or cottonseed oil or mixed with 0.9% sodium chloride), paraldehyde can be rapidly effective, especially in infants and children where venous access is limited, but it is painful at the site of injection. It is also active, albeit unpleasantly, by mouth and also by IV infusion (4–8% infusion in sodium chloride 0.9%; *Pharmacy World Sci* 1993;**15**:17–28). It may have a role in ongoing pervasive and resistant seizures (Armstrong and Battin, *J Child Neurol* 2001;**16**:915–7; Thulasimani and Ramaswamy, *Anaethesia* 2002;**57**:99–100).

Reviews: toxicology (von Burg and Stout, *J Appl Toxicol* 1991;**11**:379–81) and kinetics (Ramsay, *Epilepsia* 1989;**30**[Suppl 2]:S1–S3).

Phenytoin

Phenytoin (see also fosphenytoin) is a useful second-line to the benzodiazepines, used as 10–20 mg/kg in 0.9% saline intravenously over 15 minutes (not exceeding 50 mg/minute) for recurrent or persistent seizures. It is effective from 20–30 minutes after injection but is not effective intramuscularly. It is not an easy drug to use due to the risk of hypotension and cardiac dysrhythmias.

Review: kinetics of phenytoin IV (Ogutu et al, *Br J Clin Pharmacol* 2003;**56**:112–9).

● Unlicensed/some efficacy

Midazolam *

Continuous IV infusion can be used for status (n = 20, case series, Koul et al, *Arch Dis Childhood* 1997, **76**, 445) with 1–3 mg/hr rapidly successful in many patients (n = 20, open, Galvin and Jelinek, *Arch Emerg Med* 1987;**4**:169–72). In refractory status, an IV bolus of midazolam followed by IV infusion was effective (mean 45 minutes) in 95% of ITU patients and appeared both safe and effective in this extreme situation (n = 19, open, Ulvi et al, *Neurol Sci* 2002;**23**:177–82). It has a sudden onset of action (30–90 seconds) but care is needed as it can cause potentially fatal respiratory depression, as midazolam's half-life prolongs significantly after sustained infusion (n = 2, Naritoku and Sinha, *Neurology* 2000;**54**:1366–8). Continuous midazolam infusion has been reported to be as effective as diazepam, although in one study recurrence and mortality were higher than with diazepam infusion (n = 40, RCT, open, Singhi et al, *J Child Neurol* 2002;**17**:106–10). The IM (Towne and DeLorenzo, *J Emerg Med* 1999, **17**, 323–8) and intranasal routes (n = 47, RCT, *Br Med J* 2000;**321**:83) may also be safe, effective, more socially acceptable and convenient alternatives to IV and rectal diazepam. Buccal midazolam was more effective than rectal diazepam in a multicentre emergency-room trial (n = 177, RCT, McIntyre et al, *Lancet* 2005; **366**:205–10) and was equipotent in another study (n = 43, Baysun et al, *Clin Pediatr* [Phila] 2005;**44**:771–6).

Reviews: general (Shorvon, *Epilepsia* 1998; **39**[Suppl 1]:S15–S23; Fountain and Adams, *Clin Neuropharmacol* 1999;**22**:261–7; Molmes and Riviello, *Pediatr Neurol* 1999;**20**:259–64).

Phenobarbital

A parenteral loading dose of 10–20 mg/kg (*Am J Hosp Pharm* 1993;**50**[Suppl 5]:S5–S16) with a maintenance dose of 5–7 mg/kg/day can be used, although some feel that this bolus dose is too high and phenobarbital should not be given at a dose greater than 100 mg/min (Zeisler and Beck, *Am J Hosp Pharm* 1994;**51**:1578). It has a slow onset and causes cardiac and respiratory depression (review in *Pharmacy World Sci* 1993; **15**:17–28).

Propofol

Propofol has been used (review by Carley and Crawford, *Emerg Med J* 2002;**19**:143–4; see also Claassen *et al*, *Epilepsia* 2002;**43**:146–53), but serious doubts have been expressed about its safety, with two studies showing an increased risk of mortality (review by Niermeijer *et al*, *J Neurol* 2003;**250**:1237–40).

Thiopental (sodium thiopentone)

Induction of anaesthesia with a 2.5% solution (4–8 mg/kg) can be effective, continued with an infusion of 0.2% solution until seizure-free for 24 hours. Phenobarbital should be substituted once seizures stop, as thiopentone accumulates in fat and affects the myocardium.

Thiamine

The use of thiamine may be indicated and prevents serious complications when glucose IV is given as supportive therapy in status (Efawgse, *JAMA* 1994;**270**:854–9; Slovis and Wrenn, *JAMA* 1994;**271**:980–1).

Topiramate *

In refractory status, loading doses of topiramate (10 mg/kg/d for two days then 5 mg/kg/d) may be effective in children (n=3, Perry *et al*, *Epilepsia* 2006;**47**:1070–1; see also n=3, Bensalem and Fakhoury, *Epilepsy Behav* 2003;**4**:757–60), eg. given by nasogastric tube over 2/7 in resistant status (n=3, Kahriman *et al*, *Epilepsia* 2003;**44**:1353–6).

Valproate *

High-dose valproate IV successfully achieved seizure freedom within 15 minutes in 85% patients in a series of emergency cases (n=97, Peters and Pohlmann-Eden, *Seizure* 2005;

14:164–9) and can be given rectally and in patients with hypotension (n=13, Sinha and Naritoku, *Neurology* 2000;**55**:722–4).

■ Unlicensed/possible efficacy

Chloral hydrate

Doses of up to 30 mg/kg at four-hourly intervals given orally or rectally may be effective in resistant status, although onset may be delayed (review in *Ann Emerg Med* 1990;**19**:674–7).

Etomidate

This non-barbiturate induction agent has some anticonvulsant activity. It has a length of action of about 6–10 minutes and doses of 0.2–0.3 mg/kg IV repeated after 20 minutes have been successful. Care would be needed as etomidate may cause involuntary muscle contractions and epileptiform seizures during prolonged IV infusion.

Flumazenil

Flumazenil IV may be effective as an anti-convulsant (n=12, Savic *et al*, *Lancet* 1991; **337**:133–7). In intractable epilepsy, flumazenil may be superior to diazepam, without sedation (n=12, d/b, c/o, Sharief *et al*, *Epilepsy Res* 1993;**15**:53–60), although it may induce seizures (n=67, Schulze-Bonhage and Elger, *Epilepsia* 2000;**41**:186–92). Review by Reisner-Keller and Pham in *Ann Pharmacother* 1995;**29**:530–2.

Lidocaine

A 1% solution given as a 2–3 mg/kg bolus over two minutes can be rapidly effective (ie. within minutes) in cases refractory to other drugs (De Giorgio *et al*, *Epilepsia* 1992;**33**:913–16). The effect lasts about 30 minutes but due to the relatively short duration, a second dose is needed in about 50% of cases (Pascual *et al*, *J Neurol Neurosurg Psychiatry* 1992;**55**:49–51). If successful, IV infusion at 4 mg/kg/hour may be considered. Enhanced seizure activity after high doses and cardiac arrhythmias are potential problems and so it should be used only with caution if any form of heart block or sinus bradycardia exists as it may induce ventricular arrhythmia or complete heart block.

Propofol

Propofol has established anticonvulsant activities. There have been a number of reports of successful use by IV infusion (n = 1, Begemann et al, Epilepsia 2000;**41**:105–09). Propofol has been compared with barbiturates (n = 16) in refractory status epilepticus and a protocol for use proposed (Stecker et al, Epilepsia 1998;**39**:18–26). A retrospective chart analysis suggested propofol and midazolam were of similar efficacy in refractory status epilepticus (n = 14, Prasad et al, Epilepsia 2001;**42**:380–6).

★ No efficacy

Tiagabine *

A retrospective chart analysis suggested tiagabine was more likely to increase NCSE than reduce it (n = 90, Koepp et al, Epilepsia 2005;**46**:1625–32).

GILLES DE LA TOURETTE

see Tourette's syndrome (1.28)

1.18 INSOMNIA

Insomnia, the difficulty in initiating or maintaining sleep, is generally a symptom of a condition, not an illness itself and should always be treated as such. Insomnia can be caused by a variety of external (eg. environment) and internal stimuli (eg. psychiatric illness, stress, emotional conflict, physical illness and drugs, see 5.15), and can be transient, chronic, initial or with early morning wakening. The causes, where possible, should be determined and treated, as well as placing emphasis on sleep hygiene.

Principles of sleep hygiene:

1. Avoid excessive use of caffeine (particularly within 3–4 hours of going to bed), alcohol or nicotine. A hot milky drink at bedtime may promote sleep.
2. Do not stay in bed for prolonged periods if not asleep. Go to another dimly lit room — watching TV can have an alerting effect.
3. Avoid daytime naps or long periods of inactivity.
4. A warm bath or exercise a few hours before bedtime may promote sleep.

5. Avoid engaging in strenuous exercise or mental activity near bedtime (although sex can aid sleep).
6. Make sure that the bed and bedroom are comfortable and avoid extremes of noise, temperature and humidity.
7. Establish a regular bedtime routine, eg. going to bed at the same time and rising at the same time every morning, regardless of sleep duration.
8. Diet — carbohydrate (eg. pasta, etc) helps sleep, but not eating a big meal within about two hours of going to bed. Sugar may inhibit sleep, as may some vitamin supplements.

Role of drugs *

Assuming sleep hygiene is good, any hypnotics should always be used on a PRN basis, as tolerance may develop to the sedative effects within 2–3 weeks (especially with the benzodiazepines). Short-term use for short-term reasons is usually without problem and can be very useful and comforting for the patient. Longer-term use needs the risk:benefit analysis considered carefully. The principles of sleep hygiene should be discussed and any problems corrected before prescribing hypnotics. A meta-analysis of 22 RCTs of BDZs or zolpidem showed a consistent superiority over placebo for up to five weeks but the evidence beyond five weeks is unclear (s = 22, Nowell et al, JAMA 1997;**278**:2170–7, 86 refs). CBT (Smith et al, Am J Psychiatry 2002;**159**:5–11; n = 75, 6/52, Edinger, JAMA 2001;**285**:1856–64), temazepam or in combination have been shown to improve short-term outcomes for older people with persistent insomnia (n=78, RCT, p/c, 24/12, Morin et al, JAMA 1999;**17**:991–9; reviewed in EBMH 1999;**2**:117). Anyone who'd ever taken a hypnotic would know the differences between the Z hypnotics and the BDZs, but NICE failed to recognise this (see fervent rebuffs to NICE by Nutt, J Psychopharmacol 2005;**19**:125–7 and Alford and Verster, J Psychopharmacol 2005;**19**:129–32).

Reviews: * general (Becker, Neurol Clin 2005;**23**:1149–63; Wilson and Nutt, Prescriber 2005;**16**:29–43; Drugs Ther Perspect 2000;**15**:5–9), sleep disorders in elderly (Bain, Am J Geriatr Pharmacother 2006;**4**:168–92; Ancoli-Israel, Sleep 2000;**23**[Suppl 1]:S23–S30) and children (Stores, Prescriber 2001;**12**:29–39), maintenance therapies

(Rosenberg, *Ann Clin Psychiatry* 2006; **18**:49–56), non-drug methods of managing insomnia (Yang and Spielman, *Dis Manage Health Outcomes* 1999; **5**:209–24). use of medicinal plants (Wheatley, *J Psychopharmacol* 2005;**19**:414–21).

BNF listed

BENZODIAZEPINES

Benzodiazepines may be extremely useful in the short-term management of insomnia, helping to facilitate essential high-quality sleep. A meta-analysis of 45 RCTs indicated benzodiazepines are effective in improving sleep latency and duration but ADRs (eg. drowsiness and dizziness) are common, although methodologically these studies are flawed (meta-analysis, s = 45, n = 2672, Holbrook *et al*, *CMAJ* 2000;**162**:225–33; reviewed by Furukawa, *EBMH* 2000;**3**:81). Users of benzodiazepines and zopiclone are also at greater risk of road-traffic accidents, especially if combined with alcohol (involved in accidents, n = 19 386 over three years, Barbone *et al*, *Lancet* 1998;**352**:1331–6). Although relatively safe in overdose, BDZs (especially flunitrazepam and nitrazepam) have been implicated in 39% of drug poisoning suicides in Sweden from 1992–1996, so care is needed (Carlsten *et al*, *Scand J Public Health* 2003;**31**:224–28). Withdrawal of long-term BDZ hypnotics may improve cognitive functioning in the elderly (n = 104, d/b, one year, Curran *et al*, *Psychol Med* 2003;**33**:1223–37; comment by Furukawa, *EBMH* 2004;**7**:46, noting a high drop-out rate).

Flunitrazepam

This longer-acting benzodiazepine may have an abuse potential (Woods and Winger, *J Clin Psychopharmacol* 1997;**17**[3 Suppl 2]:S1–S57; reviewed by Druid *et al*, *Forensic Sci Int* 2001;**122**:136–41), including in combination with other drugs, and is probably under-rated in this respect, especially in forensic settings (Daderman and Edman, *Psychiatry Res* 2001; **103**:27–42).

Flurazepam

Flurazepam is a benzodiazepine with a short half-life but with longer-acting metabolites.

Predicting hypnotic dependence risk
(Tyrer, *Br Med J* 1993;**306**:706–8)

Factor	Score
Benzodiazepine hypnotic used	3
High mean dose	2
Duration of treatment > 3 months	2
Dependent personality	2
Short elimination half-life drug	2
Tolerance or dose escalation	2
Total	
Dose higher than BNF mean	
No dependence, abrupt withdrawal	= 0
Some dependence risk, withdraw over two weeks recommended	= 1–4
Strong dependence risk, withdraw over 4–12 weeks	= 5–8
High risk of dependence, withdraw gradually plus support programme	= 8–13

Loprazolam

Loprazolam is an intermediate-acting benzodiazepine with a half-life of 7–15 hours.

Lormetazepam *

Lormetazepam is an intermediate acting benzodiazepine. In depressive insomnia, lormetazepam given at 8.00 PM seems the optimum time (cf 6.00 PM and 10.00 PM), as it advances sleep without changing morning waking time (n = 38, RCT, p/c, c/o, Benedetti *et al*, *Int Clin Psychopharmacol* 2004;**19**:311–7). Short-term use has no effect on daytime vigilance or motor task performance (n = 12, RCT, d/b, c/o, Iudice *et al*, *Int J Clin Pharmacol Ther* 2002;**40**:304–9) and it may produce minimal psychomotor impairment in younger adults (n = 18, RCT, d/b, p/c, Fabbrini *et al*, *Clin Ther* 2005;**27**:78–83).

Nitrazepam

Nitrazepam is a longer-acting benzodiazepine similar to diazepam, which has active metabolites. Stable plasma levels can be attained in five days, so avoid use in the elderly.

Temazepam *

Temazepam is a shorter-acting benzodiazepine, whose abuse potential has been well recognised. 7.5 mg and 15 mg are equally effective (n = 131, RCT, d/b, Erman et al, Curr Med Res Opin 2004;**20**:441–9).

'Z' HYPNOTICS

The 'Z' hypnotics are now widely used and offer many benefits over the benzodiazepines. NICE in the UK concluded that there was nothing to chose between 'Z' hypnotics and the hypnotic benzodiazepines, a conclusion that has been hotly disputed. **Zolpidem** is potent and quick-acting (often within 15 minutes) and ideal for initiating sleep and has many fans in the pharmaceutical and medical worlds. **Zaleplon** has a similar profile. **Zopiclone** and the benzodiazepines have a slower onset but longer action. For an active comparison, in a single-dose study of zolpidem 10 mg vs zaleplon 10 mg, zolpidem was preferred by 62% of insomniacs (n = 53, RCT, d/b, c/o, Allain et al, Hum Psychopharmacol 2003;**18**:369–74). A large review concluded that the incidence of dependence with zopiclone and zolpidem is remarkably lower than hypnotic BDZs, and that they are relatively safe (n = 58, Hajak et al, Addiction 2003;**98**:1371–8).

Review: comparative tolerability of 'Z' hypnotics (Terzano et al, Drug Saf 2003;**26**:261–82), comprehensive (s = 24, n = 3909, Dundar et al, Hum Psychopharmacol 2004;**19**:305–22).

Zaleplon

Zaleplon is a pyrazolopyrimidine hypnotic, a selective full agonist at the omega-1 benzodiazepine receptor (Noguchi et al, Eur J Pharmacol 2002;**434**:21–8). It can be taken at bedtime or after the person has failed to go to sleep, because peak plasma levels occur after one hour and it has a short half-life (one hour). Zaleplon 5 mg (elderly) and 10 mg (adults) has been shown to be an effective hypnotic, with a significant reduction in sleep latency, comparable to zolpidem, but with no rebound insomnia over four weeks, or withdrawal, unlike zolpidem (n = 615, RCT, Elie et al, J Clin Psychiatry 1999;**60**:536–44). Several studies have shown a lack of residual effects the next day even when 10 mg zaleplon was taken two hours before waking, while residual effects from zolpidem have been detected five hours after a dose (n = 36, Danjou et al, Br J Clin Pharmacol

1999;**48**:367–74; n = 13, d/b, p/c, c/o, Stone et al, Br J Clin Pharmacol 2002;**53**:196–202; n = 30, p/c, c/o, Verster et al, J Clin Psychopharmacol 2002;**22**:576–83). Indeed, one study showed zaleplon 10 mg to have no or minimal residual effects, even when taken as little as an hour before waking, with 20 mg only having residual effects if taken three hours before waking, an advantage compared to zolpidem 10 mg (n = 40, RCT, d/b, p/c, c/o, Hindmarch et al, Hum Psychopharmacol 2001;**16**:159–67) and zopiclone (n = 30, RCT, s/b, p/c, c/o, Vermeeren et al, Sleep 2002;**25**:224–31). Lack of both long-term tolerance and rebound insomnia has been suggested (Dooley and Plosker, Drugs 2000;**60**:413–45). Use in the elderly also appears safe and effective (RCT, 2/52, Hedner et al, Int J Geriatr Psychiatry 2000;**15**:704–12).

Reviews: general (Richardson et al, Med Gen Med 2002;**14**:9; Israel and Kramer, Ann Pharmacother 2002;**36**:852–9; Anon, Am J Health-Sys Pharm 2000;**57**:430–31; Wilson and Nutt, Prescriber 2000;**11**:85–93 and 49–56; Patat et al, Hum Psychopharmacol 2001;**16**:369–92), extensive (Weitzel et al, Clin Ther 2000;**22**:1254–67; Dooley and Plosker, Drugs 2000;**60**:413–45), kinetics (Greenblatt et al, Clin Pharmacol Ther 1998;**64**:553–61), in the elderly (Walsh et al, Clin Drug Investig 2000;**20**:143–9) and pharmacology (Heydorn, Expert Opin Investig Drugs 2000;**9**:841–58).

Zolpidem *

Zolpidem is a imidazopyridine hypnotic which binds preferentially to the omega-1 benzodiazepine receptor. It decreases time to sleep and increases total sleep time and efficiency, but does not affect sleep architecture. It has a rapid onset of action and a short duration. It has been shown to be at least as effective as zopiclone, with less rebound on discontinuation and is better tolerated, eg. no metallic taste (n = 479, d/b, 14/7, Tsutsui et al, J Int Med Res 2001;**29**:163–77). Indeed, lack of residual psychomotor effects in one study led to suggestions that the drug be considered for use in navy fighter and other pilots (n = 12, Sicard et al, Aviat Space Environ Med 1993;**64**:371–5), and for jet-lag (n = 130, RCT, d/b, p/c, c/o, Jamieson et al, Sleep Med 2001;**2**:423–30). In a comparison of zolpidem, zopiclone and lormetazepam in elderly patients, zolpidem caused least cognitive, memory and equilibrium adverse effects and should, thus, be the preferred hypnotic in the elderly (n = 48, RCT, d/b, p/c, c/o, Allain et al, Eur J Clin Pharmacol 2003;59:179–88). In a fascinating study, zolpidem 10mg taken at night up to 3–5 times a week significantly improved overall sleep, which was sustained, with no evidence of rebound, dose escalation or withdrawal, showing that true PRN hypnotic use may be highly effective and safe (n = 199, RCT, p/c, 12/52, Perlis et al, J Clin Psychiatry 2004;65:1128–37).

Reviews: (Lee, CNS Drugs 2004; 18[Suppl 1]:17–23, 43–5; Israel and Swainston-Harrison and Keating, CNS Drugs 2005;19:65–89).

Zopiclone

Zopiclone is an established and safe non-benzodiazepine hypnotic, albeit only licensed in the UK for up to 7.5mg/d for four weeks. Zopiclone is equivalent, but not superior, to BDZs (n = 2672, meta-analysis, Holbrook et al, CMAJ 2000;162:225–33; reviewed by Furukawa, EBMH 2000;3:81). A New Zealand study concluded that the fatal toxicity for zopiclone was not significantly different to BDZs as a group, whereas alprazolam and clomethiazole had greater toxicity (Reith et al, J Toxicol Clin Toxicol 2003;41:975–80). Zopiclone may impair memory storage during sleep (n = 8, d/b, p/c, c/o, Silva et al, Neurosci Res 2003;47:241–3).

Reviews: extensive (Noble et al, Drugs 1998; 55:277–302; Hajak, Drug Saf 1999;21:457–69), kinetics (Fernandez et al, Clin Pharmacokinet 1995;29:431–41), abuse potential/dependence (Lader, J Neurol 1997;244[4 Suppl 1]:S18–S22).

OTHER HYPNOTICS

Antihistamines

Antihistamines may be effective and are often used as OTC sleep aids. Promethazine has a relatively long half-life and a low abuse potential. Diphenhydramine may have an abuse potential (de Nesnera, J Clin Psychiatry 1996;57:136–7) and has been strongly linked to cognitive impairment and decline in older hospitalised patients and is best avoided in this

patient group (n = 426, Agoustini et al, Arch Intern Med 2001;161:2091–7).

Barbiturates

Barbiturates should only be used for severe, intractable insomnia where there are compelling reasons, and only in patients already taking barbiturates (CSM warning in Curr Problems 1996;22:7). Toxicity in overdose can be high.

Chloral hydrate

Chloral has properties similar to the barbiturates and is relatively safe in the elderly as the half-life is not significantly lengthened. An abuse potential exists and it can be toxic in overdose (n = 1, Frankland and Robinson, Can J Psychiatry 2001;46:763–4).

Clomethiazole (chlormethiazole)

Clomethiazole is a thiamine derivative with sedative-hypnotic and anticonvulsant properties. It has a rapid onset of action and short half-life, even in the elderly, although they may be more sensitive to it. Dependence and abuse has been reported, but is not considered too important if the patient is not dependence prone (n = 5, Hession et al, Lancet 1979;ii:953–4). It is unsafe in overdose.

Triclofos

Triclofos is a chloral-related drug with similar actions to chloral but with less gastric irritation and a more palatable taste. Only available as a liquid in the UK.

● Unlicensed/some efficacy

Other sedative drugs at night

Other sedative drugs the patient may already be taking, especially antipsychotics and antidepressants, may be prescribed as a single dose at night. In longer-term therapy most can be given this way. It is also important to avoid the use of 'stimulating' drugs at night, eg. anticholinergics and MAOIs. Low-dose doxepin (25–50mg) has been shown to produce a mild to moderate but significant rapid and sustained improvement in insomnia compared to placebo, although rebound insomnia and side-effects were noted (n = 47, p/c, Hajak et al, J Clin Psychiatry 2001;62:453–63). Many sedative antidepressants are toxic in overdose and may disrupt REM sleep.

Mirtazapine

Insomnia is reported by 90% depressed patients, but stimulation of 5-HT$_2$ receptors is thought to underlie the insomnia and adverse changes in sleep architecture seen with SSRIs/SNRIs. Mirtazapine blocks 5-HT$_2$ receptors and may improve sleep, eg. 30 mg increased sleep efficiency and decreased wakenings (and their duration), but with no effect on REM (n = 20, RCT, d/b, p/c, 3/7, Aslan et al, Sleep 2002;25:677–9). Mirtazapine may in fact help normalise abnormal REM sleep (n = 32, Schittecatte et al, Psychiatry Res 2002;109:1–8). In depressed patients, mirtazapine produces a significant shortening of sleep-onset latency, increases total sleep time, and leads to a marked improvement in sleep efficiency (Thase, J Clin Psychiatry 1999;60[Suppl 17]:28–31; discussion 46–8). It may also significantly improve objective sleep parameters compared to fluoxetine in people with MDD and insomnia (n = 19, RCT, d/b, 8/52, Winokur et al, J Clin Psychiatry 2003;64:1224–9).

Phenothiazines

Promazine at 25–100 mg can be fairly sedative with a low abuse potential, but a significant side-effect profile.

Quetiapine *

Quetiapine 25–10 mg has been shown to improve sleep, probably at least partly through its antihistaminic effects (n = 14, RCT, d/b, p/c, 17/7, Cohrs et al, Psychopharmacology 2004;174:421–9).

Trazodone *

Trazodone may be a borderline antidepressant, but it has marked sedative effects probably via its antihistaminic effect. A review of trazodone as a hypnotic concluded that, except perhaps in depressed people, there is little or no data on efficacy or tolerability, and no dose-response data for sleep, so more research is needed before use can be considered of lower risk (review, James et al, J Clin Psychiatry 2004;65:752–5; see also Mendelson, J Clin Psychiatry 2005;66:469–76).

■ **Unlicensed/possible efficacy**

Alcohol

Alcohol causes sedation but increases slow-wave sleep, reduces and disrupts REM sleep, the diuretic effect is counter-productive and overdose can have serious consequences. Rebound arousal can occur with higher doses when blood concentrations reach zero, leading to awakening (Stradling, Br Med J 1993;306:573–5). Alcohol is thus not recommended for routine medical use. Having said that, it is used widely as self-medication and, unlike chloral, is available in a number of highly palatable formulations (eg. Adnams, Woodfordes, Chalk Hill) and in lager. Interestingly, ageing Scotch Whisky up-regulates GABA receptors more than younger or blended scotch (regardless of ethanol concentration), and is better at calming and inducing sleep (Koda et al, J Agriculture Food Chem 2003; 51:5238–44). You almost certainly read it here first — and possibly last too.

Gabapentin

In alcoholics with persistent insomnia, gabapentin may improve sleep a bit more than trazodone (n = 55, open, 6/52, Karam-Hage and Brower, Psych Clin Neurosci 2003; 57:542–4).

Lavender oil

Ambient lavender oil odour may improve sleep duration in the elderly (understandably open study; n = 4, Hardy et al, Lancet 1995;346:701).

Nicotine

Low concentrations of nicotine can cause mild sedation and relaxation and so a cigarette could help sleep in an anxious person. Higher levels cause arousal and agitation (Stradling, Br Med J 1993;306:573–5).

Paroxetine

Paroxetine 20 mg/d may be an effective treatment for primary insomnia (n = 15, open, Nowell et al, J Clin Psychiatry 1999;60:89–95), although this might be a placebo response (Musa, J Clin Psychiatry 1999;60:795).

Tiagabine *

Although tiagabine 4–6 mg was effective in helping insomnia in the elderly (n = 24, RCT, d/b, p/c, Walsh et al, Sleep 2005:**28**:673–6), a more recent trial failed to show any effect on primary insomnia in the elderly (n = 207, RCT, d/b, p/c, Roth et al, Sleep 2006;**29**:335–41).

✳ No efficacy

Caffeine
Caffeine competes with the inhibitory neuro-transmitter adenosine, causing cortical arousal and decreased sleep. 150 mg of caffeine before retiring has a marked effect on sleep latency, reduces sleep efficacy and REM periods. Its half-life of five hours means any ingested near bedtime will effect sleep latency (Stradling, Br Med J 1993;**306**:573–5). See caffeinism (1.30).

Melatonin *
The data on melatonin is mixed. Most reviews (Armour and Paton, Psychiatr Bull 2004;**28**:222–4; Bramble and Feeham, Child Adolesc Mental Health 2005;**10**:145–9) have concluded that it is not effective, the optimal dose is unknown and outcomes are poorly documented, although short-term use at least seems relatively safe. The most recent and extensive meta-analysis concluded that there was absolutely no evidence that melatonin helps any type of sleep disorder, but that it is safe during short-term use (s = 32, n = 97 + 427 + 651, RCT, Buscemi et al Br Med J 2006;**332**:385–93). Having said that, there are many people who are quite convinced of its efficacy, eg. melatonin improved sleep in major depression (n = 24, open, Dolberg et al, Am J Psychiatry 1998;**155**:1119–21), 2 mg significantly improved sleep efficiency in chronic schizophrenics with poor sleep (n = 19, RCT, Shamir et al, J Clin Psychiatry 2000;**61**:373–7), and a mean dose of 5.4 mg may have some effect on initial insomnia in medically-ill patients (n = 33, RCT, d/b, p/c, 16/7, Andrade et al, J Clin Psychiatry 2001;**62**:41–5).

MANIA AND HYPOMANIA
see Bipolar – Mania and hypomania (1.10.2)

1.19 NARCOLEPSY

Symptoms
Narcolepsy is a rare and often misdiagnosed disabling neurological disorder of excessive daytime sleepiness, sleep paralysis, hypnagogic hallucinations, cataplexy (sudden loss of muscle tone provoked by strong emotions, eg. laughter) and abnormalities in REM sleep. There is a strong genetic linkage, and normally starts in the 20s or 30s. The incidence ranges from 1 in 1000 to 10 000, but appears to be a frequently missed diagnosis. Narcolepsy is probably caused by the loss of a relatively few neurons responsible for producing the neuropeptide hypocretin. Other specific symptoms include cataplexy (an abrupt, bilateral loss of skeletal muscle tone), hypnagogic hallucinations (vivid dreams while falling asleep or waking), sleep paralysis and automatic behaviour (unconscious functioning while asleep).

Role of drugs *
The use of stimulants or modafinil is considered first-line treatment, with some antidepressants useful in some resistant cases, and the risks of pharmacotherapy are usually outweighed by the risks to the patient of vehicle crashes, work-place and other mishaps. The role of oxybate is as yet unclear. However, there is no good evidence that antidepressants are effective for narcolepsy or improve quality of life (s = 2, Vignatelli et al, Cochrane Database Syst Rev 2005;**3**:CD003724).
Reviews: * general (Thorpy, CNS Drugs 2006; **20**:43–50; Mahmood and Black, Curr Treat Options Neurol 2005;**7**:363–71), narco-lepsy-cataplexy (Mignot and Nishino, Sleep 2005; **28**:754–63).

BNF listed

Dexamfetamine
Dexamfetamine 5–50 mg/d can be highly effective, although doses of 40–60 mg/d have been shown to be more effective than lower doses (methamfetamine: n = 16, RCT, d/b, Mitler et al, Sleep 1993;**16**:306–17). If tolerance develops, drug holidays may be necessary. Although dexamfetamine is not immune from problems of chronic stimulant ingestion, many can take it for decades without apparent adverse consequences. Dexamfetamine acts by enhancing release of noradrenaline, dopamine and serotonin, but the stimulant effect appears to be mainly via dopamine.

Modafinil *

Modafinil is chemically a wake-promoting agent and is pharmacologically unrelated to stimulants. It is licensed in the UK for symptomatic relief of excessive sleepiness associated with narcolepsy, sleep apnoea and moderate to severe chronic shift work sleep disorder. Its precise mechanism of action is unknown. It significantly increases daytime sleep latency but does not suppress cataplexy. Modafinil offers advantages because of its lack of rebound phenomena after treatment withdrawal and its low abuse potential. Modafinil 600mg/d appears the maximum tolerated dose (n=32, RCT, Wong et al, J Clin Pharmacol 1999;**39**:30–40), and 200mg BD may be the optimum dose in narcolepsy, compared to 200 or 400mg once daily (n=32, RCT, d/b, 3/52, Schwartz et al, Clin Neuropharmacol 2003;**26**:252–7), with no tolerance in a 40-week follow-up, or withdrawal (RCT, 9/52, n=271, Modafinil study group, Neurology 2000;**54**:1166–75). It may also be useful for narcolepsy associated with closed-head brain injury and with sedating psychotropics (n=10, case series, Teitelman, Am J Psychiatry 2001;**158**:970–1), improving daytime wakefulness in people unresponsive to stimulants (n=150, open, 6/52, Schwartz et al, Sleep Med 2003;**4**:43–9) and for excessive daytime sedation with topiramate (Berigan, Prim Care Companion J Clin Psychiatry 2002; **4**:249–50). Splitting the doses may help promote wakefulness throughout a day compared to once-daily (s=2, n=56, RCT, d/b, Schwartz et al, J Neuropsychiatry Clin Neurosci 2005;**17**:405–12). Studies directly comparing it to amfetamines and methylphenidate, currently the preferred therapies for narcolepsy, are not yet available.
Reviews: * general (Myrick et al, Ann Clin Psychiatry 2004;**16**:101–9), mode of action (Ballon and Feifel, J Clin Psychiatry 2006;**67**:554–66; Stahl, J Clin Psychiatry 2002;**63**:467–8), pharmacokinetics (Robertson and Hellriegel, Clin Pharmacokinet 2003;**42**:123–37).

Sodium oxybate *

Sodium oxybate is now licensed in UK and many countries for cataplexy in adults with narcolepsy. Oxybate probably promotes slow (delta) wave sleep consolidating night-time sleep, increasing stage 3 and 4 sleep, reducing the onset of REM sleep. This improvement in sleep architecture (n=25, open, 10/52, Mamelak et al, Sleep 2004;**27**:1327–34) benefits daytime functioning. The starting dose is 4.5 g/d, titrated slowly every two weeks (or longer) up to 9 g/d as a BD dose (bedtime and 2.5–4 hours later, due to its short half-life). If oxybate is stopped for more than 14 days it should be retitrated, although withdrawal symptoms with therapeutic doses are minimal (n=55, Anon, J Toxicol Clin Toxicol 2003;**41**:131–5). Doses of 4.5, 6 and 9 g a night produces decreases in cataplexy attacks of 57%, 65% and 85% respectively (n=228, RCT, d/b, p/c, 8/52, Xyrem ISG, Sleep Med 2005;**6**:415–21), and a discontinuation study suggested a long-term efficacy (n=55, d/b, mean 21/12, US Xyrem MSG, Sleep Med 2004;**5**:119–23; see also n=136, RCT, d/b, p/c, 4/52, Anon, Sleep 2002;**25**:42–9). Because of its abuse potential (it is the sodium salt of gamma-hydroxybutyrate [GHB]), prescribing is limited to physicians experienced in the treatment of sleep disorders. GHB is abused for its euphoric and weight loss effects, and its amnesic effect has led to it being used as a date-rape drug (Camacho et al, Am J Drug Alcohol Abuse 2005;**31**:601–7; Gonzalez and Nutt, J Psychopharmacol 2005 **19**:195–204).
Reviews: * general (Lemon et al, Ann Pharmacother 2006;**40**:433–40), mode of action (Sills, Curr Opin Pharmacol 2006;**6**:108–13).

+ Combinations

Modafinil + tranylcypromine *

There is a case report of successful use of tranylcypromine and modafinil for refractory narcolepsy (n=1, Clemons et al, Sleep Med 2004;**5**:509–11).

● Unlicensed/some efficacy

Methylphenidate

Methylphenidate 2.5–5mg BD (up to 60mg/d) can be used (see also dexamfetamine above). Tolerance can be a problem, with drug holidays helpful. It has been considered as good as dexamfetamine (n=40, open, Zwicker et al, J Sleep Res 1995;**4**:252–5) and may have a better side-effect profile (reviewed by Challman and Lipsky, *Mayo Clin Proc* 2000;**75**:711–21).

Selegiline

Two trials have shown a potent and dose-related effect, at doses of at least 20mg/d (n = 30, RCT, Mayer et al, *Clin Neuropharmacol* 1995;**18**:306–19; n = 17, d/b, c/o, Hublin et al, *Neurology* 1994;**44**:2095–101), and may be useful in patients who get disturbing side-effects with stimulants.

■ Unlicensed/possible efficacy

Codeine

Codeine has a limited efficacy on subjective measures (n = 8, RCT, Fry et al, *Sleep* 1986;**9**:269–74), but it may occasionally be dramatically effective (n = 1, Benbadis, *Pharmacotherapy* 1996;**16**:463–5) and as effective as **pentazocine** (n = 1, eight years, *Lancet* 1981; i:92).

MAOIs

MAOIs may be useful in refractory cases, although difficult to use (eg. tranylcypromine; n = 1, Gernaat et al, *Pharmacopsychiatry* 1995; **28**:98–100).

Pentazocine

See codeine above.

SSRIs

These are generally considered less effective than tricyclics but some positive results have been reported with, eg. fluoxetine (Langdon et al, *Sleep* 1986;**9**:371–2).

Tricyclics

Clomipramine and imipramine have been used for cataplexy and sleep paralysis, particularly in stimulant-resistant or intolerant patients. Clomipramine at 10–25mg/d can be effective and may have the most specific effect on cataplexy (n = 21, open, Guilleminault et al, *Acta Neurol Scand* 1976;**54**:71–87). Side-effects from tricyclics can be considerable and rebound cataplexy can occur with abrupt withdrawal.

◆ Others

Other drugs used include benzodiazepines such as **clonazepam** (1–4mg/d; Thompson et al, *Ann Neurol* 1982;**12**:62–3), **clonidine** 150–300mcg/d (Salin-Pascual et al, *J Clin Psychiatry* 1985;**46**:528–31), **levodopa** (which may improve vigilance and performance but not capacity to fall asleep rapidly; n = 6, Boivin and Montplaisir, *Neurology* 1991;**41**:1267–9) and **propranolol** (n = 48, 18/12, Meier-Ewart et al, *Sleep* 1985;**8**:95–104; see also n = 4, Kales et al, *Ann Int Med* 1979;**91**:741).

1.20 OBSESSIVE-COMPULSIVE DISORDER (OCD)

Symptoms

OCD probably has a lifetime prevalence of 2–3%, an early onset (childhood or adolescence), and frequently becomes chronic and disabling if untreated. It is characterised by recurrent and intrusive thoughts of compulsive, stereotyped, repetitive behaviour or thoughts, eg. recurrent checking, hand-washing, etc. Functioning is impaired by obsessive thoughts and rituals. Resisting these thoughts results in heightened anxiety.

Role of drugs *

There is much evidence for the cause of OCD being related to a dysfunctional serotonin system, and SSRIs and clomipramine have been shown to be effective. The available data (meta-analyses/reviews by Ackerman and Greenland, *J Clin Psychopharmacol* 2002;**22**:309–17; Hollander and Kahn, *EBMH* 2003;**6**:23; s = 9, n = 278, RCT, b/d, Bloch et al, *Mol Psychiatry* 2006: 11:622–32) concludes that:

1. **Drug:** Only antidepressants affecting the serotonin system are effective:
   - the SSRIs as a class are similarly effective to clomipramine and both are superior to non-serotonergic drugs
   - clomipramine is perhaps slightly more effective than SSRIs
   - tricyclics (other than clomipramine) and mirtazapine seem ineffective
   - concomitant depression does not seem necessary for improvement in obsessive-compulsive symptoms.

2. **Dose:** the daily dose usually needs to be high, eg. 250–300mg clomipramine, or 60–80mg fluoxetine or paroxetine. Lower doses are unlikely to have any clinically significant effect.

3. **Duration:** Response is slow and may not occur for several weeks. Continue with the maximum tolerated dose of an SSRI for three months (25% respond given adequate dose and duration). A minimum of 1–2 years pharmacotherapy is recommended, as relapse is common on discontinuation and the risks of long-term therapy may be outweighed by the risks of relapse and its consequences.

4. **Treatment resistance:** Add an antipsychotic (best evidence for risperidone and haloperidol), although only 30% will show a meaningful response.

5. **Discontinuation:** Very gradual discontinuation over several months is recommended.

In the UK, NICE has produced guidance on OCD and uses a stepped care approach. However, it did not emphasise the need to use higher doses for prolonged periods of time. Drugs may only reduce symptomatology by 30–60%, but many patients consider this a significant benefit. Switching from an SSRI (paroxetine) to venlafaxine or vice versa if no response may be an effective strategy (n = 150, RCT, d/b, Denys et al, J Clin Psychiatry 2004;**65**:37–43; review by Bhui, EBMH 2004;**7**:114). The effects of SSRIs may be enhanced by CBT (n = 48[c = 43], O'Connor et al, Acta Psychiatr Scand 2006;**113**:408–19), especially if the CBT is added immediately after drug response (n = 96[c = 59], RCT, s/b, 12/52, Tenneij et al, J Clin Psychiatry 2005;**66**:1169–75; comment by Cottraux, EBMH 2006;**9**:53). Although clearly effective in many people when used properly, there is some doubt about the long-term outcome and efficacy of SSRIs in OCD (n = 60, 1–5 years, Alonso et al, J Clin Psychiatry 2001;**62**:535–40).

Reviews: * general (Fineberg and Gale, Int J Neuropsychopharmacol 2004;**28**:1–23; Mukhopadhyay, Prescriber 2003;**14**:39–48), WCA guidelines (Greist et al, CNS Spectr 2003, [Suppl 1], S7–S16), BAP evidence-based guidelines (Baldwin et al, J Psychopharmacol 2005;**19**:567–96), drug treatment options (Kaplan and Hollander, Psychiatr Serv 2003;**54**:1111–18; McDonough and Kennedy, Harv Rev Psychiatry 2002;**10**:127–37), antipsychotics in OCD (Fineberg et al, J Psychopharmacol 2006;**20**:97–103), algorithms for pharmacotherapy (Albert et al, Panminerva Med 2002;**44**:83–91).

BNF listed

Clomipramine

Clomipramine is clearly superior to placebo and non-serotonergic drugs (s = 11, d/b, c/o, Piccinelli et al, Br J Psychiatry 1995;**166**:424–43; see also review of meta-analyses in introduction). IV clomipramine may be effective in patients intolerant or non-responsive to oral clomipramine (n = 54, RCT, Fallon et al, Arch Gen Psychiatry 1998;**55**:918–24; n = 15, RCT, Koran et al, Am J Psychiatry 1997;**154**:396–401).

Escitalopram *

Escitalopram is now licensed for the treatment of OCD at a dose of 10–20mg/d. Escitalopram 10mg/d was as effective as (and better tolerated than) paroxetine 40mg/d and escitalopram 20mg/d was effective as early as six weeks (n = 466, RCT, d/b, p/c, 24/52, Stein et al, Curr Med Res Opin 2007;**23**:701–11). Long-term efficacy has also been shown in an open 16-week study, followed by a discontinuation phase in the 320 responders, where escitalopram had a relapse rate of 23% compared to 52% in the placebo group (n = 468, RCT, d/b, 24/52, Fineberg et al, Eur Neuropsychopharmacol 2007;**17**:480–9).

Fluoxetine

Fluoxetine has shown a significant clinical effect at 20–60mg/d, developing over 13 weeks, and continuing to be effective for at least nine months with few side-effects (eg. n = 130, RCT, p/c, 12/12, Romano et al, J Clin Psychopharmacol 2001;**21**:46–52). It may also be effective in children, but takes over eight weeks to reach full effect (n = 43, RCT, p/c, 16/52, Liebowitz et al, J Am Acad Child Adolesc Psychiatry 2002; **41**: 1431–8).

Fluvoxamine *

Fluvoxamine has been shown to be partially or very effective in several trials (eg. n = 38, d/b, p/c, 10/52, Jenike et al, Am J Psychiatry 1990;**147**:1209–15). It may be equivalent to clomipramine but better tolerated (n = 227, RCT, d/b, 10/52, Mundo et al, Hum Psychopharmacol 2001;**16**:461–8), showing a clinical effect in about 4–6 weeks, although it may not be of any additional benefit in patients non-responsive to fluoxetine or clomipramine, except where side-effects had been limiting (open, Mattes, *Am J Psychiatry* 1994;**151**:1524). Chronic OCD patients usually need additional support to maintain an acute treatment response (n = 30, seven years, Rufer et al, *Eur Arch Psych Clin Neurosci* 2005;**255**:121–8).

Paroxetine

Paroxetine is licensed for the symptoms of OCD and for relapse prevention at doses of 40–60 mg. Higher doses are necessary, particularly in acute OCD, as 20 mg/d is not effective (n = 348, RCT, d/b, p/c, 12/52, Hollander et al, *J Clin Psychiatry* 2003;**64**:1113–21). Paroxetine is equipotent to clomipramine, but better tolerated in adults (n = 406, RCT, 6/12, Zohar et al, *Br J Psychiatry* 1996;**169**:468–74) and in children with OCD (n = 20, open 12/52, Rosenberg et al, *J Am Acad Child Adolesc Psychiatry* 1999;**38**:1180–5).

Sertraline *

Sertraline is licensed for OCD in adults and also in children and adolescents (dose: 6–12 years, 25–50 mg/d; 13–17 years, use the adult dose but with no dose increases after less than a week, and a lower body weight may require lower doses). Sertraline has been shown to be effective in many studies (eg. n = 167, RCT, p/c, 12/52, Kronig et al, *J Clin Psychopharmacol* 1999;**19**:172–6), with a possible dose-response relationship, eg. 50 mg/d and 200 mg/d were more potent than 100 mg/d, but adverse effects were dose-related (n = 324, p/c, Greist, *Arch Gen Psychiatry* 1995;**52**:289–95). It appears slightly more effective than fluoxetine but was as well-tolerated in an extended OCD trial (n = 150, RCT, d/b, 6/12, Bergeron et al, *J Clin Psychopharmacol* 2002;**22**:148–54). Rapid titration of sertraline to 150 mg/d over five days may give a faster onset of action in acute OCD, with similar tolerability to slower (15 days) titration (n = 32, s/b, 12/52, Bogetto et al, *Eur Neuropsychopharm* 2002;**12**:181–6). A relapse prevention effect has been shown in a maintenance study, where the sertraline group had a lower drop-out than placebo (9% vs 24%), with lower acute exacerbations (12% vs 35%), and with lack of prominent discontinuation symptoms after cessation (n = 649, 223 completers, RCT, 6/12, Koran et al, *Am J Psychiatry* 2002;**159**:88–95; review by Soomro, *EBMH* 2002;**5**:115). High-dose sertraline (up to 400 mg/d) may be effective in refractory

OCD (n = 66, RCT, d/b, 12/52, Ninan et al, *J Clin Psychiatry* 2006;**67**:15–22).

Review: * combination and augmentation therapies (Walsh and McDougle, *Expert Opin Pharmacother* 2004;**5**:2059–67).

Antipsychotics + SSRIs/clomipramine *

Many antipsychotics have been used as SSRI-augmentation in resistant OCD. If successful, they should probably continue for at least several months, as relapse on discontinuation is high (n = 18, retrospective chart, Maina et al, *Int Clin Psychopharmacol* 2003;**18**:23–8). **Risperidone** has been shown to be effective as SSRI augmentation (eg. n = 70, RCT, 12/52, McDougle et al, *Arch Gen Psychiatry* 2000;**57**:794–801; comment by Ramasubbu, *Arch Gen Psychiatry* 2002;**59**:472–3; see also n = 16[c = 12], p/c, d/b, c/o, 9/52, Li et al, *J Clin Psychiatry* 2005;**66**:736–43), with doses of 3 mg/d more effective than lower doses (Baker, *J Clin Psychiatry* 1998;**59**:131–3). Really low-dose adjunctive risperidone (0.5 mg/d) may be effective in patients non-responsive to standard doses of fluvoxamine (n = 45, RCT, d/b, p/c, 6/52, Erzeovesi et al, *Eur Neuropsychopharmacol* 2005;**15**:69–74). Smaller studies have suggested some efficacy for **olanzapine** 5 mg/d in SSRI-resistant OCD (n = 23, 43% responders, open, Bogetto et al, *Psychiatry Res* 2000;**96**:91–8; n = 26, open, two years, Marazziti et al, *J Psychopharmacol* 2005;**19**:392–4) and produced a 25% improvement in 46% patients (n = 26, d/b, p/c, Bystritsky et al, *J Clin Psychiatry* 2004;**65**:565–8) but in the only RCT, there was no additional advantage of adding olanzapine in fluoxetine-refractory OCD patients (n = 44, RCT, p/c, 6/52, Shapira et al, *Biol Psychiatry* 2004;**55**:553–5). **Quetiapine** 300 mg/d was a successful adjunct to SSRIs in resistant OCD (n = 40, RCT, 8/52, d/b, p/c, Denys et al, *J Clin Psychiatry* 2004;**65**:1040–8) and produced significant improvement in 65% compared to none with placebo augmentation (n = 27, s/b, 8/52, Atmaca et al, *Int Clin Psychopharmacol* 2002;**17**:115–9). In another case series, however, 150 mg/d was largely ineffective as adjunctive treatment in SSRI-resistant OCD (n = 8, open, Sevincok and

Topuz, *J Clin Psychopharmacol* 2003;**23**:448–50). A small pilot study suggested **aripiprazole** may have some efficacy as monotherapy or as SSRI augmentation (n = 8, open, 8/52, Connor et al, *J Clin Psychiatry* 2005;**66**:49–51).

Buspirone + SSRIs

A trial of **fluvoxamine** and buspirone was not successful (n = 33, RCT, p/c, McDougle, *Am J Psychiatry* 1993;**150**:647–9; 819–21), but there are case reports with other SSRIs, eg. **sertraline** (n = 2, Menkes, *Br J Psychiatry* 1995;**167**:823–4; n = 1, Veivia et al, *J Pharm Technology* 1995; **11**:50–2) and **fluoxetine** (Alessi and Bos, *Am J Psychiatry* 1991;**148**:1605).

Carbamazepine + clomipramine

Carbamazepine may be useful as augmentation in refractory OCD (n = 1, Iwata et al, *J Clin Psychiatry* 2000;**161**:528–9).

Clomipramine + SSRIs

Citalopram plus clomipramine was markedly more effective than clomipramine in treatment-resistant OCD (n = 16, open, 3/12, Pallanti et al, *Eur Psychiatry* 1999;**14**:101–6).

Inositol + SSRIs

One trial showed inositol at 18 g/d to significantly reduce Y-BOCS rating scale scores (n = 13, d/b, c/o, 6/52, Fux et al, *Am J Psychiatry* 1996;**153**:1219–21) and, in another, 30% patients responded to inositol augmentation of SSRIs (n = 10, open, Seedat and Stein, *Int Clin Psychopharmacol* 1999;**14**:353–6).

Lithium + SSRIs

The only study of lithium augmentation of fluvoxamine in OCD was unable to show a clinically significant effect (n = 30, d/b, p/c, McDougle et al, *J Clin Psychopharmacol* 1991;**11**:175–84).

Mirtazapine + citalopram *

Mirtazapine 15–30 mg/d decreased the time to response to citalopram from eight weeks to four weeks, but with similar response rates from weeks 8 to 12, which could be significant in severe OCD, although a d/b study would be needed to confirm this (n = 49, s/b, 12/52, Pallanti et al, *J Clin Psychiatry* 2004;**65**:1394–9; comment by Schüle and Laakmann, *EBMH*

2005;**8**:42). In mirtazapine-responders, discontinuation led to relapse suggesting a prophylactic effect (n = 30, d/b, p/c, 8/52, Koran et al, *J Clin Psychiatry* 2005;**66**:515–20).

Pindolol + SSRIs

Pindolol 7.5 mg/d may possibly improve the response to paroxetine in multiple SSRI-resistant OCD (n = 14, d/b, p/c, 6/52, Dannon et al, *Eur Neuropsychopharmacol* 2000;**10**:165–9).

Tricyclics (combined)

Addition of desipramine to clomipramine in SSRI-resistant OCD patients did **not** enhance its action (Barr et al, *Am J Psychiatry* 1997;**154**:1293–5), but addition of nortriptyline 50 mg/d to clomipramine 150 mg/d produced a more rapid onset of action than clomipramine alone (n = 30, RCT, Noorbala et al, *J Clin Pharm Ther* 1998;**23**:155–9).

● Unlicensed/some efficacy

Citalopram

Citalopram has been shown to be as effective as fluvoxamine and paroxetine (n = 30, s/b, Mundo et al, *J Clin Psychopharmacol* 1997;**17**:267–71; review by Pato, *Int Clin Psychopharmacol* 1999;**14**[Suppl 2]:S19–S26). Very high dose citalopram (160 mg/d) may be effective in severe, resistant OCD (n = 1, Bejerot and Bodlund, *Acta Psychiatr Scand* 1998;**98**:423–4). Predictors of response include longer duration of more severe illness, no previous SSRI and an adequate dose for adequate duration (RCT, Stein et al, *Int Clin Psychopharmacol* 2001;**16**:357–61).

Venlafaxine

Venlafaxine has been shown to be as effective as paroxetine but not superior (n = 150, RCT, d/b, Denys et al, *J Clin Psychopharmacol* 2003; **23**:568–75). In one trial venlafaxine (n = 26; 225–350 mg/d) was almost as effective as clomipramine (n = 47; 150–225 mg/d) but better tolerated (n = 73, RCT, s/b, 12/52, Albert et al, *J Clin Psychiatry* 2002;**63**:1004–9), and another showed a slight positive effect for venlafaxine 225 mg/d in OCD (n = 16, d/b, p/c, 8/52, Yaryura-Tobias and Neziroglu, *Arch Gen Psychiatry* 1996;**53**:653–5). There are case reports of response in treatment-resistance, and rapidly and dramatically to 150–300mg/d (n = 3, Ananth et al, Am J Psychiatry 1995;**152**:1832; Grossman and Hollander, Am J Psychiatry 1996;**153**:576–7).

Reviews: * SNRIs in OCD (Phelps and Cates, Ann Pharmacother 2005;**39**:136–40; Dell'Osso et al, J Clin Psychiatry 2006;**67**:600–10).

■ Unlicensed/possible efficacy

Clozapine
Clozapine has been used for OCD symptoms in schizophrenia (n = 15, open, Reznik et al, Pharmacopsychiatry 2004;**37**:52–6), but an open study was unable to show any effect for clozapine in refractory OCD (n = 10, McDougle et al, Am J Psychiatry 1995;**152**:1812–4) and there are a number of reported cases of OCD actually being unmasked or induced by clozapine (Baker et al, J Clin Psychiatry 1992; **53**:439–42).

Gabapentin
Gabapentin up to 3600mg/d has been used in patients only partially responsive to fluoxetine 30–100mg/d (n = 5, open, 6/52, Cora-Locatelli et al, J Clin Psychiatry 1998;**59**:480–1).

Memantine *
Memantine 15mg/d as antidepressant augmentation may be rapidly effective in some refractory cases (n = 2, Pasquini and Biondi, Prog Neuropsychopharmacol Biol Psychiatry 2006; **30**: 1173–5) and 20mg/d produced a response over 3/52 as an adjunct to clomipramine 300mg/d and sulpiride 400mg/d, maintained over 3/12 (n = 1, Poyurovsky et al, Am J Psychiatry 2005;**162**:2191–2).

Morphine *
Rather bizarrely, once-weekly oral morphine was effective in some treatment-resistant OCD patients, unlike lorazepam or placebo (n = 23, RCT, d/b, c/o, p/c, 6/52, Koran et al, J Clin Psychiatry 2005;**66**:353–9).

Nicotine *
Nicotine chewing gum 4mg has improved treatment-resistant OCD (n = 1, Pasquini et al, Prog Neuropsychopharmacol Biol Psychiatry 2005;**29**:157–9).

Ondansetron
Ondansetron 3mg/d was effective in some OCD patients (n = 8[c = 6], open, 8/52, Hewlett et al, J Clin Psychiatry 2003;**64**:1025–30).

Oxcarbazepine
There is a case of successful use of oxcarbazepine for OCD (n = 1, McMeekin, J S C Med Assoc 2002;**98**:316–20).

Phenelzine
Phenelzine 75mg/d was shown to be equipotent as clomipramine 225mg/d in one trial (n = 30, d/b, Vallejo et al, Br J Psychiatry 1992;**161**:665–70) but, in a randomised comparison (n = 60, RCT, Jenike et al, Am J Psychiatry 1997;**154**:1261–4), phenelzine 60mg/d was shown to be inferior to fluoxetine (80mg/d) except in patients with asymmetry or other atypical obsession, and no preferential response was detected in patients with high anxiety levels.

Riluzole *
Riluzole 100mg/d appeared to have some activity as an adjunct in a treatment-resistant OCD (n = 13, open, Coric et al, Biol Psychiatry 2005;**58**:424–8).

Topiramate *
Topiramate (mean 250mg/d) may be useful as an adjunct to SSRIs in resistant OCD (n = 16, < 13/52, Van Ameringen et al, Depress Anxiety 2006;**23**:1–5).

Tramadol
There is a report of rapid reduction in OCD symptoms with 100mg/d tramadol, allowing fluoxetine to be introduced as the long-term treatment (n = 1, Goldsmith et al, Am J Psychiatry 1999;**156**:660–1).

Tricyclics (except clomipramine)
Many tricyclics have been studied and some have been shown to be superior to placebo but generally they are not as potent as clomipramine or the SSRIs, eg. imipramine (Volavka et al, Psychiatry Res 1985;**14**:85–93) and amitriptyline. Nortriptyline (Thoren et al, Arch Gen Psychiatry 1980;**37**:1281–5) has been shown to be ineffective.

◆ Others

Other drugs tried include **buspirone** (Pato et al, Am J Psychiatry 1991;**148**:127–9; extensive review in Ann Pharmacother 1992;**26**:1248–51; see also combinations), and **diphenhydramine** up to 250mg/d (n=28, d/b, c/o, 6/52, Hewlett et al, J Clin Psychopharmacol 1992;**12**:420–30).

* No efficacy

Clonazepam *

Clonazepam seems ineffective as monotherapy in treating OCD, although it may be helpful for specific sub-groups with co-morbid anxiety (n=27, d/b, p/c, 10/52, Hollander et al, World J Biol Psychiatry 2003;**4**:30–4) and as augmentation of sertraline (n=37, RCT, d/b, p/c, 12/52, Crockett et al, Ann Clin Psychiatry 2004;**16**:127–32).

Flutamide

The anti-androgen flutamide was almost completely ineffective in one trial (n=8, Altemus et al, J Clin Psychiatry 1999;**60**:442–5).

Oxytocin

Initial enthusiasm was not confirmed in a study of intranasal administration (n=3, Salzberg and Swedo, Am J Psychiatry 1992;**149**:713–4).

Tricyclics (some)

See possible efficacy section.

Trazodone

A study showed trazodone up to 300mg/d to be equipotent with placebo (n=21, d/b, c/o, 10/52, Pigott et al, J Clin Psychopharmacol 1992; **12**:156–62).

1.21 PANIC DISORDER
see also Anxiety disorder (1.6)

Symptoms

Panic disorder is usually characterised by sudden attacks of anxiety, where physical symptoms predominate, peaking within 10 minutes and with an associated fear of serious consequences, eg. heart attack. These attacks need to include four of the following: palpitations, abdominal distress/nausea, numbness/tingling, inability to breathe or shortness of breath, choking, sweating, chest pains, dizziness, depersonalisation (common), flushes/chills, fear of dying and trembling/shaking (extensive review by Johnson et al, Drugs 1995;**49**:328–44, 150 refs). The lifetime prevalence is up to 3.5%, with a point prevalence of 1.5% (males) and 2.8% (females). There is frequently a family history.

Role of drugs

In general, short-term benefits may be gained with drug therapy. The main principle is to start low and go slow (to minimise initial jitteriness), and accept that response may take some time to occur, eg. SSRIs are effective long-term with a slow onset of action, initial worsening (meta-analysis, 34 RCTs, nine open, n=2367; Bakker et al, Acta Psychiatr Scand 2002;**106**:163–7; although efficacy may have been overestimated: s=12, Otto et al, Am J Psychiatry 2001;**158**:1989–92) and some exacerbation on discontinuation. Benzodiazepines have a quicker onset of action but obvious potential problems, eg. the dependence potential and tolerance. There is insufficient data on MAOIs and buspirone. Placebo responders tend to show an early and temporary remission. Although paroxetine and clomipramine may be superior to CBT and placebo (n=131, d/b, 12/52, Bakker et al, J Clin Psychiatry 1999;**60**:831–8, MS), combined therapy is generally better than for either therapy alone, at least in the maintenance phase (CBT vs imipramine, a poorly-tolerated and less serotonergic agent; n=326, RCT, 12/12, Barlow et al, JAMA 2000;**283**:2529–36; Glass, JAMA 2000;**283**:2573–4). Relapse rates at 6–12 months can be as high as 75% on discontinuation of psychotropics, and so continued treatment and support is necessary in most patients over at least a year (Scott et al, Adv Psychiatr Treat 2001;**7**:275–82).

Reviews: * general (Roy-Byrne et al, Lancet 2006;**368**:1023–32; Kumar and Oakley-Browne, Clin Evid 2006;**15**:1438–52; Katon, N Engl J Med 2006;**354**:2360–7; Cloos, Curr Opin Psychiatry 2005;**18**:45-50, 44 refs; Kumar and Browne, EBMH 2003;**6**:34–37; Sheeham, J Clin Psychiatry 2003;**63**[Suppl 14]:17–21;), BAP evidence-based guidelines (Baldwin et al, J Psychopharmacol 2005; **19**:567–96); WCA guidelines (Pollack et al, CNS Spectr 2003;**8**[Suppl 1]:17–30), long-term (Doyle and Pollack, J Clin Psychiatry 2004;**65**[Suppl

5]:S24–S28), in older people (Flint and Gagnon, *Drugs Aging* 2003;**20**:881–91), refractory panic (Bandelow and Ruther, *CNS Spectr* 2004, **9**, 725–39; Mathew *et al, Psychopharmacol Bull* 2001; **35**:97–110; Slaap and den Boer, *Depress Anxiety* 2001;**14**:112–22), epidemiology (Batelaan *et al, Tijdschr Psychiatr* 2006;**48**:195–205).

BNF listed

Benzodiazepines *

Benzodiazepines are rapidly effective and are thus useful in people needing immediate relief (review by Kasper and Resinger, *Eur Neuropsychopharmacol* 2001;**11**:307–21). Many benzodiazepines have been studied, eg. **clonazepam** is longer-acting, with 1–2 mg/d the best balance between benefit and tolerability (n = 413, RCT, p/c, 13/52, Rosenbaum *et al, J Clin Psychopharmacol* 1997;**17**:390–400) and it may have a sustained therapeutic effect over a prolonged period (n = 67, three years, open, Nardi *et al, Psychiatry Res* 2005;**137**:61–70). Early co-administration of clonazepam with sertraline may facilitate early improvement in panic symptoms (n = 50, RCT, d/b, Goddard *et al, Arch Gen Psychiatry* 2001;**58**:681–86). **Alprazolam** (n = 23, d/b, p/c, Bond *et al, J Affect Disord* 1995;**35**:117–23) and **diazepam** have also been used (n = 241, RCT, p/c, d/b, 8/52, Noyes *et al, J Clin Psychiatry* 1996;**57**:349–55). The main problem is discontinuation, where relapse may be more common with shorter-acting benzodiazepines, eg. alprazolam (n = 50, Noyes *et al, Am J Psychiatry* 1991;**148**:517–23) so transfering to an SSRI in is advised.

Citalopram

Citalopram is licensed in the UK for panic disorder, with or without agoraphobia. The starting dose in panic disorder is 10 mg/d for one week, increasing to 20–30 mg/d as the optimum dose (n = 475, RCT, p/c, d/b, 8/52, Wade *et al, Br J Psychiatry* 1997;**170**:549–53), to a maximum of 60 mg/d. Citalopram may also control phobic symptoms in panic, especially at 20–30 mg/d (n = 475, RCT, 8/52, Leinonen *et al, J Psychiatry Neurosci* 2000;**25**:25–32). After an eight-week trial (n = 475), an optional continuation phase (n = 279) showed 20–60 mg/d citalopram to be effective and well-tolerated over one year

(n = 279, RCT, d/b, 8/52, Lepola *et al, J Clin Psychiatry* 1998;**59**:528–34). It may be quicker acting than paroxetine, but equipotent (n = 58, RCT, s/b, 60/7, Perna *et al, Pharmacopsychiatry* 2001;**34**:85–90). Escitalopram and citalopram appear equally effective in panic disorder (n = 366, RCT, d/b, p/c, 10/52, Stahl *et al, J Clin Psychiatry* 2003;**64**:1322–7, MS).

Escitalopram

Escitalopram is licensed in the UK for panic disorder, with or without agoraphobia. The initial dose is 5 mg/d for the first week, then 10 mg/d, increasing to a maximum of 20 mg/d. Escitalopram and citalopram appear equally effective in panic disorder (n = 366, RCT, d/b, p/c, 10/52, Stahl *et al, J Clin Psychiatry* 2003; **64**:1322–7, MS).

Paroxetine *

Paroxetine is licensed in the UK for panic and agoraphobia. A 10 mg/d starting dose is recommended. Several studies have shown a significant effect, eg. as effective as citalopram (n = 58, RCT, s/b, 60/7, Perna *et al, Pharmacopsychiatry* 2001;**34**:85–90) and as effective as clomipramine, but with a more rapid onset of action and less side-effects (eg. n = 367, d/b, p/c, 12/52, Lecrubier *et al, Acta Psychiatr Scand* 1997;**95**:145–52). The optimum effective dose is 40 mg/d (n = 278, d/b, p/c, Ballenger *et al, Am J Psychiatry* 1998;**155**:36–42). Continued improvement is maintained with low drop-outs (n = 176, RCT, d/b, p/c, 36/52 follow-on, Lecrubier *et al, Acta Psychiatr Scand* 1997;**95**:153–60). After 12 months treatment, a further year of paroxetine did not reduce relapse rates compared to discontinuation in panic disorder (with or without agoraphobia) (n = 143, open, three years, Dannon *et al, BMC Psychiatry* 2004;**11**:16). As with other drugs, combining with CBT is significantly more effective than placebo plus CBT in reducing the number of panic attacks, as well as being well-tolerated (n = 120, RCT, p/c, 12/52, Oehrberg *et al, Br J Psychiatry* 1995;**167**:374–9).

Tricyclics

Tricyclics are established as effective in panic disorder. They may take four weeks to start to work and 12 weeks for maximal effect. Initial jitteriness is a common problem and so it is usually necessary to start at a low dose (10–25 mg/d) and warn patients that they may feel more anxious initially (n=81, RCT, p/c, 8/52, Uhlenhuth et al, J Affect Disord 1989;**17**:261–70). **Clomipramine** has been shown to be effective at less than 100 mg/d (eg. n=180, d/b, Caillard et al, Acta Psychiatr Scand 1999;**99**:51–8) and with a biphasic response, symptoms worsening over 12 weeks before improving. It is as effective as paroxetine in panic disorder, but with a slower onset of action and more side-effects (n=367, d/b, p/c, 12/52, Lecrubier et al, Acta Psychiatr Scand 1997;**95**:145–52), and with efficacy maintained over 36 weeks in a follow-up study (n=176, RCT, Lecrubier et al, Acta Psychiatr Scand 1997;**95**:153–60). **Imipramine** is effective (vs placebo) in all studies using doses above 150 mg/d (Br J Psychiatry 1989;**155**[Suppl 6]:S46–S52). A modest dose of **trimipramine** 50 mg/d proved effective in multi-drug resistant panic disorder (n=1, Cerra, Am J Psychiatry 2006;**163**:548). Long-term maintenance is needed for most patients, especially with a high baseline BDI and who need higher doses to reach remission (n=51, RCT, Lotufo-Neto et al, J Clin Psychopharmacol 2001;**15**:13–7). Weight gain is a specific and significant adverse effect, as are dry mouth, sweating and increased heart rate, and sexual dysfunction (n=51, RCT, p/c, d/b, 12/12, Mavissakalian et al, J Clin Psychopharmacol 2002;**22**:155–61). A two-year follow-up of imipramine shows a continued and substantial prophylactic efficacy (n=18, RCT, Mavissakalian and Perel, Ann Clin Psychiatry 2001;**13**:63–7). Early detection of relapse may be a viable alternative to long-term therapy (n=51, RCT, d/b, 12/12, Mavissakalian and Perel, J Clin Psychopharmacol 2002;**22**:294–9).

+ Combinations

Olanzapine + paroxetine *
There is a case of complete remission when olanzapine was added to paroxetine (n=1, Chao, Pharmacopsychiatry 2004; **37**:239–40).

Clonazepam + paroxetine
Use of clonazepam, slowly tapered after four weeks, as an initial adjunct to paroxetine was as affective as continued clonazepam,

facilitating longer-term monotherapy (n=60, RCT, p/c, 12/52, Pollack et al, J Psychopharmacol 2003;**17**:276–82).

● Unlicensed/some efficacy

Fluvoxamine
Fluvoxamine has been compared favourably with placebo and cognitive therapy (n=55, RCT, p/c, 8/52, Black et al, Arch Gen Psychiatry 1993;**50**:44–50; n=32, RCT, d/b, c/o, Pigott et al, Arch Gen Psychiatry 1993;**50**:44–50), but not all placebo trials have shown efficacy. It may have a biphasic response, with symptoms worsening over 12 weeks before improving, although one study noted a potent anti-panic action with a relatively rapid onset (n=188, RCT, p/c, 8/52, Asnis et al, Psychiatry Res 2001;**103**:1–14).

Fluoxetine
Fluoxetine is effective when initial doses are kept very low (2.5–5 mg/d) then increased, as higher doses produce side-effects such as anxiety and over-stimulation, possibly due to serotonergic supersensitivity. Fluoxetine 20 mg/d is clearly superior to placebo over a range of symptoms in panic disorder (n=243, RCT, Michelson et al, Am J Psychiatry 1998;**155**:1570–77; RCT, p/c, 24/52, Michelson et al, Br J Psychiatry 1999;**174**:213–8). If there is no response by 6/52, it may benefit from an increase up to 60 mg/d (12/52, RCT, Michelson et al, Br J Psychiatry 2001;**179**:514–8). Once weekly fluoxetine (10–60 mg/week) has proved successful as maintenance (n=10, open, 24/12, Emmanuel et al, J Clin Psychiatry 1999;**60**:299–301).

Gabapentin *
Gabapentin 600–3600 mg/d may have anxiolytic effects in severe panic disorder (n=103, RCT, d/b, p/c, 8/52, Pande et al, J Clin Psychopharmacol 2000;**20**:467–71).

Sertraline *
Pooled data indicates that sertraline is an effective treatment for panic disorder, even in people with risk factors for poor response (n=664, s=4, d/b, Pollack et al, J Clin Psychiatry 2000;**61**:922–7) and prevents relapse of panic (n=240, RCT, d/b, p/c, 8/52, Kamijima et al, Int

Clin Psychopharmacol 2005;**20**:265–73). Early response predicts final remission, a useful aid to decision-making (n = 544, p/c, Pollack *et al*, *J Psychiatr Res* 2002;**36**:229–36). Sertraline 50-150 mg/d is equivalent in efficacy to paroxetine (40–60 mg/d) but better tolerated and easier to stop (n = 225, RCT, d/b, 12/52, Bandelow *et al*, *J Clin Psychiatry* 2004;**65**:405–13; MS; n = 183, 52 + 28/52, Rapaport *et al*, *Acta Psychiatr Scand* 2001;**104**:289–98).

■ Unlicensed/possible efficacy

Inositol

In one trial, inositol 12 g/d improved panic symptoms, whereas lorazepam did not (n = 25, d/b, p/c, c/o, 4/52, Benjamin *et al*, *Am J Psychiatry* 1995;**152**:1084–6) and was superior to fluvoxamine 150 mg/d in reducing panic attacks (n = 20, RCT, c/o, 8/52, Palatnik *et al*, *J Clin Psychopharmacol* 2001;**21**:335–9).

MAOIs

Phenelzine at 45–90 mg/d may be at least as effective as imipramine in patients with panic attacks as part of 'endogenous depression' (n = 35, open, 6/12, Buiges and Vallejo, *J Clin Psychiatry* 1987;**48**:55–9) and in atypical depression with panic attacks (n = 119, RCT, d/b, p/c, Liebowitz *et al*, *Arch Gen Psychiatry* 1988;**45**:129–37). MAOIs have fallen out of use but may be useful in resistant cases.

Mirtazapine

Mirtazapine may be a rapidly effective alternative to SSRIs for panic (n = 28, RCT, open, 12/52, Boshuisen *et al*, *Int Clin Psychopharmacol* 2001;**16**:363–8; n = 45, open, 3/12, Sarchiapone *et al*, *Int Clin Psychopharmacol* 2003;**18**:35–8). In an open trial, 60% patients showed a sustained response to mirtazapine at 16 weeks (n = 10, open, Carpenter *et al*, *Ann Clin Psychiatry* 1999;**11**:81–6). Mirtazapine was similar in efficacy and tolerability to fluoxetine in another trial (n = 27, RCT, 8/52, Ribeiro *et al*, *Braz J Med Biol Res* 2001;**34**:1303–7).

Moclobemide

In one study, the long-term effects of CBT were enhanced by concomitant moclobemide 600 mg/d (n = 55, RCT, 8/52, Loerch *et al*, *Br J Psychiatry* 1999;**174**:205–12), but moclobemide was ineffective as monotherapy. Comparisons with clomipramine (n = 135, RCT, 8/52, Kruger and Dahl, *Eur Arch Psych Clin Neurosci* 1999;**249**[Suppl 1]:S7–S10) and fluoxetine (RCT, d/b, 8/52, Tiller *et al*, *Eur Arch Psych Clin Neurosci* 1999;**249**[Suppl 1]:S19–S24) showed similar efficacy but comparator drugs may have been at sub-therapeutic doses.

Olanzapine *

Olanzapine (mean 12.3 mg/d) was remarkably effective in reducing refractory panic attacks, with 50% even being panic-free at the trial end (n = 10, open, 8/52, Hollifield *et al*, *Depress Anx* 2005;**21**:33–40).

Oxcarbazepine

Increasing an oxcarbazepine dose from 600 mg/d to 900 mg/d has successfully treated panic disorder (n = 1, Windhaber *et al*, *J Clin Psychiatry* 1997, **58**, 404–5).

Pindolol

Augmentation of SSRIs has been suggested but no evidence exists (see Mathew *et al*, *Psychopharmacol Bull* 2001;**35**:97–110).

Pramipexole

Successful augmentation of SSRIs with pramipexole up to 1.5 mg/d has been reported (n = 2, Marazziti *et al*, *Am J Psychiatry* 2001;**158**: 498–9).

Reboxetine *

Reboxetine has some efficacy but less than citalopram (n = 19, RCT, s/b, c/o, 18/52, Seedat *et al*, *Int Clin Psychopharmacol* 2003;**18**:279–84) and significantly less than paroxetine (n=68, RCT, s/b, Bertani *et al*, *Pharmacopsychiatry* 2004;**37**:206–10).

Valproate

Valproate 1500 mg/d may be useful for resistant panic disorder (eg. cases by Marazziti and Giovanni, *Am J Psychiatry* 1996;**153**:842–3; Roberts *et al*, *Am J Psychiatry* 1994;**151**:1521). Divalproex sodium (300–600 mg/d) improved affective symptoms, particularly panic, in patients with panic disorder and mood instability who had not responded to conventional therapy (n = 13 [c = 10], open, 8/52, Baetz and Bowen, *Can J Psychiatry* 1998;**43**:73–7).

◆ Others

Other drugs tried include **carbamazepine** (Tondo et al, *Am J Psychiatry* 1989;**146**:558–9; review by Keck et al, *J Clin Psychopharmacol* 1992;**12**[Suppl]:S36–S41), **clonidine** (reviewed by Puzantian and Hart, *Ann Pharmacother* 1993; **2**:1351–3), **ondansetron** (Schneier et al, *Anxiety* 1996;**2**:199–202), **propranolol** (n = 29, RCT, 6/52, Ravatis et al, *J Clin Psychopharmacol* 1991;**11**:344–50) and **trazodone** (n = 74, d/b, 8/52, Charney et al, *J Clin Psychiatry* 1986; **47**:580–6).

✱ No efficacy

Buspirone

Buspirone is not superior to placebo (d/b, c/o, *J Clin Psychiatry* 1988;**49**[8, Suppl]:S30–S36), or in combination with CBT (n = 77, RCT, Bouvard et al, *Psychother Psychosom* 1997;**66**:7–32).

Caffeine

Caffeine is anxiogenic and panic patients seem to be more sensitive to its effects (Lee et al, *Am J Psychiatry* 1988;**145**:632–5).

Venlafaxine *

Venlafaxine SR 75–225 mg/d was not significantly better than placebo in full panic disorder but generally reduced symptoms (n = 361, RCT, d/b, p/c, 10/52, Bradwejn et al, *Br J Psychiatry* 2005;**187**:352–9), although there have been cases of response reported.

1.22 POST-TRAUMATIC STRESS DISORDER (PTSD)

Symptoms

PTSD is an anxiety disorder resulting from an extreme stressful event, eg. serious threat to life or involvement of a loved one in a catastrophic event, and where a personal vulnerability exists. The person then re-experiences the event recurrently through dreams and feelings. PTSD may be quite common yet often unrecognised and may lead to significant morbidity and

mortality. The lifetime prevalence may be 1–9%. Severe trauma can produce long-lasting neurobiological changes and drugs that affect these changes may thus have a beneficial effect. Interestingly, only drugs with a significant effect on the serotonin system seem to work.

Role of drugs *

Drug treatment is still relatively poorly studied but from current data it seems that 'positive' symptoms (eg. nightmares, etc) respond better, whereas 'negative' symptoms of avoidance (eg. social withdrawal, etc) are less responsive to drugs. There is an almost total lack of response to placebo in chronic PTSD. SSRIs (eg. sertraline and paroxetine) have been shown to be effective in short-term studies (6–12/52), and for relapse prevention over 6–12/12. Higher doses of serotonergic drugs for longer periods (at least five weeks) seem necessary. Discontinuing SSRIs after 12 weeks results in a greater risk of relapse and symptom exacerbation. Long-term atypicals, non-SSRIs and AEDs may also be effective (s = 9, Davis et al, *CNS Drugs* 2006;**20**:465–76). BDZs are probably ineffective (review by Asnis et al, *Drugs* 2004;**64**:383–404).

Reviews: * general (Davidson et al, *J Neuropsychiatry Clin Neurosci* 2004;**16**:135–47; Kilic, *Acta Psychiatr Scand* 2001;**104**:409–11), BAP evidence-based guidelines (Baldwin et al, *J Psychopharmacol* 2005;**19**:567–96), pharmacotherapy (Pearlstein, *J Clin Psychiatry* 2000;**61**[Suppl 7]:S40–S43; WFSBP Guidelines, Bandelow et al, *World J Biol Psychiatry* 2002;**3**:71–99; Davis et al, *Expert Opin Pharmacother* 2001;**2**:1583–95; Hageman et al, *Acta Psychiatr Scand* 2001;**104**:411–22).

BNF listed

Paroxetine

Paroxetine is licensed for PTSD, with a standard 20 mg dose, increasing gradually to 50 mg/d if needed. Doses of 20 mg and 40 mg/d have been shown to be effective and well-tolerated in adults (both male and female) with chronic PTSD (n = 551, RCT, p/c, 12/52, Marshall et al, *Am J Psychiatry* 2001;**158**:1982–8; n = 307, d/b, p/c, 12/52, Tucker et al, *J Clin Psychiatry* 2001;**62**:960–8). It has also been used successfully for post-traumatic grief (n = 15, open, Zygmont et al, *J Clin Psychiatry* 1998;

59:241–5) and non-combat-related, chronic PTSD (n=17, open, 12/52, Marshall et al, J Clin Psychopharmacol 1998;**18**:10–8).

Sertraline

Sertraline is licensed for PTSD in women, but may not be effective in men. Two RCTs in PTSD have shown sertraline (mean dose 150mg/d) to be superior to placebo in measures of global and functional outcomes and symptom severity (n=187, RCT, 12/52, Brady et al, JAMA 2000;**283**:1837–44; critical review by Bisson, EBMH 2000;**3**:109) and at 50–200mg/d to produce a 60% response rate cf 38% with placebo (n=208, RCT, p/c, 12/52, Davidson et al, Arch Gen Psychiatry 2001;**58**:485–92). Sertraline seems particularly effective in treating psychological symptoms of PTSD, eg. anger, anhedonia, detachment and numbing as opposed to somatic symptoms, eg. insomnia and exaggerated startle response (n=400, 12/52, Davidson et al, Psychol Med 2002;**32**:661–70). Two open-label continuation studies have shown a prophylactic effect, eg. relapse rates with sertraline (5%, mean dose 137mg/d) were lower than placebo (26%) in those responding to a 12-week acute phase (n=96, open, 24/52, Davidson et al, Am J Psychiatry 2001;**158**:1974–81; review by Bisson, EBMH 2002;**5**:110, which noted that although there are major methodology concerns it is good data and suggests at least one year's treatment with sertraline should be effective). In another continuation trial, 92% who completed a 12/52 RCT maintained response over the next six months and 54% of the non-responders converted to response (n=128, open 24/52, Londberg et al, J Clin Psychiatry 2001;**62**:325–31).

Review: Schwartz and Rothbaum, Expert Opin Pharmacother 2002;**3**:1489–99.

● Unlicensed/some efficacy

MAOIs

Phenelzine may exert a notable effect on intrusive and avoidance symptoms (n=60, RCT, d/b, 8/52, Kosten et al, J Nerv Ment Dis 1991;**179**:366–70). The strong inhibitory effect on REM sleep may be contributory.

SSRIs (paroxetine and sertraline licensed) *

Fluoxetine (up to 60mg/d) was shown to be superior to placebo in civilians with PTSD (41% response), with a very low placebo response rate (n=53, RCT, p/c, 12/52, Connor et al, Br J Psychiatry 1999;**175**:17–22; see also n=131, RCT, p/c, d/b, 6/12, Martenyi et al, Br J Psychiatry 2002;**181**:315–20; comment by Butterfield, EBMH 2003;**6**:51; strong criticism by Agell, Br J Psychiatry 2003;**182**:366–7 and defence by Eli Lilly; Br J Psychiatry 2003;**182**:367–8). Fluoxetine was more effective for relapse prevention than placebo (22% vs 50%) in responders over 6/12 (n=123[c=114], open, 6/12, Davidson et al, J Clin Psychopharmacol 2005;**25**:166–9). Care may be needed initially with use in patients with co-morbid panic attacks, as fluoxetine may increase panic/anxiety (short review of fluoxetine in PTSD by Marshall et al, Am J Psychiatry 1995;**152**:1238–9), so start low and go slow. **Citalopram** was partly effective in two cases (n=2, Khouzam et al, Mil Med 2001;**166**:921–3). **Fluvoxamine** 100–300mg/d (mean 150mg) appeared to improve combat-related PTSD but not depressive symptoms (n=15, open, 14/52, Escalona et al, Depress Anxiety 2002;**15**:29–33). Dreams linked to the traumatic experience may also respond, although not insomnia (n=21, open, 10/52, Neylan et al, J Trauma Stress 2001;**14**:461–7).

Tricyclics

Amitriptyline (n=46, p/c, 8/52, Davidson et al, Arch Gen Psychiatry 1990;**4**:259–69) and **imipramine** (n=60, RCT, p/c, 8/52, Kosten et al, J Nerv Ment Dis 1991;**179**:366–70) have been shown to produce a modest and clinically meaningful effect. However, doses of 300mg/d for at least eight weeks are needed.

■ Unlicensed/possible efficacy

Antipsychotics *

Antipsychotics are generally considered to be relatively poorly effective. Lack of effect from **olanzapine** at up to 20mg/d in PTSD has been shown (n=15, RCT, d/b, p/c, 10/52, Butterfield et al, Int Clin Psychopharmacol 2001;**16**:197–203), although in people unresponsive to 12 weeks SSRI at maximum tolerated dose, addition of olanzapine was significantly superior to placebo on some specific measures, but not on the global response (n = 19, d/b, p/c, 8/52, Stein et al, Am J Psychiatry 2002;**159**:1777–9). Olanzapine augmentation of SSRIs may be useful for nightmares and insomnia in combat-related PTSD (n = 5, open, Jakovljevic et al, Acta Psychiatr Scand 2003;**107**:394–6) and sleep symptoms (n = 5, Jakovljevic et al, Acta Psychiatr Scand 2003;**07**:394–6). Olanzapine 5–10mg/d was slightly more effective than fluphenazine for combat-related PTSD and reduced psychotic symptoms, although a placebo arm would have been helpful (n = 55, open, 6/52, Pivac et al, Psychopharmacol [Berl] 2004;**175**:451–6). Augmentation with **quetiapine** may be an option (Sokolski et al, Mil Med 2003;**168**:486–9) and encouraging outcomes were seen in a small pilot study of quetiapine as adjunctive treatment in resistant PTSD (n = 20[c = 18], open, 6/52, Hamner et al, J Clin Psychopharmacol 2003;**23**:5–20). In SSRI-poorly responsive PTSD, adjunctive quetiapine (mean 216mg/d) improved all major symptoms in 45% (n = 15, open, 8/52, Ahearn et al, Int Clin Psychopharmacol 2006;**21**:29–33). Adjunctive **risperidone** in resistant combat PTSD was well-tolerated and produced a modest improvement in one study (n = 40, RCT, d/b, p/c, 5/52, Hamner et al, Int Clin Psychopharmacol 2003;**18**:1–8) and 2–4mg/d has helped decrease some psychotic and PTSD symptoms in antidepressant-resistant patients (n = 26, open, 6/52, Kozaric-Kovacic et al, J Clin Psychiatry 2005;**66**:922–7). **Aripiprazole** has been used successfully in PTSD, especially for sleep disturbances and hyperarousal (n = 5, Lambert, Int Clin Psychopharmacol 2006;**21**:185–7). **Clozapine** has been used successfully in co-morbid psychosis and PTSD (n = 1, Hamner, Am J Psychiatry 1996;**153**:841) and in treatment-resistant, abused adolescents with psychosis and PTSD (n = 6, Wheatley et al, J Clin Psychopharmacol 2004;**24**:167–73). **Levo-mepromazine** helps reduce sleep problems in PTSD (Aukst-Margetic et al, Eur Psychiatry 2004;**19**:235–6). **Ziprasidone** has been used successfully (n = 2, Siddiqui et al, J Psychiatry Neurosci 2005;**30**:430–1).

Benzodiazepines *

Although generally considered ineffective, potential anti-arousal effects can be useful and beneficial effects have been seen with **alprazolam** (n = 16, RCT, d/b, c/o, Braun et al, J Clin Psychiatry 1990;**51**:236–8) and **clonazepam** at 4–5mg/d (n = 13, open, 6/12, Gelpin et al, J Clin Psychiatry 1996;**57**:390–4), but clonazepam was largely ineffective in improving sleep disturbances and nightmares in combat-related PTSD (n = 6, 2 + 2/52, p/c, c/o, s/b, Cates et al, Ann Pharmacother 2004;**38**:1395–9). Care is needed with possible abuse, induction of depression, the potential for the release of impulsive or antisocial behaviour and severe withdrawal reactions (n = 8, Risse et al, J Clin Psychiatry 1990;**51**:206–9).

Beta-blockers/propranolol

Propranolol 40mg TDS for seven days immediately post-trauma (n = 11) has shown lower levels of PTSD symptoms than in those refusing (n = 8) propranolol (n = 19, open, Vaiva et al, Biol Psychiatry 2003;**54**:947–9).

Bupropion

In one study, bupropion decreased depressive symptoms and most patients reported global improvement, although PTSD symptoms remained mostly unchanged (n = 17, open, Canive et al, J Clin Psychopharmacol 1998; **18**: 379–83; expert consensus guidelines in J Clin Psychiatry 2000;**61**:1–76).

Buspirone

Open studies have suggested some efficacy on all symptom clusters (eg. Hamner et al, Depress Anxiety 1997;**5**:137–9), including aggression, and possibly with a rapid onset (n = 1, Duffy, Ann Clin Psychiatry 1992;**4**:193–6).

Carbamazepine

Some effect on hyperarousal, hostility and intrusive symptoms has been reported in old studies (eg. Wolf et al, Biol Psychiatry 1988;**23**:642–4) and in a case report (n = 1, Looff et al, J Am Acad Child Adolesc Psychiatry 1995;**34**:703–4).

DHEA *

7-keto DHEA has been used successfully in treatment-resistant PTSD (n = 5, Sageman and Brown, J Clin Psychiatry 2006;**67**:493–6).

Gabapentin

Successful use has been reported in a case series (n = 30, Hamner et al, Ann Clin Psychiatry 2001;13:141–6; see also n = 2, Berigan, J Clin Psychiatry 2002;63:744; n = 1, Malek-Ahmadi, Ann Pharmacother 2003;37:664–6).

Levetiracetam *

Levetiracetam (mean 2000 mg/d) may be useful as antidepressant augmentation in refractory PTSD (n = 23, retrospective, mean 10/52, Kinrys et al, J Clin Psychiatry 2006;67:211–4).

Liothyronine/triiodothyronine

Triiodothyronine 25 mcg/d has been used successfully to augment ineffective SSRI (fluoxetine or paroxetine 40 mg/d) mono-therapy (n = 5, 8/52, Agid et al, J Clin Psychiatry 2001;62:169–73).

Mirtazapine *

A number of studies have suggested an effect in some symptoms at 45 mg/d (64% response vs 20% for placebo; n = 29, RCT, d/b, p/c, 8/52, Davidson et al, Biol Psychiatry 2003;53:188–91). It was effective and well-tolerated in PTSD in Korea (n = 15, open, 8/52, Bahk et al, Hum Psychopharmacol 2002;17:341–4) and in Korean veterans (n = 100, RCT, open, 6/52, Chung et al, Hum Psychopharmacol 2004; 19:489–94). For PTSD nightmares, mirtazapine may have some significant effects, perhaps by an effect on sleep (n => 300, open, Lewis, Am J Psychiatry 2002;159:1948–9). A continuation study showed a modest enduring effect for six months (n = 15[c = 12], 24/52, Kim et al, Psychiatry Clin Neurosci 2005;59:743–7).

Oxcarbazepine

Oxcarbazepine has been used for PTSD (n = 1, Berigan, Can J Psychiatry 2002;47:973–4).

Phenytoin *

Phenytoin may have some use at anticonvulsant doses and may be associated with changes in brain structure (n = 9, open, 3/12, Bremner et al, J Clin Psychiatry 2004;65:1559–64; Bremner et al, J Psychopharmacol 2005;19:159–65).

Prazosin

Prazosin (mean dose 9.6 mg/d) may reduce nightmares in veterans with chronic PTSD if taken for at least eight weeks (n = 59, retrospective chart analysis, Raskind et al, J Clin Psychiatry 2002;63:565–8) and a mean dose of 9.5 mg/d at night was well-tolerated and superior to placebo on primary outcome measures in PTSD (n = 10, d/b, p/c, c/o, 20/52, Raskind et al, Am J Psychiatry 2003; 160:371–3).

Tiagabine

Tiagabine 8 mg/d (range 4–12 mg/d) may be worth investigating in PTSD (n = 7, open, 8/52, Taylor, J Clin Psychiatry 2003;64:1421–5; UG) and a discontinuation study in responders suggested some relapse prevention efficacy (n = 29[c = 19], open, 12/52, Connor et al, Psychopharmacol [Berl] 2006;184:21–5).

Topiramate

A naturalistic review showed a rapid effect on PTSD symptoms for add-on or adjunctive topiramate (n = 35, open, Berlant and van Kammen, J Clin Psychiatry 2002;63:15–20).

Trazodone

A small study suggested an effect (n = 6, open, Hertzberg et al, J Clin Psychopharmacol 1996;1:294–8).

Valproate

Intrusion, hyperarousal and depressive symptoms may respond to valproate (n = 16, 8/52, Clark et al, J Trauma Stress 1999;12:395–401). It has been used in combat-related PTSD (Fesler, J Clin Psychiatry 1991;52:361–4) and in civilians with non-combat-related PTSD (open, Otte et al, J Clin Psychopharmacol 2004;24:106–8).

◆ Others

Other drugs tried include **clonidine** for self-mutilatory behaviour (van der Kolk, J Affect Disord 1987;13:203–13) and as an adjunct to imipramine in Cambodian refugees (n = 9, Kinzie and Leung, J Nerv Ment Dis 1989;177:546–50), **cyproheptadine** for nightmares (eg. Brophy, Mil Med 1991;156:100–1) and low dose **lithium** (Kitchner and Greenstein, Mil Med 1985;150:378–81).

✱ No efficacy

Caffeine

Panic patients may have increased sensitivity to caffeine (Lee et al, Am J Psychiatry 1988; 145:632–5).

Flumazenil

Two studies have shown no effects (eg. Coupland et al, Biol Psychiatry 1997;41:988–90).

Naltrexone

Only non-significant subtle improvements were seen in a small, short trial (n = 8, open, 2/52, Lubin et al, Hum Psychopharmacol 2002; 17:181–5).

PSYCHIATRIC EMERGENCY, ACUTE

see Acute psychiatric emergency (1.1)

1.23 PSYCHOSIS AND SCHIZOPHRENIA

see also Catatonia (1.12)

Symptoms

Schizophrenia is a life-long fluctuating illness with a high chance of relapse. Schneider's 'First rank symptoms' are often quoted as the main diagnostic features. They include hearing thoughts spoken aloud, 'third person' hallucinations, hallucinations in the form of a commentary, somatic hallucinations, thought withdrawal or insertion, thought broadcasting, delusional perceptions and feelings, or actions experienced as being made or influenced by external agents. Schizophrenics most frequently have a lack of insight, auditory hallucinations, ideas of reference, suspiciousness, flatness of affect, voices speaking to them, delusional mood, delusions of persecution and thoughts spoken aloud.

Possible causes of schizophrenia

The dopamine hypothesis, ie. excess dopamine activity in the mesolimbic remains the most widely quoted explanation but is clearly not the whole story and there are many other theories, eg. hypofunction of the glutamate systems, particularly at the NMDA sub-type of glutamate receptor, combined dopamine hyperfunction and glutamate hypofunction (Smith et al, Am J Psychiatry 2001;158:1393–9; extensive review by

Goff and Coyle, Am J Psychiatry 2001;158:1367–77, 148 refs) and 5-HT$_2$ hyperfunction. The balance between D$_2$ and 5-HT$_2$ may be important. Abnormal connections between nerves involving amino acid neurotransmitters may be a consequence of developmentally reduced synaptic connectivity (during perinatal and adolescent periods), rather than loss of neuronal or glial cells. Antipsychotics are thought to exert a significant part of their clinical effect via blockade of mesolimbic (Farrison, Lancet 2000;356:958–9) D$_2$ receptors.

Role of drugs in schizophrenia ✱

Antipsychotics have a major role in the management of schizophrenic illnesses but the actual choice of drug is difficult. In nearly all RCTs using haloperidol as the comparator, haloperidol doses were higher than recommended even for severely ill patients, so it's not surprising some of the newer drugs look better tolerated (s = 49, Hugenholtz et al, J Clin Psychiatry 2006;67:897–903). Trials sponsored by a manufacturer nearly always favour that manufacturer's drug (see 'why olanzapine beats risperidone, risperidone beats quetiapine and quetiapine beats olanzapine', s = 42, Heres et al, Am J Psychiatry 2006;163:185–94). In a rare independent, comparison, the CATIE study has compared olanzapine (7.5–30mg/d), risperidone (1.5–6mg/d), perphenazine (8–32mg/d), quetiapine (200–800mg/d) and ziprasidone (40–160mg/d). Overall, 74% patients discontinued within 18 months, olanzapine had the lowest drop-out rate but had its known side-effects and perphenazine was as effective as the others (n = 1493, RCT, < 18/12, Lieberman et al, N Engl J Med 2005;353:1209–23). In schizophrenics who did not respond to an atypical antipsychotic, clozapine was more effective than switching to another atypical (n = 99, CATIE, McEvoy et al, Am J Psychiatry 2006;163:600–10), and switching to risperidone or olanzapine was more effective than quetiapine or ziprasidone, based on time to discontinuation (n = 444, RCT, d/b, CATIE, Stroup et al, Am J Psychiatry 2006;163:611–22). The largest independent meta-analysis of RCTs showed that clozapine appears the most superior to first generation antipsychotics (FGAs); olanzapine, risperidone and amisulpride next; with quetiapine, sertindole, ziprasidone and aripiprazole as effective as first generation antipsychotics (s = 142, Davis et al, Arch Gen Psychiatry 2003;**60**:553–64).

1. Early-onset and limitation of disease progression (see tables on first-episode psychosis) *

While still unproven and controversial, evidence is accumulating that antipsychotics such as risperidone started after the symptoms first appear, or even in a prodromal stage, prevent or delay the progression of schizophrenia (risperidone vs CBT, n = 59, 12/12, McGorry et al, Arch Gen Psychiatry 2002;**59**:921–8). There would inevitably be some drug treatment of people who would not go on to develop this illness (review by Stahl, J Clin Psychiatry 2004;**65**:1445–6).

2. Acute phase *

Many antipsychotics have an immediate calming effect, which is useful in relieving patient distress in the acute stage, and then reduce the intensity of psychotic experiences. There is little proven advantage of using higher doses of some drugs, eg. above about 12–15 mg/d of high-potency antipsychotics (eg. haloperidol) and higher doses potentially give the recipient a bad and adverse experience. Most response is likely to occur within 3–4 weeks and if little occurs by 6–8 weeks, raising doses is unlikely to help. In one study, all patients showing less than a 20% improvement in BPRS (especially positive symptoms) after seven days of oral fluphenazine 20 mg/d were still classified as non-responders at four weeks (n = 131, open, 4/52, Correll et al, Am J Psychiatry 2003;**160**:2063–5), indicating that lack of early response predicts later non-response and that objective rating scales may be a useful time-effective and cost-effective tool in decision-making.

The choice of antipsychotic in the acute phase remains an individual decision. Atypicals are not statistically better than typicals after controlling for comparator doses (23 RCT meta-regression analysis, Geddes et al, Br Med J 2000;**321**:1371–6; review by McIntosh, EBMH 2001;**4**:77), but this assumes EPS are 'minimal cost'. In this analysis, studies were only a median of 6.5/52 duration, so ADRs from longer-term use are not known (low-dose typicals vs atypicals — discussion of both sides of arguments by Taylor, Psychiatr Bull 2000;**24**:465–8). Younger patients are more likely

to discontinue an antipsychotic due to lack of response (or worsening) than side-effects, so it if works, they are more likely to take it (s = 4, RCTs, d/b, 24/52, Liu-Seifert et al, BMC Med 2005;**3**:21). 'Treatment-resistance' in the acute phase may include true resistance and those with sub-optimal treatment.

Naturalistic studies have suggested that patients most at risk of excessive antipsychotic dosing include those on depots, Afro-Americans, a history of hospitalisations and being more thought disordered (eg. n = 293, Walkup et al, J Clin Psychiatry 2000;**61**:344–8).

3. Relapse prevention

Relapse of schizophrenia occurs in around 80% of untreated schizophrenics and so maintenance therapy, which reduces relapse rates significantly, is usually an important component of the management. Sadly, it is not yet possible to accurately identify the 20% who do not relapse and, thus, do not need long-term drug therapy. If antipsychotics are stopped, relapse may be delayed for 2–6 months, with the individual often feeling better (due to reduced side-effects) before the relapse. Intermittent therapy (prodrome-based or crisis intervention) has been advocated and is generally accepted as ineffective (n = 363, RCT, Gaebel et al, Schizophr Res 2002;**53**:145–59). Side-effects, particularly the under-rated akathisia, weight gain and dysphoria, tend to reduce compliance.

Long-term antipsychotics are an important relapse-prevention strategy but it is difficult to motivate people to continue while relatively asymptomatic. While compliance and adherence are terms used, 'concordance' implies an agreement between the prescriber and patient as to the degree of drug-taking acceptable to both. In patients, this will balance the positive effects of the drug (eg. symptom suppression) and the negative effects (eg. side-effects) and finding a good reason not to relapse, eg. family, friends or job, may aid effective maintenance therapy. Schizophrenics have better adherence with atypicals over the first six months of therapy (but not at 12/12, using prescription refill records), and so interventions to improve compliance are needed for all patients (n = 288, 12/12, Dolder et al, Am J Psychiatry 2002;**159**:103–8). Compliance therapy has been shown to improve attitude, concordance and insight on an intensive one-to-one basis (n=47[c=27], RCT, 6/12, Kemp *et al, Br Med J* 1996;**312**:345–9), although some service users consider this brain-washing.

The use of high dose antipsychotic medication (Thompson, *Br J Psychiatry* 1994;**164**: 448–58)

The upper end of the dose ranges of older antipsychotics is often not clearly established and usually defined by limits of safety and the SPCs. Doses above these limits should only be used 'with caution and under specialist supervision'. 'Chlorpromazine equivalents' have been used to compare drugs or calculate total doses of multiple drugs, but maximum doses vary between drugs, and dosage equivalents are of only limited use (see *2.2.1*). The evidence and scientific rationale for the effectiveness of high doses is limited.

Main dangers of high dose antipsychotics:

1. Sudden cardiac-related death, eg. QT prolongation, Torsades de Pointes.
2. CNS toxicity, eg. CNS and respiratory depression, hypoxia, seizures.

Main uses of antipsychotics above BNF limits:

1. **Psychiatric emergency:** see 'Acute psychiatric emergency' (*Chapter 1.1*).
2. **Acute treatment:** ie. after the emergency, but before the antipsychotic takes full effect. Doses should be reduced as soon as possible once the patient has responded.
3. **Long-term treatment:** eg. in treatment-resistant schizophrenia where residual symptoms impair living or rehabilitation:
   - **as polypharmacy:** the prescribing of multiple antipsychotics is 'not recommended' as it 'may constitute a hazard' and side-effects are not minimised
   - **poor resources:** inadequate resources/environment often result in the need for more medication at higher doses.

Factors to be considered before prescribing high-dose antipsychotics:

- The diagnosis is fully confirmed and documented.
- Plasma levels are therapeutic and compliance with regimen is assured.
- Treatment duration has been fully adequate.
- Reduced doses for a trial period have been tried to rule out eg. akathisia.
- Adverse social and psychological factors have been minimised.
- Alternative antipsychotic therapies tried.

If exceeding standard antipsychotic doses, the following should be routine:

- Multidisciplinary team and patient (or advocate) discussion, obtaining valid consent if possible, making a thorough record of the decision and reasoning, including target signs and symptoms, and outcome evaluation.
- Consideration of any contraindications, eg. cardiac, age, renal, hepatic, weight, and smoking, and any interactions, eg. with tricyclics, carbamazepine, etc.
- ECG pre-treatment to exclude QTc prolongation, repeated every 1–3 months.
- Doses increased only slowly.
- Regular checks carried out on pulse, bp temperature and hydration.
- Prescription reviewed regularly and reduced after three months if no improvement.

4. Discontinuation

Many people with schizophrenia are on long-term antipsychotics (depot or oral) at the dose they received when acutely ill. With depression 'the dose that got you well keeps you well' is probably true, but this is not often the case with schizophrenia. There is abundant evidence that this may not be necessary as since continuous antipsychotic intake is 'topping-up' D2 blockade (significant D2 blockade can persist for 16 weeks after discontinuing depots and can be 30% even after six months: n = 4, Nyberg et al, Arch Gen Psychiatry 1997;**54**:953–8). Reducing doses from their acute levels may actually improve outcomes and symptoms but (and it's a big but) some people really do need higher doses long-term. This does not mean you should not try reducing doses but that care is needed to prevent unnecessary and potentially catastrophic relapses.

If reducing doses or stopping antipsychotics in someone on a high dose long-term

- Check the history carefully to see if there is clear evidence of previous illness. If so, proceed only with great caution and document carefully. A history of non-compliance without relapse is a good sign but not to be taken as confirmation that antipsychotics are not needed.
- Make only small changes each time.
- Leave for six months to assess the outcome of each change.
- Remember that the peak for relapse may be at about 3–6 months post-dose reduction or stopping.
- Make further changes only at 3–6 monthly intervals.
- Have a robust system in place for detecting early signs of relapse.
- Have a robust plan for increasing or re-introducing doses when early signs occur; to restabilise the patient.
- Remember that some people need higher doses and there is much to gain by reducing doses but, probably, more to lose should the person relapse and not be able to return to previous levels of functioning.
- Consider also the possible consequences of relapse, eg. damage to the individual and others, and previous events.

Risk factors for relapse

Medication risk factors include:

- **Drug used,** eg. rehospitalisation rates for schizophrenics discharged on atypicals (olanzapine, n = 313 or risperidone, n = 268) were similar (31% and 33% respectively) but considerably lower than those (n = 458) discharged on conventional antipsychotics (48%) over a two-year period (Rabinowitz et al, Am J Psychiatry 2001;**58**:266–9), confirmed by CATIE.
- **Doses:** there are some ethnic trends in drug responses, and doses may need to be lower in some racial groups (n = 192, 6/52, Emsley et al, J Clin Psychiatry 2002;**63**:9–14). Higher doses lead to extra ADRs and a higher risk of non-compliance.
- **Duration of untreated psychosis (DUP):** a retrospective chart analysis indicated that DUP is the best predictor of outcome, ie. those with more insidious onset and severe negative symptoms are more likely to have multiple episodes (n = 67, four years, Altamura et al, Schizophr Res 2001;**52**:29–36). See also early onset tables.
- **Unmanaged substance misuse:** this reduces anti-psychotic effects in dual diagnosis, with sooner and longer readmissions, especially in those non-compliant with drugs (n = 99, four years, Hunt et al, Schizophr Res 2002; **54**:253–64).

Review: optimal duration of prophylactic antipsychotics in schizophrenia (Bosveld-van Haandel et al, Acta Psychiatr Scand 2001; **103**:335–46).

Suicide prevention *

Around 5% of schizophrenics will commit suicide, usually near illness onset (n = 22 598, Palmer et al, Arch Gen Psychiatry 2005;**62**:247–53). A five-year retrospective study suggested both risperidone and olanzapine gave some protection from suicidality compared to other (excluding clozapine) antipsychotics (n = 756, Barak et al, Psychopharmacol [Berl] 2004; **175**: 215–9). Clozapine has a clear anti-suicide effect.

Stroke

The UK CSM recommends not using risperidone and olanzapine in elderly demented people with behavioural problems, due to an increased risk of stroke (3% vs 2% vs 1% on placebo), although the absolute risk is low, and the alternatives are not risk-free. The restriction does not apply to elderly demented people without behavioural problems. A recent study has shown no increased risk with risperidone (n = 6964) or olanzapine (n = 3421) compared to typicals (n = 1015) in the elderly without dementia (Herrman et al, Am J Psychiatry 2004; **161**:1113–5).

Reviews: * recent advances (Barnes and Joyce, Curr Opin Psychiatry 2001; **14**:25–37), GP guide (Taylor and Geddes, Prescriber 2002; **13**:31–51), adolescent schizophrenia (Hollis, Adv Psychiatr Treat 2000; **6**:83–92), genetics (Malhotra, Curr Opin Psychiatry 2001; **14**:3–7), metabolic syndrome review (Thakore, Br J Psychiatry 2005; **186**:455–6), metabolic side-effects of atypicals in children (Fedorowicz and Fombonne, J Psychopharmacol 2006; **20**:533–50), systematic review and meta-analysis of second generation antipsychotics vs low-potency first generation (n = 2320, s = 31, Leucht et al, Lancet 2003; **361**:1581–9).

PHENOTHIAZINES

Chlorpromazine

Chlorpromazine is used for a wide range of psychotic conditions but use in the elderly is problematical. IV use is not recommended unless the injection is diluted and the patient is in a supine position. Cochrane concludes that chlorpromazine remains a global 'benchmark' for schizophrenia, as a well-established, effective but imperfect treatment (Thornley et al, Cochrane Database Syst Rev 2003; **2**:CD000284).

Fluphenazine (see also depots)

An oral preparation is available but fluphenazine is usually used as a depot.

Levomepromazine (methotrimeprazine) *

This phenothiazine, related to promethazine, has significant sedative effects but causes little respiratory depression (study vs haloperidol and risperidone; n = 62, RCT, 4/52, Blin et al, J Clin Psychopharmacol 1996; **16**:38–44). Levomepromazine (range 600–1000 mg/d, mean 710 mg/d) may be more effective than

chlorpromazine in TRS (n = 38, RCT, open/d/b, 30/52, Lal et al, J Psychiatry Neurosci 2006; **31**:271–9).

Pericyazine

Pericyazine is a piperidine phenothiazine similar to thioridazine, with marked sedative and hypotensive side-effects. Use as a low-dose anxiolytic-sedative has increased with the fall of thioridazine. Little is published about the drug.

Perphenazine *

Perphenazine is a piperazine phenothiazine with a relatively short half-life (8–12 hours). Chosen as a 'typical' comparator, the CATIE study has shown perphenazine to be as effective as olanzapine, risperidone, quetiapine and ziprasidone (n = 1493, RCT, < 18/12, Lieberman et al, N Engl J Med 2005; **353**:1209–23).

Prochlorperazine

Prochlorperazine is a piperazine phenothiazine better known for its use as an antiemetic and in Ménières disease.

Promazine

Promazine is similar to chlorpromazine and retains a minor role as a non-dependence-prone hypnotic, although the potential for side-effects should not be ignored.

Thioridazine

Due to concerns about the long-known issue of QT prolongation, thioridazine is now only licensed for resistant schizophrenia, considered inappropriate for patients with a history of cardiac arrhythmias and requires a baseline ECG and serum potassium, plus monitoring throughout treatment. A dose-related increase in the risk of lengthened QT-interval has been reported, detectable at doses as low as 10 mg/d (n = 596, Reilly et al, Lancet 2000; **355**:1048–52) and an association with sudden unexplained death in psychiatric in-patients (Reilly et al, Br J Psychiatry 2002; **180**:515–22; Reilly et al, Psychiatr Bull 2002; **26**:110–2). A large observational study showed thioridazine (median 31 mg/d) and haloperidol (median 1.8 mg/d) to have similar cardiac safety (cohort study, Hennessy et al, Br J Clin Pharmacol 2000; **58**:81–7).

Antipsychotics in early onset or first episode schizophrenia/psychosis

| Aims of treatment | • Minimise deterioration or even perhaps prevent the illness developing.
• Reduce stigma from symptoms, aiming for complete, not incomplete, remission.
• Increase engagement by minimising adverse experience with medication through use of minimum effective doses. |

Principles of pharmacological management (Carpenter, *Am J Psychiatry* 2001;**158**:1771–3)

Early intervention (EI) with effective antipsychotics	• A systematic review of all available studies to May 2004 concluded that a longer duration (particularly if over two years; n = 88, Malla *et al*, *Schizophr Res* 2002;**54**:231–42; n = 157, Wunderink *et al*, *Acta Psychiatr Scand* 2006;**113**:332–9) of untreated psychosis (DUP) is consistently associated with modestly worse symptoms and functioning, and less chance of remission in people with first episode psychosis (s = 26, n = 4490, Marshall *et al*, *Arch Gen Psychiatry* 2005;**62**:975–83; comment by Perkins, *EBMH* 2006;**9**:36), and a similar review comes to the same conclusion (Perkins *et al*, *Am J Psychiatry* 2005;**162**:1785–804; Norman *et al*, *Br J Psychiatry* 2005;**187**[Suppl 48]:S19–S23). Delay in starting antipsychotics in first-episode psychosis is not necessarily neurotoxic for the brain or lead to reduced hippocampal volumes (n = 105, Ho *et al*, *Am J Psychiatry* 2005;**162**:1527–9). Structured early intervention programmes improve overall functioning and adherence but not necessarily symptoms (n = 144, RCT, 18/12, Garety *et al*, *Br J Psychiatry* 2006;**188**:37–45; comment by van Meijl, *EBMH* 2006;**9**:69). Substance misuse early in the illness has been linked with increased severity of illness (n = 232, Bühler *et al*, *Schizophr Res* 2002;**54**:234–51), and so should also be managed.
Drug dose is optimal	• Slow titration is needed — both introduction and discontinuation. The mean time to response is nine weeks (n = 118, Robinson *et al*, *Am J Psychiatry* 1999;**156**:544–9), and may be delayed longer (n = 522, RCT, median 30/52, Emsley *et al*, *Am J Psychiatry* 2006;**163**:743–45).
Patient choice is considered a high priority *	• Consider what the patient prefers (weight gain is the most unpopular side-effect and its impact on the user must not be trivialised). • Explain that there is no clear way of treating prodromal symptoms without the high risk of treating 'false positives' (Larsen *et al*, *Acta Psychiatr Scand* 2001;**103**:323–4). • Minimise 'obvious' ADRs that might make patients look different, and which reduces compliance and engagement (n = 42, Amminger *et al*, *Schizophr Res* 2002;**54**:223–30). Although EPS is a common side-effect from antipsychotics in first-episode schizophrenia, 28% untreated patients also have some EPS at baseline (n = 535, RCT, d/b, Honer *et al*, *J Psychopharmacol* 2005;**19**:277–85).
Duration of treatment is adequate	• The relapse rate over five years is high (n = 104, Robinson *et al*, *Arch Gen Psychiatry* 1999;**56**:241–7). On discontinuation, up to 78% may experience an exacerbation or relapse within one year, and 96% may do so within two years (n = 53, RCT, open, 18/12, Gitlin *et al*, *Am J Psychiatry* 2001;**158**:1835–42). Patients should be advised that not taking antipsychotics for several years will almost inevitably lead to relapse and rehospitalisation (n = 104, Robinson *et al*, *Arch Gen Psychiatry* 1999;**56**:241–7). The optimum duration of therapy is as yet unclear.
Treatment is monitored	• Older drugs have high incidence of EPS (even with low dose haloperidol; n = 57, 12/12, Oosterhuizen *et al*, *J Clin Psychiatry* 2003;**64**:1075–80), raised prolactin and adverse cognitive effects. • Newer drugs have higher incidence of weight gain (which should be dealt with early, not after it has happened) and diabetes, which needs to be screened for, monitored and managed.

Choice of antipsychotic in early onset/first episode schizophrenia/psychosis

Most trials of new drugs versus older drugs are carried out on more chronic patients rather than first-episode, and favour the newer drugs as the typical comparator doses are often inappropriately high and play down ADRs, especially weight gain (Remington, *Br J Psychiatry* 2005;**187**[Suppl 48]:S77–S84).

Risperidone   Risperidone is now a standard first choice. In the 75% who initially clinically improved, relapses were delayed longer with risperidone (mean 3.3 mg/d; median 466 days) than haloperidol (mean 2.9 mg/d; median 205 days) (n = 555, RCT, d/b, < 5 years, median 30/52, Schooler et al, *Am J Psychiatry* 2005;**162**:947–53). Cognitive functioning improves more with risperidone than haloperidol, independently of changes in symptoms, (n = 533 [c = 359], RCT, 3/12 follow-up, Harvey et al, *Am J Psychiatry* 2005;**162**:1888–95). Even low dose (1–1.8 mg/d) can produce dramatic improvements in prodromal phase or first-episode schizophrenia (n = 10, open, 12/52, Cannon et al, *Am J Psychiatry* 2002;**159**:1230–2; n = 436, open, two years, Fraile et al, *Actas Esp Psiquiatr* 2002;**30**:142–52). In a dose comparison, 2 mg/d was as effective as 4 mg/d with fewer side-effects and, although 4 mg/d (especially with slow titration; Williams, *J Clin Psychiatry* 2001;**62**:282–9; RCT, n = 183, 6/52, Emsley, *Schizophr Bull* 1999;**25**:721–9) was slightly better at 4/52, the two were similar at 8/52, so it may make little pharmacological sense in dose escalating at an early stage (n = 49, d/b, 8/52, Merlo et al, *J Clin Psychiatry* 2002;**63**:885–91).

Olanzapine *   Low dose olanzapine is preferable to haloperidol in first-episode psychosis, with superior efficacy, lower discontinuations, greater retention in treatment and reduced side-effects (n = 83, selected sub-analysis of the larger Tollefson n = 1996 study; RCT, Sanger et al, *Am J Psychiatry* 1999;**156**:79–87, MS; n = 158, open, Bobes et al, *Prog Neuropsychopharmacol Biol Psychiatry* 2003;**27**:473–81), although weight gain is a significant adverse effect (mean 15.4 kg) in first-episode psychosis (n = 263, open, two years, Zipursky et al, *Br J Psychiatry* 2005;**187**:537–43; comment by Lambert, *EBMH* 2006;**9**:72). Olanzapine (mean 9.6 mg/d) improved cognitive functioning compared to haloperidol (4.6 mg/d) using a contrived composite score, although even then the advantage was small (n = 167, RCT, d/b, 12/52, Keefe et al, *Am J Psychiatry* 2004;**161**:985–95).

Quetiapine   Low EPS, weight gain and prolactin effects make quetiapine an ideal drug of choice, but first-episode data is lacking. One small study suggested first-episode schizophrenia seems to respond well to once-daily quetiapine (mean 425 mg/d), without the need for continuously high D2 receptor blockade (n = 14, open, 12/52, Tauscher-Wisniewski et al, *J Clin Psychiatry* 2002;**63**:992–7).

Clozapine   A flexible dose study showed clozapine and chlorpromazine were equipotent at 12/12 in drug-naive first-episode schizophrenia, but clozapine was more effective at 12/52 (Lieberman et al, *Neuropsychopharmacol* 2003;**28**:995–1003). There was a 15% decrease in the odds of achieving remission for every year of untreated psychoses.

Haloperidol *   Haloperidol 2 mg/d is much better tolerated than 8 mg/d and as effective against PANSS scores (n = 40, RCT, d/b, 6/52, Oosthuizen et al, *Int J Neuropsychopharmacol* 2004;**7**:125–31). It has equivalent efficacy to olanzapine, although the high drop-out rate was high and the trial excluded more severely ill people (n = 263 [c = 83], RCT, d/b, one year, Strakowski et al, *Schizophr Res* 2005;**78**:161–9; comment by Awad, *EBMH* 2006;**9**:47). Unlike olanzapine, haloperidol is associated with reduced grey matter volume in first episode, either due to haloperidol-induced toxicity or superior olanzapine efficacy (n = 263, RCT, d/b, volunteer controlled, 24/12, Lieberman et al, *Arch Gen Psychiatry* 2005;**62**:361–70).

Reviews: general (Carpenter, *Am J Psychiatry* 2001;**158**:1771–3; Kasper, *J Clin Psychiatry* 1999;**60**[Suppl 23]:5–9; Rummel et al, *Cochrane Database Syst Rev* 2003;**4**:CD004410; Marshall and Lockwood, *Cochrane Database Syst Rev* 2004;**2**:CD004718), predictors of response (Robinson et al, *Am J Psychiatry* 1999;**156**:544–9), antipsychotics in first episode (Feetam and Donoghue, *Pharm J* 2003;**270**:405–9, 47 refs), neuropathological changes (n = 70, Cahn et al, *Arch Gen Psychiatry* 2002;**59**:1002–10), prodromal predictors of psychosis and 12/12 outcome (n = 49, Yung et al, *Schizophr Res* 2003;**60**:21–32).

Trifluoperazine

Trifluoperazine is a piperazine phenothiazine widely used as an antipsychotic and sometimes claimed to have 'activating' effects at low doses. A Cochrane review concludes trifluoperazine to be of similar efficacy to other antipsychotics (n = 1162, s = 13, Marques et al, Cochrane Data-base Syst Rev 2004;**1**:CD003545).

BUTYROPHENONES

Benperidol *

Benperidol is a potent D2 blocker marketed originally as specific for antisocial forms of sexual behaviour, with uncontrolled studies and reports claiming beneficial effects. Cochrane concludes that there is insufficient evidence to assess the drug's effectiveness, with only one poor RCT, where it was inferior to perphenazine (Leucht and Hartung, Cochrane Database Syst Rev 2005; **2**: CD003083). See 1.26.

Haloperidol (see also depots) *

Haloperidol is the prototype and standard reference butyrophenone still widely used for the treatment of acute and chronic psychosis, both orally and as an injection (aqueous and depot). Although the BNF limit is 30mg/d, there is no additional antipsychotic advantage from doses higher than 12mg/d in psychosis (eg. n = 176, RCT, d/b, 13/52, Volavka et al, Arch Gen Psychiatry 1992;**49**:354–61), and in acute mania (n = 47, RCT, d/b, Rifkin et al, Br J Psychiatry 1994;**165**:113–6). Indeed, 4mg/d may be as effective as 10mg/d and 40mg/d in newly-admitted in-patients, mostly schizophrenics (Stone et al, Am J Psychiatry 1995;**152**:1210–2). Even ultra-low doses (1–2mg/d) may be effective and well-tolerated in first-episode psychosis (n = 35, open, Oosthuizen et al, J Psychopharmacol 2001;**15**:251–5) producing 53–74% D_2 receptor occupancy, with sub-stantial clinical improvement and minimal side-effects (n = 7, Kapur et al, Am J Psychiatry 1996;**153**:948–50; n = 2, Hirsschowitz et al, Am J Psychiatry 1997;**154**:715–6). However, even low-dose haloperidol (mean 1.7mg/d) has been reported to cause as much TD as standard dose typicals (n = 57, 12/12, Oosthuizen et al, J Clin Psychiatry 2003;**64**:1075–80). Any dose

above 20mg/d should thus be the exception rather than the rule. This is illustrated by a 63% dose reduction in chronic treatment-resistant schizophrenics on high-dose haloperidol resulting in improvement of symptoms and side-effects, further improved by intensive behaviour therapy (n = 13, open, Liberman et al, Am J Psychiatry 1994;**151**:756–9). The elimination half-life in brain tissue is about 6–8 days, with significant amounts still detectable after two weeks. Thus, residual side-effects may continue for many weeks or months after stopping the drug, due to persistence of active CNS levels (Kornhuber et al, Am J Psychiatry 1999;**156**:885–90). Cochrane concludes that haloperidol is superior to placebo but that its ADRs are such that alternative antipsychotics should be prescribed (Joy et al, Cochrane Database Syst Rev 2006;**4**:CD003082). There have been some concerns over the risk of a dose-related increase in QT-interval (n = 596, Reilly et al, Lancet 2000;**355**:1048–52), especially if given by the IV, rather than IM route.

Reviews: Pharmacokinetics (Kudo and Ishizaki, Clin Pharmacokinetics 1999;**37**:435–56).

THIOXANTHENES

Flupentixol (see also depots) *

Oral flupentixol is usually used in low dose for anxiety and depression but flupentixol 5–20mg/d was as effective as olanzapine 5–20mg/d with more EPS but less weight gain (n = 28, RCT, d/b, 4/52, Gattaz et al, Pharma-copsychiatry 2004;**37**:279–85).

Zuclopenthixol (see also depots) *

Zuclopenthixol is a relatively long-acting oral antipsychotic, also available as a shorter- and longer-acting depot. In a much-needed trial of oral vs depot zuclopenthixol in people with violence and schizophrenia, violence was inversely proportional to compliance, and much lower in the depot group (n = 46, RCT, s/b, one year, Arango et al, Eur Psychiatry 2006;**21**:34–40). Cochrane concludes that oral zuclopenthixol is a viable option but needs routine anticholinergics (s = 18, n = 1578, Kumar and Strech, Cochrane Database Syst Rev 2005;**4**:CD005474).

DIPHENYLBUTYLPIPERIDINES

Fluspirilene

See depots.

Pimozide

Pimozide is licensed for chronic schizophrenia and other psychoses, especially paranoid and monosymptomatic hypochondriacal psychoses, eg. parasitosis. It is effective against a wide range of positive symptoms (Sultana and McMonagle, *Cochrane Database Syst Rev* 2000;**3**:CD001949), but with potential cardiotoxic effects (see 3.2). A review concluded that pimozide had effects on global functioning and mental state similar to other typical antipsychotics (Gray, *EBMH* 2000; **3**:117), but that any use in delusional disorders is based almost entirely on case reports.

BENZAMIDES, substituted

Review: * consensus statement on substituted benzamides in psychiatry (Racagni et al, *Neuropsychobiol* 2004;**50**:134–43).

Amisulpride *

Low dose amisulpride (related to sulpiride) blocks pre-synaptic D2 and D3 autoreceptors, higher doses blocking post-synaptic receptors, with little effect on other receptors. It is often classified as 'atypical' (or even an 'atypical' atypical: Lecrubier, *Int Clin Psychopharmacol* 2000;**15**[Suppl 4]:S21–S26). Amisulpride 50–100mg/d seems optimum for negative symptoms (eg. n = 232, d/b, p/c, Danion et al, *Am J Psychiatry* 1999;**156**:610–6; review by Moller, *Eur Arch Psychiatry Clin Neurosci* 2001;**251**:217–24). A meta-analysis showed some effect at low dose for predominantly negative symptoms and lower use of anticholinergic drugs (n = 2214, s = 18, RCT, Leucht et al, *Am J Psychiatry* 2002;**159**:180–90; caution expressed by Remington and Kapur, *EBMH* 2002;**5**:85). Another meta-analysis of four studies suggests negative symptoms respond to low-dose amisulpride (when it is an autoreceptor blocker, increasing dopamine turnover), but that the placebo response is high, the response of positive symptoms is lacking, and that at the dose necessary for positive symptom response (when it becomes

a D2/D3 blocker), its effect was essentially that of a typical agent (Storosum et al, *Schizo Bull* 2002;**28**;193–201). Amisulpride has been compared with risperidone (n = 309, RCT, d/b, 6/12, Sechter et al, *Neuropsychopharmacol* 2002;**27**;1071–81) and at 200–800mg/d is equivalent to olanzapine 5–20mg/d at 2/12, but with less weight gain (n = 377, RCT, d/b, 6/12, Martin et al, *Curr Med Res Opin* 2002;**18**:355–62) but more prolactin effects (RCT, d/b, 6/12, Mortimer et al, *Int Clin Psychopharmacol* 2004;**19**:63–9). Amisulpride 400–800mg/d may improve depressive symptoms in schizophrenia compared to risperidone and haloperidol (n = 612, 4/52, Peuskens et al, *Eur Neuropsychopharm* 2002;**12**:305–10). EPSEs and raised prolactin are generally considered to be dose-dependent. Oral bioavailability is poor. Cochrane concludes that amisulpride has a good general profile, may improve global and negative symptoms and might be more acceptable and more tolerable than high-potency conventional antipsychotics (n = 2443, RCTs = 19, Mota et al, *Cochrane Database Syst Rev* 2002;**2**:CD001357).

Reviews: general (Mortimer, *Int J Neuropsychopharmacol* 2004;**7**[Suppl 1]:S21–25; meta-analysis of RCTs by Leucht, *Int J Neuropsychopharmacol* 2004;**7**[Suppl 1]:S15-20; Green, *Curr Med Res Opin* 2002;**18**:113–7), receptor blockade (Curran and Perry, *CNS Drugs* 2002;**16**:207–11).

Sulpiride

Sulpiride is a specific dopamine (D2, plus some D3 and D4) receptor blocker, well-established in the UK (extensive review by Caley and Weber, *Ann Pharmacother* 1995;**29**:152–60).

ATYPICAL OR SECOND GENERATION ANTIPSYCHOTICS

'Atypical' is a widely-used term to describe a diverse group of antipsychotics with specific characteristics, eg. minimal EPS, lack of sedation or a fast dissociation from D2 receptors. It may be better to either consider antipsychotics on a spectrum, from typical (eg. chlorpromazine) at one end to atypical (eg. clozapine) at the other, or to base it upon a particular definition of atypicality, eg. serotonin-dopamine antagonism

(SDA), limbic specificity or a structural grouping. **Reviews of atypicals:** * terminology (Fleischacker, *Curr Opin Psychiatry* 2002;**15**:1–2), general (Anon, *Drug Ther Bull* 2004;**42**:57–60; Mortimer, *Expert Opin Invest Drugs* 2004;**13**:315–29; Moller, *World J Biol Psychiatry* 2004;**5**:9–19; Serretti *et al*, *Curr Med Chem* 2004;**11**:343–58), side-effects (Ananth *et al*, *Curr Pharm Des* 2004;**10**:2219–29), TDM (Hiemke *et al*, *Ther Drug Monit* 2004;**26**:156–60; Raggi *et al*, *Curr Med Chem* 2004;**11**:279–96), doses (Kinon *et al*, *CNS Drugs* 2004;**18**:597–616), use in non-schizophrenic conditions (Jeste and Dolder, *J Psychiatr Res* 2004;**38**:73–103) and mechanisms of action (Horacek *et al*, *CNS Drugs* 1006;**20**:389–409).

Aripiprazole *

Aripiprazole is a dopamine D2 and $5HT_{1A}$ receptor partial agonist, and a $5HT_{2A}$ receptor antagonist. It stimulates dopamine receptors but to a lower level than dopamine, while blocking endogenous dopamine (100% D2 occupancy by aripiprazole reduces dopaminergic activity to about 30%). Thus, putting it simply, when dopamine activity is high it reduces this (and hence psychotic symptoms) and, if low, will slightly increase it. There is only a minimal effect on alpha-1, H_1 and $5HT_{2C}$ receptors. In acute exacerbation of schizophrenia, aripiprazole 10 mg/d seems an effective strategy (n = 367, RCT, d/b, p/c, 6/52, Cutler *et al*, *CNS Spectr* 2006;**11**:691–702). The starting dose should be 5 mg/d if the patient is switching from another antipsychotic, increased to 10 mg/d, and then 15 mg/d as tolerated. Although 10–30 mg/d seems effective, higher doses have been used, albeit with variable success (35–60 mg/d, n = 4, Crossman and Lindenmayer, *J Clin Psychiatry* 2006;**67**:1158–9; 75 mg/d n = 1, Duggan and Mendhekar, *J Clin Psychiatry* 2006;**67**:674–5). A systematic review has concluded that aripiprazole is superior to placebo with less raised prolactin than other antipsychotics, although study attrition rates were large and poorly reported (s = 10, El-Sayeh *et al*, *Br J Psychiatry* 2006;**189**:102–8). It seems effective for relapse prevention, where 15 mg/d seems well-tolerated and effective (n = 310, RCT, p/ c, d/b, 6/12, Pigott *et al*, *J Clin Psychiatry* 2003; **64**:1048–56; comment by Mortimer, *EBMH* 2004;**7**:41 noting placebo level side-effects,

no dose titration, simple dosing, and that 30% of stable people relapsed over 6/12 when switched, and a lack of symptom reduction in more severely ill patients). Time to steady state takes one to two and maybe four weeks so don't increase doses too quickly (Uzun *et al*, *Psychiatr Danub* 2005;**17**:67–75). Cochrane concludes aripiprazole is effective, with a lower risk of akathisia, raised prolactin and QTc prolongation than other atypicals (El-Sayeh and Morganti, *Cochrane Database Syst Rev* 2006 **2**: CD004578).

Reviews: * general (Fleischacker, *Expert Opin Pharmacother* 2005;**6**:2091–101; Kinghorn and McEvoy, *Expert Rev Neurother* 2005;**5**:297–307; Naber and Lambert, *Prog Neuropsychopharmacol Biol Psychiatry* 2004;**28**:1213–9; Harrison and Perry, *Drugs* 2004;**64**:1715–36; Swainston *et al*, *Drugs* 2004;**64**:1715–36), pharmacology and mode of action (Gupta and Masand, *Ann Clin Psychiatry* 2004;**16**:155–66; Gründer *et al*, *Arch Gen Psychiatry* 2003;**60**:974–7).

Clozapine (see also *Tables 1.3–1.6*)

Clozapine is the prototype atypical antipsychotic, indicated for treatment-resistant schizophrenia and unresponsive psychotic disorders in Parkinson's disease. Before starting, patients should have a physical examination and any cardiac disease excluded.

Efficacy: Clozapine is probably effective in up to 30–50% of treatment-resistant schizophrenics (n = 268, RCT, d/b, p/c, 6/52, Kane *et al*, *Arch Gen Psychiatry* 1988;**45**:789–96). This may rise to 60% if adequate doses are given for up to 12 months, eg. a one-year study of treatment refractory or antipsychotic-intolerant schizophrenics showed that 50% of the former and 76% of the latter groups responded to clozapine over 52 weeks, the peak response occurring at 12–24 weeks (n = 84, open, Lieberman *et al*, *Am J Psychiatry* 1994;**151**:1744–52). There is probably little clinical gain in prolonging exposure to clozapine beyond eight weeks at any particular dose if no response is seen (n = 50, open, Conley *et al*, *Am J Psychiatry* 1997;**154**:1243–7). In resistant schizophrenia, clozapine was superior to risperidone on most efficacy measures, although both were well-tolerated (n = 273, RCT, d/b, 12/52, Azorin *et al*, *Am J Psychiatry*

2001;**158**:1305–13). A meta-analysis of atypicals in treatment-resistant schizophrenia indicated that clozapine has consistent superiority over typicals (efficacy and safety), but that the evidence for other atypicals in treatment-resistant schizophrenia is inconclusive (meta-analysis, n = 1916, s = 12, Chakos et al, Am J Psychiatry 2001;**158**:518–26).

Mode of action: Clozapine's mode of action is open to some debate, eg. it has a low occupancy of D_2 receptors (30–60%) and thus may act via D_1, 5-HT$_2$, ACh, 5-HT$_6$ and 5-HT$_7$ receptors and inhibition of pre-synaptic alpha-2 autoreceptors. Some D_2 limbic specificity has been detected.

Blood levels: Plasma levels may be useful in optimising therapy if poor response occurs. Plasma clozapine levels of 200–450 ng/ml have been shown to be superior to levels of 150 ng/ml and below (n = 56, VanderZwaag et al, Am J Psychiatry 1996;**153**:1579–84). Levels over 350 ng/ml (Kronig et al, Am J Psychiatry 1995;**152**:179–82) should only be reached with extreme care and blood levels may not necessarily be related to therapeutic efficacy (n = 41, Kurz et al, Br J Psychiatry 1998;**173**:341–4). Low plasma levels may occur in CYP1A2 rapid metabolisers (review by Greenwood-Smith et al, J Psychopharmacol 2003;**17**:234–8) and may account for some non-responders.

Suicide reduction: It is now reasonably well-established that clozapine may reduce suicide rates in schizophrenia. The suicide rate for schizophrenia can be as high as 1 in 10, a startling comparison with the risk of 1 in 50 for reversible agranulocytosis. The InterSePT study (n = 980, RCT, d/b, two years, Meltzer et al, Arch Gen Psychiatry 2003;**60**:82–91; comment on this ambitious and landmark study, by Volavka, EBMH 2003;**6**:93) has shown a 25% reduction in suicide events compared to olanzapine, a drug itself with possible antisuicide effects. The InterSePT study also showed that the reduced suicide rate was from clozapine's intrinsic action not from concomitant medication (supplementary analysis, Glick et al, J Clin Psychiatry 2004;**65**:679–85; see also n = 88, Meltzer and Okayli, Am J Psychiatry 1995; **152**:183–90), making a contribution to the risk:benefit analysis of clozapine. The reduction in suicidality may be due to reduction in impulsiveness and aggression (n = 44, open,

6/12, prospective, Spivak et al, J Clin Psychiatry 2003;**64**:755–60). However, another study failed to show a reduced completed suicide rate with clozapine (9.2–10.5% in each group over four years), as the reduced death rate was entirely due to reduced respiratory disorders (n = 1514 plus 2830 matched-controls, four years, Sernyak et al, Am J Psychiatry 2001; **158**:931–7; disputed by Ertugrul and Meltzer, Am J Psychiatry 2002;**159**:323–5; comment by Reinstein et al, Clin Drug Investig 2002;**22**:341–6).

Blood dyscrasias: Clozapine can cause a usually reversible neutropenia in 3–4% of patients, which may lead on to agranulocytosis in 0.8% of patients over one year, with a non-dose-related higher risk in older people and those with lower base-line wbc counts (n = 11555, Alvir et al, N Engl J Med 1993;**329**:162–7). Onset peaks around 8–10 weeks (range 0.5–24+ weeks) and treatment is thus restricted as per Table 1.2. A meta-analysis concluded the incidence of dyscrasias in long-term therapy may actually be as high as 7% (n = 2530, Wahlbeck et al, Am J Psychiatry 1999;**156**:990–9). The UK CPMS database study indicated that agranulocytosis is 2.4-fold higher in Asians compared to Caucasians, and there is an age-related increase in risk of 53% per decade, but no dose-relationship (n = 12760, Munro et al, Br J Psychiatry 1999;**175**:576–80). Clozapine is also both able to induce transient granulocytopenia without the usual rise in granulocyte colony stimulating factor (G-CSF) levels. The use of clozapine in people with a low wbc count due to benign ethnic neutropenia (BEN) may be allowed with haematologist advice. Of 53 patients rechallenged after clozapine-induced leucopenia or neutropenia, 38% had a further dyscrasia and, in most of these, it was more severe, longer-lasting and occurred more quickly than the original episode, but 55% were rechallenged successfully and remained in treatment (n = 53, Dunk et al, Br J Psychiatry 2006;**188**:255–63). The use of G-CSF in neutropenia is both effective and logical (eg. n = 1, Schuld et al, Acta Psychiatr Scand 2000; **102**:153–5; Sperner-Unterweger et al, Br J Psychiatry 1998;**173**:82–4).

Cost-effectiveness: Even with the previous high acquisition costs of clozapine in the UK (now breathtakingly reduced in UK, as a result

Clozapine UK prescribing and monitoring summary

Clozapine is indicated in the UK for treatment-resistant schizophrenia and psychosis in Parkinson's disease, ie. patients 'non-responsive' or 'intolerant' of conventional antipsychotics (*Table 1.3*). It can be dispensed on a weekly, fortnightly or four-weekly basis (*Table 1.4*), but only following a satisfactory blood result (*Table 1.5*).

TABLE 1.3: SUMMARY OF UK CLOZAPINE PRESCRIBING RESTRICTIONS

'Non-responsive'	Lack of satisfactory clinical improvements despite the use of at least two marketed antipsychotics prescribed at adequate dose for an adequate duration
'Intolerant'	The impossibility of achieving clinical benefit with conventional antipsychotics because of severe or untreatable neurological or other adverse reactions, eg. extrapyramidal or tardive dyskinesia
Patient requirements	Hospital-based originally. Normal white blood cell and differential blood counts. Enrolled with clozapine non-rechallenge database (CNRD)
Prescriber and dispensing requirements	Consultant must be registered with CNRD (clozapine non-rechallenge database). Hospital or nominated community pharmacy must be registered with CNRD

TABLE 1.4: SUMMARY OF UK CLOZAPINE MINIMUM BLOOD TEST REQUIREMENTS

Blood tests	Required frequency	Validity
Pre-treatment	Single blood screen	10 days, if satisfactory (green)
First 18 weeks of treatment First sample at three days	Weekly (usually Monday or Tuesday with result on Wednesday or Thursday)	11 days (not including day of sample) if satisfactory (green)
Weeks 19–52	Every 2 weeks if blood results have been satisfactory	21 days (not including day of sample) if satisfactory (green)
Weeks 53 onwards	Every four weeks, if 'stable haematological profile'	42 days (not including day of sample) if satisfactory (green)
Discontinuation (temporary or permanent)	Weekly (up to 18 weeks), or fortnightly (19 weeks onwards) for four weeks after completely stopping clozapine	If test result has not been, or does not go red, clozapine may be restarted. See *Table 1.6*

TABLE 1.5: SUMMARY OF UK TEST RESULTS

Results	Meaning	Action
Green	Satisfactory	Routine tests
Amber	wbc or neutrophil counts below accepted levels	Repeat test twice a week until either red or green
Red	wbc below 3000/mm^3 and/or absolute neutrophils below 1500/mm^3	Immediate cessation of therapy. Sample blood daily until patient recovered. No further prescribing allowed unless an error has occurred or consultant takes full responsibility

TABLE 1.6: SUMMARY OF TEMPORARY BREAKS IN CLOZAPINE THERAPY ADVICE

1. Dose		
Dose on discontinuation	Break	Dose on restart
Any	<48 hours	Restart on previous dose
Any	>48 hours	Restart at 12.5–25mg and build up gradually to previous dose to minimise dose-related side-effects
2. Sampling frequency		
Previous monitoring frequency	Break	Monitoring on restart
Weekly	<1 week	Weekly, no need to restart 18-week period
Weekly	>1 week	Weekly, **must** restart 18-week period
After 18 weeks		
Fortnightly	≤3 days	Fortnightly
Fortnightly	≤3 days	Weekly for six weeks, then fortnightly
Four-weekly	≤3 days	Four-weekly
Four-weekly	>3 days	Weekly for six weeks, then four-weekly
Fortnightly or four-weekly	>4 weeks	Weekly for 18 weeks, then resume on previous frequency

of Denzapine® [Denfleet] and Zaponex® [Ivax] brands joining Clozaril® [Novartis] on the British market), it could still be a very cost-effective treatment for resistant schizophrenia, but lower UK prices make this even better. Savings result almost exclusively from reduced costs of hospitalisation (Meltzer et al, Am J Psychiatry 1993;**150**:1630–8; review in Lancet 1993;**306**:1427–8; UK study n = 63, Hayhurst et al, J Psychopharmacol 2002;**16**:169–75).

Reviews: * combination therapies (Mouaffak et al, Clin Neuropharmacol 2006;**29**:28–33; Kontaxakis et al, Clin Neuropharmacol 2005; **28**:50–3), safety (Fitzsimons et al, Expert Opin Drug Saf 2005;**4**:731–44), in children (Kranzler et al, Child Adolesc Psychiatr Clin N Am 2006; **15**:135–59).

Olanzapine *

Olanzapine is licensed for the treatment of schizophrenia and relapse prevention. It blocks a wide variety of receptors, eg. $5\text{-HT}_{2A/C}$, 5-HT_3, 5-HT_6, D_{1-5}, M_{1-5}, alpha-one and H1, with some mesolimbic dopamine selectivity. The starting and main therapeutic dose is 10mg/d (range 5–20mg/d, mean 15–18mg/d). The main side-effects are somnolence and weight gain but with low EPS and a lower incidence of treatment-emergent tardive dyskinesia than haloperidol (re-analysis of data from three studies, Tollefson et al, Am J Psychiatry 1997;**154**:1248–54; n = 1714, RCT, d/b, up to 2.6 years, Beasley et al, Br J Psychiatry 1999;**174**:23–30, MS). A transient rise in prolactin levels can occur. There is a positive correlation between plasma levels and dose, and curvilinear relationship between plasma level and clinical improvement (n = 54, open, Mauri et al, Eur Psychiatry 2005;**20**:55–60) and so olanzapine levels may be useful to optimise doses and assess the influence of gender, smoking and interactions (n = 194, Skogh et al, Ther Drug Monit 2002;**24**:518–26). Many studies have shown a clinical effect, eg. where olanzapine (mean dose 15mg/d) was more effective than haloperidol (10–20mg/d) on negative symptoms (n = 335, RCT, d/b, 12/12, Tollefson and Sanger, Am J Psychiatry 1997;**154**:466–74), superior to haloperidol for all symptoms of schizophrenia, with fewer side-effects, including EPS and prolactin levels (n = 1996, d/b, 6/52, Tollefson et al, Am J Psychiatry

1997;**154**:457–65) and superior to risperidone for primary negative symptoms and with less side-effects (n = 339, d/b, 28/52, Tran et al, J Clin Psychopharmacol 1997;**17**:407–18, MS; reviewed by Cunningham Owens, EBMH 1998;**1**:55). It may also be effective for secondary negative symptoms, but not necessarily in having a direct beneficial effect on primary negative symptoms (n = 39, open, 12/52, Kopelowicz et al, Am J Psychiatry 2000;**157**:987–93). Neuropsychological changes in early phase schizophrenia during 12 months of treatment with olanzapine (5–20mg/d), risperidone (4–10mg/d), or haloperidol (5–20mg/d) showed olanzapine may have some superior cognitive effects (n = 65, Purdon et al, Arch Gen Psychiatry 2000;**57**:249–58). One (non-Lilly) study in treatment-resistant schizophrenia suggested that switching from an atypical/haloperidol to olanzapine may improve cognitive function but improve psychopathology in only 9% (n = 45, Lindenmayer et al, J Clin Psychiatry 2002;**63**:931–5). Olanzapine appeared highly effective in a relapse prevention study (n = 583, RCT, d/b, one year, Beasley et al, J Clin Psycho-pharmacol 2003;**23**:582–94, MS). Cochrane concludes that olanzapine may be effective, with low EPS and greater weight gain, but that the high drop-outs and unfamiliar rating scales make firm conclusions difficult to draw (Duggan et al, Cochrane Database Syst Rev 2005;**2**:CD001329).

Reviews: * general (Kando et al, Ann Pharma-cother 1997;**31**:1325–34), pharmacology and kinetics (Falsett, Hosp Pharm 1999;**34**:423–35, 91 refs; Callaghan et al, Clin Pharmacokinetics 1999;**37**:177–93), TDM/plasma levels, dosing and interactions (n = 71, Bergemann et al, Pharmacopsychiatry 2004;**37**:63–8).

Paliperidone * (UK launch due in 2007)

Paliperidone, the 9-hydroxy metabolite of risperidone, was licensed in USA in 2006 and is due for launch in UK in 2007. The starting and standard dose is 6mg/d, which has placebo level EPS, with no need for dose titration. The oral form uses the OROS sustained release system giving a once-daily dosage and steady plasma levels. Efficacy has been shown in a short-term study (n = 628, RCT, 6/52, Kane et al, Schizophr Res 2007;**90**:147–61) and a relapse prevention study (n = 113, RCT, d/b, p/c, 6/52, Kramer et al, J Clin Psychopharmacol 2007;**27**:6–14). An oil-based depot injection is in development and due around 2010.

Quetiapine *

Quetiapine is structurally related to clozapine and a recent meta-analysis showed it to be a good first-line antipsychotic (s = 8, Schulz et al, Schizophr Res 2003;**62**:1–12). Doses of 300–450mg/d (range 150–750mg/d) are quoted as the most effective. Doses need to be increased gradually over several days initially to reduce the incidence of postural hypotension. Many double-blind randomised trials indicate that the drug is as effective in schizophrenia as reference drugs (eg. n = 101, Peuskens and Link, Acta Psychiatr Scand 1997;**96**:265–73; n = 448, RCT, 6/52, Copolov et al, Psychol Med 2000;**30**:95–105). In schizophrenics only partially responsive to typicals, significantly more responded to quetiapine 600mg/d than haloperidol 20mg/d, and quetiapine was better tolerated (n = 288, d/b, 8/52, Emsley et al, Int Clin Psychopharmacol 2000;**15**:121–31). Quetiapine may improve cognitive functioning (n = 58, RCT, Velligan et al, Schizophr Res 2002;**53**:239–48) and negative symptoms (s = 4, n = 1106, Tandon, Hum Psychopharmacol 2004;**19**:559–63). Analysis from three RCTs has shown that the onset of action of quetiapine is significant by the end of week one (SANS and BPRS), sooner than usually expected (s = 3, n = 620, RCT, d/b, Small et al, Curr Med Res Opin 2004;**20**:1017–23). There is a huge variation in plasma levels in patients taking quetiapine (n = 62, Hasselstrom and Linnet, Ther Drug Monit 2004;**26**:486–91) and high doses have been used in TRS (Pierre et al, Schizophr Res 2005;**73**:373–5). Quetiapine shows transiently high D2 occupancy which drops rapidly over 12–14 hours, which may explain the low EPS and low prolactin elevation (n = 12, Kapur et al, Arch Gen Psychiatry 2000;**57**:553–9). Switching to once-daily quetiapine is feasible for most patients (with an SR formulation due in 2007–8), although a few may experience worsening symptoms or orthostatic hypotension (n = 21, RCT, d/b, c/o, 4 + 4/52, Chengappa et al, Can J Psychiatry 2003;**48**:187–94). Quetiapine seems to be safe and effective in psychosis in the elderly but lower doses, although higher doses perhaps in functional psychosis (n = 100 [c = 91], open, 4/52, Yang et al, J Psychopharmacol 2005; **19**:661–6). Cochrane concludes that although quetiapine is more effective than placebo, no difference could be detected against traditional antipsychotics and drop-outs, due to adverse effects, were lower with quetiapine, but still high (Srisurapanont et al, Cochrane Database Syst Rev 2004;**2**:CD000967).

Reviews: * general (Cheer and Wagstaff, CNS Drugs 2004;**18**:173–99, 139 refs; Hellewell, Hosp Med 2002;**63**:600–3), safety (Dev and Raniwalla, Drug Saf 2000;**23**:295–307), pharmacokinetics (DeVane and Nemeroff, Clin Pharmacokinet 2001;**40**:509–22), use in Parkinson's disease (Matheson and Lamb, CNS Drugs 2000;**14**:157–72), dosing strategies, including higher doses (Citrome et al, J Clin Psychiatry 2005;**66**:1512–6).

Risperidone *

Risperidone is licensed for acute and chronic psychosis. It has D_2 and 5-HT_2 blocking actions and has been shown to be effective against both positive and negative symptoms with few side-effects. It may also improve sleep in schizophrenics (cf haloperidol, n = 109, Yamashita et al, Psychiatry Res 2002;**109**:137–42).

Dose: An extensive literature analysis concluded that risperidone's optimum dose is 4mg/d, lower doses being consistently less effective and > 6mg/d having more side-effects, with less efficacy at > 10mg/d (Ezewuzie and Taylor, J Psychopharmacol 2006;**20**:86–90). Titration to 6mg/d over three days is recommended, but a slower titration has been recommended (over weeks rather than days, stabilising on 2–4mg/d initially before proceeding to higher doses), particularly in drug-naive first-episode schizophrenics and the elderly. Slow titration markedly reduces the final doses needed, EPS and the risk of non-compliance (n = 17, Kontaxakis et al, Am J Psychiatry 2000; **157**:1178–9), and may lead to better outcomes (retrospective review; n = 1056, Love et al, J Clin Psychiatry 1999;**60**:771–5; n = 96, McGorry, J Clin Psychiatry 1999;**60**:794). Even very low dose (1–2mg/d) can produce dramatic improvements in prodromal phase or first episode schizophrenia (n = 10, 12/52, open,

Cannon et al, Am J Psychiatry 2002;**159**:1230–2). In the acute phase, a rapid dose-loading regimen (1mg every 6–8 hours up to 3mg BD) has been relatively well-tolerated and is effective in acute states (n = 11, Feifel et al, J Clin Psychiatry 2000;**61**:909–11), and the availability of a quick dissolving tablet (Risperdal Quicklets® [Janssen-Cilag]) may facilitate this.

Efficacy: Risperidone has shown efficacy across a wide range of symptoms of psychosis and schizophrenia, eg. against positive and negative symptoms, disorganised thoughts, hostility and affective symptoms, and superior at four weeks and better tolerated than haloperidol (n = 67, d/b, 8/52, Wirshing et al, Am J Psychiatry 1999;**156**:1374–9). Comparisons with olanzapine have been favourable, eg. more effective than olanzapine with comparable side-effects (n = 42, open, 6/12, Ho et al, J Clin Psychiatry 1999;**60**:658–63), or lower weight gain (n = 377, RCT, Conley and Mahmoud, Am J Psychiatry 2001;**158**:765–74). Relapse prevention has now been clearly shown by a robust one-year study against haloperidol, where the risperidone group had a greater reduction in psychotic symptoms and EPS and a lower relapse rate (n = 397, average follow-up one-year, Csernansky et al, N Engl J Med 2002;**346**:16–22; comment by McIntosh, EBMH 2002;**5**:77). Risperidone (4–6mg/d, n = 153) was superior to placebo (n = 73) and quetiapine (600–800mg/d, n = 156) in acute exacerbations of schizophrenia requiring hospitalisation (n = 382, RCT, d/b, p/c, 6/52, Potkin et al, Schzophr Res 2006;**85**:254–65).

Refractory schizophrenia: Efficacy similar to clozapine has been claimed for risperidone in treatment-resistant or intolerant schizophrenia (n = 86, d/b, Bondolfi et al, Am J Psychiatry 1998;**155**:499–504; fiercely criticised by Meltzer and others, Am J Psychiatry 1999; **156**:1126–8). Other data has suggested risperidone to be only slightly less effective than clozapine, but with fewer side-effects (n = 35, open, 12/52, Lindenmayer et al, J Clin Psychiatry 1998;**59**:521–7), equivalent to clozapine on negative symptoms but not on positive symptoms (n = 29, d/b, parallel, 6/52, Breier et al, Am J Psychiatry 1999;**156**:294–8), and better tolerated and more effective than haloperidol (n = 67, d/b, Wirshing et al, Am J Psychiatry 1999;

156:1374–9). In another study in TRS, 25% responded to risperidone (mean 7mg/d) and 58% responded to clozapine (mean 520mg/d), suggesting that risperidone may be worth a try before clozapine (n = 24, Sharif et al, J Clin Psychiatry 2000;**61**:498–504).

Cognitive function: There is growing evidence for the role of poor cognitive function (especially working memory) in poor outcome of schizophrenia, and risperidone has been shown to produce an improvement in cognitive function (n = 25, Rossi et al, Acta Psychiatr Scand 1997;**95**:40–3), including against haloperidol (n = 59, Green et al, Am J Psychiatry 1997;**154**:799–804).

Reviews: TDM (therapeutic range of 25–150microg/L, n = 50, Odou et al, Clin Drug Invest 2000;**19**:283–92).

Sertindole *

Sertindole is supplied on a named-patient basis in the UK and is licensed for schizophrenia in patients who are intolerant of at least one other antipsychotic. The CHMP have now agreed to lift marketing restrictions, linked with an undertaking for Lundbeck to manage a phased re-introduction throughout Europe. Following a period of managed supply within the UK, it is expected that sertindole will be made more widely available to UK specialist clinicians. It has D_2, $5HT_2$ and alpha-1 blocking activity, the D_2 blockade having a uniquely high limbic specificity, leading to EPS equivalent to placebo at all therapeutic doses (n = 497, d/b, p/c, 8/52, Zimbroff et al, Am J Psychiatry 1997;**154**:782–91). To minimise the risk of postural hypotension, the initial dose is 4mg/d, increased by 4mg/d every 4–5 days, to 12–20mg/d (n = 16, s/b, Sramek et al, J Clin Psychopharmacol 1997;**17**:419–22). Five RCTs involving 1000 patients over eight weeks have shown clinical effectiveness in both positive and negative symptoms compared to haloperidol (review by Pickar, Lancet 1995;**345**:557–62). Slight lengthening of QTc has been shown in some patients, although no cases of ventricular arrhythmia have been seen in trials or post-marketing surveillance. This QTc prolongation has led to highly cautionary monitoring requirements. An ECG is required before and during treatment (see 3.2.1), as well as baseline serum potassium and magnesium (corrected if abnormal). Side-effects are nasal congestion, reduced ejaculatory volume, postural hypotension and dizziness and dry mouth. Cochrane concludes that sertindole is effective at 20 mg/d, and as tolerable as placebo (s = 3, n = 1104, Lewis et al, Cochrane Database Syst Rev 2005;**3**:CD001715).

Reviews: * general (Murdoch and Keating, CNS Drugs 2006;**20**:233–55; Hale et al, Int J Psychiatry Clin Pract 2000;**4**:55–62; Wilton et al, J Psychopharmacol 2001;**15**:120–6).

Zotepine *

Zotepine is a tricyclic dibenzothiepine licensed for schizophrenia in some countries. Both zotepine and its active metabolite norzotepine have a high affinity for a range of dopamine and serotonin receptor sub-types, and have some NARI activity. To minimise hypotension, the dose should be titrated from 25 mg TDS every four days to a maximum of 300 mg/d (as a TDS dose). It has been compared to haloperidol, low dose chlorpromazine and higher dose chlorpromazine 300–600 mg/d (less EPSE and greater improvement in BPRS, n = 158, RCT, 8/52, Cooper et al, Acta Psychiatr Scand 2000;**101**:218–25). Relapse prevention has been shown (n = 121, d/b, p/c, 6/12, Cooper et al, Psychopharmacol [Berl] 2000;**150**:237–43). Zotepine (mean 130 mg/d +/- 50 mg) was not superior to placebo for stable primary negative symptoms of schizophrenia, possibly due to the low-dose (n = 80, RCT, d/b, p/c, 8/52, Moller et al, Pharmacopsychiatry 2004;**37**:270-8). A meta-analysis suggested efficacy over comparator drugs, although nearly all trials were no more than 12/52 duration (s = 15, Butler et al, Int J Psychiatry Clin Pract 2000;**4**:19–27). The risk of seizures is dose-related and rises above 300 mg/d. An ECG is recommended pre-treatment in people with CHD, at risk of hypokalaemia or taking other drugs known to prolong QTc. Cochrane concludes from 10 studies that zotepine is as effective as typical and atypical antipsychotics and superior to placebo (n = 1006, Fenton et al, Cochrane Database Syst Rev 2000;**2**:CD001948; reviewed by Remington, EBMH 2000;**3**:78).

Review: Prakash and Lamb (CNS Drugs 1998;**9**:153–75, 115 refs; Cooper, Prescriber 2000;**11**:35–42).

Ziprasidone (not available in UK)

Ziprasidone is licensed in the USA and some European countries for schizophrenia, and is effective in the treatment of positive, negative and depressive symptoms of schizophrenia and schizoaffective disorder. The main side-effects are rash (5%) and orthostatic hypotension. Ziprasidone 5–20 mg has been shown to be effective in acute psychosis, and better tolerated than haloperidol IM (n = 132, 3/7, Brook et al, J Clin Psychiatry 2000;**61**:933–41), superior to placebo on PANSS with placebo level EPS (n = 278, RCT, d/b, p/c, one year, Arato et al, Int Clin Psychopharmacol 2002;**17**:207–15), in schizoaffective disorder (n = 115, RCT, d/b, p/c, 6/52, Keck et al, J Clin Psychopharmacol 2001;**21**:27–35) and effective for relapse prevention (n = 301, RCT, d/b, 28/52, Hirsch et al, J Clin Psychiatry 2002;**63**:516–23). The IM formulation is effective in doses of 10 mg IM every two hours or 20 mg IM every four hours. The maximum dose is 40 mg/d (n=79, RCT, d/b, Daniel et al, Psychopharmacol 2001;**155**:128–34). Olanzapine was superior to ziprasidone for schizophrenia symptoms, but ziprasidone was superior for weight changes and lipid profile (n = 277 + 271, RCT, d/b, 28/52, Breier et al, Am J Psychiatry 2005;**162**:1879–87). Although lorazepam may be given at the same time, the two must not be mixed in the same syringe due to compatability issues. If long-term therapy is required, oral ziprasidone should replace intramuscular administration as soon as possible.

Reviews: general (Kane, J Clin Psychiatry 2003; **64**[Suppl 19]:S19–S25; Beehham et al, J Clin Psychopharmacol 2003;**23**:229–32; Carnahan et al, Pharmacotherapy 2001;**21**:717–30, 46 refs).

DEPOT AND LONG-ACTING INJECTIONS

The major advantage of depots is assured compliance and steady plasma levels (although this may not be true in practice; n = 30, Tuninger and Levander, Br J Psychiatry 1996;**169**:618–21), with associated and proven reduction in relapses, rehospitalisation and severity of relapse. There may also be some reduction in bioavailability problems (some people metabolise antipsychotics extensively via the first-pass effect). Used properly, depots can lead to reduced relapses, low side-effects and stable therapeutic effects. By being sure of doses received, depots should be able to facilitate better downward titration of doses to reduce the incidence of side-effects. The major disadvantages include the impossibility of altering a dose if side-effects develop (eg. dystonia, NMS), patients seeing depot administration as 'being controlled', having no control over or involvement in their treatment or, worse still, as being a punishment. Many patients and families/caregivers are insufficiently educated about the pros and cons of depot administration. It is not enough just to prevent relapse with a depot.

One review (Adams et al, Br J Psychiatry 2001;**179**:290–9; reviewed by McGorry, EBMH 2002;**5**:42) concludes that depots are safe and effective and may confer a slight advantage over oral drugs in reducing relapse rates. Depot injections do, of course, also hurt, the pain declining over 10 days and this has a negative effect on patient attitude towards medication (n = 34, Bloch et al, J Clin Psychiatry 2001;**62**:855–9), although there is some evidence to the contrary (Walburn et al, Br J Psychiatry 2001;**179**:300–7).

The need for a meticulous (Z-tracking) injection technique (Belanger-Annable, Canadian Nurse 1985;**81**:1–3) and using the most appropriate preparation and dose for that individual are essential for long-term success (Muldoon, Br Med J 1995;**311**:1368).

Reviews: overview (Altamura et al, Drugs 2003; **63**:493–512; Taylor, Psychiatr Bull 1999;**23**:551–3; Kennedy and Mikhail, Lancet 2000;**356**:594), optimising the use of depots (Dencker and Axelsson, CNS Drugs 1996;**6**:367–81).

Pharmacokinetics

The tables on pp 151–153 show the plasma levels for each depot as single doses (although these have been difficult to obtain and are not reliable), and as computer-generated profiles for multiple doses (based on single-dose profiles). Surprisingly, there is still evidence of large variations in the plasma levels of haloperidol decanoate, although there was no relationship between side-effect ratings and fluctuations in plasma levels (n = 30, three years, Tuninger and Levander, Br J Psychiatry 1996;**169**:618–21).

Flupentixol decanoate
(Depixol®, Lundbeck)

Flupentixol is one of the most widely prescribed depots in the UK. It is a dopamine specific thioxanthene antipsychotic with potentially activating effects at low dose, and has been dubbed a 'partial atypical' (Kuhn et al, Fortschr Neurol Psychiatr 2000;**68**[Suppl 1]: S38–S41).

- Duration of action = 3–4 weeks.
- Peak = 7–10 days.
- Rate limiting half-life = eight days (single dose), 17 days (multiple doses).
- Time to steady state = 10–12 weeks.

Fluphenazine decanoate
(Modecate®, Sanofi-Synthelabo) *

Fluphenazine decanoate is a longer-acting phenothiazine and a four-week interval between injections is possible. The efficacy data is very limited, the 70 RCTs showing little difference between depots and oral (David et al, Cochrane Database Syst Rev 2005;**1**: CD000307). Responders have been shown to have greatest improvement with fluphenazine levels above 1.0ng/ml and doses above 0.2–0.25mg/kg/d (n=72, RCT, d/b, 4/52, Levinson et al, Am J Psychiatry 1995;**152**:765–71; n=24, Miller et al, J Clin Pharm Ther 1995;**20**:55–62). Fluphenazine 25mg every six weeks or every two weeks produces similar side-effects, symptom relief and relapse rates, but with reduced drug exposure with the longer dosage interval (n = 50, RCT, 54/52, Carpenter et al, Am J Psychiatry 1999;**156**:412–8).

- Duration of action = 1–3 weeks.
- Peak = 6–48 hours.
- Rate-limiting half-life = 6–10 days (single doses), 14–100 days (multiple doses).
- Time to steady state = 6–12 weeks (Marder et al, Br J Psychiatry 1991;**158**:658–65).

Fluspirilene
(Redeptin®, SmithKline French)

Fluspirilene is now only available in the UK as an import from Belgium, as a water-based micro-crystalline injection.

- Duration of action = 1.5 weeks.
- Peak within two days.
- Rate limiting half-life = 7–9 days.
- Time to steady state = 5–6 weeks.

Haloperidol decanoate
('Haldol Decanoate' ®, Janssen-Cilag)

Haloperidol decanoate is longer-acting and a four-week interval between injections is possible. An analysis of 13 studies suggests a maximal effect at 50 mg/4 weeks, with no evidence that doses above 100 mg/4 weeks have any additional effects (s = 6, Taylor, *Psychiatr Bull* 2005;**29**:104–7). Rates of deterioration with 50–100 mg/month were not significantly greater in one study compared to 25 mg/month, and ADRs were possibly higher (n = 105, RCT, d/b, Kane *et al*, *Am J Psychiatry* 2002;**4**:554–60; review by Marois and Roy, *EBMH* 2002;**5**:113). It is probably best reserved for chronic relapsing schizophrenics responsive to haloperidol (full review, Hemstrom *et al*, *Drug Intell Clin Pharm* 1988;**22**:290–5).

- Duration of action = six weeks.
- Peak = 3–9 days.
- Rate limiting half-life = 18–21 days (single + chronic).
- Time to steady state = 10–12 weeks at monthly dosing.

Pipothiazine
(Piportil®, JHC) *

Pipothiazine is a piperidine phenothiazine marketed in the UK as the palmitate. Cochrane concludes that although better data is needed, pipothiazine is a viable antipsychotic choice (Dinesh *et al*, *Cochrane Database Syst Rev* 2004;**4**:CD001720).

- Duration of action = 4–6 weeks.
- Peak = 9–10 days.
- Rate limiting half-life = 14–21 days.
- Time to steady state = 8–12 weeks.

Zuclopenthixol acetate
(Clopixol-Acuphase®, Lundbeck) *

Zuclopenthixol acetate is available as 'Clopixol-Acuphase' in the UK. 50–150 mg as a single dose provided a rapid and effective reduction in psychotic symptoms in 25 patients (*Curr Med Res Opin* 1990;12:58–65) over about 78 hours. The maximum cumulative dose is 400 mg over two weeks, with no more than four injections. It is a drug of choice in acute psychiatric emergency in many areas. Cochrane concludes that there is inadequate data on Acuphase and no convincing evidence

either way in APE compared to IM haloperidol (Fenton *et al*, *Cochrane Database Syst Rev* to 2004;**2**:CD00525). See also acute psychiatric emergencies (*1.1*).

- Duration of action = 2–3 days.
- Peak = 24–40 hours (n=19, Amdisen *et al*, *Psychopharmacology* [Berl] 1986;**90**:412–6).
- Rate limiting half-life = 32hrs +/- 7.

Zuclopenthixol decanoate
(Clopixol®, Lundbeck)

This is an established antipsychotic which has also been used in high dose in aggression, particularly in learning disabilities and forensic patients but is not indicated for this.

- Duration of action = 2–4 weeks.
- Peak = 4–9 days.
- Rate limiting half-life = 17–21 days (multiple doses).
- Time to steady state = 10–12 weeks.

Risperidone
(Risperdal Consta®, Janssen-Cilag) *

This novel, long-acting injection uses risperidone molecules in a synthetic and absorbable polymer microsphere base suspended in water. It is licensed for schizophrenic and other psychoses. The initial dose is 25–37.5 mg fortnightly (equivalent to oral doses of up to 2–3 mg/d), with a maximum of 50 mg every two weeks. Plasma levels are stable after 3–4th injections and maintained for 4–5 weeks after last injection then decline rapidly. D2 receptor studies show 25, 50 and 75 mg fortnightly risperidone is in the range found in patients effectively treated with 2–6 mg/d oral risperidone (n = 13, Gefvert *et al*, *Int J Neuropsychopharmacol* 2005;**8**:27–36; see also Love and Conley, *Am J Health Syst Pharm* 2004;**61**:1792–800). Risperidone levels may be lower with Consta than oral, but there is also a lower 9-OH risperidone:risperidone ratio with Consta, which may indicate higher depot doses are needed (n=78+82, Nesväg *et al*, *Acta Psychiatr Scand* 2006;**114**:21–6) and 25 mg/fortnight may be insufficient since it provides low plasma levels and possibly sub-therapeutic in vivo D2 occupancies (editorial by Taylor, *Acta Psychiatr Scand* 2006;**114**:1–2). Consta seems safe and effective, although

Depot and longer-acting injection pharmacokinetics

These graphs show the known plasma levels of the available longer-acting antipsychotic injections in the UK. The single dose kinetics are reasonably well-established for these preparations. The multiple-dose graphs are computer-generated as little or no data exists, with downward arrows indicating when injections are given. These graphs will, however, give some indication of the time to steady state, and the length of time before plasma levels fall to zero after a depot has been stopped. The 'y' axis units are not established for any of the multiple dose graphs, and there will of course be some inter-individual variation.

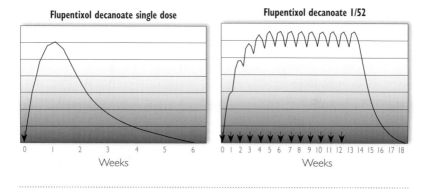

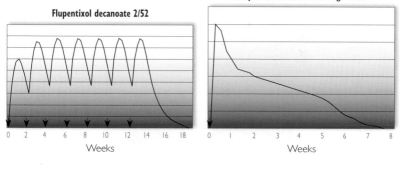

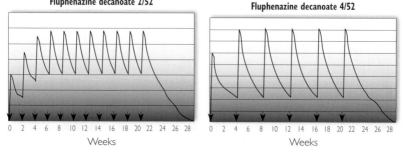

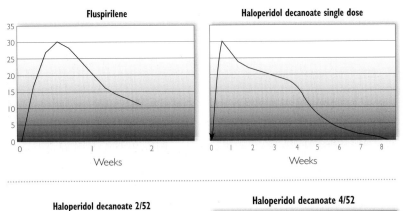

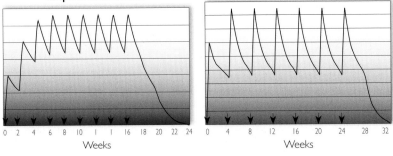

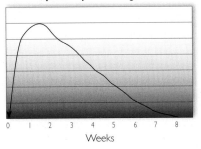

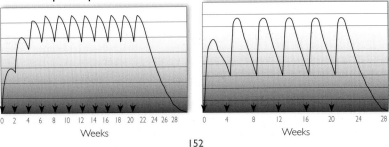

Risperidone Consta single dose

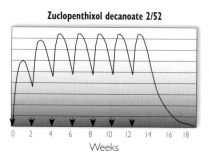

Risperdal Consta 2/52

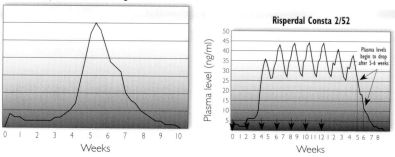

Plasma level (ng/ml)

Plasma levels begin to drop after 5-6 weeks

Weeks

Zuclopenthixol decanoate single dose

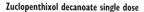

Weeks

Zuclopenthixol decanoate 1/52

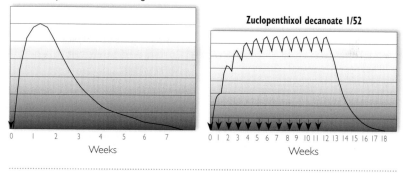

Weeks

Zuclopenthixol decanoate 2/52

Zuclopenthixol acetate single dose

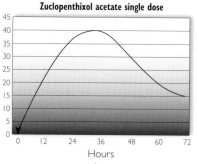

Weeks

Hours

50–75 mg had higher side effects (n = 400, RCT, d/b, p/c, 12/52, Kane et al, Am J Psychiatry 2003; **160**:1125–32). Since there is no significant drug release for 3–4 weeks, with a peak at 4–6 weeks, it is possible that a third fortnightly injection could be given before the full effect of the first is seen, and in recidivist patients, a full effect may occur only after many months of steady plasma levels. Where at all possible, patients should be pre-treated with risperidone orally for at least a few days before the injection is commenced to rule out any severe EPS, hypotension or other idiosyncratic reactions. Oral cover may be needed for the first 3–4 weeks, then tapered during weeks 4–5. Since steady state occurs about 6–8 weeks after each dose change, some have recommended dose increases only every eight weeks (Knox and Stimmel, Clin Ther 2004;**26**:1994–2002). There may be a small release of risperidone in the first few days from the surface of the granules and transient

EPSE may occur after one day (n = 3, Adamou and Hale, *Am J Psychiatry* 2004;**161**:576–7). Elimination is complete 7–8 weeks after the last injection. Switching to Consta can be done by abrupt switch from other depots without oral transition (open, 12/52, Turner *et al*, *Int Clin Psychopharmacol* 2004;**19**:241–9). The vials must be stored at 2–8°C, although can be kept at <25°C for up to seven days but should not be longer or put back in a fridge again.

Efficacy: * There have been several published reviews of Consta outcomes. In one, 65% of patients completed one year on Consta, 5% dropped out because of ADRs, and 25% suffered ADRs (n = 615, open, 12/12, Fleischacker *et al*, *J Clin Psychiatry* 2003;**64**:1250–7). Another review concludes that:

- the mean dose is 35 mg
- half of those with a good outcome at 6/12 had not yet improved by 3/12
- oral doses are needed longer than the first 3/52 (n = 50, naturalistic follow-up, Paton and Okocha, *Psychiatr Bull* 2004; **28**:12–4, IS).

In patients switching from stable oral typicals to Consta®, EPSE reduced and PANSS total scores reduced (n = 725, open, up to 50/52, van Os *et al*, *Int Clin Psychopharmacol* 2004;**19**:229–32; n = 725, open, Lasser *et al*, *Eur Psychiatry* 2004;**19**:219–25) and a naturalistic study showed 51% drop-out and moderate effectiveness (n = 100, 6/12, Taylor *et al*, *J Clin Psychiatry* 2004;**65**:1076–83), although another study concluded that the strongest prognostic indicator for early discontinuation in difficult to engage (poor complier) users appears to be switching from an oral antipsychotic, rather than a depot (n = 88, open, Patel *et al*, *Int Clin Psychopharmacol* 2004;**19**:233–9).

Reviews: * general (Ehter and Fuller, *Ann Pharmacother* 2004;**38**:2122–7).

+ Combinations

Polypharmacy with antipsychotics falls into three main categories:

- two or more drugs of the same class
- multiclass (two drugs in different classes at full dose)
- adjunctive and augmentation (low dose of one with a standard dose of another).

Appropriate reasons for the use of antipsychotic combinations include:

- Failure to respond to clozapine.
- Poor clozapine tolerance, with a second drug as augmentation of a low clozapine dose.
- As augmentation in clozapine partial response.
- Patients unwilling to stop an old drug or refusing to try clozapine.
- During a switch from one antipsychotic to another.
- When discontinuing a depot poses an unacceptable risk, eg. forensic patients.
- As a temporary measure during an acute exacerbation of illness.

Inappropriate reasons for the use of antipsychotic combinations include: *

- Confusing a sedative effect with an antipsychotic effect.
- Not waiting long enough for an antipsychotic to work (ie. at least six weeks) before making changes.
- As a substitute for failing to plan and communicate a switch, which is then never fully completed.
- Where clinical improvement occurs before a switch is completed, and the clinician 'quits while ahead' rather than risking completing the change.
- Using high doses to make up for inadequate resources and environment.

Despite widespread use of combinations (with increased ADRs and possibly reduced outcomes; n = 459 + 584, McCue *et al*, *J Clin Psychiatry* 2003; **64**:984–9), there are in fact only a very few RCTs of combination antipsychotics in schizophrenia (clozapine plus either risperidone or sulpiride) and in a retrospective case-control study multiple antipsychotics were associated with a major increase in drug exposure, adverse events and time in hospital, but with no apparent clinical gain compared to monotherapy (n = 70 pairs, Centorrino *et al*, *Am J Psychiatry* 2004; **161**:700–6). A critical review concludes there is some evidence for sulpiride, lamotrigine and E-EPA as clozapine augmentation (s = 11, n = 270, Kontaxakis *et al*, *Eur Psychiatry* 2005; **20**:409–15). Combinations should thus only be used once standard monotherapies have been found inadequate, and then with carefully monitored outcomes (clinical and adverse) and discontinued if no clear advantage is seen.

Reviews: 29 case reports, 172 case series and one double-blind study (Lerner et al, *Prog Neuropsychopharmacol Biol Psychiatry* 2004;**28**: 89–98), editorial review of the lack of evidence and trials of combinations (Stahl et al, *Acta Psychiatr Scand* 2004;**110**:241–2).

Clozapine combinations and augmentation

Clozapine + aripiprazole *

There are now many case reports of aripiprazole combined with clozapine, eg. in TRS (n = 3, Rocha and Hara, *Prog Neuropsychopharmacol Biol Psychiatry* 2006;**30**:1167–9), where it did not improve PANSS scores but there were significant decreases in weight, BMI, cholesterol and triglycerides (n = 10[c = 8], open, 6/52, Henderson et al, *Acta Psychiatr Scand* 2006; **113**:142–7). The combination has also helped negative symptoms (n = 3, Clarke et al, *J Clin Psychiatry* 2006;**67**:675–6) and significant improvement has occurred when aripiprazole was combined with low-dose (150–200 mg/d) clozapine (n = 3, Lim et al, *J Clin Psychiatry* 2004; **65**:1284–5).

Clozapine + amisulpride (see also sulpiride) *

Combining a specific D2-blocker with clozapine is a well-known strategy. There are some open studies (but no RCT yet), eg. 86% clozapine-refractory schizophrenics rated response as at least 'good' when amisulpride was added (n = 7, Agelink et al, *Am J Psychiatry* 2004;**161**:924–5), amisulpride significantly improved response to clozapine without significant additional side-effects (n = 33[c = 28], open, 6/12, Munro et al, *Acta Psychiatr Scand* 2004;**110**:292–8) and 80% improved with amisulpride 700 mg/d (range 520–980 mg/d) as adjunctive therapy (n = 15, retrospective, Lerner et al, *Clin Neuropharmacol* 2005;**28**:66–71). There are also some case reports (n = 1, George and Cowan, *Acta Psychiatr Scand* 2005;**111**:163; n = 6, Cook and Hoogen-boom, *Australas Psychiatry* 2004; **12**:74–6).

Clozapine + galantamine *

Galantamine 16 mg/d improved cognitive function in three patients when used as an adjunct to clozapine (n = 5, 8/52, Bora et al, *Clin Neuropharmacol* 2005;**28**:139–41).

Clozapine + lamotrigine

In an RCT, lamotrigine 200 mg/d added to clozapine in treatment-refractory schizophrenics improved positive and general symptoms, but not negative symptoms, the first RCT to show a non-dopamine blocking drug works in TRS (n = 34, RCT, d/b, p/c, 14/52, Tiihonen et al, *Biol Psychiatry* 2003;**54**:1241–8).

Clozapine + mirtazapine *

Mirtazapine augmentation of clozapine has improved negative symptoms (especially apathy and anhedonia) and BPRS scores (n = 24, RCT, d/b, p/c, 8/52, Zoccali et al, *Int Clin Psychopharmacol* 2004;**19**:71–6).

Clozapine + olanzapine

One patient responded to clozapine 100 mg/d and olanzapine 10 mg/d when individually neither was satisfactory (n = 1, Rhoads, *J Clin Psychiatry* 2000;**61**:678–80).

Clozapine + ondansetron

Ondansetron (4 mg BD) has enhanced the action of clozapine in treatment-refractory schizophrenic (n = 1, Briskin and Curtis, *Am J Psychiatry* 1997;**154**:1171). See also 'Unlicensed/possible efficacy'.

Clozapine + quetiapine

After six months on clozapine (200–800 mg/d), randomly selected patients had 25% of the clozapine dose openly converted to quetiapine (1 mg clozapine:2 mg quetiapine). Average weight loss was 0.22–10.5 kg after one month, and maintained, with '100% user satisfaction' reported, and improvement in those (n = 13) who had developed diabetes (n = 65, open, 10/12, Reinstein et al, *Clin Drug Invest* 1999;**18**:99–104).

Clozapine + risperidone *

The data on risperidone augmentation of clozapine is variable, with positive and negative RCTs. One RCT has shown risperidone 4–6 mg/d to improve sub-optimal clozapine response (n = 40, RCT, d/b, p/c, 12/52, Josiassen et al, *Am J Psychiatry* 2005;**162**:130–6), supporting case reports (eg. n=2, Morera et al, Acta Psychiatr Scand 1999;**99**:305–7; n=3, Raskin et al, Acta Psychiatr Scand 2000;**101**:334–6), although a moderate (four-fold) rise in prolactin levels can occur (n=40, open, Henderson et al, J Clin Psychiatry 2001;**62**:605–8). However, addition of risperidone 3 mg/d to clozapine had no significant effect in symptoms of severe schizophrenia (n=68, RCT, p/c, d/b, 8+18/52, Honer et al, N Engl J Med 2006;**354**:472–82), and in another RCT, addition of risperidone up to 6 mg/d made no difference to psychopathology or quality of life compared to placebo, although placebo looked a good treatment for PANSS positive symptom sub-scale (n=30, RCT, p/c, d/b, 6/52, Yagcioglu et al, J Clin Psychiatry 2005;**66**:63–72).

Clozapine + sulpiride

In the first RCT of combined antipsychotics, clozapine and sulpiride produced a substantially greater improvement than clozapine alone in TRS (n=24, RCT, Shiloh et al, Br J Psychiatry 1997;**171**:569–73), although the two study groups had some initial differences.

Clozapine + ziprasidone *

Addition of ziprasidone allowed a 18% reduction in clozapine dose and improved mental state in 77% patients (n=9, 6/12, Ziegenbein et al, Clin Neuropharmacol 2005;**28**:220–4).

Other antipsychotic combinations and augmentation

Amisulpride + risperidone or ziprasidone *

In a small open trial, 80% improved on the combination with amisulpride at a mean dose of 693 mg/d (n=15, open, Lerner et al, Clin Neuropharmacol 2005;**28**:66–71).

ECT + antipsychotics

This combination may be beneficial for positive (but not negative) symptoms of schizophrenia, with a 55% response rate and possible role early in an acute exacerbation of chronic schizophrenia with flupentixol (n=293, Chanpattana and Chakrabhand, Psychiatry Res 2001;**105**:107–15).

Olanzapine + quetiapine *

This combination was completely successful in a patient with raised prolactin intolerant

of clozapine, with no elevation of prolactin (n=1, Dunkley and Reveley, J Psychopharmacol 2005;**19**:97–101).

Olanzapine + sulpiride *

Sulpiride 600 mg/d augmentation of established and partially effective olanzapine had no effect on positive or negative symptoms but significantly improved depressive symptoms (n=17, RCT, 8/52, Kotler et al, Int Clin Psychopharmacol 2004;**19**:23–6).

Risperidone + olanzapine

This combination has been used with some reported success (n=5, open, Lerner et al, Clin Neuropharmacol 2000;**23**:284–6).

Valproate + antipsychotics

Reviews of valproate as an adjunct in schizophrenia have concluded that there is no proven advantage for valproate augmentation, although some studies showed inconsistent benefit and it may be useful in acute management (Basan et al, Schizophr Res 2004;**70**:33–7; Basan and Leucht, Cochrane Database Syst Rev 2004;1:4028), although one review was more positive (Citrome, Psychopharmacol Bull 2003;**37**[Suppl 2)]:S74–S88). Valproate as an adjunct to risperidone or olanzapine for acute exacerbation of schizophrenia has resulted in an earlier response of psychotic symptoms (n=249, RCT, d/b, Casey et al, Neuropsychopharmacol 2003;**28**:182–92).

● Augmentation (with drugs with no intrinsic antipsychotic activity)

Anticholinesterases (see also donepezil, galantamine + clozapine) *

Unlike donepezil (see no efficacy), rapid improvement in refractory negative symptoms of schizophrenia has been reported with **galantamine** (n=1, Rosse and Deutsch, Clin Neuropharmacol 2002; **25**:272–5), and addition of galantamine to risperidone has been clinically valuable in clozapine-intolerant chronic schizophrenics (n=2, Allen and McEvoy, Am J Psychiatry 2002;**159**:1244–5). **Rivastigmine** up to 16 mg BD has significantly improved quality of life and cognitive functioning with few ADRs (n = 16, 12/12, Lenzi et al, Clin Neuropharmacol 2003;**26**:317–21).

Benzodiazepines

Benzodiazepines have no antipsychotic effect but short-term use may reduce anxiety, tension and insomnia and high doses may have some tranquillising effects. They may also allow lower doses of antipsychotics to be used, as high doses of antipsychotics are often used for their additional sedative properties, eg. in psychotic agitation. In the acute situation, benzodiazepines have a rapid onset, are highly sedative, well-tolerated and a low EPS risk. See also 'Acute psychiatric emergency' (1.1).

Carbamazepine

Carbamazepine has been used in addition to antipsychotics to improve behaviour in over-active or aggressive schizophrenics. The effect on 'core' symptoms is likely to be secondary or small and only in schizophrenics, not schizoaffectives (n = 162, d/b, p/c, 4/52, Okuma et al, Acta Psychiatr Scand 1989;**80**:250–59). It is ineffective as maintenance (n=27, d/b, c/o, 95/7, Carpenter et al, Arch Gen Psychiatry 1991;**48**:69–72). Based on available RCTs, Cochrane could not recommend carbamazepine for routine use in schizophrenia, either as monotherapy or augmentation (Leucht et al, Cochrane Database Syst Rev 2002;**3**:CD001258) and a related systematic review and meta-analysis of the 10 RCTs (n = 283) of carbamazepine augmentation in schizophrenia failed to show any clinically significant positive effect (n = 283, Leucht et al, J Clin Psychiatry 2002;**63**:218–24). Remember also that carbamazepine will induce CYP3A4 and reduce the plasma levels of many antipsychotics.

Cicloserin

Cicloserin is a partial agonist of a glutamate receptor sub-type and addition of cicloserin 50 mg/d to typical antipsychotics, risperidone and olanzapine produced a significant reduction in negative symptoms (n = 24, d/b, p/c, c/o, 6/52, Heresco-Levy et al, Am J Psychiatry 2002; **159**:480–2; n = 9, Goff et al, Am J Psychiatry 1995;**152**:1213–15), supporting the view that glutamate function may be important in

schizophrenia. However, in a trial of clozapine-treated patients, successive placebo and increasing cicloserin doses failed to show any improvement in negative symptoms (n = 10, Goff et al, Am J Psychiatry 1996;**153**:1628–30). Dietary supplementation with high-dose glycine is a possible adjuvant treatment option.

Cox-2 inhibitors *

Celecoxib added to risperidone in resistant schizophrenia showed a significant reduction in PANSS compared to risperidone mono-therapy (n = 50, RCT, d/b, p/c, 5/52, Muller et al, Eur Arch Psychiatry Clin Neurosci 2004;**254**:14–22).

Cyproheptadine

Adding cyproheptadine 24 mg/d to haloperidol 30 mg/d significantly reduced negative symptoms (n = 30, RCT, Akhondzadeh et al, J Clin Pharm Ther 1999, **24**, 49), supporting an earlier study where 32 mg/d showed a good response in 40%, with two relapsing on withdrawal (n = 10, open, Silver et al, Biol Psychiatry 1989;**25**:502–4).

DHEA (dehydroepiandrosterone)

DHEA 100 mg/d produced significant improvements as adjunctive therapy in nega-tive, depressive and anxiety symptoms of schizophrenia, especially in women (n = 30, RCT, d/b, p/c, 6/52, Strous et al, Arch Gen Psychiatry 2003;**60**:133–41).

Dipyridamole

Combined dipyridamole (75 mg/d) and haloperidol (16–20 mg/d) was superior to haloperidol alone in schizophrenia, this possibly being via an effect on the interaction between the adenosine and dopamine systems (n = 30, RCT, Akhondzadeh et al, J Clin Pharm Ther 2000; **25**:131–8).

Folate

Folic acid 15 mg/d in addition to psychotropic drugs has been reported to significantly improve clinical response and recovery from acute psychiatric disorders (n = 123, RCT, d/b, p/c, 6/12, Godfrey et al, Lancet 1990;**336**:392–5; using methylfolate; Wing and Lee, Br J Psychiatry 1992;**160**:714–5).

Ginkgo Biloba

Ginkgo Biloba as an adjunct to haloperidol enhanced its effectiveness and reduced EPS compared to placebo (n = 109, RCT, d/b, p/c, 12/52, Zhang et al, J Clin Psychiatry 2001;**62**:878–83; comment by Knable, EBMH 2002;**5**:90).

Glycine *

High-dose glycine (0.8 g/kg/d) as add-on to olanzapine or risperidone significantly reduced negative symptoms by 23% and improved cognitive function (n = 17, RCT, d/b, p/c, c/o, 6/52, Heresco-Levy et al, Biol Psychiatry 2004;**15**:165–71; see also n = 11, RCT, Heresco-Levy et al, Br J Psychiatry 1996; **169**:610–17). Logically, the best results seem to be in patients with low pre-treatment plasma glycine levels. High-dose glycine added to antipsychotics was effective with no increase in antipsychotic levels (n = 12, RCT, Javitt et al, Int J Neuropsychopharmacol 2001;**4**:385–91). However, glycine 60 g/d had no statistically significant effects when used as augmentation of clozapine in schizophrenia (n = 30, d/b, p/c, Evins et al, Am J Psychiatry 2000;**157**:826–8).

Lamotrigine *

Lamotrigine augmentation is somewhat controversial. A number of studies have shown a positive effect in TRS, eg. augmentation of clozapine (n = 7) produced a significant reduction of BPRS, but not when augmenting risperidone (n = 3), haloperidol (n = 3), olanzapine (n = 3) or flupentixol (n = 1). A possible explanation is that enhancing glutamate transmission with NMDA antagonists produces schizophrenia-like symptoms and behavioural disruption in healthy volunteers and rodents. Pre-treatment with lamotrigine prevents this, possibly by enhancing antipsychotics or having an independent action (Large et al, Psychopharmacology [Berl] 2005;**6**:1–22). Conversely in TRS, adjunctive lamotrigine had no effect on primary end-points but improved positive symptoms using PANSS (n = 38 [c = 31], RCT, d/b, p/c, 10/52, Kremer et al, Biol Psychiatry 2004;**56**:441–6). Cochrane concludes that the available data on lamotrigine for schizophrenia is poor and no global response is detectable (s = 5, n = 537, Premkumar and Pick, Cochrane Database Syst Rev 2006;**4**:CD005962).

Reviews: * concise (Thomas et al, Int J Neuropsychopharmacol 2005;**8**:1–3), mode of action (Large et al, Psychopharmacology [Berl] 2005; **6**:1–22).

Oxcarbazepine

Oxcarbazepine has been used as an adjunctive treatment in acute schizophrenia (n = 6, open, Leweke et al, Am J Psychiatry 2004;**161**: 1130–1).

Selegiline *

Low-dose oral selegiline as antipsychotic augmentation may improve negative symptoms of schizophrenia (n = 67, d/b, p/c, 12/52, Bodkin et al, Am J Psychiatry 2005;**162**:388–90).

D-serine *

D-serine is a full agonist at glycine NMDA receptors and, when used at 30 mg/kg/d as adjunct to olanzapine or risperidone, significantly improved PANSS, 20% reduction in BRS in 35% pts, with no detrimental adverse effects (n = 39, RCT, d/b, p/c, c/o, 6/52, Heresco-Levy et al, Biol Psychiatry 2005;**15**:577–85).

SSRIs *

There has been some interest in the SSRIs as adjuvant therapy for non-core and positive symptoms. **Citalopram** has been trialled successfully for the depressive/anxiety symptoms of PANSS (RCT, Taiminen et al, Int Clin Psychopharmacol 1997;**12**:31–5) and has been shown to improve subjective well-being (n = 90, d/b, p/c, Salokangas et al, Acta Psychiatr Scand 1996;**94**:175–80) but addition of citalopram 40 mg/d to atypicals in schizophrenia had no effect on any clinical or cognition measures (n = 19, RCT, p/c, c/o, 24/52, Friedman et al, J Clin Psychopharmacol 2005;**25**:237–42). **Fluoxetine** 20 mg/d significantly improved positive and negative symptoms in conjunction with antipsychotics in two open studies of treatment-resistant schizophrenics (n = 9, open, 6/52, Goff et al, Am J Psychiatry 1990;**147**:492–4; Bachr and Ruskin, Am J Psychiatry 1991; **148**:274–5), but may increase the incidence of EPS (review: Ciraulo and Shader, J Clin Psychopharmacol 1990;**10**:48–50) and was ineffective in clozapine-treated patients (n = 33, open, p/c, 8/52, Buchanan et al, Am J Psychiatry 1996;**153**:1625–7). **Fluvoxamine** was ineffective as augmentation of risperidone-resistant schizophrenia (n = 30, open, 12/52, Takashi et al, Hum Psychopharmacol 2002;**17**:95–8; review of fluvoxamine as an adjunct by Silver, CNS Drug Rev 2001;**7**:283–304). It should only be used with clozapine with extreme care (see 4.2.3). A small study indicated that adjunctive **paroxetine** may offer sustained efficacy in treating negative symptoms of chronic schizophrenia (n = 8, open, 30/12, Jockers-Scherubl et al, J Clin Psychiatry 2001;**62**:573). **Sertraline** may be a useful adjunct for depression in schizophrenia, albeit with a relatively high drop-out rate (n = 26, d/b, p/c, 8/52, Mulholland et al, J Psychopharmacol 2003;**17**:107–12).

● Unlicensed/some efficacy

Amoxapine *

Amoxapine was equivalent to risperidone in a Mexican trial, a possible alternative where a low-cost atypical would be welcome (n = 48, RCT, d/b, 6/52, Apiquian et al, Neuropsychopharmacology 2005;**30**:2236–44), although another trial was unable to show an effect in schizophrenia (d/b, RCT, Fitzgerald et al, J Clin Psychopharmacol 2004;**24**:448–50).

Estradiol/estrogen *

In 10 women with postpartum psychosis, estradiol reversed the symptoms in 100% over two weeks, a remarkable outcome that deserves further study, say the authors (n = 10, open, 6/52, Ahokas et al, J Clin Psychiatry 2000;**61**:166–9). Transdermal estrogen was, however, unable to prevent relapse of postnatal affective psychosis when started within 48 hours of delivery (n = 29, open, 12/7, Kumar et al, J Clin Psychiatry 2003;**64**:112–8). Estrogen as an adjunct to haloperidol significantly reduced positive and general symptoms in women of child-bearing age with chronic schizophrenia (n = 32, RCT, d/b, p/c, 8/52, Akhondzadeh et al, Prog Neuropsychopharmacol Biol Psychiatry 2003;**27**:1007–12). There is also a report of daily percutaneous estradiol gel alone abolishing all psychotic symptoms in a woman whose schizoaffective psychosis appeared premenstrually (n = 1, Korhonen et al, Acta Psychiatr Scand 1995;**92**:237–8) and psychosis associated with amenorrhoea on the basis of

hypoestrogenemia responding to estrogen and progesterone (n = 1, Rettenbacher et al, J Clin Psychiatry 2004;**65**:275–7).

■ Unlicensed/possible efficacy

Bromocriptine

It has been speculated that increasing some dopaminergic function may improve negative symptoms of schizophrenia. Bromocriptine (n = 6, open, Levi-Minzi et al, Compr Psychiatry 1991;**32**:210–16), and dexamfetamine (mentioned by Breier in Curr Opin Psychiatry 1995;**8**:41–4) may decrease these negative symptoms, at least in some patient sub-groups.

Lithium

Lithium-responsive psychosis can occur and may be familial and is perhaps genetically distinct from the bulk of schizophrenias. A meta-analysis has concluded that although a few studies show some efficacy of lithium in schizophrenia, the overall results are inconclusive (n = 611, s = 20, Leucht et al, J Clin Psychiatry 2004;**65**:177–86). Cochrane also concludes that lithium is ineffective as a sole agent and augmentation is less effective than you would expect, but may potentially be useful in a few patients (n = 611, s = 20, Leucht et al, Cochrane Database Syst Rev 2003;**3**:CD003834; review by Bender and Dittmann-Balcar, EBMH 2004;**7**:104) where affective symptoms are prominent (n = 21, d/b, p/c, c/o, Terao et al, Acta Psychiatr Scand 1995;**92**:220–4; n = 5, case series, Martin et al, J Clin Psychiatry 2000; **61**:948). Lithium augmentation of clozapine may provide additional clinical benefit in schizoaffective but not schizophrenic patients, albeit with some risks (n = 20, p/c, 4/52, Small et al, J Clin Psychopharmacol 2003;**23**:223–8).

Melatonin

In one study, melatonin 2 mg/d significantly improved sleep efficiency in chronic schizophrenics with poor sleep, but not in those with better sleep efficiency (n = 19, RCT, c/o, p/c, Shamir et al, J Clin Psychiatry 2000;**61**:373–7).

Modafinil *

Modafinil 200 mg/d has produced improvements in cognitive functioning in schizophrenia (n = 20, RCT, d/b, p/c, c/o, Turner et al, Neuropsychopharmacol 2004;**29**:1363–73) and 100-200 mg/d may improve fatigue and cognitive functioning in schizophrenia (n = 11, open, 4/52, Rosenthal and Bryant, Clin Neuropharmacol 2004;**27**:38–43).

Ondansetron

Ondansetron may block raised dopamine function without sedating. There is an isolated case report of a good response at 4 mg/d in a drug-resistant patient (n = 1, White et al, Lancet 1991;**337**:1173). In a study of psychosis in advanced Parkinson's disease, 94% responded to ondansetron, with reduced hallucinations, paranoid delusions and confusion (n = 16, open, 8/52, Zoldan et al, Neurology 1995;**45**:1304–8). See also combinations.

Omega-3 Fatty Acids

There is some evidence for abnormal phospholipid metabolism in schizophrenia, and trials with PUVAs have produced inconsistent but usually favourable findings (review by Peet, Adv Psychiatr Treat 2002;**8**:223–29). There may be a bell-shaped response curve, with 2 g the optimum dose and 4 g and higher possibly counter productive (Horrobin, Am J Psychiatry 2003;**160**:188–9). E-EPA (ethyl-eicosapentaenoic acid) may be effective as adjunctive therapy for persistent psychotic symptoms (n = 40, RCT, 12/52, Emsley et al, Am J Psychiatry 2002;**159**:1696–8). However, omega-3 fatty acids have been shown to be ineffective in treating residual symptoms of schizophrenia (n = 87, RCT, 16/52, Fenton et al, Am J Psychiatry 2001;**158**:2071–4), although patients with schizophrenia may be able to improve their general psychopathology by taking a supplement that combines essential polyunsaturated fatty acids (EPUFAs) with antioxidants (n = 73, 4/12, Arvindaksham et al, Schizophr Res 2003;**62**:195–204), as long as they do not mind smelling of fish.

Tetrabenazine

Tetrabenazine has been used for the treatment of psychoses and psychoneuroses but the high incidence of side-effects makes this a relatively unsuitable drug.

◆ Others

Other drugs that have been tried include **aza-thioprine** (n = 1, Levine, Lancet 1994;**344**:59–60), high dose **beta-blockers** (propranolol: Lancet 1980;ii:627–8; nadolol up to 120 mg/d; Clin Pharm 1989;**8**:132–5), **clonidine** as augmentation (Br J Psychiatry 1988;**152**:293), **calcium-channel blockers** (such as nifedipine: Am J Psychiatry 1992;**149**:1615; and verapamil: Drug Intell Clin Pharm 1990;**24**:838–40), **dexamfetamine** (small trial, van Kammen and Bornow, Int Clin Psychopharmacol 1988;**3**:111–21), **famotidine** (n = 1, Lancet 1990;**335**:1312; review by Martinez, Ann Pharmacother 1999;**33**:742–7, 14 refs), **levodopa** (letter in Am J Psychiatry 1988;**145**:1180), **naltrexone/naloxone** (review by Welch and Thompson, J Clin Pharm Ther 1994;**19**:279–83) and **prednisone** (n = 1, Cohen et al, Lancet 1996; **347**:1228).

✱ No efficacy

Buspirone

Buspirone has various receptor activities, eg. 5-HT$_{1A}$ partial antagonism and dopamine antagonism but no improvement was seen at up to 2400 mg/d, and exacerbation of psychosis has been reported, although an occasional response has been reported (n = 1, Medrano and Padierna, Am J Psychiatry 1996;**153**:293).

Caffeine

Excess caffeine consumption can present as psychosis, increasing arousal (eg. n = 13, d/b, p/c, Lucas et al, Biol Psychiatry 1990;**28**:5–40) and may have a psychotogenic effect (n = 2, Zaslove et al, Br J Psychiatry 1991;**159**:565–7). However, moderate use of caffeine has probably little effect on anxiety, depression and psychosis (eg. n = 26, RCT, d/b, c/o, Mayo et al, Br J Psychiatry 1993;**162**:543–5).

Cannabidiol ✱

In a small case series in TRS, only one patient showed mild improvement with cannabidiol, the other two showed none (n = 3, 35/7, Zuardi et al, J Psychopharmacol 2006;**20**:683–6).

Donepezil ✱

There has been some interest in donepezil,

particularly for negative symptoms. However, a number of RCTs and other trials have shown an almost complete lack of significant affect, unlike galantamine and rivastigmine. Donepezil did not improve cognition or symptoms in community-based schizophrenics (n = 36, RCT, d/b, p/c, 8/52, Freudenrich et al, Psychopharmacol [Berl] 2005;181:358–63), had no significant effect on cognitive function at 5–10mg/d as an adjunct to risperidone (n = 36, d/b, p/c, 12/52, Friedman et al, Biol Psychiatry 2002;51:349–57) and made no difference to any rating scale in two add-on trials in schizophrenia (n = 12, RCT, d/b, p/c, c/o, 12/52, Tul et al, Int J Neuropsychopharmacol 2004;7:117–23; n = 8, d/b, c/o, 18/52, Stryjer et al, Hum Psychopharmacol 2004;19:343–6). However, some case reports have shown some effects, eg. improvements in verbal fluency but not in symptomatology (n = 1, MacEwan et al, Acta Psychiatr Scand 2001;104:469–72), improved memory (n = 1, Howard et al, J Psychopharmacol 2002;16:267–70), improved attention, learning and executive functions (n = 15, RCT, d/b, c/o, 18/52, Erickson et al, Clin Neuropharmacol 2005;28:179–84; n = 14, open, 6/12, Mazza et al, Clin Ther 2005; 156:203–9) and modest improvements in manual dexterity, memory and processing speed (n = 15, open, 6/52, Buchanan et al, Schizophr Res 2003;59:29–33).

Methylphenidate
Bolus IV methylphenidate has been used to induce an exacerbation of symptoms in an attempt to predict those people most likely to relapse when antipsychotics are discontinued (mentioned in Klein and Wender, Arch Gen Psychiatry 1995;52:429–33).

Topiramate *
Topiramate had no effect on BPRS when added to clozapine, risperidone, olanzapine or flupentixol (n = 9, open, Dursun and Deakin, J Psychopharmacol 2001;15:297–301), and a study suggested significant deterioration when added to existing antipsychotics in TRS, and so it should not be used with clozapine as anticonvulsant cover (n = 5, open, Millson et al, Am J Psychiatry 2002;159:675; n = 1, Hofer et al, J Clin Psychiatry 2003;64:1267–8). Although the risk may be significant, topiramate 300mg/d

as add-on to atypicals in TRS has reduced general PANSS psychopathological symptom scores in some (n = 26, RCT, d/b, p/c, c/o, 2x12/52, Tiihonen et al, J Clin Psychiatry 2005; 66:1012–5, IS).

Tricyclics
Tricyclics seem ineffective in treating depressive symptoms during acute psychotic episodes and may even be counterproductive (n = 58, RCT, d/b, p/c, 4/52, Kramer et al, Arch Gen Psychiatry 1989;46:922–8).

Vitamin B6
No difference in PANSS scores was detectable with B_6 supplementation in stable chronic schizophrenics (n = 15, d/b, p/c, c/o, 9/52, Lerner et al, J Clin Psychiatry 2002;63:54–8).

RAPID-CYCLING BIPOLAR DISORDER
see Rapid-cycling bipolar disorder (1.10.4)

1.24 SEASONAL AFFECTIVE DISORDER (SAD)
see also Depression (1.14), Mania and hypomania (1.10.2) and Bipolar mood disorder (1.10)

SAD is a recurrent affective disorder, predominantly major depression, but can include mania or hypomania. It has a characteristic seasonal relationship, usually autumn or winter (20 studies, Magnusson, Acta Psychiatr Scand 2000;101:176–84), for at least two or three years, with full remission at a characteristic time of the year and outnumbering any non-seasonal episodes. The incidence may be around 1–10% (eg. 2.4% in North Wales) and peaks in winter. Atypical depressive features include hypersomnia, increased appetite and weight and carbohydrate cravings. Theories for the cause include excess melatonin secretion, delayed or reduced amplitude circadian rhythms and serotonergic dysfunction. It is often undiagnosed, with about half of sufferers being given other depressive diagnoses and antidepressants (n = 1999, Michalak et al, Br J Psychiatry 2001;179:31–4). Light therapy is considered first choice for SAD (n = 96, RCT, Lam et al, Am J Psychiatry 2006;163:805–12; Golden et al, Am J Psychiatry 2005;162:656–62;

Terman, *EBMH* 2006;**9**:21), although it is not without risk, with side-effects including jumpiness (9%), headache (8%), and nausea (16%), despite a beneficial effect on improving bothersome symptoms (n = 83, open, Terman and Terman, *J Clin Psychiatry* 1999;**60**:799–808). Its effects may be dose-related (meta-analysis, Lee and Chan, *Acta Psychiatr Scand* 1999;**99**:315–23).

Role of drugs *

While phototherapy is well established, pre-liminary data from controlled trials indicates that drug treatment may also be effective, with bupropion and sertraline suggested as effective. Seasonal major depression can be prevented by starting an antidepressant early in the season while patient is still well (eg. with bupropion 150-300 mg/d; s = 3, n = 1042, RCT, p/c, Modell *et al*, *Biol Psychiatry* 2005;**58**:658–67).

Reviews: general (Magnusson, *Acta Psychiatr Scand* 2000;**101**:176–84; Magnusson and Boivin, *Chronobiol Int* 2003;**20**:189–207; Eagles, *Br J Psychiatry* 2003;**182**:174–6; Hilger *et al*, *Nerven-arzt* 2002;**73**:22–9), pathophsyiology (Lam and Levitan, *J Psychiatry Neurosci* 2000;**25**:469–80), light therapy (Golden *et al*, *Am J Psychiatry* 2005; **162**:656–62; Terman, *EBMH* 2006;**9**:21).

● Unlicensed/some efficacy

Bupropion *

Bupropion XL is licensed in USA for SAD, based on three RCTs using 150–300 mg/d where treatment was started in autumn while the patients were still well (s = 3, n = 1042, RCT, p/c, d/b, Modell *et al*, *Biol Psychiatry* 2005; **58**:658–67).

Sertraline

Sertraline (50–200 mg/d) was significantly superior to placebo in winter pattern SAD in one study (n = 187, RCT, d/b, p/c, O/P, 8/52, Moscovitch *et al*, *Psychopharmacol* [Berl] 2004; **171**:390–7).

■ Unlicensed/possible efficacy

Beta-blockers

In a trial of up to 60 mg/d propranolol administered pre-sunrise (5.30–6.00 AM), 73% of those with winter depression responded,

and those transferred to placebo showed varying degrees of relapse. The effect may be via short-term, short-acting beta-blocker-induced truncation of nocturnal melatonin secretion early morning but not in the evening (n = 33, d/b, p/c, Schlager, *Am J Psychiatry* 1994;**151**:1383–5). Atenolol appeared less effective in another trial (n = 19, d/b, p/c, c/o, Rosenthal *et al*, *Am J Psychiatry* 1988;**145**:52–6), but a small group of patients showed a sustained and substantial response.

Citalopram

Light therapy has an early onset of action and, in responders, citalopram significantly reduces relapse in the continuation phase (n = 282, p/c, 15/52, Martiny *et al*, *Acta Psychiatr Scand* 2004; **109**:230–4).

Fluoxetine

In an out-patient study, fluoxetine 20 mg/d was superior to placebo (59–34%), but was not quite statistically significant (n = 68, p/c, 5/52, Lam *et al*, *Am J Psychiatry* 1995;**152**:1765–70).

Melatonin

A small study showed that low dose melatonin taken in the early afternoon reduced depression, possibly by a 'phase shift' mechanism (n = 5, Lewy *et al*, *Psychiatry Res* 1998;**77**:57–61).

Mirtazapine

One pilot study has shown a rapid and well-tolerated effect in SAD (n = 8, open, 4/52, Hesselmann *et al*, *Hum Psychopharmacol Clin Exp* 1999;**14**:59–62).

Moclobemide

Moclobemide 300–450 mg/d was of benefit in some patients with SAD (n = 581, RCT, d/b, 6/52, Partonen and Lonnqvist, *J Affect Disord* 1996;**41**:93–9).

Modafinil *

A pilot study suggested modafinil significantly re-duces fatigue and sleepiness (n = 13 [c = 9], open, 8/52, Lundt, *J Affect Disord* 2004;**81**:173–8).

Reboxetine

A pilot study indicated a rapid and significant effect in SAD in 65% patients, including atypical symptoms in the first week (n=16, open, 6/52, Hilger et al, Eur Neuropsychopharmacol 2001;11:1–5).

St John's wort
One study showed some effect (s/b, see Kasper, Pharmacopsychiatry 1997;**30**[Suppl 2]: S89–S93).

Tranylcypromine
In a small study, 86% responded completely to tranylcypromine (mean dose 30mg/d) in winter depression (n=14, open, Dilsaver and Jaeckle, J Clin Psychiatry 1990;**51**:326–9).

✷ No efficacy

Ginkgo biloba
One study was unable to show an effect from 'Bio-Biloba' in preventing winter depression (n=27, RCT, 10/52, Lingaerde et al, Acta Psychiatr Scand 1999;**100**:62–6).

1.25 SELF-INJURIOUS BEHAVIOUR (SIB)

SIB is a self-destructive behaviour resulting in significant tissue damage, but without lethal intent. It can occur in learning disabilities (eg. Lesch-Nyhan syndrome), as well as in OCD, sadomasochism, schizophrenia and borderline personality disorder. There seems to be a variety of causes, eg. relief of dysphoria, poor impulse control and dissociation.

Role of drugs
Opiate antagonists may be useful where a reward mechanism seems to exist. There is some evidence of a serotonergic involvement. Antipsychotics seem to work mainly via a non-specific sedating mechanism.
Review: psychopharmacology of severe SIB associated with learning disabilities (Clarke, Br J Psychiatry 1998;**172**:389–94).

+ Combinations

Clozapine + clomipramine
This combination was successful in treating compulsive self-mutilation in a drug-resistant mild learning disability patient (n=1, Holzer et al, Am J Psychiatry 1996;**153**:133).

● Unlicensed/some efficacy

Antipsychotics
Antipsychotics are frequently prescribed but evidence for their efficacy is suggestive rather than conclusive. **Risperidone** was shown to be effective for up to 52 months in 75% of developmentally disabled in-patients (retrospective chart analysis, Brahm et al, Pharmacotherapy 2001;**21**:382). Low-dose **olanzapine** (5mg/d) has been used successfully for SIB (n=2, Hough, J Clin Psychiatry 2001;**62**:296–7) and **clozapine** 200mg/d has been effective in a few cases (n=2, Hammock et al, J Autism Dev Disord 2001;**31**:109–13).
Review: Janowsky et al, J Clin Psychopharmacol 2005;**25**:19–25.

Buspirone
In a trial of developmentally disabled individuals with self-injury and anxiety, 64% responded to doses of 20–45mg/d with a maximal response seen more than three weeks later (n=14, open, Ratey et al, J Clin Psychiatry 1989;**50**:382).

Lithium
Some old studies have suggested that lithium is effective in both aggression and SIB, eg. response was seen in 2–8 weeks with a lithium serum concentration of 0.7–1.0mEq/L (n=42, d/b, p/c, 4/12, Craft et al, Br J Psychiatry 1987; **150**:685–9).

Naltrexone/naloxone
There is conflicting data about the efficacy of naltrexone in SIB. Some studies show some efficacy when used in adequate dose for adequate duration, eg. 25–100mg/d orally (n=4, Sandman et al, Am J Ment Retard 1990;**95**:93–102). It may be that lower doses (eg. 10–50mg/d) are more effective and it undoubtedly helps some patients (eg. n=1, 32/52, Griengl et al, Acta Psychiatr Scand 2001;**103**:234–6; n=1 plus review, White and Schultz, Am J Psychiatry 2000;**157**:1574–82, 121 refs). Some trials have, however, shown a lack of efficacy, eg. mentally retarded and autistic adults failed to respond and, indeed, many patients worsened (n=33, d/b, p/c, c/o, Willemsen-Swinkels et al, Arch Gen Psychiatry 1995;**52**:766–73). SIB may get worse over

the first few weeks of naltrexone but then improves and so short studies could miss the effect. Although 50–100mg/d showed some improvement in hand-to-head and head-to-object SIB, the 14-day duration in the second trial and variation in behaviour made statistical evaluation invalid (n=8, d/b, Thompson et al, Am J Ment Retard 1994;**99**:85–102). There is some evidence of raised opioid peptide activity in autism, Fragile-X syndrome and other mental handicaps, which would explain the effect.

Review: Symons et al, Ment Retard Dev Disabil Res Rev 2004;**10**:193–200.

Propranolol

Propranolol may decrease SIB and response may be seen with average doses of 120mg/d which may be immediate or gradual over several weeks (review; Ruedrich et al, Am J Ment Retard 1990;**95**:110–9).

■ Unlicensed/possible efficacy

Clomipramine

Clomipramine 25–125mg/d reduced SIB target symptoms rapidly in some subjects (n=11, open, Garber et al, J Am Acad Child Adolesc Psych 1992;**31**:1157–60).

Dextromethorphan

Dextromethorphan 30mg/d successfully controlled SIB and aggression in a man with learning disabilities (n=1, Welch and Sovner, Br J Psychiatry 1992;**161**:118–20).

Fluoxetine

Some benefit (20–85% reductions in SIB) has been shown in some mentally retarded young adults (n=4, Ricketts et al, J Am Acad Child Adolesc Psychiatry 1993;**32**:865–9).

Topiramate

Topiramate 200mg/d was observed to produce remission of self-mutilation in patient with BPD (n=1, Cassano et al, Bipolar Disorders 2001;**3**:161).

1.26 SEXUAL DEVIANCY DISORDERS

Sexual deviancy disorders are abnormalities of a basic biological drive and are recognised as psychiatric syndromes. They include exhibitionism, fetishism, sexual masochism or sadism, paedophilia and voyeurism, but not rape (considered a sexual expression of aggression rather than an aggressive expression of sexuality). The main characteristic is of intense, recurrent sexual arousal and fantasies, particularly connected with inanimate objects, children, non-consenting adults or the self.

Role of drugs

Drug therapy may sometimes be a useful adjunct to other therapies, due to the chronic nature of the disease and its high and unpredictable relapse rates, but needs care and is controversial. One review (Bradford, J Sex Res 2000;**37**:248–57) suggested a treatment hierarchy of CBT, SSRIs, low-dose antiandrogen, higher dose antiandrogen, then very high dose antiandrogen. Deviant sexual behaviour is rare in women and so drug therapy is usually aimed at reducing sexual drive in men. The success of any form of treatment is highly dependent on detailed evaluations and diagnosis. Placebo-controlled studies have huge ethical complications.

Reviews: * general (Krueger and Kaplan, J Psychiatr Pract 2002;**8**:21–32), extensive pharmacological options (Bradford, J Sex Res 2000;**37**:248–57), sexual functioning (Meston and Frohlich, Arch Gen Psychiatry 2000;**57**:1012–30), treatment protocols for cyproterone, medroxyprogesterone etc (Reilly et al, Can J Psychiatry 2000;**45**:559–63).

BNF listed

Benperidol

Benperidol is a standard butyrophenone which, although used for control of deviant antisocial sexual behaviour, has no proven use other than as an antipsychotic. The only double-blind study published showed a slight reduction in sexual thoughts, but not in behaviour (Drug Ther Bull 1974;**12**:2).

Cyproterone (acetate)

Cyproterone is available in many countries to treat severe hypersexuality and sexual deviation in men. It has both antiandrogenic and antigonadotropic actions and probably acts by disrupting the receptors' response to androgens (review: Cooper, *Can J Psychiatry* 1986;**31**:73–9). It can reduce sexual interest, drive and arousal, as well as deviant fantasies and behaviour and significantly reduces some sexual behaviours in paraphilias and paedophilia (n = 19, RCT, d/b, p/c, c/o, Bradford *et al*, *Arch Sex Behav* 1993;**22**:383–402). Few proper trials support its use and there are no adequate double-blind crossover trials in learning disabilities. The onset of action may be delayed for 2–3 weeks and is reversible within 3–6 weeks of stopping. An adequate trial of four months is usually recommended. A depot injection is available on a named patient basis and a syrup can be made. Cyproterone 100mg/d rapidly cured a woman of severe sexual obsessions, maintained over two years and after discontinuation (n = 1, Eriksson, *Br J Psychiatry* 1998;**173**:351) and so may have other applications.

● **Unlicensed/some efficacy**

LHRH antagonists
Luteinising hormone-releasing hormone (gonadorelin, LHRH) antagonists can produce complete chemical castration and thus have a potent effect on sexual deviancy. A thorough review concluded that LHRH antagonists offer a treatment option for severe paraphilia, with little or no relapse if the patient remains under treatment (n = 118, s = 13, Briken *et al*, *J Clin Psychiatry* 2003;**64**:890–7). **Nafarelin** has been used for this purpose. **Flutamide**, a pure antiandrogen similar to cyproterone, has been used in conjunction with nafarelin and in one case resulted in rapid discontinuation in exhibitionism (n = 1, Rousseau *et al*, *Can J Psychiatry* 1990;**35**:338–41). **Leuprolide** acetate is an alternative (n = 1, Dickey, *Can J Psychiatry* 1992;**37**:567–9) and a depot leuprolide significantly suppressed self-reported deviant sexual interests and behaviour and was well-tolerated, although bone demineralisation occurred in 25% (n = 12, open, Krueger and Kaplan, *Arch Sex Behav* 2001;**30**:409–22). **Triptorelin** has also been used (n = 6, Thibaut *et al*, *Acta Psychiatr Scand* 1993;**87**:445–50), where depot triptorelin palmoate 3.75mg/month plus psychotherapy was effective for reducing

episodes of deviant sexual behaviours over 3–12 months in all men with severe paraphilia (n = 30, open, Rosler and Witztum, *N Engl J Med* 1998;**338**:416–22).

Medroxyprogesterone (acetate)
Medroxyprogesterone has indirect anti-androgenic activity by preventing testosterone release from the testicles (review by Cooper, *Can J Psychiatry* 1986;**31**:73–9) and increasing the metabolic clearance of testosterone, resulting in suppression of sexual arousal and libido. Adverse effects include weight gain, diabetes and DVTs, although feminisation has not been reported. Again, few proper trials have been carried out. Due to a possible central tranquillising effect, care is needed on ethical grounds (Berlin, *Bull Am Acad Psychiatry Law* 1989;**17**:233–9).

SSRIs
Low serotonin has been shown to produce increased sex-drive in animals, and so SSRIs may have a significant effect in reversing this, eg. reduced daily frequency and duration of paraphilia and related disorders has been shown (n = 26, open case series, Kafka and Hennen, *J Clin Psychiatry* 2000;**61**:664–70). A similarity between sexual deviancy and OCD has been postulated and there are case reports of the successful use of fluoxetine to decrease the intensity and intrusiveness of sexual fantasies, resulting in more conventional sexual behaviour and impulse control (eg. n = 199, Greenberg and Bradford, *Sexual Abuse* 1997;**9**:525–32). SSRI-induced anorgasmia may be a contributory factor to this effect. Controlled clinical trials are needed to confirm a definite effect.

■ **Unlicensed/possible efficacy**

Carbamazepine *
Carbamazepine has been used to treat sexual disinhibition in dementia (n = 1, Freymann *et al*, *Pharmacopsychiatry* 2005;**38**:144–5).

Gabapentin
Gabapentin has been used to treat sexual disinhibition in dementia (n = 3, Alkhalil *et al*, *Am J Ther* 2004;**11**:231–5).

Imipramine

Some improvements in paraphilic and non-paraphilic sexual addictions and depressive symptoms were noted in 90% patients treated with imipramine, fluoxetine or lithium (n = 10, Kafka, *J Clin Psychiatry* 1991;**52**:60–5).

Lithium

See imipramine.

Methylphenidate

Methylphenidate may be used cautiously to augment the effect of SSRIs in paraphilias and related disorders (n = 26, Kafka and Hennen, *J Clin Psychiatry* 2000;**61**:664–70).

Naltrexone *

Compulsive sexual behaviour has been treated with naltrexone and SSRIs (n = 2, Raymond et al, *Int Clin Psychopharmacol* 2002;**17**:201–5) and naltrexone was reported to have a positive response in 15 adolescent sexual offenders, with a therapeutic window of 50–200 mg/d. Of the six non-responders, five responded to leuprolide (n = 21, open, Ryback, *J Clin Psychiatry* 2004;**65**:982–6).

Topiramate *

Topiramate 50 mg/d reduced compulsive non-paraphilic sexual behaviours strongly triggered by environmental cues in one patient (n = 1, Khazaal and Zullion, *BMC Psychiatry* 2006; **6**:22).

Valproate *

Valproate has been a useful adjunct in bipolar sex offenders, but only for mood, not for paraphilic symptoms (open, retrospective, Nelson et al, *J Affect Disord* 2001;**64**:249–55).

1.27 SOCIAL ANXIETY DISORDER (SOCIAL PHOBIA DISORDER)
see also Anxiety disorder (*1.6*)

Introduction *

Social anxiety is the second most common phobia (incidence in USA is 5%; n = 43 093, Grant et al, *J Clin Psychiatry* 2005;**66**:1351–61; comment by Manfro, *EBMH* 2006;**9**:88) where the sufferers fear public ridicule, scrutiny and negative evaluation, with fear of making a public mistake, embarrassment or criticism. Feared

situations include public speaking, social gatherings, writing under supervision or eating and drinking in public. Anticipatory anxiety leads to impaired performance. Two sub-divisions include general and specific social phobia. This is a serious, disabling anxiety disorder associated with reduction in quality of life (n = 829, s = 3, RCTs, p/c, Stein and Kean, *Am J Psychiatry* 2000;**157**:1606–13), but is underdiagnosed with less than 5% of sufferers receiving a diagnosis (n = 3862, Katzelnick et al, *Am J Psychiatry* 2001; **158**:1999–2007). Early diagnosis and treatment may be vital (Kahalid-Khan et al, *Paediatr Drugs* 2007;**9**:227-37).

Role of drugs *

Drugs and behavioural approaches are commonly used. Serotonin reuptake inhibitors are clearly superior to placebo and are emerging as the gold standard drug therapy, with another SSRI or venlafaxine XL second-line and moclobemide, MAOIs and benzodiazepines third choice. The only predictor of response is length of treatment, which should be at least 12 weeks (Stein et al, *J Clin Psychiatry* 2002; **63**:152–5). Cochrane concludes that SSRIs have the strongest evidence, for short-term and probably the long-term (n = 36, RCT, Stein et al, *Cochrane Database Syst Rev* 2004;**4**:CD001206). The placebo response has been found to be moderately large (15 p/c studies, Oosterbaan et al, *J Psychopharmacol* 2001;**15**:199–203). CBT alone is probably more effective than fluoxetine and placebo (n = 60, RCT, d/b, 12/12, Clark et al, *J Consult Clin Psychol* 2003;**71**:1058–67; review Taylor *EBMH* 2004;**7**:75).

Reviews: * general (Schneier, *N Engl J Med* 2006;**355**:1029–36; Kaminer and Stein, *World J Biol Psychiatry* 2003;**4**:103–10; Nash, *Prescriber* 2005;**16**:17–24), BAP evidence-based guidelines (Baldwin et al, *J Psychopharmacol* 2005;**19**:567–96), symptoms, subtypes and severity (Stein et al, *Arch Gen Psychiatry* 2000;**57**:1046–52).

BNF listed

Escitalopram *

Escitalopram is licensed in the UK for social anxiety (although citalopram is not licensed). The starting dose is 10 mg/d, increased to a maximum of 20 mg/d or reduced to 5 mg/d, depending upon an individual's response.

Efficacy has been shown in a number of major trials. Escitalopram 10–20 mg/d was superior to placebo (54% vs 39% response) using the LSAS total score (n = 358, RCT, p/c, d/b, 12/52, Kasper et al, Br J Psychiatry 2005; 186:222–6; MS) and appeared effective and well-tolerated in the long-term (n = 517, RCT, d/b, p/c, 24/52, Montgomery et al, J Clin Psychiatry 2005;66:1270–8; comment by Stein, EBMH 2006;9:52). A sub-analysis of pooled data showed efficacy against all symptom dimensions (s = 2, RCT, p/c, 12/52, Stein et al, Depress Anxiety 2004;20:175–81).

Paroxetine *

Several studies show paroxetine to be superior to placebo, eg. at 20–50 mg/d reducing symptoms and avoidance (n = 187, RCT, p/c, 12/52, Stein et al, JAMA 1998;280:708–13), with 40 mg/d the optimum dose (n = 384, d/b, 12/52, Liebowitz et al, J Clin Psychiatry 2002;63:66–74). These trials had a high drop-out rate, and so some caution over the confidence in the studies has been expressed (Dahl, EBMH 1999;2:53; Prescrire Int 2003;12:137–9). Two other RCTs have shown an effect from paroxetine 20–50 mg/d from four weeks onwards (n = 290, RCT, 12/52, Baldwin et al, Br J Psychiatry 1999;175:120–6; review by Wilson, EBMH 2000;3:41; n = 92, RCT, Allgulander, Acta Psychiatr Scand 1999;100:193–8). Paroxetine 10–50 mg/d is also effective and well-tolerated for social anxiety in children and adolescents (8–17) (n = 322, RCT, p/c, d/b, 16/52, Wagner et al, Arch Gen Psychiatry 2004;61:1153–62). Lack of response at eight weeks does not necessarily predict long-term lack of response and so a minimum of 12 weeks treatment is necessary (review, s = 3, Stein et al, J Clin Psychiatry 2002;63:152–5). It may be effective for relapse prevention (n = 323[c = 257], RCT, p/c, Stein et al, Arch Gen Psychiatry 2002;59:1111–8).

Venlafaxine *

Venlafaxine XL is now licensed for moderate to severe generalised social anxiety disorder (n = 279[c = 173], RCT, d/b, p/c, 12/52, Liebowitz et al, J Clin Psychiatry 2005;66:238–47). The standard dose is 75 mg/d. It is as effective and as well-tolerated as paroxetine 20–50 mg/d (n = 434, RCT, d/b, p/c, 12/52,

Allgulander et al, Hum Psychopharmacol 2004; 19:387–96; n = 413[c = 318], RCT, p/c, d/b, 12/52, Liebowitz et al, Arch Gen Psychiatry 2005;62:190–8). 75 mg/d appears as effective as 150–225 mg/d (n = 386, d/b, p/c, 6/12, Stein et al, Psychopharmacol [Berl] 2004;177:280–8). Lower doses may be useful in children and adolescents (n = 293, RCT, p/c, 16/52, March et al, Biol Psychiatry 2007;62:1149–54).

Combinations

Paroxetine + clonazepam

Unlike panic disorder, combining a BDZ with paroxetine did not lead to a quicker response in social anxiety (n = 28[c = 19], d/b, p/c, 10/52, Seedat and Stein, J Clin Psychiatry 2004; 65:244–8).

• Unlicensed/some efficacy

Benzodiazepines

The BDZs have a rapid onset, good tolerability and flexible dosing, but cause sedation, lack of coordination and long-term use has some potential risks. **Diazepam** may be ineffective (n = 31, d/b, c/o, s/b, James and Savage, Am Heart J 1984;108:1150–5), but **alprazolam** (n = 65, 12/52, Gelernter et al, Arch Gen Psychiatry 1991;48:938–45) is equivalent to other treatments and **clonazepam** has been widely studied (review by Jefferson, J Clin Psychiatry 2001;62[Suppl 1]:S50–S53) and appears safe and effective.

Cycloserine *

D-cycloserin may be effective as a 'when required' drug an hour before public speaking (n = 27, RCT, d/b, p/c, Hofmann et al, Arch Gen Psychiatry 2006;63:298–304).

Gabapentin

Gabapentin (900–3600 mg/d) was well-tolerated and significantly reduced symptoms in one trial (eg. n = 69, RCT, d/b, p/c, 14/52, Pande et al, J Clin Psychopharmacol 1999;19:341–8).

Mirtazapine *

Mirtazapine seemed effective and well-tolerated in women with social anxiety but not comorbid psychiatric illness (n = 66[c = 60],

RCT, d/b, p/c, 10/52, Muehlbacher et al, J Clin Psychopharmacol 2005;**25**:580–3; comment by Mörtberg, EBMH 2006;**9**:75), supporting an earlier pilot study with a 41% response rate (n = 14, open, 12/52, van Veen et al, Int Clin Psychopharmacol 2002;**17**:315–7).

Moclobemide

Moclobemide has been compared favourably with phenelzine (n=78, RCT, d/b, 24/52, Versani et al, Br J Psychiatry 1992;**161**:353–60), building up to 600mg/d over two weeks and maintained for twelve weeks to produce a therapeutic effect (Nutt and Bell, Adv Psychiatr Treat 1997;**3**:79–85). Another trial showed some efficacy but the advantage over placebo was relatively small and not significant (n = 77, p/c, Schneier et al, Br J Psychiatry 1998;**172**:70–7), and it was not effective at up to 900mg/d (n=523, p/c, 12/52, Noyes et al, J Clin Psychopharmacol 1997; **7**:247–54).

Phenelzine

Phenelzine (mean dose 66mg/d) was effective in 85% patients with refractory social anxiety (n=7, open, Aarre, Nord J Psychiatry 2003;**57**:313–5) and in a complex trial, phenelzine was slightly superior to Group CBT, and both were superior to placebo (n = 133, 12/52, Heimberg et al, Arch Gen Psychiatry 1998;**55**:1113–4; reviewed by Thyer, EBMH 1999;**2**:80).

Pregabalin

Pregabalin 600mg/d was effective and well-tolerated in social anxiety, whereas 150mg/d and placebo were ineffective (n = 135, RCT, d/b, p/c, 10/52, Pande et al, J Clin Psychopharmacol 2004;**24**:141–9, MS). In a comparative study, it was as effective as lorazepam 2mg TDS (n=271, RCT, d/b, p/c, 4/52, Feltner et al, J Clin Psychopharmacol 2003;**23**:240–9, MS; see also Pary, EBMH 2004;**7**:17).

SSRIs (paroxetine, escitalopram and venlafaxine are licensed, see above and fluoxetine in next section) *

Citalopram 40mg/d appears well-tolerated and as effective (75% response) as moclobemide (n=71, RCT, s/b, 8/52, Atmaca et al, Hum Psychopharmacol 2002;**17**:401–5), supported by additional reports (eg. n = 22, open, Bouwer and Stein, J Affect Disord 1998;**49**:79–82; Varia et al, Prog Neuropsychopharmacol Biol Psychiatry 2002;**26**:205–8). Improvement in social anxiety symptoms may lag behind depression resolution, and may need more than 12 weeks for full response (n=21, open, 12/52, Schneier et al, Depress Anxiety 2003;**17**:191–6). **Fluvoxamine** may have some role, eg. 200mg/d (mean dose) was superior to placebo in one study (n=92, RCT, Stein et al, Am J Psychiatry 1999;**156**:756–60), the CR version was superior to placebo in another (n=279, RCT, p/c, 12/52, Davidson et al, J Clin Psychopharmacol 2004;**24**:118–25), and it has been used for clozapine-induced social phobia (n = 12, open, 12/52, Pallanti et al, J Clin Psychiatry 1999;**60**:819–23; but see drug interactions). It may be useful long-term if the person has responded to short-term treatment (n = 112, 24/52 extension, Stein et al, Int J Neuropsychopharmacol 2003;**6**:317–23). **Sertraline** is licensed in several countries for social anxiety and at up to 200mg/d was more effective than placebo in one well-designed flexible-dose trial, although the exclusion criteria were unclear (n = 204, RCT, 20/52, van Ameringen et al, Am J Psychiatry 2001;**158**:275–81; review by Pieters, EBMH 2001;**4**:91). In another trial, sertraline was significantly more effective than placebo (n=415, RCT, d/b, p/c, 12/52, Liebowitz et al, J Clin Psychiatry 2003;**64**:785–92). Its efficacy may be enhanced by combination with exposure therapy (n=387, RCT, d/b, 24/52, Blomhoff et al, Br J Psychiatry 2001;**179**:23–30). Sertraline may be effective long-term, but relapse may occur on discontinuation (n=375, RCT, p/c, d/b, one year, Haug et al, Br J Psychiatry 2003;**182**:312–8).

■ Unlicensed/possible efficacy

Botulinum toxin *

Severe axillary hyperhydrosis has been treated with botulinum toxin, significantly improving overall disability (n = 40, RCT, p/c, 8/52, Connor et al, J Clin Psychiatry 2006;**67**:30–6).

Bupropion

Bupropion has been used (n = 10, open, 12/52, Emmanuel et al, Depress Anxiety 2000; **12**:111–3).

Levetiracetam *

A pilot study showed levetiracetam to have a significant effect on symptoms at up to 3 g/d (n = 20, open, 8/52, Simon et al, J Clin Psychiatry 2004;**65**:1219–22) and a small RCT showed 500–3000 mg/d was numerically, but not statistically, superior to placebo (n = 16, RCT, d/b, p/c, 7/52, Zhang et al, J Psychopharmacol 2006;**20**:551–3).

Tricyclics

One small open trial showed a low response and a high drop-out from side-effects (n = 15, open, 8/52, Simpson et al, J Clin Psychopharmacol 1998;**18**:132–5).

* No efficacy

Beta-blockers *

There is no evidence for efficacy, except perhaps in people where management of tremor is essential, eg. musicians (eg. nadolol; n = 31, d/b, c/o, s/b, James and Savage, Am Heart J 1984;**108**:1150–5). Pindolol 15 mg/d was no more effective than placebo in augmenting SSRI treatment of generalised social phobia (n = 14, d/b, p/c, c/o, 4/52, Stein et al, Am J Psychiatry 2001;**158**:1725–7). However, illicit self-medication with propranolol (up to 320 mg/d) has been reported (n = 1, Fontanella, Rev Bras Psiquiatr 2003;**25**:228–30), with symptoms manageable with adjunctive paroxetine, so maybe it does work, but at higher doses.

Fluoxetine

A large pilot study failed to show that fluoxetine up to 60 mg/d was superior to placebo, although the latter had an unusually high response rate (n = 60, RCT, d/b, 14/52, Kobak et al, J Clin Psychopharmacol 2002;**22**:257–62).

St John's wort *

SJW was not superior to placebo in one trial (n = 40, RCT, p/c, 12/52, Kobak et al, J Clin Psychopharmacol 2005;**25**:51–8).

Valproate

A small study showed complete ineffectiveness of valproate at up to 1500 mg/d (n = 16, mentioned by Jefferson, J Clin Psychiatry 2001; **62**[Suppl 1]:S50–S53).

1.28 TOURETTE'S SYNDROME (GILLES DE LA TOURETTE)

see also OCD (1.20) and Self-injurious behaviour (1.25)

Symptoms

The main diagnostic symptoms of this hereditary disorder include multiple tics, vocal tics (grunts, snarls and obscenities), stereotyped movements (jumping and dancing), overactivity, learning difficulties and emotional problems. It occurs in 1–5 per 10000 of the population and is more common in males. It has an onset at 5–6 years, beginning with respiratory or vocal tics with grunting or barking noises. Psychiatric co-morbidity is common, eg. OCD, anxiety, depression and ADHD.

Role of drugs

If the condition is affecting the person's abilities to function, drug therapy may be useful. Low starting doses, gradual increases and adequate trials are necessary. Pimozide and haloperidol are the only two drugs licensed in USA.

Reviews: general (Kossoff and Singer, Paediatr Drugs 2001;**3**:355–63; Robertson and Stern, Br J Hosp Med 1997;**58**:253–5), pharmacological options (Silay and Jankovic, Expert Opin Emerg Drugs 2005;**10**:365-80; Jimenez-Jimenez and Garcia-Ruiz, Drugs 2001;**61**:2207–20).

BNF listed

Haloperidol

Haloperidol 0.5–40 mg/d was the licensed drug of choice and remains a treatment option. Side-effects may be limiting and its efficacy has been questioned (n = 22, p/c, d/b, Sallee et al, Am J Psychiatry 1997;**154**:1057–62). See also pimozide and nicotine chewing gum.

Pimozide

Pimozide 1–20 mg/d may be as effective as haloperidol in some patients, with less side-effects. An ECG is essential monitoring (see 3.2.1). Two trials have shown pimozide 1–20 mg/d to be superior to haloperidol, eg. in children with Tourette's and ADHD (n = 66, open, Sallee et al, Acta Psychiatr Scand 1994;**90**:4–9; n = 22, p/c, d/b, Sallee et al, Am J Psychiatry 1997;**154**:1057–62).

● Unlicensed/some efficacy

Clonidine

Clonidine 0.1–0.6 mg/d may be as effective as haloperidol in some patients. In one trial, clonidine was more effective than placebo (n = 47, d/b, *Arch Gen Psychiatry* 1991;**48**:324–8), but in a later trial of clonidine (up to 0.2 mg/d) and desipramine (up to 100 mg/d) in children with both ADHD and Tourette's syndrome, desipramine was superior to clonidine in reducing ADHD and tic symptoms (n = 37, d/b, p/c, c/o, Singer et al, *Pediatrics* 1995;**95**:74–81). Clonidine or methylphenidate alone and in combination are effective for ADHD with co-morbid tics (n = 16, RCT, p/c,16/52, TSSG, *Neurology* 2002;**58**:527–36; review by Goldberg, *EBMH* 2002;**5**:122).

Lorazepam

Lorazepam 1.5–10 mg/d may be useful as adjuvant therapy.

Risperidone

There are now a number of studies showing a significant effect. Risperidone (mean dose 2.5 mg/d) was clearly superior to placebo on global assessment of Tourette symptoms (n = 48, RCT, d/b, p/c, Dion et al, *J Clin Psychopharmacol* 2002;**22**:31–9), and a mean dose of 3.8 mg/d was at least as effective as pimozide (mean 2.9 mg/d), but was much better tolerated (n = 50, d/b, 12/52, Bruggeman et al, *J Clin Psychiatry* 2001;**62**:50–6). Risperidone (mean 2.5 mg/d) may also be useful for the short-term management of tics in Tourette's (n = 34, RCT, d/b, p/c, 8/52, Scahill et al, *Neurology* 2003;**60**:1130–5). Risperidone may have a similar efficacy to clonidine over a wide range of symptoms (n = 21, RCT, d/b, 8/52, Gaffney et al, *J Am Acad Child Adolesc Psychiatry* 2002;**41**:330–6). There are reports of response in multiple drug-resistant Tourette's syndrome and OCD responding rapidly to risperidone 6 mg/d (Giakas, *Am J Psychiatry* 1995;**152**:1097–8; Shulman et al, *Neurology* 1995;**45**:1419; n = 38, 4/52, Bruun and Budman, *J Clin Psychiatry* 1996;**57**:29–31).

Sulpiride

Sulpiride 200–400 mg/d has been used, and has been considered by some as a treatment of choice, although there is no literature about it.

＋ Combinations

Naltrexone + codeine

Sequential use of naltrexone (100–300 mg/d) and codeine phosphate (15–120 mg/d) has proved effective (n = 2, McConville et al, *Lancet* 1994;**343**:601). See also naltrexone/opiate antagonists.

■ Unlicensed/possible efficacy

Amisulpride *

Successful use of amisulpride has been reported (n = 1, Fountoulakis et al, *Ann Pharmacother* 2004;**38**:901).

Aripiprazole *

Aripiprazole has been used with some success (n = 6, retrospective, 12/52, Murphy et al, *Int J Neuropsychopharmacol* 2005;**8**:489–90), including for tics (Kastrup et al, *J Clin Psychopharmacol* 2005;**25**:94–6), with 10–20 mg/d dramatically and rapidly effective in some patients (n = 11, Davies et al, *Hum Psychopharmacol* 2006;**21**:447–53; Bubl et al, *World J Biol Psychiatry* 2006;**7**:123–5; Constant et al, *Int J Neuropsychopharmacol* 2006;**9**:773–4; n = 2, open, Padala et al, *Prim Care Companion J Clin Psychiatry* 2005;**7**:296–9). It may dramatically reduce tics with minimal side-effects (n = 1, Dehning et al, *Am J Psychiatry* 2005;**162**:625).

Buspirone

Drug-resistant Tourette's has been treated successfully with buspirone 30 mg/d (n = 1, Dursun et al, *Lancet* 1995;**345**:1366–7).

Cannabinoids

In a survey of people with Tourette's who had tried marijuana, 82% reported a reduction or complete remission in motor and vocal tics, urges and OCD symptoms (n = 17, Muller-Vahl et al, *Acta Psychiatr Scand* 1998;**98**:502–6), and an RCT showed that THC doses of up to 10 mg/d showed significant trends in favour of THC on a variety of measures, with no reported adverse effects (n = 24, RCT, d/b, 6/52, Muller-Vahl et al, *J Clin Psychiatry* 2003;**64**:459–65).

Fluoxetine

81% patients with OCD in Tourette's syndrome had improved symptoms on fluoxetine (n = 32, open, *Neurology* 1991;**41**:872–4). A potential effect for fluoxetine has been suggested in children with OCD symptoms in Tourette's (n = 11, Kyrlan *et al, Clin Neuropharmacol* 1993; **16**:167–72).

Levetiracetam *

When used for tics, levetiracetam 1–2 g/d produced some improvement in all patients in a pilot study (n = 60, open, Awaad *et al, Mov Disorder* 2005;**20**:714–8).

Methadone

Up to 110 mg/d has been used successfully in one treatment-resistant case (Meuldijk and Colon, *Am J Psychiatry* 1992;**149**:139–40).

Methylphenidate

Methylphenidate can aggravate tics or be associated with their appearance (Klein and Wender, *Arch Gen Psychiatry* 1995;**52**:429–33), but one study has shown that some tics are significantly worse, although generally these are not to the extent of contraindicating a trial, eg. in ADHD with Tourette's (Gadow *et al, Arch Gen Psychiatry* 1995;**52**:444–55). See clonidine.

Nicotine

Transdermal nicotine (7 mg/d) has been shown to be superior to placebo as an adjunct to haloperidol (n = 70 [c = 56], d/b, p/c, Silver *et al, J Clin Psychiatry* 2001;**62**:707–14; n = 6, Silver and Sanberg, *Lancet* 1993;**342**:182). A further study has shown that a single transdermal nicotine patch (7 mg/24 hours) shows a significant effect over 1–2 weeks, with considerable individual variation (n = 16, open, Silver *et al, J Am Acad Child Adolesc Psychiatry* 1996;**35**:1631–6). Nicotine chewing gum is an alternative that enhanced the symptomatic effects of haloperidol when used in combination (n = 10, open, McConville *et al, Am J Psychiatry* 1991;**148**:793–4). Long-term use has obvious problems, but PRN usage may help to minimise this.

Olanzapine *

In a small study, olanzapine (mean 14.5 mg/d)

improved aggression and tics in Tourette's, albeit with significant weight gain (n = 10, RCT, s/b, 10/52, Stephens *et al, J Child Adolesc Psychopharmacol* 2004;**14**:255–66; see also n = 10, open, 8/52, Budman *et al, J Clin Psychiatry* 2001;**62**:290–4; n = 1, Bhadrinath, *Br J Psychiatry* 1998;**173**:366). It may be as effective but better tolerated than pimozide (n = 4, d/b, c/o, one year, Onofrj *et al, J Neurol* 2000;**247**:443–6).

Ondansetron *

In haloperidol-resistant Tourette's, ondansetron 24 mg/d significantly improved tic severity on one rating scale but not on another (n = 30, RCT, d/b, p/c, 3/52, Toren *et al, J Clin Psychiatry* 2005;**66**:499–503).

Paroxetine

Paroxetine may have a role in the treatment of episodic rage in Tourette's, where 76% patients had reduced or absent rage episodes (n = 45, open, 8/52, Bruun and Budman, *J Clin Psychiatry* 1998;**59**:581–4).

Pergolide

One trial showed pergolide (up to 300 mcg/d) to be safe and effective in children with Tourette's disorder, chronic motor or vocal tic disorder (n = 245, RCT, 6/52, Gilbert *et al, Neurology* 2000;**54**:1310–6).

Selegiline

Selegiline was just significantly superior to placebo in children with Tourette's syndrome and ADHD (n = 24, d/b, p/c, c/o, Feigin *et al, Neurology* 1996;**46**:965–8).

Topiramate

There have been cases of Tourette's syndrome responding to topiramate up to 200 mg/d (n = 2, Abuzzhab and Brown, *Am J Psychiatry* 2001;**158**:968).

◆ Others

Other drugs used include **calcium-channel blockers** (verapamil and nifedipine, but not diltiazem; n = 2, Walsh *et al, Am J Psychiatry* 1986; **143**:1467–68), **clomiphene** (*Postgrad Med J* 1987;**63**:510), **nifedipine** (Berg, *Acta Psychiatr Scand* 1985;**72**:400–1; Goldstein, *J Clin Psychiatry*

1984;**45**:360), and **pentazocine** (*Clin Pharm* 1985; **4**:494).

1.29 TRICHOTILLOMANIA
see also OCD (*1.20*)

Symptoms
Trichotillomania presents as impulsive pulling out of the person's own hair (scalp, eyebrows, and eyelashes, as well as pubic, chest and other hair), resulting in noticeable hair loss. It is associated with OCD, and can occur in the presence of learning disability, anxiety, depression, schizophrenia and borderline personality disorder. It may result in relief of tension, can be episodic or chronic, and is more common in females.

Role of drugs *
A range of psychological and behaviour therapies are used and may be most effective when combined with pharmacotherapy. Drug therapy is still unproven and trials need to be of at least 8–10 weeks duration to prove or disprove an effect in an individual case. Combining pharmacology and behavioural treatments may give better outcomes (n = 63, Keuthen et al, *Am J Psychiatry* 1998;**155**:560–1). HRT (habit reversal training) combined with sertraline is more effective than either approach alone (n = 24, RCT, d/b, Dougherty et al, *J Clin Psychiatry* 2006;**67**:1086–92). One trial showed that CBT was more effective than clomipramine, and both were superior to placebo (n = 23, RCT, 9/52, Ninan et al, *J Clin Psychiatry* 2000;**161**:47–50). Dermatological help is beneficial.

Reviews: diagnosis (Hanna, *Child Psychiatry Hum Dev* 1997;**27**:255–68), general (Hautmann et al, *J Am Acad Dermatol* 2002;**46**:807–21; Papadopulos et al, *Int J Dermatol* 2003;**42**:330–4; Nuss et al, *Cutis* 2003;**72**:191–6; Hautmann et al, *J Am Acad Dermatol* 2002;**46**:807–21; Walsh and McDougle, *Am J Clin Dermatol* 2001;**2**:327–33; Diefenbach et al, *Clin Psychol Rev* 2000;**20**:289–309).

+ Combinations

Olanzapine + SSRI
Symptom improvement has been reported when olanzapine 10mg/d was added to fluoxetine 40mg/d (n = 1, Potenza et al, *Am J Psychiatry* 1998;**155**:1329–30). Olanzapine

1.25–7.5mg/d has been used with some success as augmentation of citalopram in refractory cases (n = 4, Ashton, *Am J Psychiatry* 2001;**158**:1929–30).

Risperidone + fluvoxamine
Resistant trichotillomania has responded to risperidone augmentation of fluvoxamine (n = 1, Gabriel, *Can J Psychiatry* 2001;**46**:285–6).

● Unlicensed/some efficacy

Clomipramine
Several studies (eg. n = 13, d/b, c/o, 10/52, Swedo et al, *N Engl J Med* 1989;**321**:497–501) have shown clomipramine in doses of around 180mg/d to be effective in some patients with trichotillomania. Some patients non-responsive to fluoxetine have then responded to clomipramine (eg. Naylor and Grossman, *J Am Acad Child Adolesc Psychiatry* 1991;**30**:155–6).

■ Unlicensed/possible efficacy

Bupropion *
Bupropion 300mg/d (but not 150mg/d) has produced almost complete resolution of symptoms in one treatment-resistant case (n = 1, Bhanji and Margolese, *J Clin Psychiatry* 2004;**65**:1283).

Citalopram
Citalopram may be safe in trichotillomania, with modest but significant improvements (n = 14, open, 12/52, Stein et al, *Eur Arch Psychiatry Clin Neurosci* 1997;**247**:234–6).

Escitalopram *
Escitalopram 10mg/d produced complete remission in a 10-year-old boy (n = 1, Bhatia and Sapra, *Eur Psychiatry* 2004;**19**:239–40).

Fluoxetine
Fluoxetine appears minimally effective, the doses required are high (up to 80mg/d) and if response occurs, relapse is not uncommon. Behavioural therapy was superior to fluoxetine, which was no better than placebo in one study (n = 43, RCT, 12/52, van Minnen et al, *Arch Gen Psychiatry* 2003;**60**:517–22) and another study failed to show an effect on hair pulling at up to

80mg/d on any of the measures used (n=23, d/b, c/o, 31/52, Streichenwein and Thornby, *Am J Psychiatry* 1995;**152**:1192–6) but there are some reports of response (eg. Winchel *et al*, *J Clin Psychiatry* 1992;**53**:304–8; n=21, RCT, d/b, c/o, 18/52, Christenson, *Am J Psychiatry* 1991;**148**:1566–71). It is generally considered second-line to clomipramine.

Fluvoxamine

Some potential use has been reported in reducing overall distress but not hair pulling (n=21, open, 12/52, Stanley *et al*, *J Clin Psychopharmacol* 1997;**17**:278–83).

Haloperidol

Haloperidol has been used successfully as augmentation of SSRIs (n=9, open, Van Ameringen *et al*, *J Affect Disord* 1999;**56**:219–26).

Inositol

Inositol, a glucose isomer with notable effects on serotonin, was well-tolerated and effective in reducing hair pulling in patients unwilling to take or intolerant of SSRIs (n=3, Seedat *et al*, *J Clin Psychiatry* 2001;**62**:60–1).

Lithium

80% patients tried on lithium showed reduced hair pulling and some hair regrowth, possibly via an effect on aggressive behaviour (n=10, open, 14/12, Christenson *et al*, *J Clin Psychiatry* 1991;**52**:116–20).

Olanzapine *

Olanzapine monotherapy up to 10mg/d has produced a significant reduction in hair pulling and anxiety, with 22% achieving full remission (n=18, open, 3/12, Stewart and Nejtek, *J Clin Psychiatry* 2003;**64**:49–52), and it has been successfully used to augment fluoxetine (n=2, Srivastava *et al*, *Aust NZ J Psychiatry* 2005; **39**:112–3).

Quetiapine

There is one case report of response (Khouzam *et al*, *Psychiatry* 2002;**65**:261–70).

■ **Others**

Other drugs tried include **paroxetine** (n=1, Reid,

Am J Psychiatry 1994;**151**:290), **pimozide** as SSRI augmentation (eg. *J Clin Psychiatry* 1992;**53**:123–6) and **trazodone** (eg. Sunkureddi and Markovitz, *Am J Psychiatry* 1993;**150**:523–4).

1.30–31 OTHER DRUG-RELATED TOPICS

1.30 CAFFEINISM

Caffeine consumption at 250–500mg/d is regarded as moderate use. Caffeinism is estimated to start at a consumption of between 600mg and 750mg/d, with above 1000mg/d well into the toxic range. 12mcg/mL is the US Olympic Committee upper limit for caffeine levels (*Am J Hosp Pharm* 1990;**47**:303). Caffeine dependence displays features of a typical psychoactive substance dependence, ie. withdrawal, continued use despite caffeine-induced problems, tolerance and persistent desire or unsuccessful attempts to cut down or control use (n=16, Strain *et al*, *JAMA* 1994;**272**:1043–8). Caffeine withdrawal is a DSM-IV diagnosis and thus should be taken seriously. Sudden withdrawal can produce headaches (52%), rebound drowsiness, fatigue/lethargy and depression (n=62, d/b, 4/7, Silverman *et al*, *J Psychopharmacol* 1991;**5**:129–34; *N Engl J Med* 1992;**327**:1109–14; review by Dews *et al*, *Food Chem Toxicol* 2002;**40**:1257–61), with many other effects reported. Positive effects of moderate amounts include increased alertness and vigilance and reduced fatigue.

Symptoms of caffeinism (acute or chronic)

Adverse effects of low to moderate doses: Diuresis, increased gastric secretion, fine tremor, increased skeletal muscle stamina, mild anxiety, negative mood, palpitations and nervousness.

Adverse effects of high doses: Chronic insomnia, persistent anxiety, restlessness, tension, irritability, agitation, tremulousness, panic, poor concentration, confusion, disorientation, paranoia, delirium, tremor, muscle twitching and tension, convulsions, vertigo, dizziness, tinnitus, auditory and visual hallucinations, facial flushing, hyperthermia, hypertension, nausea, vomiting, abdominal discomfort, headaches, tachypnoea and disturbed sleep.

Adverse consequences: There is some contradictory evidence about the effect of caffeine on people with mental health problems. Clearly, high doses can cause significant effects. Acute high doses (10mg/kg) significantly increase arousal and have a psychotogenic effect in schizophrenics (n=13, d/b, Lucas et al, Biol Psychiatry 1990;**28**:35–40). Schizophrenics often have higher caffeine intakes and average intake should be routinely monitored (Rihs et al, Eur Arch Psychiatry Clin Neurosci 1996;**246**:83–92) as it can exacerbate schizophrenia (n=2, Mikkelsen, J Clin Psychiatry 1978;**39**:732–6). Ward studies have shown that 'chronic caffeine use created clinically significant levels of anxiety and tension that could be reduced by decreasing caffeine consumption'. Caffeinism can precipitate or exacerbate psychosis and make these more resistant (n=2, Zaslove et al, Br J Psychiatry 1991;**159**:565–7) to drug treatment, especially antipsychotics. The clinical signs of affective diseases can be modified. 150mg of caffeine at bedtime has been shown to have a marked effect on sleep latency, total sleep time and reduced sleep efficacy and REM periods. Consumption may be influenced by some genetic factors (n=1934 twin study, Kendler and Prescott, Am J Psychiatry 1999;**156**:223–8). Conversely, there are reports of lack of correlation between caffeine consumption and anxiety and depression, with no changes when a ward moved to decaffeinated products (n=26, d/b, c/o, Mayo et al, Br J Psychiatry 1993;**162**:543–5), and little difference in behaviours between caffeinated and decaffeinated periods (Koczapski et al, Schizophr Bull 1989;**15**:339–44). Withdrawal of caffeine from a group of severely retarded and highly disturbed patients produced no improvement in sleep patterns, but reintroduction was accompanied by a highly significant increase in ward disturbances (2/52, Searle, J Intellect Disabil Res 1994;**38**:383–91), which may explain the contraindictions in evidence.

Methods of caffeine reduction

1. Recognition of the problems of excess consumption (>750mg/d) caffeine and the likely benefits of reduction.
2. Identification of all current caffeine sources and the pattern of consumption.
3. Implement a planned gradual reduction, eg. making weaker drinks, taken less often, increasing use of caffeine-free equivalent drinks (particularly at 'usual' drinking times of the day), using half-caffeine coffee, or mixing

caffeine and decaffeinated coffee to give a lower strength.
4. Use of analgesia (caffeine-free, of course) for withdrawal headaches.
5. Setting a target for consumption, which will not need to be complete abstinence, eg. caffeine drinks only at set times in the day, eg. on rising, etc.

Intake can be calculated thus:

Source	Caffeine content	
	per 100 ml	per container
Brewed coffee	55–85 mg	140–210 mg/cup
Instant coffee	35–45 mg	85–110 mg/cup
Decaf. coffee	2 mg	5 mg/cup
Cocoa	3 mg	7 mg/cup
Brewed tea	25–55 mg	55–140 mg/cup
Coca-cola	11 mg	36 mg/can
Pepsi cola	7 mg	22 mg/can
Milk chocolate		22 mg/100 g
Hedex seltzer		60 mg/sachet
Aqua ban		100 mg/tablet
A cup is taken as being 250 ml		

Causes

Patients may drink large quantities of tea and coffee to relieve thirst/dry mouth caused by tricyclic and phenothiazine side-effects, and caffeine is more attractive and less fattening than wine gums. In-patient settings, especially in the evening, often build in caffeine consumption.

Reviews: general (Smith, Food Chem Toxicol 2002;**40**:1243–55; Glass, JAMA 1994;**272**:1065–6), withdrawal (Juliano and Griffiths, Psychopharmacology (Berl) 2004;**176**:1–29), in psychiatric patients (Kruger, Psychol Rep 1996;**78**:915–23).

1.31 ELECTROCONVULSIVE THERAPY (ECT)

ECT was first used in its current form in 1938 (Linington and Harris, Br Med J 1988;**297**:1354–5). It is effective for rapid and short-term improvement in severe depression where other treatments have proven ineffective or life is threatened. The risks are higher in pregnancy, older people and in children. It is also used in mania (especially manic delirium), more rarely catatonia and drug-resistant Parkinsonism. ECT is probably superior to, or at least as effective as, antidepressants and tends to be quicker-acting in severely depressed patients, although there remains some dispute about this. ECT may be better than drugs for the short-term treatment of acute depression (n = 256, s = 6, UK ECT Group, *Lancet* 2003;**361**:799–808; comment by Bauer, *EBMH* 2003;**6**:83). Combining maintenance ECT with antidepressants has been suggested as improving outcomes in patients who have responded to acute treatment with ECT, compared to antidepressants only (n = 58, retrospective chart review, Gagné et al, *Am J Psychiatry* 2000; **157**:1960–5).

ECT facilitates monoaminergic transmission by increasing receptor sensitivity and increasing the turnover and release of noradrenaline (Ottosson et al, *Biol Psychiatry* 1985;**20**:933–46).

High-risk patients: These include those with severe cardiovascular disease, arrhythmias, pacemakers, obstructive pulmonary disease, asthma, pregnancy, osteoporosis, cerebral tumours, hydrocephalus and multiple sclerosis. If the patient has hypertension, sublingual nifedipine 20 minutes prior to ECT attenuates the hypertensive response (n = 5, Wells et al, *Anaesth Intensive Care* 1989;**17**:31–3).

Premedication: Atropine or glycopyrrolate can be used as antimuscarinics occasionally, mainly in patients with cardiovascular risks (n = 19, Bouckoms et al, *Convulsive Therapy* 1989;**5**: 48–55).

Muscle relaxants: Suxamethonium is used to prevent fractures that can occur during the procedure secondary to the tonic-clonic muscular contractions (n = 52, d/b, Konarzewski et al, *Anaesthesia* 1988;**43**:474–6).

Induction agents: * **Propofol** is now widely used since methohexital was withdrawn. It is well-tolerated and short-acting with quick recovery, but shortens seizure length by up to 25% (Adams, *Anaesthesia* 1989;**44**:168–9), may effect seizure threshold and may be associated with bradycardia and hypotension. Some small studies indicate that seizure duration does not affect overall efficacy (n=66, Mitchell et al, *Aust NZ J Psych* 1991;**25**:255–61; n = 20, d/b, Fear et al, *Br J Psychiatry* 1994;**165**:506–9), although ECT courses may be prolonged. **Etomidate** is short-acting, has a rapid recovery, less hypotension than propofol and may lengthen seizure duration compared to methohexital and propofol (Ilivicky et al, *Am J Psychiatry* 1995, **152**, 957–8). It may

perhaps cause convulsions pre-ECT (n = 1, Nicoll and Callender, *Br J Psychiatry* 2000;**177**:373), is painful at the injection site, has a high incidence of extraneous muscle movements, and rarely causes adrenocortical dysfunction with repeated doses (a major concern which limits use with longer courses) although it can be successful (n = 3, Benbow et al, *Psychiatr Bull* 2002;**26**:351–3). Inhaled **sevoflurane** has been used successfully as an induction agent for ECT (n = 5, Palmer et al, *Psychiatr Bull* 2004;**28**:326–8). **Sodium thiopentone** has little documented effect on seizure threshold or duration but the longer duration of action can delay recovery (a particular problem in the elderly).

Maintenance: ECT has been used at two-, three- and then four-weekly intervals for six months to prevent relapse (reviews by Andrade and Kurinji, *J ECT* 2002;**18**:149–58; Gupta, *Am J Psychiatry* 2001;**158**:1933–4; n = 43, Russell et al, *J ECT* 2003 **19**:4–9).

Reviews: * comprehensive review (Scott, *Adv Psychiatr Treat* 2005;**11**:150–6), in the elderly (Flint and Gagnon, *Can J Psychiatry* 2002;**47**:734–41), systematic review (s = 115, Wijeratne et al, *Med J Aus* 1999;**171**:250–4), induction agents (Freeman, *Psychiatr Bull* 1999;**23**: 740–1) and running an ECT department (Russell, *Adv Psychiatr Treat* 2001;**7**:57–64).

Drug considerations

Antipsychotics *

Antipsychotics lower the seizure threshold and would be expected to lead to seizures at lower ECT doses. A review of ECT with antipsychotics in schizophrenia concluded that the data was sparce but that the combination appeared to be safe and effective (review by Braga and Petrides, *J ECT* 2005;**21**:75–83).

Benzodiazepines

Benzodiazepines may lessen the improvement with unilateral ECT (Abrams, *Br J Psychiatry* 1992;**161**:129–30; Green, *Br J Psychiatry* 1992;**161**:717–8; n = 124, Jha and Stein, *Acta Psychiatr Scand* 1996;**94**:101–4). They may reduce the effectiveness of ECT, even several months after treatment is stopped, probably by raising the seizure threshold, having an effect on seizure duration, the number of submaximal seizures or by increasing the number of treatments needed.

Bupropion

Use with ECT has been reported (n = 2, Kellner et al, J Clin Psychopharmacol 1994; **14**:215–6), as has prolonged seizures when used with lithium and venlafaxine (n = 1, Conway and Nelson, J ECT 2001; **17**:216–8).

Caffeine

Caffeine 240 mg IV has been used to augment seizure duration (reported by the ideally named Coffey et al, Am J Psychiatry 1990; **147**:579–85) or 300–1000 mg orally (n = 30, Ancill and Carlyle, Am J Psychiatry 1992; **149**:137), as has 125 mg IV during treatment (Jaffe and Dubin, Am J Psychiatry 1992; **149**:1610). A small study showed a complex effect which deserves a full study to determine the optimum dose and timing (Francis et al, Am J Psychiatry 1994; **151**:1524–6). Cases of cardiac dysrhythmia have been reported in the elderly, so care is needed (n = 3, Jaffe et al, Convuls Ther 1990; **6**:308–13).

Carbamazepine

Logic would dictate that since carbamazepine is an anticonvulsant it would have an effect on reducing seizures (as for benzodiazepines). A small retrospective study showed that in seven patients taking either valproate or carbamazepine, seizure durations were slightly shorter but that this appeared to have no dramatic effect on either the efficacy or side-effects of ECT (n = 7, Zarate et al, Ann Clin Psychiatry 1997; **9**:19–25).

Ciprofloxacin *

There is a case of prolonged seizures related to concurrent ciprofloxacin 1 g/d (n = 1, Kisa et al, J ECT 2005; **21**:43–4).

Clozapine

The UK SPCs recommend suspending clozapine for 24 hours pre-ECT to reduce the risk of unwanted seizures. A review showed ECT (2–20 sessions) with clozapine (mean 518 mg/d, range 200–900 mg/d) to probably be safe and with short-term efficacy (72% showing marked initial improvement but only in 23% beyond 4/12) in resistant cases (n = 22, Havaki-Kontaxaki et al, Clin Neuropharmacol 2006; **29**:52–6; see also n = 36, Kupchik et al, Clin Neuropharmacol 2000; **23**:14–16). Many may benefit but adverse events occur in 17%, including prolonged seizures (n = 1, Bloch et al, Br J Psychiatry 1996; **169**:253–4), and supraventricular tachycardia (Beale et al, Convul Ther 1994; **10**:228–31). Not omitting doses is, however, a risky strategy, especially with higher doses of clozapine where the seizure threshold may be significantly lower.

Donepezil *

There is a single case report of adverse reaction (n = 1, Bhat et al, Int J Geriatr Psychiatry 2004; **19**:594–5), but a trial showed a single dose might reduce recovery times and improve cognitive deficits (t/b, RCT, Prakash et al, J ECT 2006; **22**:163–8).

Duloxetine *

There were no apparent problems with ECT in a patient taking olanzapine and duloxetine (n = 1, Hanretta and Malek-Ahmadi, J ECT 2006; **22**:139–41).

Flumazenil

Effective ECT was only possible in a benzodiazepine-dependent depressed woman when the anticonvulsant effect of clonazepam was reversed by flumazenil 0.1 mg (n = 1, Berigan et al, Am J Psychiatry 1995; **152**:957).

Ibuprofen *

Ibuprofen 600 mg/d 90 minutes before ECT may reduce the frequency and severity of post-ECT headache (n = 34, RCT, p/c, d/b, Leung et al, J Clin Psychiatry 2003; **64**:551–3), although Kessler thinks their data shows that it might actually increase seizure duration (Kessler, J Clin Psychiatry 2004; **65**:442).

Ketamine

Enhanced ECT seizure duration has been reported (mentioned in review by Weiner et al, 1991; **14**:857–67).

Lamotrigine *

A case series in bipolar depression showed lamotrigine did not interfere with ECT and appeared safe (n=9, Penland and Ostroff, *J ECT* 2006;**22**:142–7).

Lithium *

The use of lithium with ECT has been reported to cause severe memory loss, neurological abnormalities and a reduced antidepressant effect, although a retrospective study showed no increase in side-effects or other problems (n=31, Jha et al, *Br J Psychiatry* 1996;**168**:241–3; see also n=12 and review, Dolenc and Rasmussen, *J ECT* 2005;**21**:165–70), although there are reports of one each of prolonged seizure, serotonin syndrome and focal seizure with ECT and lithium at sub-therapeutic levels (n=3, Sartorius et al, *World J Biol Psychiatry* 2005;**6**:121–4). It has been suggested that ECT facilitates lithium toxicity, possibly by releasing lithium from cells, producing a pure toxicity. Elderly patients may be more susceptible to this combination. Some sources recommend discontinuing lithium 48 hours before ECT to prevent this neurotoxicity and not re-starting for several days after the last treatment (Ferrier et al, *Adv Psychiatr Treat* 1995;**1**:102–10). A review of the pros and cons of the use of lithium in ECT (Lippmann and El-Mallakh, *Lithium* 1994;**5**:205–9) concluded that there must be clear indications for concurrent use of both treatments. However, discontinuing lithium would risk discontinuation effects and be potentially dangerous (see lithium in *1.10*).

MAOIs *

MAOIs are normally contraindicated with surgery as they can interact with opiates but a review has concluded there is no dangerous interaction between MAOIs and ECT (n=4, Dolenc et al, *J ECT* 2004;**20**:258–61).

Mirtazapine

An open study indicated that there were no problems with mirtazapine, either started before or during a course of ECT (n=19, Söderström, poster, XI World Congress Psychiatry, August 1999, Germany). There are cases of successful and uneventful use (n=2, Farah, *Convul Ther* 1997;**13**:116–7).

Moclobemide

As a precaution, the manufacturers recommend suspending moclobemide for 24 hours pre-ECT, although there is no data on its use with ECT.

Naloxone

Naloxone has no detectable effect (Rasmussen et al, *Convuls Ther* 1997;**13**:44–6).

Olanzapine *

There were no apparent problems with ECT in a patient taking olanzapine and duloxetine (n=1, Hanretta and Malek-Ahmadi, *J ECT* 2006;**22**:139–41).

Rivastigmine

There is one case of a course of eight ECTs being successful with the person taking rivastigmine throughout (n=1, Zink et al, *J ECT* 2002;**18**:162–4).

SSRIs

A small study showed a significantly longer seizure duration in patients taking SSRIs compared to other antidepressants (n=13, Potokar et al, *Int J Psychiatr Clin Pract* 1997;**1**:277–80), although an earlier review did not support the theory that **fluoxetine** causes prolonged seizures (n=12, *Convul Ther* 1989;**5**:344–8). There are reports of prolonged seizures with ECT and **paroxetine** and in a rater-blinded comparison seizure length was twice as long in those taking paroxetine (n=14, Curran, *Acta Psychiatr Scand* 1995;**92**:239–40). There are several reports of prolonged seizures with **fluvoxamine** and ECT and Duphar recommend a four-day interval between stopping fluvoxamine and giving ECT. There is only limited experience with ECT and **sertraline** or **citalopram**.

Sumatriptan *

Sumatriptan has been used to prevent post-ECT headaches (White et al, *Headache* 2006;**46**:692).

Theophylline

Theophylline (related to caffeine) at 100–400mg IV has been reported to facilitate ECT seizures in previously resistant patients (n=7, Leentjens et al, Convuls Ther 1996;12:232–7). There are reports of status epilepticus and increase in seizure duration with concomitant ECT.

Trazodone *

A prolonged seizure duration has been reported (n=1, Lanes and Ravaris, Am J Psychiatry 1993;150:525), although low-dose use did not produce any problems in one retrospective study (n=100, Krahn et al, J Clin Psychiatry 2001;62:108–10).

Tricyclics

Combined tricyclic and ECT therapy is often used and seems to present no routine problems. The use of anaesthetics could enhance the risk of cardiac arrhythmias and hypotension.

Valproate

A small retrospective study showed that in patients taking either valproate or carbamazepine, seizure durations were slightly shorter but that this appeared to have no dramatic effect on the efficacy, or side-effects of ECT (n=7, Zarate et al, Ann Clin Psychiatry 1997;9:19–25).

Venlafaxine

When propofol is used as an anaesthetic, venlafaxine seems safe with ECT at doses of up to 300mg/d but, at higher doses, the possibility of asystole cannot be excluded (n=13, Gonzalez-Pinto et al, J Neuropsychiatry Clin Neurosci 2002;14:206–9). Prolonged recovery and unstable blood pressure has been reported in an elderly woman (Jha and Tomar, Int J Geriatr Psychiatry 2002;17:979–80).

Zopiclone

Reduced seizure length has been reported with 7.5–15mg of zopiclone the previous night (n=2, Tobiansky, J Psychopharmacol 1991; 5:268–9) and so is best avoided.

SELECTING DRUGS, DOSES AND PREPARATIONS

TABLE 2.1.1: HYPNOTICS — RELATIVE SIDE-EFFECTS

Class	Drug	Usual night dose mg/d	Adult max dose mg/d	Elderly max dose mg/d	Elim half-life (hours) adult	elderly	G/I upset	Hang-over	Depen-dence po-tential
Shorter-acting benzodiazepines									
Ia	Loprazolam	I	2	7	10	24	○	●	●
Ia	Lormetazepam	I	1.5+	<Ad	10	14	○	●	●
Ia	Temazepam	10–20	40	20	5–11	14+	○	●	●●
Longer-acting benzodiazepines									
Ib	Flunitrazepam	I	2	I	35	35	○	●●	●
Ib	Flurazepam	15	30	15+	47–95	?	○	●●●	●●
Ib	Nitrazepam	5	10	5	18–36	40+	○	●●●	●
Chloral and derivatives									
2	Chloral betane	707	5 tabs	<Ad?	7–10	Same	●●●	●	●
2	Triclofos	I g	2 g	I g	?	?	●	?	?
Other hypnotics									
3	Clomethiazole#	N/A#	2 caps#	Same	4–5	Same	○	●	●●
4	Promethazine	25	50	–	10–19	10–19	○	○	○
5	Zaleplon	10	10	5	2	3	○	○	○
6	Zopiclone	75	75	<Ad	3.5–6	8	●	●	●
7	Zolpidem	5	(10)	10	2(2–3)	Longer	○	○	○

Classes
Ia = Shorter-acting or minimally-accumulating benzodiazepines
Ib = Longer-acting or accumulating benzodiazepines
2 = Chloral and derivative
3 = Clomethiazole (chormethiazole)
4 = Antihistamine
5 = Pyrazolopyrimidine
6 = Imidazopyridine
7 = Cyclopyrrone

Side-effects
●●● = Marked effect
●● = Moderate effect
● = Mild effect
○ = Little or nothing reported
? = No information available

Other abbreviations
Nightly dose = Suggested usual dose for an adult in the UK SPC
Adult maximum dose = Suggested maximum adult hypnotic dose in the UK SPC
Elderly maximum dose = Suggested maximum elderly hypnotic dose in the UK SPC

= I capsule is therapeutically equivalent to 5 ml syrup (I cap = 192 mg clomethiazole base, and 5 ml syrup = 157 mg clomethiazole base). Indicated for severe insomnia in the elderly only.

TABLE 2.1.2: ANTIDEPRESSANTS — RELATIVE SIDE-EFFECTS

Drug	Adult oral max dose mg/d	Elderly oral max dose mg/d	Relative side-effects (most will be dose-related)						
			Anti-cholinergic	Cardiac	Nausea ‡	Sedation	Overdose §	Pro-convulsant	Sexual dysfunction
Tricyclics									
Amitriptyline	200	75	●●●	●●●	●●	●●●	●●●	●●	●●
Amoxapine	300	150	●●●	●	●	●●●	●●●	●●●	●
Clomipramine	250	75	●●●	●●	●●	●●	●	●●	●●●
Dosulepin (dothiepin)	150	75	●●	●●	○	●●●	●●●	●●	●●
Doxepin	300	<Ad	●	●●	●	●●	●●	●	●●
Imipramine	300	50	●●	●●	●●	●●	●●	●●	●●
Lofepramine	210	<Ad	●●	●	●●	●	○	○	●●
Maprotiline	150	75	●●	●●	●●	●	●●●	●●●	●●
Nortriptyline	150	50	●●	●	●●	●	●●	●	●●
Trimipramine	300	<Ad	●●●	●●	●	●●	●●	●	●●
SSRIs									
Citalopram	60	40	○	○	●●●	○	●	○	●●
Escitalopram	20	<20	○	○	●●	○	○	○	●●
Fluoxetine	(20)	(80)	○	○	●●	○	○	○	●●
Fluvoxamine	300	300	●	○	●●●	●	○	○	●
Paroxetine	50	40	○	○	●●	○	○	○	●●●
Sertraline	200	200	○	○	●●	○	○	○	●●
MAOIs									
Isocarboxazid	60	<Ad	●●	●●	●●	○	●●	○	●
Phenelzine	90	(90)	●	●●	●●	●●	●●●	○	●●
Tranylcypromine	CA30	(30)	●	●	●	●●	●●●	○	●

TABLE 2.1.2: CONT

Drug	Adult oral max dose mg/d	Elderly oral max dose mg/d	Relative side-effects (most will be dose-related)						
			Anti-cholinergic	Cardiac	Nausea ‡	Sedation	Overdose §	Pro-convulsant	Sexual dysfunction
Others									
Bupropion/amfebutamone (U)	-	-	●	○	●	○	●●	●●●	○
Duloxetine	120	Caution	○	○	●●	●	?	?	●●
Flupentixol	3	2	●●	○	○	●	●	?	●
Mianserin	90+	<Ad	●	○	○	●●●	○	○	●●
Mirtazapine	45	45	○	○	○	●●	○	●●	●
Moclobemide	600	600	●	○	●	○	○	?	○
Reboxetine	12	NR	●	●	●	○	○	○	●●
Trazodone	600	+300	●	●	●●	●●	●	○	●●
Tryptophan	6g	6g	○	○	●	●●	●	○	○
Venlafaxine	375	375	○	●●	●●	●	●●	●	●●

Side-effects

●●● = Marked effect
●● = Moderate effect
● = Mild effect
○ = Little or minimal effect
? = No information or little reported
U = Unlicensed in UK for depression

Other abbreviations

‡ = Typical serotonergic side-effect
Adult max dose = Maximum adult antidepressant dose in UK SPC
Elderly max dose = Maximum elderly antidepressant dose as stated in UK SPC. Most state that half the adult dose may be sufficient
Overdose § = Based on UK Fatal Toxicity Index (Henry et al, Br J Med 1995;**310**:221–48). For review of epidemiology and relative toxicity of antidepressant drugs in overdose see Henry (Drug Safety 1997;**16**:374–90, 92 refs)

TABLE 2.1.3: ANTIDEPRESSANTS — PHARMACOKINETICS AND RECEPTOR EFFECTS

Drug	Major active metabolites	Half-life (hours)	Peak plasma conc (hours)	Transmitter/receptor profile 5-HT	NA/NE	DA
Tricyclics						
Amitriptyline		8–24	6	+++	++++	+
	Nortriptyline	18–96	(4–5)	+	++++	+
Amoxapine		8	1–2	+	+++	+
	7+8-hydroxyamoxapine		–	–	Weak	–
Clomipramine		17–28	2.5	+++	+	–
	Desmethylclomipramine	>36	4–24	+	+++	–
Dosulepin (dothiepin)	Desmethyldothiepin	14–40	3	+	+	+
		22–60	2			–
Doxepin		8–24	4	+	+	–
	Desmethyldoxepin	30–72	-	+++		–
Imipramine		4–18	2	+++	+	–
	Desipramine	12–24	(4–5)	+	++++	–
Lofepramine		1.6	1–2	+	++++	–
	Desipramine	12–24	(4–5)	+	++++	–
Maprotiline		12–108	8–24	+	+++	–
	Desmethylmaprotiline					–
Nortriptyline		18–96	(4–5)	+	+++	–
Trimipramine	(Desmethyltrimipramine)	7–23	3	+	+	+
Selective serotonin reuptake inhibitors (SSRIs)						
Citalopram		33	2–4	++++	–	–
Escitalopram		30	2–4	++++	–	–
Fluoxetine		24–140	6–8	++++	–	+
	Norfluoxetine	168–216	–	+	–	–
Fluvoxamine	None	13–22	2–8	+++	–	–
Paroxetine	None	24	6	++++	+	–
Sertraline		25–36	4–10	+++	–	–
	Desmethylsertraline	66–109	8–12	+	–	–

TABLE 2.1.3: CONT

Drug	Major active metabolites	Half-life (hours)	Peak plasma conc (hours)	Transmitter/receptor profile		
				5-HT	NA/NE	DA
Monoamine oxidase inhibitors						
Isocarboxazid		NK	2–3	↑	↑	↑
Phenelzine		1.5	2–3	↑	↑	↑
Tranylcypromine		2.5	2–3	↑	↑	↑
Others						
Duloxetine	NK	8–17	6	+++	+++	–
Flupentixol		35	3–8	–	–	–
Mianserin		12–29	1–3	0	0	+
	Desmethyl-8-hydroxy					
Mirtazapine	None	20–40	1–3	+++	↑	
Moclobemide	None	1–2	1	↑	↑	↑
Reboxetine	NK	13	2	0	+++	0
Trazodone		3–7	½–2	++#	0	0
	mCPP			A		
Venlafaxine $		1–2	5(2–7)	+++§	+++§	+§
	Desmethylvenlafaxine			10(8–13)		

Abbreviations

++++	=	Marked potency	++	=	Minor potency
+++	=	Moderate potency	+	=	Minimal

Other abbreviations

$	=	Dose-dependent reuptake inhibitors (see CI)
A	=	Potent postsynaptic 5-HT agonist
NA/NE	=	Noradrenaline or norepinephrine
↑	=	Cytoplasm levels increase
5-HT	=	5-hydroxytryptamine or serotonin
#	=	Also potent central 5HT antagonist
A	=	Potent post-synaptic 5-HT agonist

TABLE 2.1.4: ANTIPSYCHOTICS — RELATIVE SIDE-EFFECTS

Drug	Adult oral max dose mg/d	Elderly oral max dose mg/d	Relative side-effects (most will be dose related)								
			Anti-cholinergic	Cardiac	EPSE	Hypo-tension	Sedation	Minor O/D	Weight gain	Prolactin	Procon-vulsant
Phenothiazines											
Chlorpromazine	1000	<Ad	●●●	●●	●●	●●●	●●●	●●	●●●	●●●?	●●
Levomepromazine (methotrimeprazine)	1000	NR	●●●	●●	●●?	●●●	●●●	●●	?	●●●?	●●?
Promazine	800	<Ad	●●	●●	●	●●	●●	●●	?	●●●?	●●?
Pericyazine	(300)	<Ad	●	●●●	●	●●	●●	●●	?	●●●?	●●?
Thioridazine	600	<Ad	●●	●●●	●	●●	●●	●	●●	●●●?	●?
Fluphenazine	CA20	CA10	●	●●	●●●	●	●	●	●●	●●●?	●●?
Perphenazine	24	<Ad	●	●●	●●●	●	●●	●●	●●●	●●●?	●?
Trifluoperazine	–	<Ad	○	●	●●●	●	●	●●	?	●●●?	●
Others											
Benperidol	1.5	<Ad	?	?	?	●	●●	?	?	●●●?	●?
Haloperidol	30	30	●	●●	●●●	●	●●	●	●	●●●	●?
Flupentixol	18	<Ad	●●	○	●●●	○	●	●	●	●●?	●?
Zuclopenthixol	150	<Ad	●	●	●●●	●	●●	●●	?	●●?	○?
Pimozide	20	<Ad	●	●●●	●	●	●	?	○	●●●?	●
Amisulpride	1200	1200	○	○	●●●	○	●	○	●	●●●?	●?
Sulpiride	2400	2400	●	○	●●	○	●	●	●	●●	○?
Loxapine	250	–	●●	●	●●●	●	●●	●●●	●	●●●?	●●●
Depots ◆											
Fluphenazine decanoate (D)	100–2/52	<Ad	●●	●●	●●●	●	●●	●	●	●●●?	●
Pipotiazine palmitate (D)	200–4/52	<Ad	●●	●●	●●	●	●	?	?	●●●?	●●?
Haloperidol decanoate (D)	300–4/52	<Ad	●	●	●●●	●	●	●	●	●●●	●
Flupentixol decanoate (D)	400–1/52	<Ad	●●	○	●●	○	●	●?	?	●●?	●?
Zuclopentixol decanoate (D)	600–1/52	<Ad	●●	●	●●●	●	●●	●●	?	●●?	○?

TABLE 2.1.4: CONT

Drug	Adult oral max dose mg/d	Elderly oral max dose mg/d	Relative side-effects (most will be dose related)								
			Anti-cholinergic	Cardiac	EPSE	Hypo-tension	Sedation	Minor O/D	Weight gain	Prolactin	Procon-vulsant
Depots ◆											
Fluspirilene (D)	20–1/52	<Ad	●	●	●●●	●●	●●	?	?	●●● ?	●
Risperidone (D)	50–2/52	25–2	○	○	●●	●	?	?	●	●●	○
Atypicals											
Clozapine	900	(900)	●●●	●●●	○	●	●●●	?	●●●	○	●●●
Olanzapine	20	20	●	○	○	○	●●	○	●●●	○	●●
Quetiapine	750	<Ad	●	●	○	●	●●	●	●	●	●●
Risperidone	(16)	4	○	○	●	●	?	?	●	●●	●
Zotepine	300	150	●●	●●	●	●●	●●	?	●●● ?	●●● ?	●●
Sertindole	(20)	(20)	○	●●	○	○	○	○	●	○	○
Ziprasidone (not UK)	–	–	○	●●	○	○	○	?	○	○	○
Aripiprazole	30	30	○	●	○	○	○	?	●	○	○

Side-effects
- ●●● = Marked effect
- ●● = Moderate effect
- ● = Mild/transient effect
- ○ = Little or minimal effect
- ? = No information or little reported

Other abbreviations
- Adult max dose = Maximum adult oral antipsychotic dose as stated in UK SPC. May be lower for other indications
- Elderly max dose = Maximum oral antipsychotic dose in the elderly as stated in UK SPC. Most state that a starting dose of half to a quarter of the adult dose should be adequate, with smaller dose increments
- ◆ = 2–200 means 200mg every 2 weeks. 400–1 means 400mg every week, etc

185

TABLE 2.1.5: ANTIPSYCHOTICS — PHARMACOKINETICS AND RECEPTOR EFFECTS

Drug/group	Receptor blockade (5)										$5HT_{2a}{:}D_2$ affinity ratio	Half-life (hours)	Time to peak (oral) (2) hours	Main metabolite(s)
	D_1	D_2	D_3	D_4	$5HT_{1A}$	$5HT_{2A}$	M_1	α-1	α-2	H_1				
Phenothiazines														
Chlorpromazine	++	+	++	+		+++	++	+++	+	++	10:1	6(2–119)	3(IM 1–4, IV 2–4)	Many
Fluphenazine HCl	++	+++	+++	++		++	+	++	O	+	1:2	FHCl 33 FD 14–27/7	FHCl 3	Some, unclear if active
Fluphenazine decanoate														
Levomepromazine	++	++	+++	?		+++	+++	+++	O	+++	5:1	15–30	1–3	Some, unclear if active
Pericyazine (3)	++?	+?	++?	+?		+++?	+++?			++?		NK	NK	NK
Perphenazine	++	++	NK	?		+++	+	++		+++	2:1	10(8–12)	4–8	Some, unclear if active
Thioridazine	++	+	++	+		+++	+++	+++	+	+	5:1	21–24	NK	Mesoridazine
Trifluoperazine	++	++	NK	+	+	+++	+	+++	+	+	2:1	24	2–4	Several
Others														
Benperidol	+?	+++	+?	+?		+?	O?	+?	+?	++?	NK	8	2	1% unchanged in urine
Haloperidol HCl	++	+++	+++	+		++	+	++	O	+	1:25	HHCl2 (10–38), HD21/7	2–6	Hydroxy-haloperidol
Haloperidol decanoate														
Flupentixol HCl												22–36 D 3–7/7(L)	FHCl 3–6 FD 3–10/7	Inactive
Flupentixol decanoate														
Zuclopenthixol HCl	++	+++	+	NK		+++	++	++	NK	++	1:3	20	ZHCl 3–4 ZD 5–7 days ZA 24–48	Inactive
Zuclopenthixol decanoate														
Zuclopenthixol acetate														
Sulpiride	O	+++	+	O		O	O	O	O	O	1:50	6–8	2–6	Nil
Amisulpride	O	+++	+++	O		O	O	O	O	O		12–17	1–4	Nil
Loxapine	++	+	NK	O		+++	++	+++	O	+++	7:1	4(1–14)	1	Several, low potency
Pimozide	+	+++	+++	+		+++	+	+++	+	O	1:5	53–55	6–8	Some, unclear if active
Fluspirilene	NK	NK	NK	NK	NK	NK	NK	NK	NK	NK	NK	32–>300	1–48	Inactive

TABLE 2.1.5: CONT

Drug/group	Receptor blockade (5)										5HT$_{2a}$:D$_2$ affinity ratio	Half-life (hours)	Time to peak (oral) (2) hours	Main metabolite(s)
	D$_1$	D$_2$	D$_3$	D$_4$	5HT$_{1A}$	5HT$_{2A}$	M$_1$	α-1	α-2	H$_1$				
Atypicals														
Aripiprazole	O	++++	O	O	PAg	AAnt	O	O	O	O	N/A	75(31–146)	3–7	None known
Clozapine	++	+++4	++	+++	+	+++	+++	+++	++	+++	20–30:1	4–12	2–3	Norclozapine
Olanzapine	++	+++4	+	++	+	+++	+++	++	+	+++	50:1	30(21–54)	3–6	Inactive
Quetiapine	O	++	+	NK	++	++	O	++	O	+++	1:1	6	1.5	2 major active
Risperidone	+	+++	+	+	++	+++	O	+++	+++	++	8–11:1	20–30	1	Hydroxyrisperidone
Sertindole	+	+++4	+	+		+++	O	+++	O	+	100:1	55–90	10	Dehydrosertindole
Ziprasidone	O	++	+	O	+	++	O	+	O	O	3:1	7	4–5	Many
Zotepine	+++	+++	+++	++	++	+++	++	+++	+++	+++	4:1	14–24	1 and 10–12	Norzotepine (inactive)

Receptor binding: +++ = High affinity; ++ = Moderate; + = Low; O = Very low; NK = Not known; ? = Possible; PAg = Partial agonist with very high affinity; AAnt = Antagonist
Additional ref: Siloh, Nutt and Weizman (2000) *Atlas of Psychiatric Pharmacotherapy*, Martin Duntiz, London (very colourful and useful)

1. Flupentixol decanoate's half-life is longer (up to 17 days) on continuous administration
2. Time to oral peak may vary with food
3. Receptor-binding studies for pericyazine have not been published, but it has been reported to have some differences to chlorpromazine
4. Sertindole, olanzapine and clozapine appear to have some D2 limbic selectivity
5. Inclusion of a receptor may give some guide to therapeutic action and adverse effects
6. There is a considerable degree of variation between published sources, depending upon how the results are presented, whether they are single studies or averages, the receptor sources, assay type, etc. These figures should be taken only as a guide, eg. there is little, or nothing published about fluspirilene or pericyazine

TABLE 2.1.6: ANXIOLYTICS — RELATIVE SIDE-EFFECTS

Class	Drug	Usual dose mg/d	Adult max dose mg/d	Elderly max dose mg/d	Half-life (hours) adult (+ range)	elderly	Hang-over	Depen-dence po-tential
Shorter-acting benzodiazepines								
Ia	Loprazolam	I	3	0.75	14(6–20)	L	●	●
Ia	Clonazepam	2	20	I	30 (20–60)	Same	●●	●●
Ia	Lorazepam	4	4	<Ad	12(8–25)	Same	●●●	●●●
Ia	Oxazepam	30	120	80	8(5–15)	Same	●●●	●●
Longer-acting benzodiazepines								
Ib	Chlordiazepoxide	30	100	<50	12(6–30)	L	●●●	●●
Ib	Clobazam	30	60	20	18(9–77)	L	●	●●
Ib	Clorazepate	15	15?	<Ad	PD	L	●●●	●●
Ib	Diazepam	6	30	15	32(21–50)	L	●●●	●●
Beta-blockers								
2	Oxprenolol	80	80	80	4#(3–6)	Same	●	○
2	Propranolol	80	120	–	2#(1–2)	Same	●	○
Other anxiolytics								
3	Busipirone	30	45	45	7(2–11)	Same	○	○
4	Pregabalin	300	600	<600	6	L	○	○

Classes
Ia = Shorter-acting or minimally-accumulating benzodiazepines
Ib = Longer-acting or accumulating benzodiazepines. These also have metabolites which enhance their
length of action
2 = Beta-blockers
3 = Azapirone (Azaspirodecanedione)
4 = Anticonvulsant

Side-effects
●●● = Marked effect ○ = Little or nothing reported
●● = Moderate effect ? = No information available
● = Mild effect

Other abbreviations
Adult maximum dose = Suggested maximum dose in the UK SPC. Most recommend
treatment for up to four weeks
Elderly maximum dose = Suggested maximum in the elderly in the UK SPC. Most state that half
the adult dose should be adequate
# = Pharmacological action longer than half-life suggests
L = Longer
The data on the previous pages is based on a large number of papers. Note was taken of presentation of data,
equivalence of dose used, etc. When non-comparable papers are excluded, there is a surprisingly high level of
consistency on reported relative side-effects. Individuals response may, of course, vary widely. Many effects may
be dose-related.

2.2 SWITCHING OR DISCONTINUING PSYCHOTROPICS

Switching psychotropics can be achieved using a variety of methods, varying in rate, overlap, gap and complexity. These are summarised in the graphs and comments shown. Those remarks specifically relating to antipsychotics are marked with #.

Switch 1: Drug-free interval
(Discontinue first drug, leave drug-free interval, introduce second drug.)
Advantages:
1. Minimises combined ADRs.
2. Low relapse risk, if the patient is relatively stable and the gap is not prolonged.
3. Minimal interaction potential.
4. Side-effects from the second drug are less likely to be confused with discontinuation effects from first drug.
5. Anticholinergic drug doses can be titrated as needed. #
6. Ideal (but often impractical) for switches to clozapine to reduce additive myelosuppressive potential. #
7. Low medication error potential.
Disadvantages:
1. Takes time, which delays the desired relief of symptoms or side-effects and may extend in-patient stays. #
2. Potential for relapse during the gap and changeover (probably rare).
3. Early relapse might be interpreted as lack of efficacy of the second drug.

Switch 2: No interval
(Stop first drug, start second immediately.)
Advantages:
1. Straightforward.
2. Low medication error potential.
3. Appropriate for in-patient settings with better supervision.
4. Appropriate where an acute severe reaction to a drug has occurred, eg. statutory abrupt withdrawal of clozapine due to a blood dyscrasia. #
5. Sometimes acceptable for high-risk switches to clozapine to reduce additive myelosuppressive potential, but retaining antipsychotic cover. #

TABLE 2.2.1: SWITCHING PSYCHOTROPICS

Switch 1: Drug-free interval (safest)

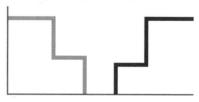

Switch 2: No interval (generally preferred)

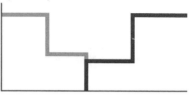

Switch 3: Partial overlap (usually acceptable)

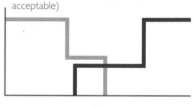

Switch 4: Full overlap (risks NMS or serotonin syndrome and combined ADRs)

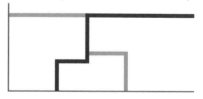

Switch 5: Incomplete (never finished, resulting in default polypharmacy, avoid)

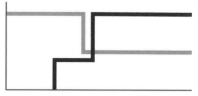

Disadvantages:

1. May raise unrealistic expectations from the patient and family of a rapid improvement on the second drug.
2. Combined ADRs may occur, albeit short-lived.
4. Potential for drug interactions if the first drug has a long half-life, eg. fluoxetine.
5. Rapid discontinuation of the first drug may produce higher relapse rates, eg. antipsychotics.
6. Discontinuation effects from the first drug might be interpreted as side-effects of the second, eg. some antipsychotics.

Switch 3: Partial overlap

(Add new drug, either at standard dose or quickly titrated upwards, while slowly tapering the first drug.)

Advantages:

1. Appropriate when side-effect relief is needed but there is a high relapse risk.
2. No sudden changes occur, which might destabilise the patient.
3. This switch may be unavoidable for depot to oral switches, where plasma levels of depot will decline slowly. #
4. Useful for switches from a high potency antipsychotic to an atypical, or from a low potency drug where cholinergic rebound may occur. Either way, anticholinergic cover can be retained for several weeks. #

Disadvantages:

1. If the taper is too quick, two drugs may be given at sub-therapeutic doses.
2. Combined ADRs may occur.
3. Potential for drug interactions, especially with antidepressants.
4. Potential for medication errors if not planned fully in advance — involve carers and patient if patient is at home.
5. High potential for polypharmacy if the switch is never completed, eg. if the patient is discharged and the message is not passed on, or the patient improves and there is a reluctance to discontinue the first drug and possibly destabilise the patient. #

Switch 4: Full overlap

(Add new drug to therapeutic dose and then slowly taper previous drug.)

Advantages:

1. Safest if relapse prevention is of greatest concern.
2. Most appropriate if the patient has recently (eg. < 3 months) recovered from acute relapse with the first drug.
3. Low risk of discontinuation effects of the first drug.
4. If depot to oral antipsychotic switch, this may be the lowest risk opportunity to assess compliance with oral drugs. #
5. Slow taper is possible and is better for drugs with a high anticholinergic activity.

Disadvantages:

1. Combined ADRs may occur (but not necessarily with antipsychotics, Gardner et al, Can J Psychiatry 1997;**42**:430–1).
2. Potential severe reactions, eg. NMS or serotonin syndrome.
3. Potential for drug interactions.
4. Potential for medication errors if not planned and completed fully.
5. High potential for polypharmacy if switch never completed, eg. if discharged and message not passed on, or patient improves and there is a reluctance to discontinue the first drug and possibly destabilise the patient. #

Switch 5: Incomplete

(Add new drug to therapeutic dose and then never stopping previous drug.)

'Default polypharmacy' should be avoided. The advantages of long-term monotherapy are that one is better able to judge the effectiveness of any given drug accurately and medication regimens are simple and not confused by polypharmacy (extensive review, Weiden et al, J Clin Psychiatry 1998;**59**[Suppl 19]:36–49). Monotherapy should thus always be tried first and if at some time later a rational, planned and assessed polypharmacy is tried then that is reasonable. See 1.23 for a discussion on combined antipsychotics.

2.2.1 SWITCHING OR DISCONTINUING ANTIPSYCHOTICS

Reviews: switching from typicals to atypicals (Taylor, CNS Drugs 1997;**8**:285–92), general (Weiden et al, J Clin Psychiatry 1997;**58**[Suppl 10]:63–72, 60 refs; Amery and Marder, Int J

Psychiatry Clin Pract 1998;**2**:S43–S49), discontinuing antipsychotics (Tranter and Healy, *J Psychopharmacol* 1998;**12**:401–6).

2.2.1.1 GENERAL ADVICE ON SWITCHING ANTIPSYCHOTICS

Reasons for switching antipsychotics include (Weiden et al, *J Clin Psychiatry* 1997;**58**[Suppl 10]: S63–S72):

1. Persistent positive (distressing and disruptive) symptoms.
2. Persistent negative (restrictive and burdening) symptoms.
3. Relapse despite compliance.
4. Persistent distressing adverse effects such as EPS, akathisia, hyperprolactinaemia, poor self-image and sexual dysfunction.
5. Oral to depot or other formulation change.

Risks of discontinuing (or switching) antipsychotics (review and guidance, Keks et al, *CNS Drugs* 1995;**4**:351–6):

1. Cholinergic rebound (eg. nausea, vomiting, restlessness, anxiety, insomnia, fatigue, malaise, myalgia, diaphoresis, rhinitis, paraesthesia, GI distress, headaches, nightmares). It may occur after discontinuation, if a second drug has less anticholinergic effects or if anticholinergic drugs are withdrawn too soon (Luchins et al, *Am J Psychiatry* 1980;**137**:1395–8). It can be severe but tends to be brief and predictable.
2. Withdrawal dyskinesias, eg. extrapyramidal symptoms, rebound akathisia (which may be confused with anxiety or psychosis, Dufresne and Wagner, *J Clin Psychiatry* 1988;**49**:435–8), rebound dystonia and worsening tardive dyskinesia (Glazer et al, *Biol Psychiatry* 1989;**26**:224–33). Withdrawal EPS may partly be related to cholinergic rebound, and have been reported in mentally 'healthy' people taking metoclopramide as an antiemetic (see Tranter and Healy, *J Psychopharmacol* 1998;**12**:401–6), and can be minimised by slow tapering (n = 81, d/b, p/c, Battegay, *Compr Psychiatry* 1966;**7**:501–9).
3. Other discontinuation symptoms, eg. NMS (Spivak et al, *Acta Psychiatr Scand* 1990;**81**:168–9).
4. Relapse or destabilisation — this may

present an unacceptable risk to the patient. Relapse rates of up to 50% at six months after abrupt discontinuation have been reported (n = 1210, Viguera et al, *Arch Gen Psychiatry* 1997;**54**:49–55). Gradual discontinuation reduces this risk (reviewed by Tranter and Healy, *J Psychopharmacol* 1998;**12**:401–6). True relapses tend to occur from 1–6 months after abrupt withdrawal of oral drugs (eg. Prien et al, *Br J Psychiatry* 1968;**115**:679–86) and 3–6 months with depots (Wistedt, *Acta Psychiatr Scand* 1981;**64**:65–84), probably due to persistence of the drug at receptor level (Cohen et al, *Arch Gen Psychiatry* 1988;**45**:879–80). There may be a particular problem with clozapine, where relapse or rebound psychosis can be more severe (eg. Baldessarini et al, *Arch Gen Psychiatry* 1995;**52**:1071–2, see also 2.2.1.4).

5. Anxiety or stress from the switch causing symptom flare-up.
6. Medication errors.
7. The replacement drug being less effective than the former, or having different but still unacceptable side-effects, resulting in premature abandonment and an inadequate trial of the new drug.

General principles for switching antipsychotics:

1. Ensure a treatment target is set and measured (take care that the key aims of a switch are not easier and less risky to achieve by, eg. dose or timing adjustment of the first drug).
2. Avoid switches coinciding with major life stress events.
3. Avoid switching after a change in treatment team. Allow full assimilation into the new treatment team first.
4. Avoid switching within 3–6 months of recovery from a drug which was successfully used to treat a major relapse.
5. In patients previously non-compliant with oral drugs now stable for under a year on a depot (Weiden et al, *J Clin Psychiatry* 1997;**58**[Suppl 10]:63–72).
6. If possible, slowly taper the first antipsychotic, probably over at least eight weeks, as this reduces the risk of relapse (Wyatt, *Arch Gen Psychiatry* 1995;**52**:205–8) and emergent extrapyramidal and psychotic symptoms.

7. Slowly taper any anticholinergic, which may also be allowed to continue for a time after the drug has been discontinued. Reintroduce if necessary for any emergent symptoms.
8. Monitor mental and physical state regularly (particularly during the first month).

Before switching to atypicals:

1. Warn about possible ADRs (eg. weight gain, short-term sedation, diabetes, implications of reduced prolactin inhibition).
2. Discuss the need for an adequate trial and the need to complete the switch.
3. Agree how to define success or failure, and the chances thereof.
4. Warn that the new drug isn't perfect — that one is swapping one set of side-effects for another.

2.2.1.2 SPECIFIC DRUG SWITCHES

NMS has been reported during many antipsychotic switches, eg. from haloperidol to risperidone (n=1, Reeves *et al*, *Ann Pharmacother* 2001;**35**:698–701).

1. Phenothiazine to phenothiazine:
Get the dose equivalent right, then switches 2 or 3 are probably reasonable.

2. Phenothiazine to D2-blocker:
Get the dose equivalent as best as possible, then switches 2 or 3 are probably reasonable but beware of cholinergic rebound (nausea, vomiting, restlessness, anxiety, insomnia, fatigue, GI distress) and stronger D2-blockade leading to additional EPSE.

3. Phenothiazine/D2-blocker to typical depot:
Studies have shown this is usually relatively straightforward if done carefully, remembering that typical depots peak plasma levels may vary (see *Table 2.2.2*) and so reduce doses accordingly. Beware of additive EPSEs.

3a. Oral antipsychotic to typical depot:
Anecdotal evidence shows that the change can usually be made uneventfully (eg. review in *Clin Pharmacokinet* 1985;**10**:315–33), although

TABLE 2.2.2: SWITCHING ANTIPSYCHOTICS

From \ To	Pheno-thiazines	D2 blockers	Typical depots	Aripip-razole	Cloza-pine	Olanza-pine	Risperi-done	Risperi-done consta	Quetia-pine
Pheno-thiazines	RT (1)	RT (2)	RT (3)	RT (4,16)	Care (5,16)	NOP (6,16)	RT (7)	RT (8)	RT (9,16)
D2 blockers	RT (10)	RT (11)	RT (3)	RT (4,16)	Care (5,16)	NOP (6,16)	RT (7)	RT (8)	RT (9,16)
Typical depots	RT (12)	RT (12)	RT (12)	RT (4,12,16)	Care (5,12,16)	RT (6,12,16)	RT (7,12)	RT (8,12)	RT (9,12,16)
Aripiprazole	RT (4)	RT (4)	RT (4)		Care (4)	RT (4)	RT (4)	RT (4)	NOP (4)
Clozapine	Care (5)	Care (5)	Care (5)	RT (4)		Care (6)	RT (5)	RT (8)	RT (9)
Olanzapine	NOP (13)	NOP (13)	NOP (13)	RT (4,13)	Care (5,13)		RT (7,13)	RT (8,13)	NOP (9,13)
Risperidone	RT (14)	RT (14)	RT (14)	RT (4,14,16)	Care (5,14,16)	NOP (6,14,16)		RT (8,14)	NOP (9,14,16)
Risperidone Consta	RT (8)	RT (8)	RT (8)	RT (8,16)	Care (8,16)	RT (8,16)	RT (8)		RT (8,16)
Quetiapine	NOP (15)	NOP (15)	NOP (15)	RT (4,15)	Care (5,15)	NOP (6,15)	RT (7,15)	RT (8,15)	

NOP = No obvious problems
RT = Read text
Care = Great care needed, also read text

there are no formal studies. Converting to the same drug as a depot should present no great problems if doses are chosen carefully (eg. switch 3, see also 2.2.1.4).

3b. Altering the frequency of a typical depot:
Such a change should present no great problems, provided antipsychotic levels do not drop too low or rise too high.

3c. Changing from one typical depot to another typical depot:
No significant problems are usually experienced (Soni et al, Acta Psychiatr Scand 1992;**85**:354–9) and a direct exchange from one depot to another can often be made uneventfully (eg. switch 3).

3d. Combined oral antipsychotic plus depot to depot alone:
This can be an unusually difficult procedure and relapses may occur more frequently with this change when compared to other changes. Relapses can occur particularly in the first 3–4 months, when antipsychotic levels can be inadvertently sub-therapeutic (Soni et al, Acta Psychiatr Scand 1992;**85**:354–9). Any change should probably be done verging on the side of caution, eg. increasing the depot dose, then reducing the oral dose later.

3e. Switching from oral fluphenazine to depot fluphenazine:
If transferring from oral fluphenazine, multiply the total daily oral dose by 1.2 and administer as fluphenazine decanoate IM every one to two weeks. Accumulation occurs and so the dosing interval may be increased to every three weeks or so after four to six weeks of therapy (Ereshefsky et al, J Clin Psychiatry 1984;**45**:50). Concomitant oral therapy should be limited to the initial period or during times of decompensation.

3f. Switching from oral haloperidol to depot haloperidol:
If transferring from stabilised oral haloperidol to haloperidol depot, multiply the total daily oral dose by 15–20, to a maximum of 300mg monthly, preferably much lower. Accumulation occurs and so the decanoate dose should be decreased by 25% a month until the minimum effective dose is achieved. The average maintenance dose appears to be about 100mg every four weeks. Elderly patients or those stabilised on less than 10mg/d oral haloperidol should receive haloperidol decanoate in an IM dose that is 10–15 times the oral dose every

four weeks. Concomitant oral therapy should be limited to the initial period or during times of decompensation.

4. Anything to aripiprazole:
In a comparison of three methods of switching to aripiprazole (abrupt, double-cross-taper and abrupt start and gradual discontinuation), outcomes and side-effects were similar in all three groups (open, o/p, 8/52, Casey et al, Psychopharmacol [Berl] 2003;**166**:391–9). Aripiprazole strongly binds to dopamine receptors, displacing almost every other antipsychotic and stimulating receptors to about 30% activity. The clinical effect of aripiprazole will start rapidly, and so a gradual cross-titration may be useful in some circumstances, as the brain may essentially go from minimal dopamine activity to 30%, which might be quite a shock. Starting at 5mg/d may be appropriate in many people. Warn women about the possible normalisation of prolactin and the need for adequate oral contraception if necessary.

5. Clozapine

5a. Switching to clozapine:
Care would be needed with the increased risk of dyscrasias with phenothiazines and delayed clearance of depots (especially Risperdal Consta®, Janssen-Cilag). Ideally, a previous drug should be completely withdrawn before clozapine is started, including depots (eg. switch 1), but this is not always practical. Clozapine is a very sedative and hypotensive drug, so care is needed with additive effects — start with the usual gradual dose titration but monitor carefully. Warn women about possible normalisation of prolactin and the need for adequate oral contraception if necessary. Pharmacokinetic interactions are unlikely (see 4.2.2).

5b. Switching from clozapine:
Converting clozapine to other antipsychotics seems particularly problematic (n=30, RCT, Shiovitz et al, Schizophr Bull 1996;**22**:591–5). Relapse after clozapine discontinuation seems to be of a higher incidence, may be more rapid (Shore, Schizophr Bull 1995;**21**:333–7) and withdrawal symptoms may be more severe (n=10, open, 12/52, Still et al, Psychiatr Serv 1996;**47**:1382–4) than with other drugs. For gradual discontinuation of clozapine, it is best to simultaneously introduce and escalate the doses of another antipsychotic.

6. Switching to olanzapine:

Additive EPSE, hypotension and drug interactions are unlikely to occur and so switch 3 is usually suitable with care. Due to a lesser effect on prolactin, unexpected (but, in these particular cases, welcome) pregnancies have been reported a couple of months after a switch from typicals to olanzapine, despite no contraceptive use for 4–5 years (n = 2, Neumann and Frasch, *Nervenarzt* 2001;**72**:876–8).

6a. Risperidone to olanzapine:

In a comparison of four different typical/risperidone to olanzapine switches in partially remitted, clinically stable schizophrenic outpatients, the most successful method was starting 10mg olanzapine then gradually discontinuing the original drug. The next most successful was gradual introduction/gradual discontinuation; and probably best for elderly/frail patients. Most dropouts (usually sleep-related) were with abrupt discontinuation (switch 2) and gradual olanzapine introduction (n = 209, 82% completed, open, Kinon et al, J Clin Psychiatry 2000;**61**:833–40).

6b. Depots to olanzapine:

There has been a three-month trial (which may have been of inadequate duration) of switching of clinically stable schizophrenics on depots, either continuing the depot or transferred to olanzapine over 4/52. After 3/12 those transferring to olanzapine were clinically improved and all preferred olanzapine, so a four-week switch is clinically viable (n = 26, RCT, open, 3/12, Godleski et al, J Clin Psychiatry 2003;**64**:119–22).

6c. Clozapine to olanzapine:

An open study of a clozapine to olanzapine switch by patients wishing to avoid blood monitoring, eight of 19 successfully completed the switch (using switch 4) and the others required restabilising on clozapine (n = 19, Henderson et al, J Clin Psychiatry 1998;**59**:585–8). In patients responsive to clozapine but suffering adverse effects, a slow cross-titration over at least two weeks to olanzapine may be successful in about 90% patients (n = 20, open, 24/52, Littrell et al, J Clin Psychiatry 2000;**61**:912–15; Lilly part-funded).

6d. Others to olanzapine:

An open study (one year, with five-year follow-up) showed that in resistant schizophrenia, switching to olanzapine may be successful (n = 25, open, Karagianis et al, Curr Med Res Opin 2003;**6**:47–80), with both a direct switch (2) and tapered switch (3), over 2/52, having equivalent outcomes, both therapeutic (67–74% successful) and for adverse effects (n = 108, RCT, open, 6/52, Lee et al, J Clin Psychiatry 2002;**63**:569–76).

7. Other antipsychotics to oral risperidone:

Hypotension may occur, so gradual dose titration over at least 3/7 (or longer if possible) to 4mg/d is recommended. Additive hypotension with low potency drugs may occur during a switch. A sudden switch (along with gradual withdrawal of anticholinergics) may be successful in about 60% patients, but a more gradual switch and dose escallation is preferable (n = 36, Kirov et al, Acta Psychiatr Scand 1997;**95**:439–43). A review of switching to risperidone recommended reducing the existing antipsychotic dose, then over-lapping risperidone with the existing therapy, rather than making an abrupt switch (Borison et al, Clin Ther 1996;**18**:592–607). Risperidone may be a suitable replacement if introduced before slow clozapine withdrawal, ie. switch 4 (Zimbroff, Am J Psychiatry 1995;**152**:1102).

8. Various to/from Risperdal Consta®

8a. Switching to risperidone long-acting injection (Risperdal Consta):

It is important to understand the release kinetics of Consta before deciding a switch strategy, ie.

| | | | | | TABLE 2.2.3: SUMMARY OF ANTIPSYCHOTIC INJECTIONS |
Drug	Peak (days)	Usual frequency	Main duration	Depot half-life	Time to steady state from first dose
Flupentixol	7–10	2/52	2–4/52	7/7	10–12/52
Fluphenazine	1–2	2–4/52	3–4/52	14/7	6–12/52
Fluspirilene	1–2	1/52	1/52	?	5–6/52
Haloperidol	3–9	4/52	4/52	21–28/7	10–12/52
Pipothiazine	9–10	4/52	4/52	21–28/7	8–12/52
Zuclopenthixol	4–9	2/52	2–4/52	7/7	10–12/52
Risperidone	35	2/52	2–3/52	?	12/52

therapeutic levels are not reached until week 4 (ie. just before the 3rd injection) but only reach optimum in weeks 5–6 (ie. after the 3rd injection). Assessment of the response to oral risperidone is strongly recommended before giving the first injection, then giving oral for 3–4 weeks, or more. Consta may have the best chance of success if the person has been shown to respond to oral risperidone first.

8b. Oral antipsychotics to Risperdal Consta®:

Continue for three weeks after starting Consta, then discontinue step-wise during week 4 (preferably through time-limited prescriptions to avoid polypharmacy).

8c. Typical depot to Risperdal Consta®:

The manufacturers recommend starting Consta one week before the last fortnightly injection, with an oral drug available if the risk of relapse is high. Alternatively, switch on the depot due date, supplementing with oral risperidone for 3–4 weeks.

8d. Oral risperidone to Consta®:

Continue risperidone for three weeks, then gradually discontinue in week 4.

8e. Consta® to others:

The last dose of Consta will finally stop releasing risperidone about six weeks later, so wait until then and introduce the new drug gradually from about day 42.

9. Anything to quetiapine:

Quetiapine has a short receptor half-life so warn women about a possible normalisation of prolactin and the need for adequate oral contraception if necessary.

9a. Phenothiazine to quetiapine:

Switch 3 may be reasonable, but be aware of additional initial postural hypotension, so a slightly slower dose titration or additional monitoring might be prudent.

9b. D2-blocker to quetiapine:

Switch 2 or 3 should be tolerable, as receptor blockade with quetiapine is quite different to that of standard D2-blockers.

9c. Typical depot to quetiapine:

Switch 2 should be tolerable, starting quetiapine when the next depot dose is due.

9d. Aripiprazole to quetiapine:

Quetiapine will not displace aripiprazole from receptors so the onset of quetiapine's action will be dependent upon the rate at which aripiprazole leaves dopamine and serotonin receptors.

9e. Clozapine to quetiapine:

Switches 2, 3 or 4 should be tolerable, depending on the reason for the switch. The two have been used together to help reduce weight gain.

9f. Olanzapine to quetiapine:

Any switch should be acceptable.

9g. Risperidone to quetiapine:

Switch 2 or 3 should be tolerable.

10. D2-blockers to phenothiazines:

Switches 2 or 3 should be considered first.

11. D2-blocker to D2-blocker:

Consider switches 1–3 first, bearing in mind the potential for NMS and additional EPSE.

12. Typical depots

12a. Depot typicals to others:

Stop the depot and introduce the next drug when the next depot dose would have been due, remembering that a slow decay in depot plasma levels may occur so beware of adding the new drug too quickly. Depots are occasionally given more often than strictly necessary.

12b. Typical depot to typical depot:

This is not usually a problem, with a direct switch often possible.

13. Olanzapine to another antipsychotic:

There are no apparent problems with stopping olanzapine suddenly, so any switch should be possible.

14. Risperidone to another antipsychotic:

There are few obvious problems with stopping or switching risperidone (eg. interactions), except the standard potential for NMS, prolactin warning and additive EPS if switching to a phenothiazine or D2-blocker. Switches 2 or 3 should be possible.

15. Quetiapine to another antipsychotic:

There are few obvious problems with stopping or switching quetiapine (except perhaps NMS), so switches 2 or 3 should be OK.

16. Prolactin warning:

Warn women about the possibility of currently raised prolactin (particularly with D2-blockers) causing amenorrhoea, and normalisation of prolactin with the new drug and, if necessary, the need for adequate oral contraception.

17. Amisulpride:

For a general, waffly review on switching to amisulpride, see Peuskens (*Curr Med Res Opin* 2002; **18**[Suppl 3]:S23–S28).

18. Discontinuing antipsychotics:

Withdrawal symptoms (eg. tardive psychosis and dyskinesias) have been reported upon abrupt discontinuation (eg. n = 1, Alphs and Lec, *J Clin Psychiatry* 1991;**52**:346–8) eg. cholinergic, rebound headache, restlessness, diarrhoea, nausea and vomiting (Lieberman, *Psychosomatics* 1981;**22**:253–4). In 1006 schizophrenics withdrawing from antipsychotics abruptly, the risk of relapse reached 25% in 10 weeks and 50% within 30 weeks, with little additional relapse risk up to 3.7 years. With gradual withdrawal, the risk of relapse was lower (n = 1210, retrospective, Viguera et al, *Arch Gen Psychiatry* 1997;**54**:49–55). For a comprehensive and fascinating review of neuroleptic discontinuation syndrome, see Tranter and Healy (*J Psychopharmacol* 1998; **12**:401–6).

2.2.1.3 ANTIPSYCHOTIC DOSE EQUIVALENTS

The antipsychotic dose(s) of each drug within each heading of this section are approximately equivalent to others under the same heading (eg. perphenazine 24 mg/d is equivalent to chlorpromazine 300 mg/d and to flupentixol 60 mg 2/52), based on the references indicated. There is, however, a genuine lack of agreement about antipsychotic equivalents. This is mainly because the four methods of assessing antipsychotic equivalence (clinical studies, non-clinical/receptor binding studies, median effective doses and manufacturer's information) can produce up to a five-fold difference in the equivalents than recommended, particularly true in the case of high-potency antipsychotics. Ranges quoted here are thus unweighted for individual variation and are valid, but imprecise.

For example, antipsychotics (excluding some atypical drugs) displace ligands from dopamine receptors (particularly D2 receptors) at a rate that highly correlates with their antipsychotic potency (eg. Peroutka and Snyder, *Am J Psychiatryiatry* 1980;**137**:1518–22) and so roughly equivalent antipsychotic doses can be calculated. However, some dose relationships, eg. haloperidol, are unlikely to be linear and sedation and anxiety may not be directly related to dopamine blockade (reviewed by Hilton et al, *Psychiatr Bull* 1996;**20**:359–62). High-potency drugs, eg. haloperidol and fluphenazine, have the highest quoted variance, over 1000% in some cases. This may lead to prescribing in higher doses than necessary (Dewan and Koss, *Acta Psychiatr Scand* 1995;**91**:229–32). Additionally,

higher doses of antipsychotics tend to be used to control disruptive behaviour rather than just to control psychotic symptoms (Peralta et al, *Acta Psychiatr Scand* 1994;**90**:354–7).

The third way to assess equivalence is to use median effective doses (ED50) and near maximal effective doses (ED85 to ED95) for the antipsychotics (systematic review and meta-analysis, Davis and Chen, *J Clin Psychopharmacol* 2004;**24**:192–208; review by Woods, *EBMH* 2004;**7**:106).

Median and near maximal daily dose		
Drug	**ED 50**	**ED 85–95**
Oral:		
Chlorpromazine	150 mg	400–450 mg
Fluphenazine	–	< 6.9 mg
Haloperidol	0.5–2 mg	3.5–10 mg
Trifluoperazine	–	10–15 mg/d
Amisulpride	50 mg	200 mg
Aripiprazole	< 1.5	10 mg/d
Clozapine		> 400 mg
Olanzapine	9 mg	> 16 mg
Quetiapine	80–215 mg	150–600 mg
Risperidone	2 mg	4 mg
Sertindole	10 mg	12–20 mg
Depots		
Fluphenazine dec	–	25 mg/fortnight
Risperidone Consta	15 mg/mon	50 mg/mon

Using the percentage of the maximum dose has been proposed as an alternative, but is also imprecise, as maximum doses may not be equivalent, eg. is flupentixol decanoate 400 mg a week really equivalent to 50 mg a week of fluphenazine decanoate? Defined daily doses (DDDs) are an alternative to CPZ equivalents, but don't really match up as they assume optimum doses are being used, which isn't always the case (Rikcken et al, *J Clin Psychopharmacol* 2003;**23**:657–9).

Antipsychotic equivalence is specifically quoted here and the doses are as accurate as data allows but to avoid any confusion you must consider the following:

1. Antipsychotic equivalence should not be confused with sedation, which in some cases,

TABLE 2.2.4: ANTIPSYCHOTIC DOSE EQUIVALENTS

Oral	mg/d (+ range)
Chlorpromazine	100mg (25–50mg IM or 250mg rectally)
Fluphenazine	2mg (1.25–5mg)
Levomepromazine	NK
Pericyazine	24mg
Perphenazine	8mg (7–15mg)
Prochlorperazine	15mg (14–25mg)
Promazine	100mg (50–200mg)
Thioridazine	100mg (75–104mg)
Trifluoperazine	5mg (2–8mg)
Benperidol	2mg
Haloperidol	3mg (1–5mg) or 1.5mg IM/IV for doses up to 20mg
Flupentixol	2mg
Zuclopenthixol	25mg (25–60mg) up to 150mg/d
Pimozide	2mg (25–60mg) up to 150mg/d
Amisulpride	100mg (40–150mg)
Sulpiride	200mg (200–333mg)
Clozapine	100mg (30–150mg)
Olanzapine	NK
Quetiapine	NK
Zotepine	NK
Risperidone	1.5mg (0.5–3mg)
Depot	**mg/week**
Fluphenazine	5–10mg (1–12.5mg)
Pipothiazine	10mg (5–12.5mg)
Haloperidol	15mg (5–25mg)
Flupentixol	10mg (8–20mg)
Zuclopenthixol	100mg (40–100mg)
Fluspirilene	2mg (NE)
Risperidone	12.5mg (25mg/fortnight)

Bioavailability from oral haloperidol is about 50% of IM, with IV approximately equivalent to IM.

Key:

NE = Not fully established

90mg (75–100) = Recommended average dose + ranges quoted in the literature. The wider the range, the greater the uncertainty about the exact equivalent

---

The actual dose of a new drug required =

$$\frac{\text{Current total daily (oral) or weekly (depot) dose of the existing drug}}{\text{Equivalent dose stated for the existing drug in that form}} \times \text{equivalent dose of the new drug as stated in that table}$$

eg. haloperidol (with a relatively low sedative effect) causes confusion over equivalence. Indeed, there may be no extra antipsychotic effect from haloperidol above 8–12 mg/d (see 1.10.4).

2. With some drugs there may not be a linear relationship between the dose and antipsychotic effect.

3. Dose frequency with depots may be important as the first pass effect may reduce the effective doses of oral preparations.

4. If using a 'broad-spectrum' drug (eg. the so-called 'dirty' drugs, such as chlorpromazine) and converting to a D2 receptor selective drug (eg. flupentixol, sulpiride, etc), the use of conversion tables may not thus be appropriate and may result in enhanced side-effects or over-dosage.

5. Differing half-lives may complicate the calculations and final dose recommendation.

6. Haloperidol and fluphenazine seems a particular problem.

7. These equivalent doses are not necessarily equivalent in terms of maximum doses.

8. For 'atypicals', therapeutic doses are better defined and so no equivalent doses are appropriate. You should always check your answer against the SPC to ensure an inappropriately high dose is not inadvertently considered (review, Atkins et al, Psychiatr Bull 1997;**21**:224–6).

Reviews: general (Peroutka and Synder, Am J Psychiatry 1980;**137**:1518–22; Anon, Am J Psychiatry 1990;**147**:258–60 + refs; Remington et al, Am J Psychiatry 1998;**155**:1301–2; Dewan and Koss, Acta Psychiatr Scand 1995;**91**:229–32 (excellent review); Schwartz and Brotman, Drugs 1992;**44**:981–92; Hilton et al, Psychiatr Bull 1996; **0**:359–62).

2.2.1.4 POST-SWITCHING ANTIPSYCHOTIC ISSUES

(Based on an extensive review by Weiden et al, J Clin Psychiatry 1998;**59**[Suppl 19]:36–49.)

Assessing response:

1. For all drugs, aim for a minimum of three months at full therapeutic dosage.

2. Be cautious of any significant gains (eg. reduced side-effects) within 6/52 of the last drug stopping, as drug concentrations at receptor level may outlast plasma levels (see haloperidol, 1.27).

3. Even if gains occur, make sure a full therapeutic trial is achieved, as discontinuation of the previous drug will lead to a gradual loss of its side-effects (including cognitive impairment), which may be interpreted as improvement.

4. If gains occur, it has been suggested to delay discontinuing any anticholinergic and/or antiakathisia drugs until during the second month.

5. Raised prolactin levels may take over 3/12 to resolve, so women need to be warned about this, and to ensure they have adequate contraceptive cover.

6. If positive changes occur, the patient should be cautioned not to risk relapse by 'over-doing it'.

Managing a sub-optimum response to a switch:

1. No improvement by 6/52 — exclude non-compliance with the switch, substance misuse and inadequate dosage. Try to work towards 12/52 at full dose.

2. Some response by 6/52 — don't get too excited, continue to 12/52.

3. Partial response between 6/52 and 12/52 — consider an increase in dose, and try to go for a 6/12 trial.

4. Initial response followed by worsening of positive symptoms — check worsening is not actually improvement (eg. previous positive symptoms hidden by the patient now surfacing), try to restabilise and aim for 12/52 at full dose.

Long-term issues:

1. With improvements in insight, increased psychosocial support and monitoring will be needed to reduce the risk of post-psychotic depression and self-harm.

2.2.2 SWITCHING BENZODIAZEPINES

Switching benzodiazepines may be advantageous for a variety of reasons, eg. to a drug with a different half-life pre-discontinuation. While there is broad agreement in the literature about equivalent doses, clonazepam has a wide variety of reported equivalences and particular care is needed with this drug. Inter-patient variability and differing half-lives means the figures can never be exact and should be interpreted using your own pharmaceutical knowledge.

be the same as those necessary to prevent withdrawal symptoms.

References:

Br J Pharm Pract 1989;11:106–10

Murphy and Tyrer, Br J Psychiatry 1991;158:511–6

Bezchlibnyk-Butler et al, Clinical Handbook of Psychotropic Drugs. 4th edn. Hogrefe and Huber, Toronto

Cowen, Adv Psychiatr Treat 1997;3:67

TABLE 2.2.5: BENZODIAZEPINE EQUIVALENT DOSES

See note in introduction regarding half lives

Diazepam	5 mg (oral, im, or iv)
Alprazolam	0.5 mg
Bromazepam	3 mg
Chlordiazepoxide	15 mg (10–25 mg)
Clobazam	10 mg
Clonazepam	0.5 mg (0.25–4)
Clorazepate	7.5 mg (7.5–10)
Flunitrazepam	0.5 mg
Flurazepam	7.5–15 mg
Loprazolam	0.5–1 mg
Lorazepam	0.5–1 mg at 4 mg/d
	2 mg at 5 mg/d
Lormetazepam	0.5–1 mg
Nitrazepam	5 mg (2.5–20 mg)
Oxazepam	15 mg (15–40 mg)
Temazepam	10 mg

2.2.3 SWITCHING ANTICHOLINERGICS

See 6.5 about the overall indications for the use of anticholinergics. Equivalent doses are:

Benzatropine	1 mg
Biperiden	2 mg
Orphenadrine	50 mg
Procyclidine	2 mg
Trihexyphenidyl (benzhexol)	2 mg

(Saklad, personal communication)

2.2.4 SWITCHING DRUGS OF ABUSE OR DEPENDENCE

Switching drugs of abuse/dependence, usually to methadone, is a common treatment strategy. The following table may be of some use, although caution is obviously necessary regarding, eg. the potency of individual amples of street drugs etc. Many dose equivalents are also derived from analgesic equivalents, which may not necessarily

TABLE 2.2.6: METHADONE EQUIVALENT DOSES

Narcotics		
Drug	Quantity	Methadone
Actified compound	100 mg	6 mg
Buprenorphine	0.3 mg	2.5 mg
Codeine linctus	100 ml	20 mg
Codeine phosphate	15 mg	1 mg
Diamorphine BP	10 mg	10 mg
Diamorphine inj[4]	5 mg	10 mg
Diconal	1 tablet	5 mg
Dihydrocodeine	30 mg	2.5 mg
Dr Collis Brown	100 ml	10 mg
Gee's linctus	100 ml	10 mg
Morphine inj	10 mg	10 mg
Morphine oral	15 mg	10 mg
MST tablets	10 mg	3.25 mg
Palfium	5 mg	5–10 mg
Pentazocine	25 mg	2 mg
Pethidine tabs/inj	50 mg	5 mg
Street heroin	¼ g*	20 mg
Street morphine	¼ g*	15 mg

* This is obviously highly variable depending upon its purity

2.2.5 SWITCHING OR DISCONTINUING ANTIDEPRESSANTS

Switching from one antidepressant to another, either for reasons of side-effects, safety or lack of efficacy, can be problematical and present unexpected problems for the unwary. It is often necessary to leave gaps of drug-free days, eg. the 14-day gap after stopping an MAOI before starting another antidepressant is well known. However, other problems may occur and clinicians must be aware of these to avoid unnecessary adverse events.

Factors that must be considered before choosing a switch regimen:

- Speed at which the switch is needed, eg. with less urgency a more cautious regimen can be used. Since many drugs are used in combination, faster switches can obviously be made, but additional monitoring is recommended.
- Current dose of the first drug.
- Individual drugs and their effects, neurotransmitter effects, kinetics, etc.
- Individuals susceptibility to (additive) side-effects.

Potential problems:

- Cholinergic rebound, eg. headache, restlessness, diarrhoea, nausea and vomiting (Lieberman, *Psychosomatics* 1981;**22**:253–54) from withdrawal of drugs blocking cholinergic receptors, eg. tricyclics.
- Antidepressant withdrawal or discontinuation symptoms (see 13)
- Serotonin syndrome, for drugs affecting serotonin (see 6.7).
- Interaction between the two drugs, eg. altered drug levels from altered metabolism (see 4.3).
- Discontinuation effects from the first drug being interpreted as side-effects of the second.

Switching drugs 'with care' means:

- Drop and stop first drug.
- Leave a gap of a few days if possible.
- Warn the patient about potential complications and what to do about them, eg. serotonin syndrome, cholinergic rebound, toxicity and discontinuation.

I. MAOI–MAOI

A two-week gap is recommended, especially if the MAOI is changed to tranylcypromine. The literature for tranylcypromine recommends leaving at least a seven-day gap after stopping other antidepressants, then starting tranylcypromine at half the usual dosage for one week. Careful observation is essential. An open study of switching MAOIs with less than a 14-day gap showed that only one patient suffered adverse events, indicative of either

How to use *Table 2.2.7*:

i. Look down the vertical column headed 'from' and find the drug, or drug group, the patient is currently taking.

ii. Follow that line along until you come to the column of the drug, or drug group to which you wish to change.

iii. The details there give the current known information. For further details look up the reference number quoted.

Example: Changing from tranylcypromine to a tricyclic requires a 14-day drug-free gap (reference 9), but changing from a tricyclic to tranylcypromine only requires a seven-day drug-free gap (reference 9).

tranylcypromine withdrawal or a mild serotonin syndrome. A shorter gap may be feasible with full dietary control, good compliance and close monitoring (n=8, Szuba *et al*, *J Clin Psychiatry* 1997;**58**:307–10). However, since deaths have been reported with such a switch (eg. n=1, Bazire, *Drug Intell Clin Pharm* 1986;**20**:954–56), caution is recommended.

2. SSRI–TCA

Fluoxetine, paroxetine and fluvoxamine (but probably not citalopram, escitalopram and sertraline at standard doses) can double or triple tricyclic levels (particularly of amitriptyline, imipramine, nortriptyline and clomipramine), by CYP2D6 inhibition and so great care is needed. Prescribing both drugs together over a change-over period is not advised unless the drugs and doses are chosen carefully and specific care is taken.

Ideally, 'drop-and-stop' before starting the next drug is recommended.

Factors to be considered with an SSRI-tricyclic switch:

- Speed at which the switch is needed, eg. faster switches can obviously be made, but additional monitoring, eg. tricyclic levels and cardiac status is recommended.

TABLE 2.2.7: SWITCHING ANTIDEPRESSANTS

NSPR=No significant problems reported, careful cross-taper; OP=Occasional problems; SSP=Serotonin syndrome possible

In the header: **To** drugs are grouped as MAOIs (Hydrazines, Tranylcypromine) and SSRIs (Citalopram/escitalopram, Fluvoxamine, Fluoxetine, Sertraline, Paroxetine). ■ = not applicable (same drug). Duloxetine[1], Bupropion[10], Moclobemide[10].

From ↓ \ To →	Hydrazines	Tranylcypromine	Tricyclics	Citalopram/ escitalopram	Fluvoxamine	Fluoxetine	Sertraline	Paroxetine	Trazodone	Bupropion	Moclobemide	Venlafaxine	Duloxetine	Mirtazapine	Mianserin	Reboxetine
Hydrazines	■	■	7-14/7[9]	14/7[1]	14/7[1]	14/7[1]	14/7[1]	14/7[1]	14/7[10] or care	7/7[10]	7/7[7] with care	14/7[16]	14/7[6]	2/52[7]	14/7[1]	2/52[7]
Tranylcypromine	■	■	14/7[9]	14/7[1]	14/7[1]	14/7[1]	14/7[1]	14/7[1]	14/7[10]	7/7[10]	7/7[1,9] with care	14/7[16]	14/7[6]	2/52[7]	14/7[1]	2/52[7]
Tricyclics	NSPR[4]	Care[2]	■	Care[2]	Great care[2]	Great care[2]	Care[2]	Great care[2]	NSPR[10]	NSPR[2]	NSPR[15]	Variable[6]	SSP[6]	NSPR[12]	NSPR	NSPR[17]
Citalopram/ escitalopram	7/7[7]	7/7[7]	Care[2]	■	SSP[5]	SSP[5]	SSP[5]	SSP[5]	Care[3,6]	NSPR[10]	7/7[14]	Care[6]	SSP[6]	NSPR[12]	NSPR	NSPR[17]
Fluvoxamine	7/7[7]	7/7[7]	Great care[2]	SSP[5]	■	2/52[8]	SSP[5]	SSP[5]	Care[3,6]	NSPR[10]	4-5/7[14]	Care[6]	SSP[6]	NSPR[12]	NSPR	NSPR[17]
Fluoxetine	5/52[7]	5/52[7]	Great care for 28/7[7]	SSP[5]	SSP[5]	■	SSP[5]	SSP[5]	Care[6]	NSPR[10]	4-5/7[14]	Care[6]	Care SSP[6]	NSPR[12]	NSPR	NSPR[14]
Sertraline	7/7[7]	7/7[7]	Care[2]	SSP[5]	SSP[5]	SSP[5]	■	SSP[5]	Care[3,6]	NSPR[10]	4-13/7[14]	Care[6]	SSP[6]	NSPR[12]	NSPR	NSPR[17]
Paroxetine	14/7[7]	14/7[7]	Great care[2]	SSP[5]	SSP[5]	SSP[5]	SSP[5]	■	Care[3,6]	NSPR[10]	4-5/7[14]	Care[6]	SSP[6]	NSPR[12]	NSPR	NSPR[17]
Trazodone	7/7[6,7]	7/7[6,7]	OP[13]	Care[3,6]	Care[3,6]	Care[6]	Care[3,6]	Care[3,6]	■	NSPR	NSPR[6,8]	Care[6]	SSP[6]	NSPR[12]	NSPR	NSPR[17]
Bupropion[10]	7/7[10]	7/7[10]	Care	NSPR[10]	NSPR[8]	NSPR[10]	NSPR[10]	NSPR[10]	NSPR	■	NSPR	NSPR	SSP[6]	NSPR[12]	NSPR	NSPR[17]
Moclobemide[10]	NSPR[7]	NSPR[7]	OP[15]	NSPR[8]	NSPR[8]	NSPR[8]	NSPR[8]	NSPR[8]	NSPR[6,8]	NSPR	■	NSPR	SSP[6]	NSPR[12]	NSPR	NSPR[17]
Venlafaxine	7/7[16]	7/7[16]	NSPR[16]	NSPR[8]	NSPR[8]	NSPR[10]	NSPR[8]	NSPR[10]	NSPR	NSPR	NSPR[16]	■	SSP[6]	NSPR[12]	NSPR	NSPR[17]
Duloxetine	5/7[6]	5/7[6]	SSP[5]	SSP[5] care	SSP[5]	SSP[5]	SSP[5]	SSP[5]	SSP[5]	SSP[5]	SSP[5]	SSP[5]	■	NSPR	NSPR	NSPR[17]
Mirtazapine	7/7[7]	7/7[7]	NSPR[12]	NSPR[12]	NSPR[12]	NSPR[12]	NSPR[12]	NSPR[12]	NSPR[12]	NSPR[12]	NSPR[16]	NSPR[12]	NSPR	■	NSPR[12]	NSPR[17]
Mianserin	14/7[1]	14/7[1]	NSPR	NSPR	NSPR	NSPR	NSPR	NSPR	NSPR	NSPR	NSPR[16]	NSPR	NSPR	NSPR[12]	■	NSPR[17]
Reboxetine	1/52[7]	1/52[7]	NSPR[17]	NSPR[17]	NSPR[17]	NSPR[17]	NSPR[17]	NSPR[17]	NSPR[17]	NSPR[17]	NSPR[17]	NSPR[17]	NSPR[17]	NSPR[17]	NSPR[17]	■
Just plain stopping[17]	Over 4/52[17]	Over 4/52[17]	Over 4/52[17]	Over 4/52[17]	Over 4/52[17]	Reduce to 20mg/d then stop	Over 4/52[17]	Over 4/52[17] or longer	Over 4/52[17]	Over 4/52[17]	Over 4/52[17]	Over 4/52[17] or longer	Over 4/52[17] or longer	Over 4/52[17]	Over 4/52[17]	Over 4/52[17]

- SSRI dose — CYP2D6 inhibition is dose-related for most drugs, eg. paroxetine, fluoxetine.
- Tricyclic — stronger serotonin reuptake inhibitors are more likely to produce serotonin syndrome (eg. clomipramine), and tertiary tricyclics (eg. imipramine, amitriptyline, clomipramine) are also metabolised by CYP3A3/4 and CYP1A2, which are inhibited by fluvoxamine.
- P450 status of the patient ie slow or rapid metaboliser (see 4.2).
- Individual susceptibility to tricyclic and SSRI side-effects.

Main potential problems (see introduction for more details):
- Cholinergic rebound.
- Tricyclic/SSRI discontinuation symptoms (see reference 13).
- Serotonin syndrome (see 6.7).
- Increased tricyclic levels via CYP2D6 inhibition by SSRIs (see 4.3.1).

Suggested switch regimens:

Tricyclic to fluoxetine, paroxetine or fluvoxamine: Taper tricyclic dose to around 25–50mg/d, start SSRI at usual starting dose and discontinue tricyclic over next 5–7 days, with careful observation.

Main potential problems (see above for details): Serotonin syndrome, raised tricyclic levels by P450 inhibition, cholinergic rebound or tricyclic withdrawal.

Tricyclic to citalopram, escitalopram or sertraline: Taper tricyclic as above, but there is a much lower potential for interactions so problems are less likely. A serotonin syndrome has been reported with sertraline and amitriptyline (Alderman et al, Ann Pharmacother 1996; **30**:1499–500).

Fluoxetine to tricyclic: Stop fluoxetine, wait several days for peak levels to fall, then add the tricyclic **cautiously at low dose** and build up slowly. Care is needed for up to four weeks as the interaction potential via 2D6 inhibition may be prolonged (see 4.3.2). An abrupt switch from fluoxetine 20mg/d to amitriptyline 50–100mg/d resulted in 14% dropping out due to adverse reactions, the rest tolerating the switch (Rutten et al, MI).

Main potential problems (see above for details): Serotonin syndrome (especially with drugs such

as clomipramine) and higher tricyclic levels via CYP2D6 inhibition.

Paroxetine to tricyclic: Leave a gap if possible or taper paroxetine dose to about 10mg/d, and introduce the tricyclic at low dose. After several days, discontinue paroxetine and increase tricyclic dose to therapeutic levels.

Main potential problems (see above for details): Paroxetine withdrawal (see reference 17), serotonin syndrome (especially with drugs such as clomipramine) and higher tricyclic levels via CYP2D6 inhibition.

Fluvoxamine to tricyclic: As paroxetine.

Main potential problems (see above for details): Fluvoxamine withdrawal (rare, see reference 17), serotonin syndrome (especially with drugs such as clomipramine) and higher tricyclic levels via CYP1A2 and 3A3/4 inhibition (especially with tertiary tricyclics).

Citalopram, escitalopram or sertraline to tricyclic: If necessary, reduce to minimum doses of citalopram (20mg/d), escitalopram (10mg) or sertraline (50mg/d). Stop the SSRI and introduce the tricyclic, titrating dose upwards as tolerated. With standard doses of these SSRIs, few problems should be seen.

Main potential problems (see above for details): SSRI withdrawal (rare, see reference 17), serotonin syndrome (especially with eg. clomipramine) and higher tricyclic levels via CYP2D6 inhibition (low risk).

3. Trazodone–others

Trazodone and **fluoxetine** have been used together but risks include enhanced sedation (eg. n=8, Nirenberg et al, J Clin Psychiatry 1992;**53**:83), serotonin syndrome (n=1, George and Godleski, Biol Psychiatry 1996;**39**:384–5) and slightly raised trazodone levels (see 4.3.2.2). A serotonin syndrome with low dose trazodone added to **paroxetine** (n=1, Reeves and Bullen, Psychosomatics 1995;**36**:159–60) would indicate the need for similar care. For **citalopram**, there is a report of lack of a pharmacokinetic interaction, with no changes in plasma levels (n=40+41 controls; Prapotnik et al, Int J Clin Pharmacol Ther 2004;**42**:120–4). There is no information on changing from trazodone to **sertraline** but a gradual switch, with close observation of the patient would seem sensible for all SSRIs. See 5.

4. Tricyclic–tricyclic

No significant problems have been reported but a gradual switch is recommended as per normal practice.

5. SSRI–SSRI

Any combination of SSRIs could precipitate a serotonin syndrome (see 6.7). Thus, careful observation initially and a gentle change over is recommended. A washout period would further minimise the possibility of problems. An example of potential problems has been shown in a report of a 'therapeutic substitution', where outpatients were abruptly swapped from **fluoxetine to sertraline** (20mg:50mg respectively dose substitution). 63% swapped successfully but 37% failed, including 18% with intolerable adverse effects (nervousness, jitters, nausea and headache), suggestive of a serotonin-like syndrome (n=54, Stock and Kofoed, *Am J Hosp Pharm* 1994;**51**:2279–81). One study showed that abrupt switching from **fluoxetine to paroxetine** produced an increased level of side-effects such as insomnia, nausea, dry mouth, nervousness and tremor in the immediate switch group when compared to a two-week washout, which was well-tolerated (n=240, d/b, Kreider et al, *J Clin Psychiatry* 1995;**56**:142–5). However, paroxetine had no effect on the kinetics of fluoxetine and norfluoxetine in another study (n=9, Dominguez et al, *J Clin Psychopharmacol* 1996;**16**:320–3).

6. Duloxetine–others

Duloxetine is relatively new to the UK market. Similar caution to that with venlafaxine should be exercised with duloxetine until more information is available.

7. MAOIs–SSRIs

The time to wait between stopping an SSRI and starting an MAOI depends upon the respective SSRI. The literature for tranylcypromine recommends leaving at least a seven-day gap after stopping other antidepressants, then starting tranylcypromine at half the usual dosage for one week. The literature also recommends a two-week gap from an SSRI before an MAOI is started but this appears only to be strictly correct for paroxetine.

Fluvoxamine to MAOI: fluvoxamine has a short half-life and so isocarboxazid/phenelzine may be started 4–5 days after stopping fluvoxamine (4–5 x half-life) or seven days for tranylcypromine.

Paroxetine to MAOI: two-week gap (MI).

Fluoxetine to MAOI: a serotonin syndrome has been reported when tranylcypromine was started six weeks after fluoxetine was stopped, due to persistence of norfluoxetine (but not fluoxetine) in the blood (letter in *Am J Psychiatry* 1993;**150**:837). Since several reported interactions exist, it might be better to allow six weeks after stopping fluoxetine before starting an MAOI (*Drug Ther Bull* 1990;**28**:334). Some isocarboxazid literature recommends a gap longer than two weeks.

Sertraline to MAOI: a one-week gap should elapse before starting an MAOI. A serotonergic syndrome has been reported with sertraline and tranylcypromine (see SSRI interactions 4.3.2). The manufacturer suggests that a two-week gap between sertraline and MAOI therapies would be prudent.

Trazodone to MAOI: the literature recommends a one-week gap. In one study, combined treatment did not show hypertensive reactions but an increase in side-effect severity, eg. sedation, postural hypotension etc occurred (n=13, Nierenberg and Keck, *J Clin Psychopharmacol* 1989;**9**:42).

Moclobemide to MAOI: moclobemide has a half-life of 14 hours and so stopping moclobemide one day and starting another antidepressant the next day is adequate.

Mirtazapine to MAOI: a one-week wash-out period is recommended by the manufacturers.

MAOI to SSRIs: a two-week gap (*Drug Ther Bull* 1990;**28**:33–4) has been suggested but longer may be safer as a severe serotonin syndrome has been reported with a two-week gap between stopping tranylcypromine and starting fluoxetine (n=1, Ruiz, *Ann Emerg Med* 1994;**24**:983–5), even although tranylcypromine has a relatively short action (ie. reversible MAO inhibition).

MAOI to trazodone: the literature recommends a two-week gap after stopping trazodone before MAOIs (see also trazodone to MAOI above).

MAOI to moclobemide: a gap is not needed

between stopping an MAOI and starting moclobemide, provided MAOI dietary restrictions are maintained for 10–14 days.

MAOI to mirtazapine: a two-week wash-out period is recommended.

8. Moclobemide–SSRIs

Due to a lack of clinical information, the manufacturers of fluoxetine recommend that normal MAOI procedures be observed for moclobemide, and so a two-week gap after stopping moclobemide is stated. This would appear over-cautious and Roche recommended that when changing to an SSRI only an 8–12 hour gap is needed.

9. Tricyclics–MAOIs

These have been used together uneventfully (see 1.14) but have also interacted (see 4.3.4). **MAOIs to tricyclic:** a 10–14-day gap is often recommended (isocarboxazid '1–2 weeks') particularly if imipramine, clomipramine or tranylcypromine are involved. Using initial low doses of the tricyclic is essential.

Tricyclic to MAOI: A one-week gap is recommended and is advisable particularly if imipramine, clomipramine or tranylcypromine are involved. Low doses of the MAOI is essential.

10. Bupropion

Studies in animals demonstrate that the acute toxicity of bupropion is enhanced by the MAOI phenelzine. Bupropion is contraindicated with MAOIs. Coadministration of bupropion with drugs that are metabolised by CYP2D6 (eg. tricyclics, paroxetine and fluoxetine) should be approached with caution and should be initiated at the lower end of the dose range of the concomitant medication. If bupropion is added to the treatment regimen of a patient already receiving a drug metabolised by CYP2D6, the need to decrease the dose of the original medication should be considered, particularly for those with a narrow therapeutic index.

11. Tryptophan–others

Adding tryptophan to therapy is far more common than switching to tryptophan, and so behavioural and neurological toxicity has been reported with concomitant high dose tryptophan and MAOIs and so initial observation and care would seem advisable. With SSRIs, cases of central toxicity, agitation and nausea have occurred with the combination and are suggested as likely to occur with all SSRIs, and the possibility of a serotonergic syndrome developing considered.

12. Mirtazapine–others

Mirtazapine has multiple routes of metabolism (CYP2D6, 3A4 and 1A2) so switching problems will be unlikely in terms of P450 inhibition. The only recommendation is for MAOIs (see 7). Fluoxetine 20–40 mg/d has been switched abruptly to mirtazapine 15 mg/d, without problems (n = 40, Preskorn et al, Biol Psychiatry 1997;**41**:96S), although serotonin syndrome has been reported during a cross-over switch to venlafaxine (n = 1, Dimellis, World J Biol Psychiatry 2002;**3**:167).

13. Trazodone–tricyclics

There are two isolated cases of hypomania after an abrupt change from trazodone to imipramine (n = 2, Haggerty and Jackson, J Clin Psychiatry 1985;**5**:342–3) so care is needed with the switch.

14. SSRIs–moclobemide/others

The literature recommends a gap of 4–5 half-lives after stopping an SSRI before starting moclobemide, as serotonin syndromes have been reported (see 4.3.3.3). However, in a study where up to 600 mg/d moclobemide was added to established fluoxetine therapy, there was no change in the number, intensity, or type of adverse events. Fluoxetine markedly inhibited the metabolism of moclobemide but did not lead to excessive accumulation, and there was no evidence of the development of a 'serotonin syndrome' (n = 18, RCT, p/c, Dingemanse et al, Clin Pharmacol Ther 1998;**63**:403–13).

Citalopram/escitalopram to moclobemide: a seven-day gap is recommended.

Fluoxetine to moclobemide: with fluoxetine's long half-life, the gap should be as much as six weeks if five times the half-life of norfluoxetine is calculated. A gap of three weeks together with careful monitoring would seem a reasonably practical figure. See also above, where no clinically significant problem was apparent and a shorter gap may be appropriate.

Fluvoxamine to moclobemide: a three-day gap is recommended (but see above).

Paroxetine to moclobemide: a five-day gap is recommended (but see above), although paroxetine's half-life can be longer in the elderly.

Sertraline to moclobemide: with the long half-life of desmethylsertraline, the gap should be up to 13 days, but five and seven days is recommended by Roche and Pfizer respectively (but see above).

Fluoxetine to bupropion: in fluoxetine non-responders, a switch to bupropion yielded 35% responders and 25% partial responders (n = 29, 12 + 8/52, open, Fava et al, Ann Clin Psychiatry 2003;**15**:17–22).

Fluoxetine to reboxetine: in fluoxetine non-responders, abrupt switch to reboxetine was well-tolerated (n = 128, open, Fava et al, J Clin Psychopharmacol 2003;**23**:365–9).

15. Tricyclics–moclobemide

Tricyclic to moclobemide: a gap is recommended if the tricyclic concerned is a 5-HT reuptake inhibitor. Roche only mention clomipramine needing a seven-day gap (study by Laux et al, Psychopharmacology Berlin 1988;**96**[Suppl]:230) although theoretically amitriptyline (five-day gap) and imipramine (four-day gap) might be included as well. However, healthy volunteers taking either clomipramine 100mg/d or amitriptyline 75mg/d for at least a week, were swapped abruptly to moclobemide (150mg first day, 300mg/d thereafter) or placebo. There was no increase in incidence or severity of side-effects nor any significant pharmacokinetic interaction between the drugs (n = 24, d/b, p/c, Dingemanse et al, J Clin Psychopharmacol 1995;**15**:41–48).

Moclobemide to tricyclic: abrupt switching from moclobemide to tricyclics appears well-tolerated (n = 13, open, Becker et al, Psychiatr Prax 1989;**16**[Suppl 1]:S44–S47) but switching to clomipramine may cause some problems (open, Luax et al, Psychopharmacology 1988;Suppl **96**: S230).

16. Venlafaxine–others

MAOI to venlafaxine: Wyeth recommend a 14-day gap between stopping an MAOI and starting venlafaxine. This is appropriate as there are a number of reports of interactions, eg. extreme agitation, diaphoresis, rapid respiration and raised CPK, eg. after a 37.5mg dose of venlafaxine seven days after phenelzine 45mg/d was stopped (Phillips and Ringo, Am J Psychiatry 1995;**15**:1400–1) and serotonin syndrome (eg. n = 4, Diamond et al, Neurology 1998;**51**:274–6). In the first reported case, the reaction did not occur a further seven days later and strongly suggests that a 14-day gap is indeed required.

Venlafaxine to MAOI: the manufacturers recommend a seven-day gap (see above).

Tricyclic to venlafaxine: five times the tricyclic's half-life should be allowed as a wash-out time before starting venlafaxine (MI). For some tricyclics this would require leaving a 2–3-week gap, an unnecessarily extended period. Wyeth, however, have no evidence of any problems.

Venlafaxine to other drugs: no information.

Other drugs to venlafaxine: no information.

17. Withdrawal or discontinuation

Adverse discontinuation events have been reported for many antidepressants. Such symptoms are not, however, indicative of dependence, which usually requires three of the following:

- tolerance
- withdrawal symptoms
- use greater than needed
- inability to reduce doses
- excessive time taken procuring drug
- primacy of drug taking over other activities
- continued use despite understanding of adverse effects.

Discontinuation symptoms have a number of characteristics, eg. they usually start within 1–2 days of stopping and resolve within 24 hours of restarting the drug, and are more common with longer courses or higher doses. They can occur with missed doses and about 30% of patients on SSRIs have dosing lapses of two or more days, long enough to produce discontinuation symptoms in patients on some short-acting SSRIs (n = 82, 3/12, Meijer et al, Br J Psychiatry 2001;**179**:519–22), but not fluoxetine (Curr Prob

2000;**26**:11–12). The *UK Drug and Therapeutics Bulletin* (1999;**37**:49–52) recommends:
- after less than eight weeks treatment, withdraw over 1–2 weeks
- after 6–8 months treatment, taper over a 6–8-week period
- after long-term maintenance treatment, reduce the dose by 25% every 4–6 weeks.

Options for the management of antidepressant withdrawal symptoms include:
1. Reduce the dose stepwise every week or so, stabilising between reductions, eg. paroxetine 20 mg/d, 10 mg/d, then 10 mg alternate days (but not less frequently). Use of the syrup, gradually diluted, may also be effective.
2. Transfer to a long half-life drug, eg. fluoxetine (care with switching), then reduce (clomipramine case, Benazzi, *Am J Psychiatry* 1999 **156**:661–2; venlafaxine case, Giakas and David, *Psychiatr Ann* 1997;**27**:85–92).
3. Treat the emerging syndrome symptomatically, eg. nausea, headache and diarrhoea have been managed with ondansetron (n=1, Raby, *J Clin Psychiatry* 1998;**59**:621–2) and ginger root (Schechter, *J Clin Psychiatry* 1998;**59**:431–2).

Reviews: recognition, prevention and management of antidepressant withdrawal syndromes (Haddad, *Drug Safety* 2001;**24**:183–97), general (Haddad, *J Clin Psychiatry* 1998;**59**:541–8; Healy, *Prescriber* 2002;**13**:91–9).

Main withdrawal symptoms

Tricyclics: cholinergic rebound, eg. headache, restlessness, diarrhoea, nausea and vomiting (Lieberman, *Psychosomatics* 1981;**22**:253–4), flu-like symptoms, lethargy, abdominal cramps, sleep disturbance and movement disorders.

MAOIs: psychosis, hallucinations, disorientation, catatonia (n=2, Liskin et al, *J Clin Psychopharmacol* 1985;**5**:46–7), irritability, hypomania (Rothchild, *J Clin Psychopharmacol* 1985;**5**:340–1), nausea, sweating, palpitations, nightmares and delirium (Liebowitz et al, *Am J Psychiatry* 1978;**135**:1565–6).

SSRIs: dizziness, vertigo/lightheadedness, nausea, fatigue, headache, sensory disturbance, 'electric shocks' in the head, insomnia, abdominal cramps, chills, flu-like symptoms, increased dreaming, anxiety/agitation and volatility, but not caused by anything else, eg. physical illness or other drugs.

Reviews: SSRI withdrawal (Healy, *Prescriber* 2002;**13**:91–9; Zajecka et al, *J Clin Psychiatry* 1997; **58**:291–7).

Specific drugs

Comparative data: There have been a number of comparative studies between SSRIs. Interruption for 5–8 days of maintenance therapy produced few discontinuation symptoms with fluoxetine (long half-life), some with sertraline and most with paroxetine (n=242, RCT, d/b, 4/52, Rosenbaum et al, *Biol Psychiatry* 1998;**44**:77–87; study funded by Lilly). In another study, suddenly discontinuing fluoxetine showed slightly more dizziness and somnolence at weeks 2–4, but no difference at week 6 compared to continuous treatment (n=395, RCT, 12/52, Zajecka et al, *J Clin Psychopharmacol* 1998;**18**:193–97; review, Kendrick, *EBMH* 1999;**2**:31). A third study of a five-day interruption showed increased symptoms after a second missed dose with paroxetine, with impaired functional performance at five days, sertraline with less pronounced changes, and fluoxetine with no significant symptoms (n=107, RCT, Michelson et al, *Br J Psychiatry* 2000;**174**:363–8).

Citalopram: even rapid discontinuation appears only to produce mild and transient effects (n=225, RCT, d/b, 10/52, Markowitz et al, *Int Clin Psychopharmacol* 2000;**15**:329–33).

Escitalopram: see citalopram.

Fluoxetine: fluoxetine has a long half-life and discontinuation problems are rare eg. isolated cases of extreme dizziness 3–14 days after fluoxetine stopped (Einbinder, *Am J Psychiatry* 1995;**152**:1235), of severe, dull, aching pain in the left arm after abrupt withdrawal, which remitted after reintroduction (n=1, Lauterbach, *Neurology* 1994;**44**:983–4) and of reversible delirium (Kasantikul, *J Med Assoc Thailand* 1995;**78**:53–4).

Fluvoxamine: a slow withdrawal may be preferred (Szabadi, *Br J Psychiatry* 1992;**160**:283–4).

Paroxetine: * paroxetine has been associated with more discontinuation reports than other SSRIs. A retrospective chart analysis showed that about 10% people may get a significant discontinuation syndrome, it is more common with rapid withdrawal and is more common in people who got adverse reactions early in treatment (n=385, Himei and Okamura, *CNS Drugs* 2006;**20**:665–72). Case reports include fever, severe fatigue, headache, nausea, vomiting and agitation and electrical shock-like sensations (Frost and Lal, *Am J Psychiatry* 1995;**152**:180). It has presented as stroke (n=2, Haddad *et al*, *J Psychopharmacol* 2001;**15**:139–41) and confused with dosulepin side-effects during a switch (n=1, Haddad and Qureshi, *Acta Psychiatr Scand* 2000;**102**:466–8). This phenomenon may be more frequent because paroxetine has a short half-life (using French Pharmacovigilance database; Trenque *et al*, *Pharmacoepidemiol Drug Safety* 2002;**11**:281–3) and inhibits its own CYP2D6 metabolism. This dissipates much quicker than fluoxetine and sertraline (n=45, RCT, open, Liston *et al*, *J Clin Psychopharmacol* 2002;**22**:169–73) and, as concentrations fall, less inhibition occurs and levels fall quicker, leading to a more rapid drop. Discontinuation symptoms tend to resolve in a few days or on reintroduction of paroxetine. The CSM recommends tapering if withdrawal symptoms occur, ie. stop if problems occur then restart and taper over 12 weeks, with either half-tablet doses or alternate day (but not less frequently) therapy. However, even a four-week gradual dose reduction may not prevent significant symptoms of vertigo, light-headedness and gait instability, so care is needed (n=5, Pacheco *et al*, *Br J Psychiatry*1996;**169**:384).

Sertraline: discontinuation reactions are relatively uncommon, eg. fatigue, cramps, insomnia (which resolved on restarting and where tapering over 14 weeks was successful: Louie *et al*, *Am J Psychiatry* 1994;**151**:450–51), electrical shock-like sensations and postural hypotension (n=1, Amsden and Georgian, *Pharmacotherapy* 1996;**16**:684–6). Abrupt sertraline 100mg/d discontinuation has been enhanced by buspirone 15mg/d (n=1, Carrazana *et al*, *Am J Psychiatry* 2001;**158**:966–7).

Duloxetine: * the UK SPC states that duloxetine should be tapered over no less than two weeks, reduced by half on alternate days. Symptoms of abrupt withdrawal have been reported to occur in 44% people stopping duloxetine (cf 23% for placebo), with dizziness (12%), nausea, headache, paraesthesia, vomiting, irritability and nightmares the most common. Resolution occurred in a week in 65% (s=6, Perahia *et al*, *J Affect Disord* 2005;**89**:207–12). Patients switching from SSRIs or venlafaxine have less nausea when starting than those starting *de novo*; immediate switching may be well-tolerated, although fluoxetine

was surprisingly excluded from this Lilly study and would pose particular problems (n=155, Wohlreich *et al*, *Ann Clin Psychiatry* 2005;**17**:259–68, MS).

Mirtazapine: a withdrawal hypomania has been reported (n=1, MacCall and Callender, *Br J Psychiatry* 1999;**175**:390; see also n=1, Berigan, *Prim Care Companion J Clin Psychiatry* 2001; **3**:143).

Moclobemide: a discontinuation syndrome may present with influenza-like symptoms. Sertraline may not modify the symptoms, suggesting a different mechanism (n=1, Curtin *et al*, *J Psychopharmacol* 2002;**16**:271–2).

Nefazodone: electrical sensations, dizziness and nausea have been reported.

Reboxetine: no withdrawal or discontinuation syndrome has been observed in studies with reboxetine, with few additional effects on abrupt withdrawal.

St. John's wort: a withdrawal syndrome has been reported (Dean *et al*, *Ann Pharmacother* 2003;**37**:150).

Tryptophan: many patients had their tryptophan stopped abruptly after it was withdrawn from the market in UK without apparent serious withdrawal problems, other than recurrence of depression.

Venlafaxine: * If used for more than six weeks, withdrawal over at least a week is recommended by the manufacturers. The UK SPC mentions withdrawal reactions from abrupt cessation, dose reduction or tapering of venlafaxine. This can include fatigue, nausea, vomiting, dizziness, dry mouth, diarrhoea, insomnia, nervousness, confusion, paraesthesia, sweating, vertigo, headache (eg. n=1, Mayr and Bonelli, *Ann Pharmacother* 2003;**37**:1145–6), electric shock-like symptoms (eg. n=2, Reeves *et al*, *Pharmacother* 2003; **23**:678–81) and mania (n=1, Fava and Mangelli, *Int J Neuropsychopharmacol* 2003;**6**:89–90). Other symptoms include abdominal distension and congested sinuses (n=1, resolving within 12 hours of restarting, Farah and Lauer, *Am J Psychiatry* 1996;**153**:576), gastrointestinal upset (which responded to reintroduction and then slow reduction over 1–4 weeks, n=3, Louie *et al*, *Am J Psychiatry* 1996;**153**:1652) and classic SSRI-type discontinuation symptoms (eg. confusion, headache, agitation, abdominal distension and sweating) occurring 16 and 20 hours after stopping (n = 2, Agelink et al, Am J Psychiatry 1997;**154**:1473–4; review of similarity to SSRI symptoms, n = 13, Boyd, Med J Aus 1998;**169**:91–2). Discontinuation effects may also adversely effect driving abilities (Campagne, Med Gen Med 2005;**7**:22). An outpatient study showed that seven of the nine patients discontinuing sustained-release venlafaxine reported the emergence of adverse reactions, compared to two of the nine stopping placebo (n = 9, d/b, p/c, Fava et al, Am J Psychiatry 1997;**154**:1760–2). It may not prevented by maprotiline, but resolved by sertraline (n = 1, Luckhaus and Jacob, Int J Neuropsychopharmacol 2001;**4**:43–4).

2.3 WEIGHT CHANGES WITH PSYCHOTROPIC DRUGS

Importance

Drug-induced weight gain is a potential threat to health, lowers self-esteem and the social embarrassment caused may lead to non-concordance (and hence risks relapse). Patients may become easily out-of-breath, have to spend money on new clothes (when already short of money), get embarrassed and often won't go out as a consequence. It's great to be as welcoming as the Angel of the North but being the same size rather takes the edge off it.

The available data is difficult to compare due to the non-equivalence of collection and presentation. Some body weight gain is common with many psychotropic drugs and, although in most instances the gain is not 'clinically' significant (although it may be significant to the individual), the gain induced by some drugs, such as lithium and atypical antipsychotics, can be clinically significant. Risk factors for weight increase have not yet been well characterised, although in general it is greatest in individuals with a past and/or family history of obesity (Ackerman and Nolan, CNS Drugs 1998;**9**:135–51, 96 refs), co-morbid binge-eating, a greater number of depressive episodes, treatment with medications associated with weight gain and low exercise (Keck and McElroy, J Clin Psychiatry 2004;**64**:1426–35). The FDA definition of 'clinically significant' weight gain is 7% or greater increase over baseline weight.

A review of the relationship between mood disorders and obesity (McElroy et al, J Clin Psychiatry 2004;**65**:634–51) concludes:

- children and adolescents with MDD may be at increased risk of being overweight
- bipolars have elevated rates of overweight and obesity
- obese people seeking weight loss treatments have a greater incidence of depression
- atypical depression is more associated with weight gain than typical depression
- obesity is associated with depression in females
- most overweight people in the community do not have mood disorders.

There is, thus, an overlap between mood disorders and obesity, but it may be coincidental.

Reviews: general (Schwartz et al, Obes Rev 2004;**5**:115–21), treatment options (Schwartz et al, Obes Rev 2004;**5**:233–8), aetiology (Virks et al, Obes Rev 2004;**5**:167–70), mechanisms (Zimmermann et al, J Psychiatr Res 2003;**37**:193–220).

2.3.1 ANTIPSYCHOTICS *

Table 2.3.1 provides an active comparison between drugs, but does not include all antipsychotics.

Most weight is gained during the first 12–16 weeks of therapy, although it can still continue for six months and can be maintained for at least two years. It can also be more marked during in-patient stays, perhaps due to lower physical activity. A large US survey (schizophrenics n = 570, non-schizophrenic comparators n = 97819) showed male schizophrenics to be as obese as the general population, but female schizophrenics to be as, or more obese than the general population, suggesting that weight gain is a significant problem particularly for females taking antipsychotics (Allison et al, J Clin Psychiatry 1999;**60**:215–20). Initial antipsychotic response to clozapine and lower BMI were associated with subsequented long-term weight gain as measured over eight years (n = 96 [c = 55], retrospective, Bai et al, Am J Psychiatry 2006;**163**:1276–9). Regular dietician visits, self-directed diet and weight loss as a treatment goal are the most effective strategies for reduction of antipsychotic-induced weight gain (n = 53, O'Keefe et al, Am J Psychiatry 2003;**64**:907–12).

Reviews: general (Russell and Mackell, CNS Drugs 2001;**15**:537–51; Allison et al, Am J Psychiatry 1999;**156**:1686–96), comparative re-

TABLE 2.3.1: RELATIVE WEIGHT GAIN WITH ANTIPSYCHOTICS

Drug	Long-term change †	Range (95% CI)	Change at 10/52 ‡
Perphenazine	5.8	0.4–11.1	–
Clozapine	5.7	4.3–7	4 (2.7–5.3)
Chlorpromazine	4.2	2.9–5.4	2.1 (0.9–3.4)
Olanzapine	4.2	3.7–4.6	3.5 (3.3–3.7)
Sertindole	2.9	2.7–3.2	3 (1.8–5.2)
Thioridazine	2.8	1.6–4	3.4 (1.8–5.2)
Quetiapine	2.5	< 1.5–3.5	(0?)
Risperidone	1.7	1.4–2	2 (1.6–2.4)
Fluphenazine	1.1	0.1–2.2	0.4 (-0.7–1.5)
Non-drug controls	0.8	0.1–1.6	1.3 (0.8–1.8)
Loxapine	0.7	-2.6–3.9	–
Polypharmacy	0.5	0.2–0.7	1.2 (0.4–2.1)
Haloperidol	0.5	0.2–0.8	0.5 (0.1–1)
Ziprasidone	0.3	-0.3–0.8	0 (-0.5–0.6)
Trifluoperazine	0.3	-0.9–1.5	–
Placebo	-1	-1.8–0.1	0.4 (-1.3–1.5)
Pimozide	-2.7	-9.3–3.9	

(Allison et al, Am J Psychiatry 1999;**156**:1686–96, 96 refs, review by Fenton, EBMH 2000;**3**:58; n = 427, Brecher et al, In J Psychiatr Clin Pract 2000;**4**:287–91)
† longer-term weight change in kg (random effects mode)
‡ weight change at 10 weeks (fixed effects mode)
Please bear in mind that this is aggregated date, so is subject to error, weight was often measured at a different time and there may be a dose-relationship and a huge inter-individual variation.

view (Wetterling, Drug Safety 2001;**24**:59–73, 93 refs), atypicals and weight gain (Nasrallah, Psychoneuroendocrinology 2003;**28**[Suppl 1]:S83–S96).

Management
See Chapter 6.

2.3.2 ANTIDEPRESSANTS

Weight change in depression is well known and weight loss or gain can be part of the presenting symptoms. Although weight gain with antidepressants may be the reversal of a pre-treatment weight loss in some people (although heavier people are more likely to gain weight if they become depressed; n = 68, Psychiatr Res 1991;**38**:197–200), the main cause with tricyclics seems to be a decreased metabolic rate (Fernstein et al, Biol Psychiatry 1985;**20**:688–92),

a lesser known but important and relevant effect. There is also an association with tricyclics that have strong antihistaminic actions. Pooled data shows that more obese patients tend to lose more weight and that weight loss is directly proportional to baseline weight. Underweight people may tend to gain weight (review in Clin Pharm 1989;**8**:727–33). Raised TNF-alpha (tumour necrosis factor) cytokinase levels are predictive of weight gain with psychotropics, but leptin isn't with mirtazapine or venlafaxine (n = 20, open, Kraus et al, Pharmacopsychiatry 2002;**35**:220–5).

SSRIs

Overall, there is a tendency with SSRIs for weight loss over the first six weeks, then gradually to regain this over six months, and then many may gain weight over the longer-term (reviewed by

Sussman and Ginsberg, *Psychiatr Ann* 1998;**28**:89–97). In the short-term, SSRIs may increase the metabolic rate, suppress appetite, and increase basal body temperature (n = 20, RCT, p/c, Bross and Hoffer, *Am J Clin Nutrition* 1995;**61**:1020–5). Fluoxetine acute therapy is associated with modest weight loss (n = 839, Michelson et al, *Am J Psychiatry* 1999;**156**:1170–6) and in a trial of obese patients, fluoxetine 60mg/d produced greater weight loss than placebo until 20 weeks, when this tended to wear off and the advantage of fluoxetine over placebo at 52 weeks was not clinically significant (n = 458, RCT, Goldstein et al, *Int J Obesity* 1994;**18**:129–35). Paroxetine has a slight clinically insignificant weight loss potential (*J Psychopharmacol* 1990;**4**:300; n = 71, Christiansen et al, *Acta Psychiatr Scand* 1996;**93**:158–63) although one study showed 30% of 61 patients gained 1–4kg (n = 151, RCT, d/b, 6/52, Ohrberg et al, *Acta Psychiatr Scand* 1992;**86**:437–44). A three-way clinical trial showed significant weight gain over six months with paroxetine, but not sertraline or fluoxetine (n = 284, RCT, 26–32/52, Fava et al, *J Clin Psychiatry* 2000;**61**:863–67). Fluvoxamine causes a non-significant weight loss (*J Psychopharmacol* 1990;**4**:299) at 100–150mg/d over six months (Harris and Ashford, *Br J Clin Res* 1991;**2**:81–8). Sertraline may have a limited weight gain effect. No significant weight changes have been reported with citalopram (Milne and Goa, *Drugs* 1991;**41**:450–77), although carbohydrate craving and weight gain has been reported, particularly early on in treatment (n = 18, Bouwer and Harvey, *Int Clin Psychopharmacol* 1996;**11**:273–8).
Review: general (Fava, *J Clin Psychiatry* 2000;**61** [Suppl 11]:37–41).

Tricyclics

Weight gain with tricyclics is well-documented but is not as well known or appreciated as it should be. The two main causes are drug-induced carbohydrate craving (Paykel, *Br J Psychiatry* 1973;**123**:501–7) and a decreased metabolic rate (Fernstein et al, *Biol Psychiatry* 1985;**20**:688–92), rather than improved mood. Little comparative data is available, but weight gain has been reported with amitriptyline (89% of patients; see also n = 73, Christiansen et al, *Acta Psychiatr Scand* 1996;**93**:158–63) and nortriptyline (67%) in one

of the few comparative studies (Fernstrom and Kupfer, *Psychiatr Res* 1988;**26**:256–71). It has also been reported with almost all tricyclics eg. imipramine (n = 128, Frank et al, *J Affect Disord* 1990;**20**:165–72) and clomipramine (n = 129, RCT, 6/52, Guelfi et al, *Br J Psychiatry* 1992; **160**:519–24).

MAOIs and RIMAs

With the MAOIs, weight gain may be related to reduced blood glucose concentrations stimulating hunger or through central mechanisms. Weight gain is very rare with tranylcypromine and weight loss is more likely (n = 198, retrospective, Rabkin et al, *J Clin Psychopharmacol* 1985;**5**: 2–9). Phenelzine is the most widely implicated (45 reports, including 32 of over 15 lbs added). 15% of 62 patients on moclobemide gained weight, although overall there was a mean 0.1 kg weight loss in all patients (n = 129, RCT, 6/52 Guelfi et al, *Br J Psychiatry* 1992;**160**:519–24).

Other antidepressants *

Venlafaxine is usually associated with weight loss (eg. Anon, *J Clin Psychiatry* 1993;**54**:119–26). Loss of appetite and weight has been reported in the available trials of **duloxetine**. Unusual appetite and weight gain has been reported with **mianserin** (Harris and Harper, *Lancet* 1980;i:590). There are only rare reports of weight changes with **trazodone** (Barnett et al, *J Clin Psychopharmacol* 1985;**5**:161–4), but not with **reboxetine**. Increased appetite and weight gain has been reported in patients treated with **mirtazapine**. One study showed increased appetite but without significant weight changes (n = 90, RCT, p/c, d/b, Claghorn and Lesem, *J Affect Disord* 1995;**34**:165–71) and another showed a slightly higher incidence than with amitriptyline (n = 150, RCT, d/b, p/c, Smith et al, *Psychopharmacol Bull* 1990;**26**:191–6). Overall, the incidence of weight gain with mirtazapine in all trials combined seems to be about 12%, with weight loss in 3% (review of mirtazapine weight-gain mechanisms; n = 14, Laimer et al, *J Clin Psychiatry* 2006;**67**:421–4).

Management of antidepressant-induced weight gain

See *Chapter 6*.

2.3.3 MOOD STABILISERS

There is a high prevalence of obesity in bipolar patients, especially with drug treatment (44% gain > 5 kg), so chose drugs unlikely to worsen this (n = 50, Fagiolini et al, J Clin Psychiatry 2002;**63**:528–33). Many factors are, however, involved, eg. male gender, hypertension, arthritis (n = 644, McElroy et al, J Clin Psychiatry 2002;**63**:207–13) and drug-induced changes in food preference, especially high-energy fluids and carbohydrates, and so dietary advice is essential (n = 89, Elmslie et al, J Clin Psychiatry 2001;**62**:486–91).

Review: weight gain with mood stabilisers (Nemeroff, J Clin Psychiatry 2003;**64**:532–9).

Lithium

Weight gain, the second most common reason for non-compliance, is reported to occur in around 33% people (perhaps up to 65%, n = 70, open, Vendsborg et al, Acta Psychiatr Scand 1976;**53**:139–47), of which 25% are probably obese (review: Sachs and Guille, J Clin Psychiatry 1999;**60** [Suppl 21]:16–9). Weight increase occurs predominantly during the first two years of treatment, more often in people already overweight and may be more common in women than men. Increased thirst has been noted in 89% and strongly correlates with weight gain. Increased hunger/food intake has not been directly shown (J Psychopharmacol 1990;**4**:303) and so the predominant mechanism may be increased intake of high-calorie drinks. Thyroid status should also be assessed, as a possible contributory cause. Lithium also increases insulin secretion, which may lead to more adipose tissue being produced, contributing to BMI gain. Weight gain may positively correlate with increased leptin levels (n = 15, 8/52, Atmaca et al, Neuropsychobiology 2002;**46**:67–9). Lithium-induced weight gain has been disputed by Armong (n = 42, open, Br J Psychiatry 1996;**169**:251–2) in a study that showed no significant weight gain, even if taken with concomitant antipsychotics and antidepressants, a surprising finding. One study showed a non-significant BMI increase, with 27% actually showing a reduced BMI (n = 117, Mathew et al, Acta Psychiatr Scand 1989;**80**:538–40).

Management

Counselling, eg. use plain/low-calorie beverages, along with normal sodium intake, dietary advice

and monitoring, particularly during the first year, may be adequate (general review by Baptista et al, Pharmacopsychiatry 1995;**28**:35–44).

Carbamazepine

Studies have show that 43% may gain some weight (n = 70, Corman et al, Can J Neurol Sci 1997;**24**:240–4) and 8% may gain over 5 kg (n = 490, RCT, p/c, d/b, Mattson et al, NEJM 1992;**327**:765–71). This may be due to increased appetite, and is reversed by discontinuation but not by dieting (n = 4, Lampl et al, Clin Neuropharmacol 1991;**14**:251–5).

Valproate *

Weight gain with valproate is recognised as a common ADR and the literature says that weight gain can be marked and progressive. In a study against lamotrigine, significant weight gain (mean 12 lb) occurred by week 10 and was maintained (n = 68, 32/52, Biton et al, Neurology 2001;**56**:172–7). Insulin resistance/hyperinsulinemia may be contributory, but leptin might not be involved independently (n = 81, survey, Pylvanen et al, Epilepsia 2002;**43**:514–7), although higher serum leptin and insulin levels were found in 15 patients becoming obese after one year of valproate, compared to the 25 who did not gain weight (n = 40, Verrotti et al, Neurology 1999;**53**:230–3; n = 20, RCT, 3/12, Demir and Aysun, Pediatr Neurol 2000;**22**:361–4). People who developed obesity with valproate (37%) have raised leptin, ghrelin and adiponectin, hormones involved in regulating balance between energy consumption and expenditure (n = 80, Greco et al, Neurology 2005;**65**:1808–9).

2.3.4 BENZODIAZEPINES

Alprazolam has been reported to cause increased appetite and weight gain in healthy male volunteers (n = 17, Haney et al, Psychopharmacology 1997;**132**:311–14). Weight gain has been reported with clobazam during one study (Ananth et al, Curr Ther Res 1979;**26**:119–26).

2.3.5 ANTICONVULSANTS

Reviews: mechanisms (Jallon and Picard, Drug Saf 2001;**24**:969–78; Biton, CNS Drugs 2003;**17**:781–91).

Gabapentin

In a study of high-dose gabapentin over at least 12 months, 23% patients gained more than 10% of their baseline weight, 15 gained 5% to 10%, 16 had no change and three lost 5% to 10%. Weight was gained in months 2 and 3 and tended to stabilise after 6–9 months, although the doses of gabapentin remained unchanged (n = 44, DeToledo et al, Ther Drug Monit 1997;**19**:394–6). A mean weight gain of 6.9kg (range 3.2–14.5kg) has been noted (n = 11, open, Gidal et al, Ann Pharmacother 1995;**29**:1048).

Lamotrigine

In a study against valproate, weight gain with lamotrigine was low (1.3 +/- 11lb) at week 10 (n = 68, 32/52, Biton et al, Neurology 2001;**56**:172–7), with no change from baseline in other studies (n = 122, open, <5years, Morrell et al, Epilepsy Res 2003;**54**:189–99; n = 38, RCT, d/b, 32/52, Biton et al, J Child Neurol 2003;**18**:133–9).

Levetiracetam *

Levetiracetam at normal doses is weight neutral (n = 970, s = 4, RCT, p/c, Gidal et al, Epilepsy Res 2003;**56**:121–6), but four cases of considerable weight loss (2.3–7 kg/month) have been reported (Hadjikoutis et al, Br Med J 2003;**327**:905) and weight gain is mentioned in the UK SPC.

Oxcarbazepine

Weight gain has been reported as a relatively frequent side-effect.

Pregabalin

The UK SPC notes increased weight.

Tiagabine

Adjunctive tiagabine may have no significant effect on body weight (n = 349, Hogan et al, Epilepsy Res 2000;**41**:23–8).

Topiramate

Topiramate has been reported to produce weight loss eg. a dose-related weight loss occurred in 50% patients in a trial in bipolar disorder, with a mean 14.2 lb weight loss (n = 76, open, Ghaemi et al, Ann Clin Psychiatry 2001;**13**:185–9) and, compared to lithium and valproate, it produced an average of 1.2 kg weight loss (n = 214, open, chart, Chengappa et al, Clin Ther 2002;**24**:1576–84). It has even been abused to try to increase weight loss (n = 1, Colom et al, J Clin Psychiatry 2001;**62**:475–6). The effect appears dose-related, with average amounts lost ranging from 1.1 kg/1.5% (up to 200mg/d) to 5.9 kg/7% (800mg/d or above). The effect peaks at 12–15 months, is greater in people with higher starting weights and is at least partially reversible (MI). Topiramate (mean 135mg/d) may produce a modest loss in SSRI-induced weight gain (n = 15, open, 10/52, Van Ameringen et al, J Clin Psychiatry 2002;**63**:981–4), although it obviously has its own side-effects.

Vigabatrin

Weight gain may occur in 5–40% patients prescribed vigabatrin long-term.

Zonisamide *

Zonisamide may cause weight loss, substantial in rare cases (SPC).

2.3.6 OTHER DRUGS

No significant weight changes have been seen in clinical trials with **acamprosate**. A retrospective study showed weight loss with **methylphenidate** to occur more with heavier children and recommended that BMI percentile curves are used as the best measure of weight changes (study and review, Schertz et al, Pediatrics 1996; **98**:763–9). A mean body weight loss of 0.5 kg occurred with **atomoxetine** in 6–12-week studies with some normalisation over the longer-term (UK SPC). Weight loss may occur with bupropion, with 28% treated losing greater than 5lb, but weight gain occurred in 9% patients (MI). Modest weight losses have been seen with long-term **bupropion** SR (n = 423, p/c, one year, Croft et al, Clin Ther 2002;**24**:662–72).

PSYCHOTROPICS IN PROBLEM AREAS

3

3.1 BREAST-FEEDING

	LOWER RISK	MODERATE RISK	HIGHER RISK
Antipsychotics	Sulpiride[5]	Amisulpride[5] Flupentixol[4] Haloperidol[6] Loxapine[8] Phenothiazines (low dose only)[7] Zuclopenthixol[4]	Aripiprazole[2] Clozapine[3] Olanzapine[2] Phenothiazines HD[7] Quetiapine[2] Risperidone[1] Sertindole[2] Ziprasidone[2] Zotepine[2]
Antidepressants	Flupentixol LD[4] Moclobemide[16] Tricyclics[12] (most) Tryptophan[16]	Amoxapine[16] Mianserin[16] Mirtazapine[11] SSRIs[9] St John's wort[16] Trazodone[13]	Doxepin?[12] Duloxetine[10] MAOIs[15] Maprotiline[12] Reboxetine[14] Venlafaxine[10]
Anxiolytics and hypnotics	Benzodiazepines LD[17] Chloral[21] Temazepam LD[17] Zolpidem[19]	Benzodiazepines HD[17] Beta-blockers[20] Clomethiazole[21]	Buspirone[18] Zaleplon[19] Zopiclone[19]
Anticonvulsants	Carbamazepine[22] Phenytoin[24] Valproate[23]	Acetazolamide[28] Benzodiazepines[17] Vigabatrin[27]	Ethosuximide[28] Gabapentin[26] Lamotrigine?[26] Levetiracetam[27] Oxcarbazepine[22] Phenobarbital[25] Pregabalin[27] Tiagabine[27] Topiramate[27] Zonisamide[27]
Others		Anticholinergics[30] Atomoxetine[34] Disulfiram[31] Methadone[35] Sodium oxybate[33]	Acamprosate[31] Anticholinesterases[29] Buprenorphine[35] Bupropion[36] Lithium?[32] Memantine[29] Methylphenidate[34] Modafinil[33]

GENERAL PRINCIPALS *

1. All psychotropics pass into milk, so no decision is risk-free. Milk levels are usually around 1% of maternal plasma levels, but there have been few formal studies.

2. Breast milk is more acidic than plasma, so basic compounds may be retained and concentrations accumulate. Protein binding may also be a factor (in general, drug binding to milk proteins is less than to plasma proteins). The higher lipid content of the hind milk (second half of feed) makes it likely to have a higher drug concentration than the first half (fore milk).

3. Drugs should be avoided if the infant is pre-mature, or has renal, hepatic, cardiac or neurological impairment. Neonates (and particularly premature infants) are at greater risk from exposure to drugs via breast milk, because of an immature excretory function and the consequent risk of drug accumulation.

4. Avoid sedating drugs and those with long half-lives. Avoid drugs known to cause serious toxicity in adults or children. Drugs licensed for use in infants do not generally pose a hazard. It is best to avoid long-acting preparations, especially those of drugs likely to cause serious side-effects (eg. antipsychotic agents), as it is difficult to time feeds to avoid significant amounts of drug in breast milk. Avoid new drugs if a therapeutically equivalent alternative that has been more widely used is available.

5. Choose a regimen and route of administration which presents the minimum amount of drug to the infant. Since nearly all psychotropics can be given as a once daily dose, this should be implemented as a single daily dose just before the infant's longest sleep period feed (eg. peak milk concentrations after oral administration: amitriptyline 1.5 hours, imipramine 1 hour, moclobemide <3 hours, sertraline 8–9 hours, fluvoxamine 4 hours), minimising actual concentration and maximising clearance before the next feed.

6. If a mother was taking a drug during pregnancy, it will not usually be necessary to switch drugs during breast-feeding, as the amount to which the infant is exposed will be less than that in utero.

7. Adverse effects will often be dose-related, so use the minimum effective maternal dose.

8. Polypharmacy may lead to enhanced adverse effects in the infant. Avoiding interacting drugs that raise plasma levels (even if asymptomatically) is essential. Multiple drug regimens may pose an increased risk, especially when adverse effects such as drowsiness are additive.

9. Drug effects on the development of the infant's brain are not clear and so monitor biochemical and behavioural parameters, especially if the infant shows signs of possible psychotropic side-effects (eg. sedation, tremulousness, colic) and take appropriate action, eg. dose reduction, drug change, etc.

10. Avoid unnecessary drug use and limit the use of over-the-counter (OTC) products.

A robust assessment of the balance of benefit to risk for a mother–child pair requires data both on the drug's passage into breast milk and its effects in infants: there is rarely enough information available about new drugs to allow such an assessment to be made.

Reviews: * pharmacokinetic overview and thera-peutic implications (Spigset and Hagg, *CNS Drugs* 1998;**9**:111–34), general (McElhatton, *Prescriber* 1999;**10**:101–17), extensive (Burt *et al*, *Am J Psychiatry* 2001;**158**:1001–9; 124 refs), practical recommendations for treating mood disorders during lactation (Eberhard-Gran *et al*, *CNS Drugs* 2006;**20**:187–98).

3.1.1 ANTIPSYCHOTICS

Reviews: general (Tenyi *et al*, *Paediatr Drugs* 2000;**2**:23–8; recommends monotherapy at low dose has the lowest risk, polytherapy at higher doses is not recommended).

1. * The UK SPC for **risperidone** states that women should not breast-feed. In two cases risperidone the milk:plasma ratio was <0.5 with a relative infant dose lower than the 10% level of concern (n=2, Ilett *et al*, *Ann Pharmacother* 2004;**38**:273–6) and in another, milk levels were 10 times higher than in the maternal serum but no adverse effects were seen in the infant and development was normal (n=1, Aichhorn *et al*, *J Psychopharmacol* 2005;**19**:211–3; see also Hill *et al*, *J Clin Psychopharmacol* 2000;**20**:285–6).

2. * There is no data on **aripiprazole**. **Olanzapine** is excreted in breast milk, with infants exposed to about 1% of a maternal dose of olanzapine (below the 10% nominal level of concern), with no adverse effects or detectable infant plasma levels, so appears relatively safe (n=7, Gardiner *et al*, *Am J Psychiatry* 2003;**160**:1428–31; see also n=3, Goldstein *et al*, *J Clin Psychopharmacol*

2000;**20**:399–403; n = 5, Croke *et al, Int J Neuropsychopharmacol* 2002;**5**:243–7; n = 1, Ambresin *et al, J Clin Psychopharmacol* 2004;**24**:93–5). The UK SPC recommends not breast-feeding while taking olanzapine. For **quetiapine**, a case series showed undetectable levels in milk, with low or undetectable levels in the infant's serum, the authors concluding that quetiapine posed only a low-level risk (n = 6, Misri *et al, J Clin Psychopharmacol* 2006;**26**:508–11). In other case reports, milk levels at an oral dose of 200 mg/d were at a maximum of 0.43% of the weight-adjusted maternal dose and fell to pre-dose levels within two hours, appearing to be too small for significant pharmacological effects (n = 1, Lee *et al, Am J Psychiatry* 2004;**161**:1715–6). **Sertindole** is excreted in rat's milk but no human data exists so should not be used, as it would be expected to be excreted in milk. **Zotepine** and norzotepine may be secreted into breast milk (where milk levels can reach 50% of maternal plasma levels) and is incompatible with breast-feeding mothers. There is no data on **ziprasidone**.

3. **Clozapine** is contraindicated as animal studies suggest it is excreted into milk and so risks agranulocytosis in the infant. In the close study of one mother, there was some accumulation of clozapine in breast milk (possibly due to higher lipid concentrations), and so doses must be kept low (Barnas, *Am J Psychiatry* 1994;**151**:945) and the infant's plasma monitored if breast-feeding is essential. There are reports indicating that babies experience sedation if mothers take clozapine and breast-feed.

4. A study showed that 0.6 mcg/kg or 1–2% of the maternal **flupentixol** dose might reach the infant and thus is probably safe at low dose, eg. <2 mg/d (n = 6, Matheson and Skjaeraasen, *Eur J Clin Pharmacol* 1988;**35**:217–20). Higher doses of **zuclopenthixol** (n = 6, Aaes-Jorgensen *et al, Psychopharmacology* [Berlin] 1986;**90**:417–8) and flupentixol can produce drowsiness in the child.

5. A **sulpiride** dose of 100 mg/d to the mother is likely to give the child less than 1 mg/d. No adverse effects have been reported at higher doses (n = 28, p/c, d/b, 4/52, Ylikorkala *et al, Br Med J* 1982;**285**:249–51). There is no information for **amisulpride**.

6. **Haloperidol** is excreted into breast milk but levels are probably low (eg. n = 1, Whalley *et al, Br Med J* 1981;**282**:1746–7), although infant levels may be the same as adults. Some element of delayed development has been detected (n = 5, Yoshida *et al, Psychol Med* 1998;**28**:81–91) and so the infant must be monitored carefully.

7. High doses of **phenothiazines** can produce drowsiness in the infant. **Chlorpromazine** has an inconsistent milk/plasma ratio, and drowsiness and lethargy are possible but not inevitable (Wiles *et al, Br J Clin Pharmacol* 1978;**5**:272–3). With careful monitoring it should be safe although some element of delayed development has been suggested (n = 3, Yoshida *et al, Psychol Med* 1998;**28**:81–91). In one case report the amount of **perphenazine** passed to an infant was about 0.1% of the adult dose in terms of mcg/kg body weight (Olesen *et al, Am J Psychiatry* 1990;**10**:1378–9), and this drug may become 'trapped' in milk due to its physiochemical properties.

8. **Loxapine** and its metabolites have been shown to appear in breast milk but no data on the potential effects is known.

3.1.2 ANTIDEPRESSANTS

Exposure to antidepressants through breast milk does not generally appear to affect infants' weight, but infants have significantly lower weight if the mother has a depression lasting longer than two months (n = 78, naturalistic, 18/12, Hendrick *et al, J Clin Psychiatry* 2003;**64**:410–12), so there is a risk of not treating depression. In a review wittily entitled a 'pooled analysis of antidepressant levels in… breast milk' the conclusion was that fluoxetine produces the highest proportion (22%) of infant levels above 10% of the average maternal level, citalopram next at 17%, and that nortriptyline, paroxetine and sertraline may be the preferred choices, with citalopram relatively safe if doses are minimised (s = 67, Weissman *et al, Am J Psychiatry* 2004;**161**:1066–78).

9.* Treatment with the **SSRIs** seems to be compatible with breast-feeding, although fluoxetine should probably best be avoided during lactation, unless also used during pregnancy. One study suggested that paroxetine (n = 16), fluvoxamine (n = 4) and sertraline (n = 30) produce minimal exposure to infants when taken by nursing mothers (Hendrick *et al, Br J Psychiatry* 2001;**179**:163–6), although Angell (*Br J Psychiatry* 2002;**180**:85–6) did not agree with this conclusion.

Citalopram, escitalopram and demethylcitalopram are excreted into milk. In one study, the mean combined dose (4.4–5.1% as citalopram equivalents) transmitted to infants was below the 10% notional level of concern, and infant levels appear low or undetectable (n=11, Heikkinen *et al*, *Clin Pharmacol Ther* 2002;**72**:184–91). Another showed infant plasma concentrations to be very low or absent, with no adverse effects (n=7, Rampono *et al*, *Br J Clin Pharmacol* 2000;**50**:263–8) and a prospective, observational, cohort study was unable to show any significant clinical events in mothers who took citalopram and breastfed (n=43, Lee *et al*, *Clin Pharmacol Ther* 2002;**71**:43). In eight women taking escitalopram 10mg/d, the total dose reaching the infants was about 5% with no apparent adverse effects, and in the infants tested (n=5), plasma levels were mostly below that detectable (Rampono *et al*, *Br J Clin Pharmacol* 2006;**62**:316–22). These data support the safety of the use of citalopram in breast-feeding women, provided doses are optimised.

Fluoxetine (s=11, n=190, Burt *et al*, *Am J Psychiatry* 2001;**158**:1001–9) plasma levels in the infant may range from undetectable to one of 340ng/ml, but with no clear associations between maternal dose, age and plasma levels. Plasma levels peak in breast milk at about eight hours post-dose and are dose-related, with 20mg/d or less producing low infant serum levels (n=19, Hendrick *et al*, *Biol Psychiatry* 2001;**15**:775–82), and probably less than 10% of the adult therapeutic dose of fluoxetine (on a mg/kg basis) reaches the infant. This is considered low enough for women to continue breast-feeding (Nulman and Koren, *Teratology* 1996;**53**:304–8; careful study, n=10 pairs, Suri *et al*, *Biol Psychiatry* 2002;**52**:446–51), with no developmental effects likely (n=4, Yoshida *et al*, *Br J Psychiatry* 1998;**172**:175–9). Mean estimated infant exposures are 2.4–3.8% of the maternal plasma level (n=11 + 10 controls, Heikkinen *et al*, *Clin Pharmacol Ther* 2003;**73**:330–7). There is clearly some significant interpatient variability and adverse effects have been observed in breast-fed infants, eg. colic. Considering the potential for accumulation, careful monitoring of the infants is mandatory, especially in neonates exposed to these drugs *in utero* (n=14, Kristensen *et al*, *Br J Clin Pharmacol* 1999;**48**:521–7).

Fluvoxamine levels in milk and infant plasma appear low in the few reported cases. The estimated daily intake by an infant is probably about 0.5% of the maternal dose (100 or 200mg/d), thought to be of little risk, with no concerns about development up to 21 months (n=1, Yoshida *et al*, *Br J Clin Pharmacol* 1997;**44**:10–11; n=2, Kristensen *et al*, *J Hum Lact* 2002;**18**:139–43; n=1, Hägg *et al*, *Br J Clin Pharmacol* 2000;**49**:286–8).

Paroxetine has been well studied and maternal doses of 10–50mg/d are found in milk, but at highly variable levels (sample n=108, range 2–101 ng/ml). In 25 mother–infant sample sets, paroxetine was detected in all but one milk sample, but undetectable (ie. <0.1 ng/ml) in the infant's serum, with no adverse events reported (n=24, Misri *et al*, *J Clin Psychiatry* 2000;**61**:828–32). Hind-milk concentrations may be 78% higher than foremilk (also seen in 16 mother and infant pairs, Stowe *et al*, *Am J Psychiatry* 2000;**257**:185–9). No adverse reactions were reported in another study (n=6, open, Ohman *et al*, *J Clin Psychiatry* 1999;**60**:519–23).

Sertraline and metabolite generally appear only at low levels in the infant (probably less than 2% of the maternal dose per day; n=10, Dodd *et al*, *Hum Psychopharmacol* 2000;**15**:161–4), unlikely to cause any significant adverse effects (n=8, Kristensen *et al*, *Br J Clin Pharmacol* 1998;**45**:453–7). Peak sertraline levels occur in milk at around 8–9 hours after the last dose, and discarding this peak reduces the infant's intake by 18% (n=26, 186 samples, Stowe *et al*, *J Clin Psychiatry* 2003;**64**:73–80). Higher levels have been reported rarely (Wisner *et al*, *Am J Psychiatry* 1998;**155**:690–2), as have rare withdrawal reactions in breast-fed children after the mother has abruptly stopped sertraline (Kent and Laidlaw, *Br J Psychiatry* 1995;**167**:412–3), implying that sertraline may appear in breast milk at levels sufficient to suppress withdrawal after birth, especially at higher doses eg. 200mg/d (eg. n=12, Stowe *et al*, *Am J Psychiatry* 1997;**154**:1255–60). Platelet 5HT uptake in the infants appears unaltered (n=14 mother–infant pairs, Epperson *et al*, *Am J Psychiatry* 2001;**158**:1631–7).

10. * The total dose of **venlafaxine** and O-desmethylvenlafaxine (OMV) ingested by breast-fed infants is probably usually around 6.4%, which is lower than the 10% notional level of concern but still needs monitoring (n=6 mothers, seven

infants, Ilett et al, Br J Clin Pharmacol 2002;**53**:17–22), as there may be enough in milk to attenuate withdrawal symptoms (Koren et al, J Obstet Gynaecol Can 2006;**28**:299–302). Other data suggests that venlafaxine can be metabolised by infants, with no detectable adverse effects or apparent developmental issues (n = 2, Hendrick et al, Am J Psychiatry 2001;**158**:2089–90). **Duloxetine** is excreted into breast milk in animal studies but no human data is available so it is not recommended at the moment.

11.* In a careful study of breast-feeding mothers, a maximum of 1.5% of the adult **mirtazapine** dose (median 38 mg/d) reached the infants and of the four infants tested, only one had detectable plasma levels, the authors concluding that mirtazapine is relatively safe (n = 8, Kristensen et al, Br J Clin Pharmacol 2006;**63**:322–7). Hindmilk levels are slightly higher than foremilk (n=1, Klier et al, Am J Psychiatry 2007;**164**:348–9).

12. **Tricyclic antidepressants** should be used with care, but it does not seem warranted that breast-feeding should be discontinued completely, as significant tricyclic levels have not been detected in neonatal serum (except for doxepin and maprotiline). One study has indicated that for tricyclics about 1% of the maternal dose/kg reaches the infant, with only minute amounts in the infant serum, no acute toxic effects and no evidence of developmental delay (n = 10, Yoshida et al, J Affect Disord 1997;**43**:225–37). For imipramine, a milk/plasma ratio of 0.05–0.08, based on high dose samples, would lead to 0.1% of the maternal daily dose appearing in milk. **Amitriptyline**/nortriptyline levels in the infant are probably very low (Breyer-Pfaff, Am J Psychiatry 1995;**152**:812–3). Two studies, including 12 mother–baby pairs, showed no detectable **nortriptyline** in the infant serum, despite some unusually high maternal plasma levels, although two infants had detectable levels of 10–hydroxy metabolites. None of the infants showed any adverse effects and so the risk could be considered very low (Wisner and Perel, Am J Psychiatry 1996;**153**:295). In two studies of a five-year follow-up of children who had received dothiepin/**dosulepin** via breast milk, no detectable adverse effects on cognitive development were detectable (compared to a variety of controls, n = 30 + 36 controls, Buist and Janson, Br J Psychiatry 1995;**167**:370–3), and the drug is unlikely to be a significant hazard for the infant (n = 5, Ilett et al,

Br J Clin Pharmacol 1992;**33**:635–9). Case reports suggest that the infant may receive only up to 3.7% of the mother's **clomipramine** dose (n = 1, Pons et al, Clin Pharmacokinetics 1994;**27**:270–89), with no adverse effects (n = 4, Wisner et al, J Clin Psychiatry 1995;**56**:17–20). **Maprotiline** is present in milk in significant amounts so should not be used (Drug Ther Bull 1983;**21**:48). **Doxepin** has a longer-acting metabolite N-desmethyldoxepin, which may accumulate in breast-fed infants, causing severe drowsiness and respiratory depression (near fatal case at 75 mg/d in eight–week-old baby: Matheson et al, Lancet 1985;ii:1124; n = 1, Frey et al, Ann Pharmacother 1999;**33**:690–3). However, other reports failed to detect any effects in the infant with maternal doxepin doses of 150 mg/d (eg. Kemp et al, Br J Clin Pharmacol 1995;**20**:497–9; Wisner et al, Am J Psychiatry 1996;**153**:1132) and so metabolic differences could explain these.

The general recommendation is to observe the child carefully for sedation and respiratory depression. A tricyclic with a short half-life for itself (and any active metabolites) would appear to be the best option. It has been recommended that amitriptyline and imipramine are the preferred tricyclics (review by Duncan and Taylor, Psychiatr Bull 1995;**19**:551–2).

13. With **trazodone**, a 50 mg single-dose study showed that 1% passed into the milk (n = 6, Verbeck et al, Br J Clin Pharmacol 1986;**22**:367–70). More information on, eg. metabolites is needed, but it would appear to be of low risk. Drowsiness and poor feeding have been reported (n = 1, Yapp et al, Ann Pharmacother 2000;**34**:1269–72; n = 2, Dodd et al, Clin Psychopharmacol 2000;**20**:717–8). Caution is thus advised.

14. **Reboxetine** is excreted in milk in rats but no human data exists so the drug should be avoided.

15. Minimal data is available for the **MAOIs**. **Tranylcypromine** is excreted in breast milk but levels are not thought to be significant. Some sources state that MAOI levels in milk are too small to affect the child, but this has not been supported by any studies other than with tranylcypromine.

16.* In six lactating women, 0.06% of a single dose of **moclobemide** was excreted unchanged in the milk. It would seem unlikely this amount would produce adverse effects in the baby (Pons et al, Br J Clin Pharmacol 1990;**29**:27–31). **Mianserin** 40–60 mg/d may produce only low milk and infant plasma levels with no untoward effects (Buist et al, Br J Clin Pharmacol 1993;**36**:133–4). In a prospective study, there was no significant problems in infants whose mothers took **St. John's wort** while breast-feeding; there was no decrease in milk production or infant weight over the first year (n = 33 + 134 controls, Lee et al, J Clin Psychiatry 2003;**64**:966–8), and in a thorough study, hyperforin was only detected at low levels in milk, with infant exposure 0.9–2.5% of the maternal dose, comparable with other psychotropics and it thus appears relatively safe (n = 5, Klier et al, J Clin Psychiatry 2006;**67**:305–9). However, if possible, it should probably be avoided in breast-feeding. There are no known problems with **tryptophan**.

3.1.3 ANXIOLYTICS AND HYPNOTICS

17.* Since **benzodiazepines** are excreted in breast milk, they should probably not be given to lactating mothers (eg. Curr Prob 1997;**23**:10). Repeated doses of long-acting benzodiazepines can produce lethargy and weight loss but low and single doses are probably of low risk, provided the infant is monitored for drowsiness. Oxazepam seems to be preferable to diazepam in lactating women but, as with all anxiolytic benzodiazepines, infants should be observed for signs of sedation and poor suckling. **Diazepam**, **oxazepam**, **lorazepam**, **lormetazepam**, **nitrazepam** and **flunitrazepam** have all been shown in breast milk, and **alprazolam** withdrawal has been reported (n = 1, Anderson and McGuire, Drug Intell Clin Pharm 1989;**23**:614). Infant **temazepam** levels have been reported to be below detection levels at maternal doses of 10–20 mg/d and no adverse effects have been seen (Lebedevs et al, Br J Clin Pharmacol 1992;**33**:204–6). Very little **midazolam** appears to reach breast milk (n = 5, Nitsun et al, Clin Pharmacol Ther 2006;**79**:549–57).

18. **Buspirone** should be avoided, based on excretion studies in rats, although there is no specific human data to show adverse effects.

19. **Zaleplon** is excreted in breast milk, and should not be administered to breast-feeding mothers, although the actual amount likely to be transferred may be very low, eg. 0.017% of the maternal dose (n = 5, Darwish et al, J Clin Pharmacol 1999;**39**:670–4). **Zopiclone** is contraindicated in breast-feeding as it is excreted

in appreciable amounts (up to 50% of maternal levels: n = 12, Matheson et al, Br J Clin Pharmacol 1990;**30**:267–71). Single occasional doses of 7.5 mg are probably of low risk as accumulation is unlikely. The AAPCD considers **zolpidem** compatible with breast-feeding, as it is found only in minute amounts in milk due to its low lipophilic properties and rapid onset and excretion. In one study of women taking a (high) stat dose of 20 mg, 0.76–3.88 mg of zolpidem was excreted into breast milk, nearly all within three hours of the dose (n = 5, Pons et al, Eur J Clin Pharmacol 1989;**37**:245–8). A low dose at bedtime and avoiding breast-feeding for the next few hours would minimise the potential effect on an infant.

20. For **beta-blockers**, the amounts excreted into breast milk are probably too small to effect the baby (<0.1% of maternal doses), but could produce bradycardia and hypoglycaemia in high doses.

21. **Clomethiazole** is excreted in insignificant amounts, based on IV and oral studies in pre-eclampsia (Acta Psychiatr Scand 1986;**73**[Suppl 329]:185–8). An infant might ingest active amounts and although the sedative effects of this could be relevant they are unlikely to be harmful. **Chloral hydrate** is excreted in breast milk and the sedation caused in the infant makes this a precaution, although only minimal sedation after large feeds has been reported (Adv Drug React Bull 1976;Dec:212). The American Academy of Pediatrics recommends that chloral can safely be used in lactating mothers, as do the authorities in many European countries.

3.1.4 ANTICONVULSANTS

Breast-feeding should be encouraged as bonding is especially important in epileptic mothers (Brodie, Lancet 1990;**336**:426–7). An extensive review (Hägg and Spigset, Drug Safety 2000;**22**:425–40, 88 refs) of anticonvulsant use during lactation concluded that:

- carbamazepine, valproate and phenytoin are compatible with breast-feeding
- ethosuximide, phenobarbital and primidone should be regarded as potentially unsafe and close clinical monitoring of the infant is recommended
- data on the newer drugs is too sparse for reliable recommendations

- occasional or short-term treatment with benzodiazepines could be considered compatible with breast-feeding, although maternal diazepam treatment has caused sedation in suckling infants after short-term use. During long-term use of benzo-diazepines, infants should be observed for signs of sedation and poor suckling.

Review: * general (Pennell, *Neurology* 2003; **61** (Suppl 2):S35–42; Bar-Oz et al, *Paediatr Drugs* 2000;**2**:113–26).

22. **Carbamazepine** has been classed by the AAPCD as compatible with breast-feeding, as levels have been found to be relatively low. This is, however, based only on case reports in epilepsy, with few reports when used as a mood stabiliser. The half-life is longer in infants, with levels in milk ranging from 7% to 95% of the mother's serum, but probably usually around 10%. There are cases of adverse effects in the infant (n = 1, Merlob et al, *Ann Pharmacother* 1992;**26**:1563–5; n = 1, Frey et al, *Eur J Pediatr* 1990;**150**:136–8) and several of poor feeding. The mother should be informed of the potential signs of hepatic dysfunction and CNS effects (review, Chaudron and Jefferson, *J Clin Psychiatry* 2000;**161**:79–90). **Oxcarbazepine** is excreted into breast milk, the breast milk/plasma ratio for drug and metabolite being about 0.5, similar to carbamazepine (n = 1, Bulla et al, *Eur J Clin Pharmacol* 1988;**34**:311–3), and it is currently contraindicated.

23. **Valproate** has been classified by the AAPCD as compatible with breast-feeding, based on case reports in epilepsy. Infant serum levels usually range from 5–12% but can range from undetectable to 40% of the mother's serum level (n = 16, van Unruh et al, *Ther Drug Monit* 1984;**6**:272–6). In six mother–infant pairs, where infant exposure was exclusively during breast-feeding, mothers had valproate levels in the usual range for bipolar (39–79 mcg/mL) but the infants had low levels (0.7–1.5 mcg/mL), thus presenting a relatively low risk compared to the risk of relapse in the mother (n = 6, Piontek et al, *J Clin Psychiatry* 2000;**61**:170–2). Valproate thus appears relatively safe, although with the small but finite risk of haematological effects (Stahl et al, *J Pediatr* 1997;**130**:1001–3). Care and careful counselling is needed for higher doses (review, Chaudron and Jefferson, *J Clin Psychiatry* 2000;**161**:79–90).

24. Small quantities of **phenytoin** are excreted in breast milk, peaking at three hours, and have been considered clinically safe (*Adv Drug React Ac Pois Rev* 1982;**1**:255–87).

25. Larger doses of **phenobarbital** and **primidone** may accumulate in breast milk. This may cause unacceptable drowsiness and lead to the need to stop or at least reduce breast-feeding.

26. * Extensive passage of **lamotrigine** into breast milk occurs, and with a slow elimination in the newborn. Lamotrigine is metabolised by glucuronidation, which is immature in neonates and may lead to accumulation, with concentrations in the infant possibly reaching levels at which pharmacological effects could be expected. In one report, the milk to maternal serum ratio was a consistent 0.6, with infant serum levels of 23–33% of the maternal serum levels. This is probably of low risk provided all remain alert to the potential for life-threatening rashes (n = 3, Ohman et al, *Epilepsia* 1998;**39** [Suppl 2]:21; review, Chaudron and Jefferson, *J Clin Psychiatry* 2000;**161**:79–90). In three cases, infant plasma levels were 30% (range 20–43%) of the maternal level, the fourth was undetectable, so some variation occurs but care is definitely needed (n = 4, Liporace et al, *Epilepsy Behav* 2004;**5**:102–5). **Gabapentin** crosses into breast milk. In six mother–baby pairs, gabapentin levels were estimated to be 12% of the mother's plasma level, but with no adverse effects detected (n = 6, Ohman et al, *Epilepsia* 2005;**46**:1621–4; review, Chaudron and Jefferson, *J Clin Psychiatry* 2000;**161**:79–90).

27. * Animal studies indicate **levetiracetam** is excreted into breast milk and, since unusually high levels can occur (Pennell, *Neurology* 2003;**61**[6 Suppl 2]:S35–S42), breast-feeding is not recommended. **Pregabalin** is excreted into milk in animal studies but no human data exists so is not recommended (SPC). **Topiramate** and **tiagabine** are not recommended as no human information is currently available. A small study suggested that the quantity of **vigabatrin** ingested through milk is small, at around 1–3% of the daily dose (n = 2, Tran et al, *Br J Clin Pharmacol* 1998;**45**:409–11). **Zonisamide** appears in breast milk, 41–57% being transferred, with a half-life in the two infants of 61–107 hours respectively (n = 2, Kawada et al, *Brain Dev* 2002;**24**:95–7; see also Shimoyama et al, *Biomed Chromatogr* 1999;**13**:370–2), similar to the mother's plasma

level. The UK SPC recommends avoiding breast-feeding during therapy and for one month afterwards.

28. **Ethosuximide** is excreted in breast milk, with detectable infant levels. Very low doses of **acetazolamide** may be transferred by breast milk.

3.1.5 OTHERS

29. There is no information available on **donepezil**, **galantamine** and **rivastigmine**, so should not be used in breast-feeding mothers. Human data is lacking but **memantine** is lipophilic and so is probably excreted into breast milk.

30. There is no data for **anticholinergics**.

31. No information is available to date on **disulfiram** in breast milk and so use must be with great caution. There is the possibility of interactions with alcohol in paediatric medicines (see 4.7.1). **Acamprosate** is excreted in the milk of lactating animals and so the literature states that use in breast-feeding is a contraindication. No human data is available.

32. * **Lithium** has been classified by the AAPCD as contraindicated in breast-feeding since 1989 but this is based on limited information. Breast milk levels may be approximately 40% (range 24–72%), with infant serum having levels 5–200% of the mother's serum concentrations and there have been old case reports of adverse events (eg. hypotonia and lethargy, possibly due to reduced renal clearance), although many of these may have been multifactorial. A recent systematic study, however, has shown relatively low milk and lower infant plasma levels with no serious or persistent adverse events noted, the authors suggesting there is a need to reassess this widespread contraindication, provided careful; monitoring is carried out (n=10 mother-infant pairs, Viguera et al, Am J Psychiatry 2007;**164**:342–5). There is wide interindividual variability of the dose reaching an infant, and so informed choice, with careful monitoring (eg. TDM of milk or infant plasma), considering poorer renal excretion and fluid balance/electrolytes and use of low doses, may help if the risk of bipolar relapse is high if stopping lithium (Moretti et al, Ther Drug Monit 2003;**25**:364–6).

Review: Chaudron Jefferson, J Clin Psychiatry 2000;**161**:79–90.

33. * **Modafinil** is contraindicated in breast-feeding. **Sodium oxybate** is not recommended but there is no human data available (SPC).

34. * In one report, no **methylphenidate** was detectable in breast milk 20–21 hours after the last dose of a plain tablet (probably because methylphenidate's short half-life of 2–3 hours) so breast-feeding before a morning dose should have a low risk (n=1, Spigset et al, Am J Psychiatry 2007;**164**:348). The UK SPC recommends caution for **atomoxetine**.

35. * **Methadone** at maintenance doses reduces the risk of poor quality street drugs being used and has been used successfully in breast-feeding. A 12–mother study showed that the amount of methadone in breast milk was measurable but low (insufficient to prevent the development of a neonatal absence syndrome in seven infants; see also n=8 pairs, Begg et al, Br J Clin Pharmacol 2001;**52**:681–5), infant plasma levels were below the limit of detection in seven infants, and no adverse effects attributable to methadone were noted. The conclusion was that breast-feeding should not be discouraged in women on a methadone maintenance program (Wojnar-Horton et al, Br J Clin Pharmacol 1997;**44**:543). Stopping opiates is also dangerous as withdrawal reactions can damage the fetus more than methadone (for effect on the child in the first year, see Arch Dis Childhood 1989;**64**:235–45) and compared to formula milk, breast-feeding reduces the severity of neonatal abstinence syndrome, delays withdrawal symptom onset and decreases the need for interventions (n=190, Abdel-Latif et al, Pediatrics 2006;**117**:1163–9). **Buprenorphine** is excreted in rat's milk, may inhibit lactation and is contraindicated in breast-feeding (UK SPC). In the one study, milk levels were considered to be low (n=1, 10 samples, Grimm et al, Ther Drug Monit 2005;**27**:526–30).

36. * **Bupropion** and metabolites accumulate in breast milk at higher levels than the mother's plasma and there is a report of an infant developing seizures from bupropion ingested via breast milk (n=1, Prescrire Int 2005;**14**:144), although other reports indicate that bupropion is not detectable in the infant's plasma (n=1, Briggs et al, Ann Pharmacother 1993;**27**:431–3; n=2 pairs, Baab et al, J Clin Psychiatry 2002 **63**:910–1).

3.2 CARDIOVASCULAR DISEASE

	LOWER RISK	MODERATE RISK	HIGHER RISK
Antipsychotics	Amisulpride[5] Flupentixol[4] Olanzapine[2] Quetiapine[2] Sulpiride[5] Zuclopenthixol[4]	Aripiprazole[2] Haloperidol[6] Loxapine?[28] Phenothiazines[7] Risperidone[1]	Clozapine[3] Pimozide[8] Sertindole[2] Thioridazine[7] Ziprasidone[2] Zotepine[2]
Antidepressants	Duloxetine[10] Mianserin[16] Mirtazapine[11] St John's wort[16] SSRIs[9] Trazodone[13] Tryptophan[16]	MAOIs[15] Moclobemide[16] Reboxetine[14]	Tricyclics (especially dosulepin)[12] Venlafaxine[10]
Anxiolytics and hypnotics	Benzodiazepines[17] Buspirone[18] Zaleplon[19] Zolpidem[19] Zopiclone[19]	Beta-blockers[20] Chloral hydrate[21] Clomethiazole[21]	
Anticonvulsants	Benzodiazepines[17] Gabapentin[26] Lamotrigine[26] Pregabalin[27] Tiagabine[27] Topiramate[27] Vigabatrin[27] Valproate[23]	Barbiturates[25] Carbamazepine[22] Oxcarbazepine[22] Paraldehyde[28] Phenytoin[24]	Fosphenytoin[24]
Others	Acamprosate[31] Memantine[29]	Anticholinergics[30] Anticholinesterases[29] Atomoxetine[34] Bupropion[36] Dextroamfetamine[35] Lithium[32] Methadone[37] Methylphenidate[34] Modafinil[33] Sodium oxybate[33]	Disulfiram[31]

GENERAL PRINCIPALS (ADAPTED FROM *MAUDSLEY GUIDELINES*)

1. Polypharmacy should be avoided where possible, particularly with drugs likely to effect cardiac rate and electrolyte balance.

2. Awareness of QT prolongation is increasing, and so care is essential with drugs likely to increase the QT interval.

3. Avoid drugs specifically contraindicated, eg. thioridazine.

4. Start low and go slow is, as ever, good advice. Rapid dose escalation should be avoided.

Psychotropics in specific cardiac conditions

Angina

Avoid drugs causing orthostatic hypotension, which may exacerbate angina. Avoid drugs causing tachycardia, eg. phenothiazines, clozapine and risperidone. Trazodone and tricyclics are best avoided, although most other antidepressants are thought to be of relatively low risk.

Arrhythmias

SSRIs are first choice antidepressants and are preferred to the tricyclics because of their lack of antiarrhythmic/proarrhythmic potential (*Drugs Ther Perspect* 1998;11:11–3). Avoid phenothiazines, butyrophenones and pimozide. Sulpiride and olanzapine seem of low risk.

Congestive heart failure (CHF)

For chronic stable CHF, avoid beta-blockers and take care with drugs causing orthostatic hypotension, eg. phenothiazines, clozapine, risperidone, tricyclics, etc. For acute CHF, the cause will indicate which drugs are safer to use. Remember that lithium plus diuretics need extra care.

Hypertension

Drugs causing orthostatic hypotension should be monitored closely. Avoid MAOIs. Hypertension can occur with venlafaxine (high dose), clozapine and sometimes with tricyclics and antipsychotics.

Myocardial infarction (MI)

If essential, use SSRIs (except perhaps fluvoxamine), trazodone or mianserin. Avoid high-dose antipsychotics, phenothiazines and pimozide. Butyrophenones, thioxanthenes and benzamides are safer.

Reviews: cardiac effects of psychotropics (Chong *et al, Ann Acad Med Singapore* 2001;**30**:625–31), psychotropics and the heart (O'Brien and Oyebode, *Adv Psychiatr Treat* 2003;**9**:414–23).

QTc prolongation

Many antipsychotics are known to affect cardiac conduction, with a class IA antiarrhythmic-like effect. One way this manifests itself is by lengthening of the QT interval. This may then lead onto torsade de pointes, which may be asymptomatic or, in rare cases, may lead on to ventricular fibrillation and sudden death. The QT interval shortens with increased heart rate, and so a rate-correct value QTc is usually used. A QTc prolonged to about 450ms is considered of some concern, and above about 500ms to be of an unquantifiable risk of leading to torsade de pointes which may be fatal, so should prompt review and possibly action. QTc varies markedly throughout the day, and so serial readings are necessary for accurate assessments.

Risk factors for antipsychotic-induced QTc prolongation:

- Recent introduction of an antipsychotic, dose increase or high doses (including overdose).
- Receiving other medicines associated with QT prolongation, including eg. some antiarrhythmic drugs, vasodilators, tricyclics, antipsychotics, macrolide and fluoroquinolone antibiotics, antimalarials, ketoconazole and antihistamines.
- Underlying cardiac disease eg. heart -failure, angina and cardiac myopathy.
- Bradycardia or 2nd or 3rd degree heart block.
- Personal or family history of QTc prolongation, ventricular arrhythmias or torsade de pointes.
- Severe renal or hepatic impairment.
- Elderly or malnourished.
- History of heavy alcohol consumption or substance misuse.
- Electrolyte imbalance, especially hypokalaemia.
- Undergoing restraint and/or severe stress.
- Slow drug metabolisers.
- Female (QT prolongation may occur more frequently).

If a prolonged QT interval is predictable, monitoring of electrolytes and ECG may be indicated, but interpretation is dependent upon the timing (time since last dose, diurnal variation, postprandial state).

Review: Harrigan *et al, J Clin Psychopharmacol* 2004;**24**:62–9.

3.2.1 ANTIPSYCHOTICS

Antipsychotic use in schizophrenia has been associated with increased rates of cardiac arrest, ventricular arrhythmia and death. One review has concluded that the greatest risk of prolonged QTc is from thioridazine, followed by pimozide, sertindole, droperidol and haloperidol, some with ziprasidone (but no evidence of progression to torsade de pointes) and none from olanzapine, quetiapine or risperidone (Glassman and Bigger, *Am J Psychiatry* 2001;**158**:1774–82). Interestingly, thioridazine (except perhaps at high dose) had no greater risk than haloperidol in a Medicaid cohort study (n = 95632 + 29086 controls, Hennessy *et al*, *Br Med J* 2002;**325**:1070–2).

Reviews: cardiovascular adverse effects of antipsychotics (Buckley and Sanders, *Drug Safety* 2000;**23**:215–28; 80 refs), QTc prolongation (Vieweg, *J Clin Psychiatry* 2002;**63**[Suppl 9]:18–24), QTc, torsade de pointes and sudden death (Haddad and Anderson, *Drugs* 2002;**62**:1649–71) and antipsychotics and QTc prolongation (Taylor, *Acta Psychiatr Scand* 2003;**107**:85–95; 136 refs).

1. **Risperidone** should be used with caution due to orthostatic hypotension; low doses slightly drop bp and increase heart rate. It is best to introduce it slowly over several weeks. In one study (Medicaid cohort study, n = 95, 632 + 29086 controls, Hennessy *et al*, *Br Med J* 2002; **325**: 1070–2), risperidone was the only drug that had higher rates than haloperidol for cardiac arrest and ventricular arrhythmia, especially at lower dose. The authors concluded that this was due to the frailest patients being given lowest doses.

2. * **Aripiprazole** may cause orthostatic hypotension and so should be used with caution in known CV disease, cerebrovascular disease and hypotension. Postural hypotension has been seen infrequently with **olanzapine**. Blood pressure monitoring is recommended periodically in patients over 65. One study showed that olanzapine (mean 14 mg/d) produced fasting triglyceride levels raised by a mean of 60 mg/dL (37%) (n = 25, 12/52, Osser *et al*, *J Clin Psychiatry* 1999;**60**:767–70), which, since triglycerides are a significant risk factor for exacerbation of CHD, needs care (Grundy, *Am J Cardiol* 1998;**81**[4A]:18B–25B). An increase in the QTc interval has only been seen rarely, eg. data from four RCTs showed the risk of QTc > 450 msec was approximately the same as at baseline, suggesting a minimal effect on QTc prolongation and hence fatal arrhythmias (n = 2700, Czekalla *et al*, *J Clin Psychiatry* 2001;**62**:191–8). The literature for **quetiapine** recommends caution with drugs known

to prolong the QTc interval and in patients with cardiovascular disease or conditions predisposing to hypotension. Trials have not shown sustained changes in the QTc interval and it would thus seem to be of low risk. Orthostatic hypotension is more common in the elderly, especially initially. **Sertindole** lengthens the QT interval and is contraindicated in people with a history of significant cardiovascular disease, congestive heart failure, cardiac hypertrophy, arrhythmia or bradycardia (< 50 bpm) and congenital prolonged QT (> 450 msec in men, > 470 msec in women). A review of its cardiac effects suggested that a counter-balancing mechanism may reduce the risk of proarrhythmic activity from prolonged QTc (Lindstrom *et al*, *Int J Neuropsychopharmacol* 2005;**8**:615–29). Trials are underway to obtain naturalistic and comparative data. **Ziprasidone** causes a well-publicised, dose-related prolongation of QTc interval (mean 10 msec), so should not be used in anyone with a known prolonged interval, recent MI or heart failure (review, Taylor, *CNS Drugs* 2003;**17**:423–30). It can cause a mean increase in heart rate of 1.4 bpm. **Zotepine** causes a dose-related QTc interval prolongation and caution is necessary in patients with CHD and with other drugs known to cause QTc prolongation. Increased heart rate can occur so care in angina pectoris is necessary. Orthostatic hypotension can occur initially in treatment, so bp measuring is recommended. Caution is necessary in severe hypertension. Unlike other antipsychotics, it tends to cause a slight shortening of the QTc interval.

3. * **Clozapine** has well-established cardiac side-effects, eg. tachycardia and postural hypotension (particularly early in treatment) and the literature (*Curr Probs Pharmacovig* 2002;**28**:8) has warned that with clozapine:

- patients who develop clozapine-induced cardiomyopathy (data mining study, Coulter *et al*, *Br Med J* 2001;**322**:1207–9) should not be re-exposed to clozapine
- it should only be started if severe heart disease has been excluded through a full history, examination and possibly an ECG
- myocarditis most commonly occurs in the first two months
- persistent tachycardia at rest, especially during first two months, should be followed up and the patient observed for other signs of cardiomyopathy/myocarditis

- ECG changes should be referred to a cardiologist for evaluation
- It should be discontinued in anyone where cardiomyopathy or myocarditis is suspected.

One study showed that 13% patients had cardiac abnormalities before and 31% after starting clozapine. Risk factors included increased age (but less so if there was a normal ECG with other antipsychotics). Prolonged QTc was dose-dependent, often corrected itself in time, occurred mostly during the initial stages of treatment, was mostly benign, and pathological prolongation of QTc was rare (n=61, Kang et al, J Clin Psychiatry 2000;**61**:441–6). A number of case series in Australia have shown a strong association with potentially fatal myocarditis (n=15, five occurring within five weeks of starting) and cardiomyopathy (n=8) in physically healthy young adults (from Australian database of 8000, Kilian et al, Lancet 1999;**354**:1841–5) and, in the USA, myocarditis (n=28, 18 fatal) and cardiomyopathy (n=41, 10 fatal: La Grenade et al, NEJM 2001;**345**:224–5). A 10-year naturalistic study also showed patients on clozapine were at risk of death from cardiovascular disease secondary to obesity, diabetes, hypertension and hyperlipidaemia (n=96, 10 years, Henderson et al, J Clin Psychiatry 2005;**66**:1116–21). Regular ECG monitoring, especially at higher doses, may be very valuable (review of myocarditis and CV toxicity by Wooltorton, Can Med Assoc J 2002;**166**:1185–6).

4. Cardiac disease is a literature precaution for **flupentixol** and **zuclopenthixol**.

5. * The literature for **amisulpride** states QTc prolongation can occur (eg. in overdose; n=4, Isbister et al, Med J Aust 2006;**184**:354–6), and it is now contraindicated with drugs that could cause torsade de pointes. There are no specific problems reported with **sulpiride**.

6. **Haloperidol** may have the risk of occasional arrhythmias and so the use of high dosage with non-responders is cautioned. Prolonged QT-interval has been reported with haloperidol (n=596, Reilly et al, Lancet 2000;**35**:1048–52), although it appeared of no greater risk than thioridazine in a Medicaid cohort study (n=95 632 + 29 086 controls, Hennessy et al, Br Med J 2002;**325**:1070–2).

7. Some ECG abnormalities have been reported with **phenothiazines**, eg. tachycardia, T-wave abnormalities, ST depression, QT prolongation and right bundle branch block. **Thioridazine** is contraindicated in patients with a history of cardiac arrhythmias or at risk of problems. Dose-related increases in risk of lengthened QT-interval have been reported, detectable at doses as low as 10mg/d (n=596, Reilly et al, Lancet 2000;**355**:1048–52). **Levomepromazine** (metho-trimeprazine) causes orthostatic hypotension that can, on occasion, be prolonged and profound. Sudden death has also been reported.

8. **Loxapine** can increase the pulse rate and produce transient hypotension. With **pimozide**, the UK CSM has had many reports of serious or fatal cardiac reactions to pimozide, and they recommend (Curr Prob 1995;**21**:2):

i. Start at 2–4mg/d. Increase by 2–4mg/d weekly (max 20mg/d).

ii. Perform ECG pre-treatment. C/I if a prolonged QT interval or a history of arrhythmia is noted.

iii. Repeat ECG annually. Review if the QT interval is lengthened.

iv. Avoid concurrent treatment with other antipsychotics (including depots), tricyclics and other QT interval-prolonging drugs (eg. some anti-malarials, antiarrhythmics, astemizole and diuretics).

3.2.2 ANTIDEPRESSANTS *

Depression is an independent risk factor for mortality in patients with CHD and for the development of heart disease (review by Ward et al, Curr Opin Psych 2003;**16**:221–5), with no prognostic difference between self-reported or clinically diagnosed depression (s=20, n=11,018, Barth et al, Psychosom Med 2004;**66**:802–13; comment by Maggi, EBMH 2005;**8**:66). Depression may be very poorly detected after MI (n=85, Luutonen et al, Acta Psychiatr Scand 2002;**106**:434–9). Depressed patients are at greater risk of myocardial infarction and vice versa, and, during the first six months post-infarction, patients who become depressed have a five-fold increase in mortality (Frazure-Smith et al, JAMA 1999;**270**:1819–25). Depressed patients are less likely to follow recommendations to reduce their cardiac risk during recovery from a myocardial infarction (n=204, survey, Ziegelstein et al, Arch Intern Med 2000;**160**:1818–23) and are less likely to comply with antihypertensives (n = 496, one year, Wang et al, J Gen Intern Med 2002;**17**:504–11). There is a strong association between the use of tricyclic antidepressants and cardiac events (especially IHD with dosulepin; n = 933 + 5516 controls, Hippisley-Cox et al, Br Med J 2001;**323**:666–9; Cohen et al, Am J Med 2000;**108**:2–8), but not with SSRIs, where the risk has actually been shown to be reduced by 65% compared to non-users (n = 143, Kimmel et al, J Am Heart Ass 2001;**104**:1894–8). Treatment of depression in this vulnerable group is thus of singular importance as, although the use of antidepressants in cardiac disease has risks, so does not using them (n = 2847, Penninx et al, Arch Gen Psych 2001;**58**:221–7).

Reviews: * general (Roose and Spatz, Drug Safety 1999;**20**:459–65, 25 refs), antidepressant cardiac side-effects (Sala et al, Curr Opin Investig Drugs 2006;**7**:256–63).

9. * Despite some reported cases of cardiac effects (eg. a plasma-level related potential for conduction problems, eg. AV block, QTc prolongation, etc; n = 114, Rodriguez de la Torre et al, Ther Drug Monit 2001;**23**:435–40), the **SSRIs** are generally considered safer to use in cardiac disease (eg. n = 456, Guy and Silke, J Clin Psychiatry 1990;**51**[Suppl 13]:37–9; review by Glassman et al, JAMA 1993;**269**:2673–5), with robust data accumulating to support this. In a recent major study, **sertraline** was shown not to increase cardiac events in depressed patients with unstable angina or recent MI, and may even cut cardiac deaths post-MI by about 10% (n = 369, RCT, Glassman et al, JAMA 2002;**288**:701–9). Indeed, SSRIs may provide some protection against myocardial infarction, with the relative reduction in platelet serotonin reuptake caused by SSRIs being the reason for the risk reduction (n = 1080 + 4356, three years, Sauer et al, Circulation 2003;**108**:32–6).

Similarly, a naturalistic study in severely ill (sub-acute cardiac rehabilitation unit) elderly cardiac patients showed that **paroxetine**, **sertraline** and **fluoxetine** had little adverse effect on cardiac state and appeared relatively safe and effective, but care was needed with drug interactions (n = 17, Askinazi, Am J Psychiatry 1996;**153**:135–6). Several open trials have indicated **fluoxetine** up to 60mg/day to have no significant adverse cardiac effects in patients

with pre-existing CHF, conduction disease and/or ventricular arrhythmia (n = 27, average age 73, open, 7/52, Roose et al, Am J Psychiatry 1998;**155**:660–6). In another study, fluoxetine 20mg/d produced a modest reduction in bp, and patients with pre-existing, stable cardiovascular disease (including hypertension) showed no significant bp change (n = 796, 12/52, Amsterdam et al, J Clin Psychopharmacol 1999;**19**:9–14). Rare cases of, eg. atrial fibrillation, bradycardia and syncope have been reported. **Paroxetine** may increase cholesterol (LDL-C) concentrations by around 11%, which might increase the risk of CHD in vulnerable individuals (n = 18, Lara et al, J Clin Psychiatry 2003;**64**:1455, IS). **Citalopram** (and presumably **escitalopram**) have no significant reported effect on blood pressure, cardiac conduction or heart rate (Milne and Goa, Drugs 1991;**41**:450–77), but exacerbation of pre-existing bradycardia has been reported (eg. Myth et al, Acta Psychiatr Scand 1992;**86**:138–45), as has occasional postural dizziness (review of citalopram cardiac safety: Rasmussen et al, J Clin Psychopharmacol 1999;**19**:407–15).

10. * **Venlafaxine** has a dose-dependent effect on supine diastolic blood pressure, clinically significant at high doses (> 200–300 mg/d), probably as a result of noradrenergic potentiation (3% incidence at less than 100mg/d, 7% for 150–200mg/d and 13% above 300mg/d). In the UK, venlafaxine is no longer subject to excessive MHRA and SPC restrictions, as:

- it is only contraindicated in patients with an identified high risk of a serious cardiac ventricular arrhythmia or with uncontrolled hypertension (but is NOT contraindicated in controlled hypertension). There is a caution for use in established cardiac disease that may increase the risk of ventricular arrhythmias.
- no baseline ECG is needed
- regular bp is recommended.

Duloxetine causes no QTc prolongation nor major cardiac effects but is contraindicated in uncontrolled hypertension.

11. Although hypertension, hypotension and tachycardia have been reported with **mirtazapine**, the incidences of 6%, 4% and 2% respectively are the same as placebo (n = 150, RCT, d/b, p/c, 6/52, Smith et al, Psychopharmacol Bull 1990;**26**:191–6). No ECG changes have been observed in

reported trials, or bp and heart rate changes in a depressed in-patient trial (n = 251, RCT, 6/12, Zivkov and Jongh, *Hum Psychopharmacol* 1995;**10**:173–80). Mild dizziness and vertigo was noted in two patients in one trial, although treatment continued (van Moffaert *et al, Int Clin Psychopharm* 1995;**10**:3–9). Mirtazapine would seem to be relatively safe.

12. **Tricyclics** produce orthostatic hypotension (and hence occasional myocardial infarction), have antiarrhythmic actions (quinidine-like) in high dose and antimuscarinic actions (raising heart rate). Thus, tricyclics should only be used with caution in patients with ischaemic heart disease, ventricular arrhythmia, angina, recent MI and hypertension. Indeed, a case-control primary care study indicated that the odds ratio for developing IHD was significantly raised for patients who had ever received a TCA (even adjusting for other factors), with a further specific, significant and dose-related association with **dosulepin** (n = 922 with IHD, 5516 controls, Hippisley-Cox *et al, Br Med J* 2001;**323**:666–9). SSRIs are thus generally considered safer. In patients with recurrent chest pain but normal coronary angiograms, **imipramine** therapy over 9–33 months produced no symptoms of a pro-arrhythmic effect, a slightly prolonged corrected QT interval and reduced chest pain (n = 58, Cannon *et al, NEJM* 1994;**330**:1411–7). Conversely, in 24 patients with major depression compared with 24 controls, 150 mg/d of **amitriptyline** increased heart rate from 78 bpm to 93 bpm, and all other heart rate analysis parameters significantly worsened (Rechlin *et al, Psychopharmacology* 1994;**116**:110–4). **Nortriptyline** has significant effects on cardiac vagal function and should only be used with care in IHD (n = 44, Yeragani *et al, Neuropsychobiology* 2002;**46**:125–35), especially in men who may be more susceptible to its cardiac side-effects (n = 78, 6/52, Pomara *et al, Prog Neuropsychopharmacol Biol Psychiatry* 2001;**25**:1035–48). **Doxepin**-induced torsade de pointes tachycardia has been reported (Alter *et al, Ann Intern Med* 2001;**135**:384–5).

13. Reversible ventricular tachycardia (n = 1, Vitullo *et al, Chest* 1990;**98**:247–8) and QT prolongation has been reported with **trazodone** overdose (Levenson, *Am J Psychiatry* 1999;**156**:929–70), but is generally considered of low risk.

14. **Reboxetine** increased baseline heart rate in 20% of patients in short-term trials. Orthostatic

hypotension occurs with increasing frequency at higher doses.

15. **Isocarboxazid, phenelzine** and **tranylcypromine** are contraindicated in severe cardiac disease.

16. Many cases of hypertension have been reported with **moclobemide** (eg. Boyd, *Lancet* 1995;**346**:1498), so monitoring bp may be useful. Occasional hypertension with tyramine in patients with pre-existing labile hypertension has also occurred (*Acta Psychiatr Scand* 1990;**360** [Suppl]:69–70), and so caution in cardiac disease would be sensible. **St John's wort** does not affect heart rate variability, unlike amitriptyline 75 mg/d (n = 12, RCT, d/b, c/o, 14/7 per arm, Siepmann *et al, Br J Clin Pharmacol* 2002;**54**:277–82). There are no apparent problems with **mianserin** and **tryptophan**.

3.2.3 ANXIOLYTICS AND HYPNOTICS

17. **Benzodiazepines** are relatively safe but contraindicated in acute pulmonary insufficiency. One study in elderly patients showed that temazepam (up to 30 mg/d) caused a fall in systolic blood pressure and an increase in heart rate (n = 12, Ford, *Br J Clin Pharmacol* 1990;**29**:61–7).

18. **Buspirone** may have some cardiac effects, eg. rare cases of hypertension and tachycardia.

19. There are no apparent problems with **zaleplon**, **zolpidem** and **zopiclone**.

20. The use of **beta-blockers** would depend upon the nature of the cardiac disease.

21. **Clomethiazole** is contraindicated in acute pulmonary insufficiency and should be used with care in chronic pulmonary insufficiency. **Chloral** is contraindicated in severe cardiac disease.

3.2.4 ANTICONVULSANTS

22. Cardiovascular effects from **carbamazepine** are uncommon but cardiac conduction changes, hypertension and atrio-ventricular block (Labrecque et al, *Am J Psychiatry* 1992;**149**:572–3) have been reported. There is a case of a patient with a permanent dual-chamber pacemaker, where carbamazepine elevated ventricular and atrial thresholds, thus making the pacemaker ineffective (Ambrosi *et al, Lancet* 1993;**342**:365). Patients on oxcarbazepine with cardiac insufficiency and secondary heart failure should have regular weight measurements to help detect any fluid retention.

There is a new UK SPC warning that care is needed in patients with pre-existing conduction disturbances.

23. There are some rare reports of cardiac effects with **valproate**, but no specific cautions.

24. **Phenytoin** has many cardiac effects and is a useful third-line treatment in cardiac arrhythmias. It is, however, contraindicated in sinus bradycardia, sino-atrial block, second and third degree A-V block and patients with Adams-Stokes syndrome. Severe cardiovascular ADRs have been reported with **fosphenytoin** IV, including asystole, VF and cardiac arrest, mostly within 30 minutes of an injection. The literature thus recommends (*Curr Prob Pharmacovig* 2000;**26**[May]:1):

- monitoring heart rate, bp and respiration during the infusion
- observing for at least 30 minutes after the infusion ends
- as hypotension may occur at recommended doses and rates, reduction of the dose or rate may be necessary
- reducing the loading dose and/or infusion rate by 10–25% in the elderly or those with hepatic or renal impairment.

25. * IV **barbiturates** can cause hypotension. As there is no evidence that **primidone** causes QT-prolongation (and may actually shorten it), it may be the drug of choice in patients with QT-prolongation (Christidis *et al*, *Seizure* 2006; **15**:64–6).

26. There is no evidence of any problems with **gabapentin** in cardiac disease. ECG monitoring is recommended in cases of **lamotrigine** overdose (Buckley *et al*, *Lancet* 1993;**342**:1552–3).

27.* No significant changes in ECG, blood pressure or heart rate have been noted in initial clinical trials with **topiramate, vigabatrin** and **tiagabine** but **pregabalin** has a caution for use in severe congestive heart failure (SPC).

28. There have been reports of hypotension and tachycardia in young children given IV **paraldehyde** (Sinal and Crowe, *Pediatrics* 1976;**57**:158).

3.2.5 OTHERS

29. **Anticholinesterases** may cause bradycardia so care is needed with the use of **donepezil** in patients with sick sinus syndrome or other conduction conditions. Heart block has been reported with donepezil, and so the UK SPC has

recommended considering this before prescribing (*Curr Prob Pharmacovig* 1999;**25**:7). Analysis of four studies indicated that **rivastigmine** appears not to cause adverse ECG effects (n = 2149, d/b, p/c, 26/52, Morganroth *et al*, *J Clin Pharmacol* 2002;**42**:558–68), although rare cases of syncope and angina pectoris have been noted in trials. **Galantamine** would appear relatively safe but caution is advised in people with cardiovascular conditions, eg. sick sinus syndrome or other supraventricular cardiac conduction disturbances. There is little data on **memantine** in cardiac disease and use should be only with caution.

30. **Anticholinergics** should be used with caution, particularly in those with a tendency to tachycardia. Sinus bradycardia has been reported with **benzatropine** (Voinov *et al*, *Am J Psychiatry* 1992;**149**:711) and **benzhexol/trihexyphenidyl** (n = 1, Blumensohn *et al*, *Drug Intell Clin Pharm* 1986;**20**:786–7).

31. **Disulfiram** is contraindicated in the presence of cardiac failure, coronary artery disease, previous history of CVA and hypertension. The Antabuse-alcohol reaction can cause cardiac arrest even in healthy adults. There are no known problems with **acamprosate**.

32. **Lithium** rarely causes clinical problems although cardiac failure and sick sinus syndrome are contraindications. Usually benign cardiovascular side-effects may occur in 20–30% patients. The main problems with lithium can be T-wave flattening (or possibly inversion), ventricular ectopics, congestive myopathy, bradycardia (Farag *et al*, *Lancet* 1994;**343**:1371), ECG changes and conduction disturbances, eg. sinus node dysfunction (Terao *et al*, *Acta Psychiatr Scand* 1996;**93**:407–8). An analysis, however, of 827 patients (Ahrens *et al*, *J Affect Disord* 1995;**33**:67–75) showed that deaths from cardiac-related causes were no different in people taking lithium than in the general population, and so, despite the above reported problems, lithium can be considered not to have a significant risk in this situation (reviewed by Ananth, *Lithium* 1993;**4**:167–79). A pre-treatment ECG is very useful, especially in elderly people.

33. * **Modafinil** is contraindicated in severe hypertension and arrhythmia and used with caution in patients with concurrent heart disease. Monitor heart rate and blood pressure if used in moderate hypertension (MI; discussion by Heitmann *et al*, *Clin Pharmacol Therapy*

1999;**65**:328–35). **Sodium oxybate** contains a significant dose of ...er... sodium (0.75 g in 4.5 g dose) and so dietary restriction of sodium might be considered in hypertension and heart failure (SPC).

34. * The manufacturers caution to monitor bp in hypertensive patients taking **methylphenidate**. **Atomoxetine** is associated with modest increases in bp (mean <5 mm Hg) and pulse (mean < 10 bpm), which stabilise over two years (UK SPC), so use with caution in hypertension or CV disease. Recent UK MHRA guidance is that atomoxetine should be used with caution in those with prolonged QT or a family history of QT prolongation, and care when used with other drugs that produce QT prolongation, drugs that can cause electrolyte disturbances and those that inhibit cytochrome CYP2D6. QTc prolongation has been seen with atomoxetine overdose (n = 1, Sawant and Daviss, *Am J Psychiatry* 2004; **161**:757).

35. There is little evidence of developing hypertension with **dexamfetamine**, although regular bp testing has been recommended (ASDA, *Sleep* 1994;**17**:348–51).

36. **Bupropion** may cause small rises in supine blood pressure (RCT, n = 58, Kiev *et al*, *Ann Clin Psychiatry* 1994;**6**:107–15), but tends not to cause significant conduction complications, or to exacerbate ventricular arrhythmias and has a low rate of orthostatic hypotension (n = 36, open trial in patients with depression and pre-existing heart disease, Roose *et al*, *Am J Psychiatry* 1991;**148**:512–6). Infrequent occurrences of orthostatic hypotension, tachycardia, stroke and vasodilation have been reported with bupropion. Significant cardiac conduction prolongation does not seem to occur (review: Roose, *Am Heart J* 2000;**140**[4 Suppl]:S84–S88).

37. * The MHRA issued a warning in May 2006 that **methadone** can risk lengthening the QT interval and recommends cardiac monitoring at doses of more than 100 mg/d. **Buprenorphine** can cause postural hypotension.

3.3 DIABETES

	LOWER RISK	MODERATE RISK	HIGHER RISK
Antipsychotics	Amisulpride[5] Aripiprazole[2] Butyrophenones[6] Loxapine[8] Pimozide[8] Risperidone[1] Sulpiride[5] Thioxanthenes[4] Ziprasidone[2]	Clozapine[3] Phenothiazines[7] Quetiapine[2] Sertindole[2] Zotepine[2]	Olanzapine?[2]
Antidepressants	Duloxetine[10] Moclobemide[16] Reboxetine[14] SSRIs[9] Trazodone[13] Tryptophan[16] Venlafaxine[10]	Fluoxetine[9] Mianserin[16] Mirtazapine[11] Tricyclics[12]	MAOIs[15]
Anxiolytics and hypnotics	Benzodiazepines[17] Buspirone[18] Chloral[21] Clomethiazole[21] Zaleplon[19] Zolpidem[19] Zopiclone[19]	Beta-blockers[20]	
Anticonvulsants	Acetazolamide[28] Barbiturates[25] Benzodiazepines[17] Carbamazepine[22] Ethosuximide[28] Gabapentin[26] Lamotrigine[26] Oxcarbazepine[22] Pregabalin[26] Vigabatrin[27]	Phenytoin[24] Topiramate[27] Tiagabine[27] Zonisamide[27] Valproate[23]	
Others	Acamprosate[31] Anticholinergics[30] Anticholinesterases[29] Atomoxetine[33] Buprenorphine[35] Lithium[32] Memantine[29] Methadone[35] Methylphenidate[33] Modafinil[33]	Bupropion[34] Disulfiram[31] Sodium oxybate[33]	

3.3.1 ANTIPSYCHOTICS *

There is an increased risk of diabetes with all antipsychotics (*Eur Neuropsychopharmacol* 2006; **16**:187–94), but especially some of the atypicals, eg. in a huge study of people taking antipsychotics (41% on typicals and 59% on atypicals [of which 48.4% were on olanzapine, 43.7% on risperidone, 5.3% on clozapine and 4.2% on quetiapine]), those on atypicals were 9% more likely to have diabetes than those on typicals. The prevalence was significantly increased for **clozapine**, **olanzapine** and **quetiapine** but not for **risperidone** (n = 38 632, Veterans, Sernyak *et al*, *Am J Psychiatry* 2002; **159**:561–6). In another study in non-diabetic schizophrenics, glucose tolerance tests showed elevated plasma glucose (compared to placebo or typicals) at all time points for olanzapine, partly raised for clozapine and only raised with risperidone compared to untreated non-schizophrenics, indicating an adverse effect by some atypicals on glucose regulation (n = 79, Newcomer *et al*, *Arch Gen Psychiatry* 2002; **59**:337–45). In another study of diabetics, antipsychotics worsened metabolic control and doubled the need for insulin, especially in the first two years (n = 2585, Spoelstra *et al*, *J Clin Psychiatry* 2004; **65**:674–8).

In 2004, four US medical organisations recommended that patients taking atypicals (clozapine, olanzapine, quetiapine, risperidone, aripiprazole and ziprasidone) should be monitored for signs of the development of diabetes, obesity and hypercholesterolaemia, eg. screen before starting and noting risk factors (including obesity, diabetes, weight, blood pressure and cholesterol levels). Olanzapine is stated to be most likely to increase the risk of weight gain, diabetes and lipid disorders.

1. There appears to be only a clinically insignificant effect from **risperidone** on blood biochemistry (n = 38 632, Veterans, Sernyak *et al*, *Am J Psychiatry* 2002; **159**:561–6) and is probably the least likely of the atypicals to exacerbate or cause diabetes (Gianfrancesco *et al*, *J Clin Psychiatry* 2002; **63**:920–30; n = 38 632, Veterans, Sernyak *et al*, *Am J Psychiatry* 2002; **159**:561–6; n = 79, Newcomer *et al*, *Arch Gen Psychiatry* 2002; **59**:337–45).

2.* **Aripiprazole** is not thought to have any problems in diabetes. With **olanzapine**, 5000 pts

with baseline non-fasting glucose levels of ≤7.8/L, the incidence of raised glucose (≥11 mmol/L, suggestive of diabetes) was 1% (cf 0.9% placebo). Raised levels (8.9–11 mmol/L; suggestive of hyperglycaemia) were 2% with olanzapine (cf 1.6% placebo) and so hyperglycaemia or exacerbation of pre-existing diabetes is in the 'very rare' spontaneous event (<0.01%) category in the UK SPC, although post-marketing surveillance in the UK has shown the incidence of diabetes mellitus to be about 1 in 1000 (eight cases in sample of 8858, Biswasl *et al*, *J Psychopharmacol* 2001; **15**:265–71). There is, however, a significantly increased diabetes risk (UK CSM warning: *Curr Probs* 2002; **28**:3), eg. a population-based study showed that while there was a slight increase in risk with risperidone (odds ratio 2.2), the greatest risk was with olanzapine (odds ratio of 5.8 cf. conventionals or non-antipsychotic treated; n = 19 637, Koro *et al*, *Br Med J* 2002; **325**:243–5). A cohort study indicated that the incidence of new-onset diabetes was about 1%, but 20% higher with olanzapine than risperidone, and 90% higher in the first three months of treatment (n = 33 946, three years, Caro *et al*, *J Clin Psychiatry* 2002; **63**:1135–9). Olanzapine is also associated with a wide range of metabolic abnormalities, eg. weight gain, elevated levels of insulin, leptin and blood lipids (triglycerides and cholesterol), as well as insulin resistance (possibly the predominant mechanism; n = 10, Ebenbichler *et al*, *J Clin Psychiatry* 2003; **64**:1436–9; IS), even in non-obese individuals (n = 24, Henderson *et al*, *J Clin Psychiatry* 2006; **67**:789–97). One study showed that olanzapine (mean 14 mg/d) produced fasting triglyceride levels raised by a mean of 60 mg/dL (37%) (n = 25, 12/52, Osser *et al*, *J Clin Psychiatry* 1999; **60**:767–70), which needs care since triglycerides are a risk factor for precipitation or exacerbation of diabetes (Grundy, *Am J Cardiol* 1998; **81**(4A):18B–25B). Olanzapine may also precipitate or unmask diabetes in susceptible patients (n = 237, Koller and Doraiswamy, *Pharmacotherapy* 2002; **22**:841–52). Routine quarterly glucose monitoring is recommended with olanzapine, regardless of pre-existing diabetes (n = 590, Wirshing *et al*, *J Clin Psychiatry* 2002; **63**:856–65; review by Mir and Taylor, *Int Clin Psychopharmacol* 2001; **16**:63–74).

There is evidence for a slightly increased risk of diabetes with **quetiapine** (n = 38 632, Veterans, Sernyak *et al*, *Am J Psychiatry* 2002; **159**:561–6).

Sertindole may modify insulin and glucose responses and may require adjustments to hypoglycaemic drug doses. Occasional hypoglycaemia and hyperglycaemia have been reported with **zotepine**. Short-term treatment with **ziprasidone** appears to have little effect on glucose levels, and it may actually lower serum cholesterol and triglyceride levels (n = 37, 6/52, open, Kingsbury et al, J Clin Psychiatry 2001;**62**:347–9).

3. * Elevated insulin levels and diabetes have been shown with **clozapine** (n = 41, Melkersson et al, J Clin Psychiatry 1999;**60**:783–91), and a dose-related effect noted, indicating a probable influence on insulin secretion and a causal relationship (n = 384, FDA MedWatch, Koller et al, Am J Med 2001;**111**:716–23). One survey showed that 23% clozapine patients (with no PMH) had elevated plasma glucose (n = 121, Sernyak et al, J Clin Psychiatry 2003;**64**:605–8), and another study showed that clozapine impairs glucose control, independent of changes in insulin sensitivity and BMI (n = 20, open, 4/12, Howes et al, Am J Psychiatry 2004;**161**:361–3). There is also a study showing a non-significant increase in the number of people having or developing type 2 diabetes mellitus and/or impaired glucose tolerance on clozapine compared to depot antipsychotics (n = 130, Hagg et al, J Clin Psychiatry 1998;**59**:294–9). A further study has indicated that patients on clozapine experience significant weight gain and lipid abnormalities (eg. raised serum triglycerides) and have an increased risk (52% over five years) of hyperglycaemia and of diagnosed diabetes mellitus (37% over five years). Weight increase, surprisingly, was not a significant risk factor for developing diabetes (n = 82, naturalistic, five years, Henderson et al, Am J Psychiatry 2000;**157**:975–81, including lengthy discussion of possible mechanisms, similar findings of raised triglycerides in a similar study: n = 222, Gaulin et al, Am J Psychiatry 1999;**156**:1270–2). Addition of quetiapine has been suggested as a possible management option (n = 65, open, 10/12, Reinstein et al, Clin Drug Invest 1999;**18**:99–104). Routine glucose monitoring is recommended with clozapine, regardless of pre-existing diabetes (n = 590, Wirshing et al, J Clin Psychiatry 2002;**63**:856–65; review by Mir and Taylor, Int Clin Psychopharmacol 2001;**16**:63–74).

4. Lack of relationship between serum levels of **zuclopenthixol** (n = 9) and plasma insulin has been shown (Melkersson et al, J Clin Psychiatry 1999;**60**:783–91). The UK SPC for **flupentixol** notes that control of diabetes may be impaired.

5. There are no apparent problems with **sulpiride** and **amisulpride**.

6. There are no apparent problems with **haloperidol**.

7. * The 22 diabetics in a large study of **chlorpromazine** did not show any significant modifications to blood sugar levels. Five patients developed diabetes but all five appeared prone to diabetes, eg. overweight, family history, etc. (n = 850, Schwarz and Munoz, Am J Psychiatry 1968;**125**:253–5). A case-control study of cases of newly-treated diabetes indicated a modest and significant increased risk with **chlorpromazine** and **perphenazine** (n = 7227 + 6780, Wang et al, J Clin Psychopharmacol 2002;**22**:236–43) but lack of relationship between serum levels of perphenazine (n = 12) and plasma insulin has been shown (Melkersson et al, J Clin Psychiatry 1999;**60**:783–91). Many phenothiazines cause weight gain and appetite stimulation which wouldn't help diabetic control.

8. There are no apparent problems with **pimozide** nor **loxapine**.

3.3.2 ANTIDEPRESSANTS

Depression in diabetics may be as common as 27% and sertraline has been recommended as the drug of choice, with the SSRIs being generally preferred to tricyclics in a thorough review (Goodnick et al, J Clin Psychiatry 1995;**56**:128–36). SSRIs may even decrease serum glucose levels by up to 30% and cause anorexia (reducing body weight), and may enable diabetics to control hunger and eating better, via their serotonergic effects, unlike the tricyclics, which often have an appetite-raising effect. Health outcomes among patients with type 1 and type 2 diabetes appear to be poor for those also suffering from depression, possibly due to poorer self-care or an effect on the HPA axis. Outcomes improve with treatment for the depression (n = 276 + 199, Ciechanowski et al, Gen Hosp Psychiatry 2003;**25**:246–52; meta-analysis, s = 24, Lustman et al, Diabetes Care 2000;**23**:934–42).

9. * No dose changes are recommended with **citalopram/escitalopram.** Citalopram has no significant effect on insulin sensitivity in women of

reproductive age (n = 32, RCT, open, 8/52, Kauffman et al, Gynecol Endocrinol 2005;**21**:129–37), and no changes in glycaemic control were seen in another trial (Sindrup et al, Clin Pharmacol Ther 1992;**52**:547–52). Diabetics may become hypoglycaemic during **fluoxetine** treatment (Drug Ther Bull 1990;**28**:33) and its side-effects, eg. tremor, nausea, sweating and anxiety may be mistaken for hypoglycaemia. Most problems have been reported with the more common non-insulin dependent diabetes mellitus (NIDDM, type 2 disease, adult-onset) rather than the insulin dependent form (IDDM, type 1 disease, juvenile-onset). If fluoxetine is used, counsel about this effect, note a possible loss of hypoglycaemic awareness (n = 1, Sawka et al, J Pediatr 2000;**136**:394–6) and regularly check serum glucose levels (review by Salmon, Psychiatr Bull 1995;**19**:553–4). Fluoxetine has been shown to effectively reduce the severity of depression in diabetics with a trend towards better glycaemic control, so it's not all bad news (n = 60, RCT, p/c, 8/52, Lustman et al, Diabetes Care 2000;**23**:618–23). There is a case of **fluvoxamine**-induced acute hyperglycaemia in a diabetic patient (n = 1, Oswald et al, Int J Neuropsychopharmacol 2003;**6**:85–7). Little is reported with **paroxetine**. There have been no major reports of problems with **sertraline**, and maintenance sertraline seems safe and effective in diabetes with a positive effect on the diabetes itself (n = 152, RCT, d/b, p/c, Lustman et al, Arch Gen Psychiatry 2006;**63**:521–9). Sertraline has been recommended as the antidepressant of choice in diabetes (Goodnick et al, J Clin Psychiatry 1995;**56**:128–36). There are, however, cases of hypoglycaemia associated with sertraline (eg. n = 1, Takhar and Williamson, Can J Clin Pharmacol 1999;**6**:12–4; n = 1, Pollak et al, Ann Pharmacother 2001;**35**:1371–4) and raised glucose levels in a diabetic (n = 1, Sansome and Sansome, Int J Psychiatr Med 2003;**33**:103–5).

10. There is no published evidence of problems with **venlafaxine** or **duloxetine**.

11.* **Mirtazapine** does not seem to influence glucose homeostasis (n = 14, Laimer et al, J Clin Psychiatry 2006;**67**:421–4). The manufacturers of mirtazapine recommend care, although this is purely a 'class labelling' precaution.

12. **Tricyclics** may adversely affect diabetic control as they increase serum glucose levels by up to 150%, increase carbohydrate craving

and reduce the metabolic rate, but are generally considered safe unless the diabetes is very brittle. Hypoglycaemia has been associated with maprotiline (n = 1, Isotani and Kameoka, Diabetes Care 1999;**22**:862).

13. There are no apparent problems with trazodone.

14. There are no apparent problems with **reboxetine**.

15. **MAOIs** may decrease serum glucose levels by up to 35% due to a direct influence on gluconeogenesis (Goodnick et al, J Clin Psychiatry 1995;**56**:128–36). Diabetes is a UK SPC precaution for **isocarboxazid**.

16. There is a case of **mianserin** dose-related hyperglycaemia in a non-diabetic woman (Marley and Rohan, Lancet 1993;**342**:1430–1). **Moclobemide** 600mg/d did not modify the effect of glibenclamide on plasma glucose and insulin levels in healthy individuals (Amrein et al, Psychopharmacology 1992;**106**:S24–S31).

3.3.3 ANXIOLYTICS AND HYPNOTICS

17. There is a case of a diabetic presenting with a reduction in insulin requirements after discontinuing **clonazepam** (n = 1, Wagner et al, Diabetes Care 1999;**22**:2099).

18. There are no apparent problems with **buspirone**.

19. There are no apparent problems with **zaleplon**, **zolpidem** and **zopiclone**.

20. **Propranolol** may prolong the hypoglycaemic response to insulin and may effect hypoglycaemic episodes.

21. There are no apparent problems with **clomethiazole** or **chloral hydrate**.

3.3.4 ANTICONVULSANTS

22. There is an isolated report of **carbamazepine**-induced urinary retention in two diabetic patients, where withdrawal improved the condition (Steiner and Birman, Neurology 1993;**43**:1855–6). There are no apparent problems with **oxcarbazepine**.

23. **Valproate** may give false positives in urine tests for diabetes. Protein binding of valproate may be lower in diabetes (Doucet et al, Eur J Clin Pharmacol 1993;**45**:577–9).

24. Hypoglycaemia has been reported with **phenytoin** and glucose metabolism can be affected.

Protein binding of phenytoin may be lower in diabetes (Doucet *et al, Eur J Clin Pharmacol* 1993;**45**:577–9).

25. There are no apparent problems with the **barbiturates**.

26.* There are no apparent problems with **lamotrigine** or **pregabalin**. Blood glucose fluctuations have been reported with **gabapentin** (eg. n = 1, Penumalee *et al, Am J Kid Dis* 2003;**42**:E3–5).

27.* No information is available on **topiramate, zonisamide** and **tiagabine**.

28. There are no apparent problems with **ethosuximide**. Hyperglycaemia has been reported with **acetazolamide** in diabetics and prediabetics, but probably not in non-diabetic patients, so some care may be necessary.

3.3.5 OTHERS

29. There are no apparent problems with **donepezil** or **galantamine**, but diabetes mellitus is a precaution for **rivastigmine**. No effect with **memantine** has been reported.

30. There are no known problems with the **anticholinergic agents**.

31. The literature for **disulfiram** recommends caution in diabetes mellitus. There are no apparent problems with **acamprosate**.

32. There is no problem with **lithium** in diabetes, but many patients on lithium develop polyuria and polydipsia, a diabetes insipidus-like syndrome via an effect on cAMP and vasopressin. This can be controlled by ensuring an adequate fluid and salt intake. There is a case of increased clearance of lithium in a patient with persistent hyperglycaemia, probably due to the subsequent osmotic diuresis increasing renal clearance (n = 1, Cyr *et al, Ann Pharmacother* 2002;**36**:427–9). Lithium may also increase insulin secretion.

33.* There are no apparent problems with **methylphenidate** or **atomoxetine** but a transient loss of appetite may occur. There is no information on **sodium oxybate** and no apparent problems with **modafinil**.

34. Animal studies suggest some risks with **bupropion** and so caution is needed with use in type 2 diabetics (El-Dakhakhny *et al, Arzneimittel-forschung* 1996;**46**:667–9).

35.* There are no precautions for the use of **buprenorphine** in diabetes (UK SPC), nor **methadone**, although the sugar-free liquid would be the presentation of choice for the latter.

3.4 EPILEPSY

	LOWER RISK	MODERATE RISK	HIGHER RISK
Antipsychotics	Amisulpride[5] Aripiprazole[2] Haloperidol[6] Pimozide[8] Quetiapine[2] Risperidone?[1] Sulpiride[5] Zuclopenthixol[4]	Olanzapine[2] Phenothiazines (most)[7] Sertindole[2] Ziprasidone[2]	Chlorpromazine[7] Clozapine[3] Loxapine[8] Zotepine[2]
Antidepressants	MAOIs[15] Moclobemide?[16] Reboxetine[14] SSRIs[9] Tryptophan[16]	Duloxetine[10] Mianserin[16] Mirtazapine[11] Trazodone[13] Tricyclics (most)[12] Venlafaxine[10]	Amoxapine[12] Maprotiline[12]
Anxiolytics and hypnotics	Benzodiazepines[17] Beta-blockers[20] Chloral[21] Clomethiazole[21] Zaleplon[19] Zolpidem[19] Zopiclone[19]	Buspirone[18]	
Others	Acamprosate[24] Anticholinergics[23] Modafinil[26]	Anticholinesterases[22] Atomoxetine[26] Disulfiram[24] Lithium[25] Memantine[22] Methylphenidate[26]	Bupropion[27] Sodium oxybate [26]

GENERAL PRINCIPALS* (Pisani et al, Drug Safety 2002;**25**:91–110, 166 refs)

Risk factors for psychotropic-induced seizures:

- History of epilepsy (inc. febrile seizures) in the patient or their family.
- Neurological abnormalities (inc. brain injury, angioma cavernous, blood-brain barrier abnormality).
- Cerebral arteriosclerosis.
- Elderly.
- Reduced drug clearance.
- Pre-existing EEG alterations.
- Physical illness (eg malignant hypertension).
- Polypharmacy.

Practical recommendations in pre-existing epilepsy:

- Use anticonvulsants with psychotropic properties where possible (eg. carbamazepine, lamotrigine or valproate).
- Avoid high-risk drugs.
- Start low and go slow, monitoring plasma levels and EEG where possible.
- Keep dosing simple and avoid polypharmacy.

3.4.1 ANTIPSYCHOTICS

General principals

1. Keep the daily dose as low as possible; the proconvulsive effect may be dose-related.

2. Take extra care where risk factors exist, including head trauma, previous seizure history and concomitant drugs (especially other antipsychotics). The most susceptible patients are those with a history of epilepsy, a condition that predisposes to epilepsy and those withdrawing from central depressants, eg. benzodiazepines and alcohol.

3. Use lowest risk drugs unless essential.

4. Use a slow rate of introduction and withdrawal. Anticonvulsant cover may be appropriate.

5. Dose changes should be small and gentle.

6. Avoid antipsychotics having more antihistaminic, antiserotonergic, sedative and antiadrenergic effects, which may have a greater seizure threshold lowering effect.

Review: * general (Hedges et al, Drugs Today [Barc] 2003;**39**:551–7).

1. There is little adverse information about **risperidone**. Pre-marketing trials showed a seizure incidence of 0.3% (n = 2607).

2. * In pre-marketing trials, seizures occurred in only 0.1% patients taking **aripiprazole**, but should probably still be used with caution in epilepsy. The literature for **olanzapine** states that it should be used cautiously in patients with a history of seizures. Unexplained seizures (ie. patients without reported risk factors) occurred in up to 0.88% patients during pre-marketing trials (n = 2500). There may be a slightly higher risk of seizures in people over 65. The incidence of seizures during **quetiapine** trials has been equivalent to placebo. **Sertindole** should be used with caution in patients with a history of seizures, as an incidence of seizures of 1% (n = 2194) was shown in clinical studies. **Zotepine** has an established dose-related proconvulsive effect. It should not be used in patients with a personal or family history of epilepsy. The risk of seizures is dose-related and rises particularly above 300 mg/d (open, n = 129, Hori et al, Jpn J Psychiatry Neurol 1992;**46**:161–7). Seizures occurred in 0.4% patients during pre-marketing trials with **ziprasidone** (many with confounding factors), but it would be wise to use with caution in epilepsy.

3. **Clozapine** can cause dose-related seizures, the risk rising from 1% (< 300 mg/d), through 2.7% (300–600 mg/d) to 4.4% (> 600 mg/d). EEG changes occur in 75% people on clozapine, with up to 40% having paroxysmal discharges (reviewed by Pacia and Devinsky, Neurology 1994;**44**:2247–9). A more rapid dose-titration increases the risk. Many centres use valproate as routine anticonvulsant cover at higher doses of clozapine. See also 4.2.2 and 6.3.

4. **Zuclopenthixol** may have only mild to moderate effects, with few adverse reports, and may be one of the drugs of choice.

5. There are no known problems with **amisulpride**, but a spontaneously resolving generalised convulsion occurred after a 3 g overdose (Tracqui et al, Hum Exp Toxicol 1995;**14**:294–8). **Sulpiride** may be a reasonable choice, with a few cases of convulsions reported and only minimal EEG effects, although care is recommended in unstable epilepsy.

6. **Haloperidol** may have only mild to moderate effects, and may be a lower risk drug.

7. **Fluphenazine** may have a low proconvulsive effect (JAMA 1980;**244**:1460–3), although status epilepticus has been reported (n = 1, Leksowski, Psychiatr Pol 1983;**17**:445–7). The incidence of seizures with **chlorpromazine** may be 9% at doses above 1 g/d and 0.5% at less than 1 g/d and is best avoided.

8. **Pimozide** may have a low effect as, although it may enhance spike activity at low dose, it may not do so at higher dose (Oliver et al, Arch Gen Psychiatry 1982;**39**:206–9). **Loxapine**, however, lowers the seizure threshold and can cause convulsions even at normal doses.

3.4.2 ANTIDEPRESSANTS *

Unless a large scale trial is carried out (unlikely), the safest antidepressant in epilepsy will remain unknown. All patients require an individual assessment of their risk factors and recognition that there is a dose-dependent relationship between antidepressants and seizures. A **slow rate of introduction** reduces the risk. **Lamotrigine** has proved useful for interictal depression (n = 13, open, Kalogjera-Sackellares and Sackellares, Epilepsy Behav 2002;**3**:510–6), as well as in bipolar depression. In a post-hoc analysis of patients with MDD and TLE, antidepressants were effective, with no serious ADRs and no increase in seizures with citalopram, reboxetine and mirtazapine (n = 75, RCT, Kuhn et al, Epilepsy Behav 2003;**4**:674–9).

Reviews: Curran and de Pauw, Drug Saf

1998;**18**:125–33, 60 refs; Pisani *et al*, *Epilepsia* 1999;**40**[Suppl 10]:S48–S56.

9. * Serotonin function is unlikely to be of major importance in the genesis of seizures and so **SSRIs** are likely to have a low proconvulsive effect. **Citalopram** and **escitalopram** have not been reported to interact with anticonvulsants or to have a proconvulsive effect, and has been used for interictal depression without an increase in seizure frequency or severity (n = 43, 8/52, Hovorka *et al*, *Epilepsy Behav* 2000;**1**:444–7; n = 75, RCT, Kuhn *et al*, *Epilepsy Behav* 2003;**4**:674–9). **Fluoxetine** has a probable seizure incidence of 0.2%, similar to other antidepressants. In an open study of 17 patients with complex partial seizures (with and without secondary generalisation), the addition of fluoxetine in six resulted in the disappearance of seizures and a 30% reduction in the other 11 (n = 17, open, add-on, Favale *et al*, *Neurology* 1995;**45**:1926–7). **Fluvoxamine** probably has a low proconvulsive effect, although this has been disputed (Vincenti, *Lancet* 1990;**336**:947) and there have been some literature reports of fits. **Paroxetine** appears to have a minimal potential for producing seizures at clinically useful doses (Sedgwick *et al*, *J Psychopharmacol* 1987;**1**:31–4). Seizures have occurred rarely in trials and no cause-effect relationship has been proven (Milne and Goa, *Drugs* 1991;**41**:450–77). With **sertraline**, seizures occurred in early clinical trials at a similar frequency to placebo and only in people with a history of seizures.

10. Seizures have been reported in 0.26% of patients treated with **venlafaxine** during clinical trials and so a slow introduction and withdrawal is recommended. For **duloxetine**, there is a UK SPC caution for epilepsy but no reported problems as such.

11. One grand mal seizure has been reported in a patient with a history of seizures receiving **mirtazapine** at a high dose of 80mg/d during a trial. More definite information would be needed before a cause-effect link could be made. Care and monitoring would thus be standard.

12. All **tricyclics** seem to lower the seizure threshold, with **amitriptyline** reputed to be the most proconvulsive and **doxepin** possibly of lowest risk. TDM of tricyclics minimises the risk of toxicity (review by Preskorn and Fast, *J Clin Psychiatry* 1992;**53**:160–2). There is a high incidence of literature reports of convulsions with

maprotiline (Edwards, *Lancet* 1979;**ii**:1368–9) plus some EEG abnormalities (*Am J Med Genetics* 1988;**1**:369–73) and should be avoided. A slow rate of introduction reduces the risk (*Psychol Med* 1977;**7**:265–70).

13. The literature for **trazodone** was recently changed to include care in epilepsy, and to avoid abrupt changes in dose.

14. **Reboxetine** may be particularly useful in epilepsy with a low interaction potential and a spontaneous incidence of seizures of <0.2% (n = 1500), with no seizures in overdose.

15. **MAOIs** are generally not considered epileptogenic at therapeutic doses (n = 198, retrospective, Rabkin *et al*, *J Clin Psychopharmacol* 1984;**4**:270–8). MAOI-induced myoclonic jerks (review by Lieberman *et al*, *J Clin Psychopharmacol* 1985;**5**:221–8) and serotonin syndrome can occasionally be interpreted as seizures.

16. There have been no reports of problems with **moclobemide** or **tryptophan** in epilepsy to date. **Mianserin** is often quoted as being relatively safe in epilepsy (n = 40, Edwards and Glen-Bott, *Br J Clin Pharmacol* 1983;**15**:299S–311S). One study of 84 overdoses of 1 g or more showed no convulsions (*Curr Med Res Opin* 1980;**6**:44). Seizures have been reported at therapeutic doses of **amoxapine** although the literature states that this only occurs outside the recommended dosage range.

3.4.3 ANXIOLYTICS AND HYPNOTICS

17. For **benzodiazepines** in epilepsy, see *1.17*.

18. Animal studies show **buspirone** to have no anticonvulsant activity. The literature states buspirone to be contraindicated in epilepsy but there is no evidence that it is actually epileptogenic.

19. A weak anticonvulsant activity for **zopiclone** has been shown (Julou *et al*, *Pharmacol Biochem Behav* 1985;**23**:653–9). **Zolpidem** is not reported to have any anticonvulsant activity. There is no data on **zaleplon**.

20. There are no apparent problems with the **beta-blockers**.

21. For **chloral hydrate** and **clomethiazole**, see *1.17.1*.

3.4.4 OTHERS

22. **Cholinomimetics** may have some potential

for causing seizures so care is needed with **donepezil** in pre-existing seizure activity. Care should be exercised with the use of **rivastigmine** in patients predisposed to seizures. There has been no increase in the incidence of convulsions with **galantamine** in clinical trials. A single case report with **memantine** suggests it should only be used with caution.

23. There are no problems reported with the **anticholinergic** agents.

24. The literature for **disulfiram** recommends caution in epilepsy. The manufacturers report no known problems with **acamprosate** in epilepsy.

25. **Lithium** has a marked epileptogenic activity in overdose, but probably has no effect at standard dose. **Carbamazepine** and **valproate** may be suitable alternatives.

26. * **Methylphenidate** is not associated with significant risk at therapeutic doses (mentioned in Zaccara et al, Drug Saf 1990;**5**:109–51), but the literature suggests caution. **Sodium oxybate** has been reported to cause seizures and use is not recommended in epilepsy (SPC). The MHRA guidance is that **atomoxetine** should be introduced with caution in patients with a history of seizure and discontinuing considered if seizures start or increase in frequency. There are no apparent problems with **modafinil**.

27. **Bupropion** has some epileptogenic activity (literature warning: Curr Prob Pharmacovig 2001; **27**:5). The risk of seizures is about 4 in 1000, and there appears to be a correlation between plasma concentration and the risk for seizures. Doses should not exceed 450 mg/d (although new-onset seizures can occur at therapeutic doses up to 450 mg/d, eg. Pesola and Avasarala, J Emerg Med 2002;**22**:235–9), no single dose should be above 200 mg and doses should not be increased at more than 150 mg/d. It should be contraindicated in people with a history of seizures and concurrent eating disorder, known CNS tumor, and if abruptly withdrawing from benzodiazepines or alcohol. Other risk factors include concomitant use with any drug known to lower the seizure threshold, alcohol abuse, history of head trauma, diabetes treated with hypoglycaemics or insulin, and the use of stimulants or anorectics.

3.5 GLAUCOMA (narrow-angle)

	LOWER RISK	MODERATE RISK	HIGHER RISK
Antipsychotics	Butyrophenones[2] Risperidone[3] Sertindole[2] Sulpiride[3] Thioxanthenes[2]	Aripiprazole[2] Clozapine[2] Loxapine[2] Phenothiazines[1] Ziprasidone[2] Zotepine[2]	Olanzapine[3]
Antidepressants	Flupentixol[5] MAOIs[5] Moclobemide[5] Trazodone[5] Tryptophan[5] Venlafaxine[5]	Duloxetine[5] Mirtazapine[5] SSRIs[5]	Tricyclics[4]
Others	Acamprosate[6] Benzodiazepines[6] Caffeine[8] Clomethiazole[6] Disulfiram[6] Gabapentin[6] Lithium[6] Lofexidine[6] Memantine[10] Naltrexone[6] Phenobarbital[6] Phenytoin[6] Tiagabine[6] Valproate[6] Vigabatrin[6]	Atomoxetine[9] Anticholinergics[10] Carbamazepine[6] Dexamfetamine[7] Methylphenidate[9] Topiramate[6]	

Narrow-angle glaucoma (also called angle closure glaucoma or narrow angle glaucoma) occurs in eyes with a narrow anterior chamber angle, where drainage of the aqueous fluid through the anterior chamber angle is reduced or blocked. Drugs with anticholinergic properties have the potential to either induce narrow-angle glaucoma or to worsen it. Although the degree of anticholinergic effect of a drug is of relevance, the individual's susceptibility to those effects is of greater importance (review by Lam et al, Curr Opin Ophthalmol 2007;**18**:146–51).

GENERAL RECOMMENDATIONS
Patients with shallow anterior chamber and/or narrow angles, or with previously diagnosed glaucoma may be treated with drugs with anticholinergic properties provided intraocular pressure is monitored, an ophthalmologist is involved and information is given on the symptoms of acute-angle closure, with a recommendation to stop the drug and seek medical attention immediately should those symptoms occur. In a patient with a shallow anterior chamber and narrow angles an ophthalmologist would normally perform an iridotomy or some type of drainage surgery to allow drug use. Treatment with miotic therapy, eg. pilocarpine may not necessarily protect the patient with narrow angles against drug-induced angle closure. Indeed, pilocarpine itself has been reported to rarely cause pupillary block (Zimmerman et al, Ophthalmology 1981;**88**:85–8).

The main symptoms of acute narrow-angle glaucoma are blurred vision, 'coloured halos' around bright lights, intense pain, lacrimation, lid oedema, red eye, nausea and vomiting (review by Oshika, *Drug Saf* 1995;**12**:256–63). The incidence rises with age due to the aging process, eg. thickening of the lens. The peak effect from a drug on intraocular pressure can occur within 5–24 hours (or sooner) (Lieberman and Stoudemire, *Psychosomatics* 1987;**28**:145–8).

3.5.1 ANTIPSYCHOTICS

1. **Phenothiazines** are weak anticholinergics so some potential for problems exists. Screening for glaucoma has been recommended before initiating therapy (Reid et al, *Int Pharmacopsych* 1976;**11**:163–74), although several studies have shown no detectable narrow-angle glaucoma in, eg. 100 patients taking **thioridazine**, 98 on **fluphenazine** and 99 on **chlorpromazine** (Applebaum, *Arch Ophthalmol* 1963;**69**:578–80). Thus, there is need for routine care (see introduction). There are a few case reports of single high-dose injection of IV or IM chlorpromazine producing a transient decrease in intraocular pressure (mentioned in review by Bristow and Hirsch, *Drug Saf* 1993;**8**:136–48, 76 refs).

2. *Other antipsychotics with similar anticholinergic effects would include **clozapine**, **loxapine**, **flupentixol**, **zotepine** and **zuclopenthixol**. No information is available on **ziprasidone**, **aripiprazole** or **sertindole**.

3. Antipsychotics with little or no anticholinergic effect must still be considered to have a potential for problems, albeit probably at a low level, eg. **sulpiride**, **haloperidol** and **risperidone**. **Olanzapine**, is, however, contraindicated in narrow-angle glaucoma.

3.5.2 ANTIDEPRESSANTS

4. **Tricyclics** generally have a greater anticholinergic effect than phenothiazines. If patients are at risk of narrow-angle glaucoma, pre-treatment examination by an ophthalmologist is recommended. Patients with a narrow anterior chamber angle who are receiving glaucoma treatment or who have had laser treatment should have few problems provided care (see introduction) is taken (Oshika, *Drug Saf* 1995;**12**:256–63). There is a report of

four patients with narrow angles all developing acute-angle closure glaucoma with **imipramine** (Ritch et al, *Arch Ophthalmol* 1994;**112**:67–8), and with **clomipramine**, exacerbated by postural hypotension (Schlingemann et al, *Lancet* 1996;**347**:465). A survey by Reid and Blouin (*Psychosomatics* 1976;**17**:83–5) showed no abnormal intraocular pressures in patients taking tricyclics, even in combination with **phenothiazines**. A postal survey of ophthalmologists and psychiatrists indicated that occasional, probably drug-induced, cases had been seen, most frequently associated with **amitriptyline** (review by Lieberman and Stoudemire, *Psychosomatics* 1987;**28**:145–8). See general recommendations.

5. *Antidepressants which can cause dilation of the pupil include the **SSRIs**, **mirtazapine**, **moclobemide**, **trazodone** (case of aggravated angle-closure glaucoma with low-dose trazodone: Pae et al, *Psych Clin Neurosci* 2003;**57**:127–8) and **MAOIs**. There is a possible case with **fluoxetine** in a patient sensitive to anticholinergic effects and with a positive family history (Ahmad, *DICP Ann Pharmacother* 1991;**25**:436). Uveal effusions and bilateral angle-closure glaucoma have been reported with **escitalopram** (n=1, Zelefsky et al, *Am J Ophthalmol* 2006;**141**:1144–7) and acute angle-closure glaucoma with complete recovery from **citalopram** (n=1, Croos et al, *BMC Ophthalmol* 2005;**5**:23). Acute narrow-angle glaucoma associated with **paroxetine** has been reported (n=7, Eke and Bates, *Br Med J* 1997;**14**:1387), as has aggravation of narrow-angle glaucoma by **fluvoxamine** (n=1, Jimenez-Jimenez et al, *Ann Pharmacother* 2001;**35**:1565–6). There is limited experience with **reboxetine** but the literature recommends close supervision. Raised intraocular pressure or narrow-angle glaucoma is a warning in the UK SPC for **venlafaxine**, and bilateral acute narrow-angle glaucoma has been reported as developing rapidly with venlafaxine (n=1, Ng et al, *Med J Aust* 2002;**176**:241). Mydriasis has been reported with **duloxetine**, so caution is necessary in patients with raised intraocular pressure or at risk of acute narrow-angle glaucoma.

3.5.3 OTHERS

6. *There are no reported problems with any of the mood stabilisers, anxiolytics, hypnotics

or anticonvulsants, except **topiramate**, which has a particular problem. There are reports of reversible acute secondary narrow-angle glaucoma (n = 86, Fraunfelder et al, Ophthalmology 2004;**111**:109–11; n = 1, Sachi and Vijaya, J Postgrad Med 2006;**52**:72–3) occurring within a month of starting treatment, and of bilateral angle-closure glaucoma (n = 1, Levy et al, Can J Ophthalmol 2006;**1**:221–5; n = 1, Mansoor and Jain, Acta Ophthalmol Scand 2005;**83**:27–8; n = 1, Coats, J AAPOS 2003;**7**:303; Noentert et al, Neurology 2003;**61**:1306; discussion of possible mechanisms: Craig et al, Am J Ophthalmology 2004;**137**:193–5). The UK SPC notes that symptoms usually start within the first month and include decreased visual acuity and/or ocular pain. If this occurs, topiramate should be discontinued as soon as clinically feasible and appropriate measures to reduce intraocular pressure (see also Curr Probs 2002;**28**:4).

7. **Amfetamine** causes a transient rise in intraocular pressure, which is not associated with closure of the angle.

8. **Caffeine** has been reported to cause a transient rise in intraocular pressure, which is not associated with closure of the angle. Average daily intakes of more than 180 mg/d caffeine (not a lot by the author's standards) may cause a clinically significant elevation of intraocular pressure (n = 28, Avisar et al, Ann Pharmacother 2002;**36**:992–5).

9. * **Methylphenidate** causes a transient rise in intraocular pressure but which is not associated with closure of the angle. There is a single case of uneventful use of methylphenidate in a 55-year-old male with ADHD and primary open-angle glaucoma well-controlled by pilocarpine and betaxolol (Bartlik et al, Arch Gen Psychiatry 1997; **54**:188–9). The UK SPC lists glaucoma as a contraindication for **atomoxetine**.

10. * **Anticholinergics** are contraindicated in narrow-angle glaucoma. There is a case of angle-closure glaucoma after discontinuing **donepezil** (n = 1, Enzenauer and Bowers, J Geront A Biol Sci Med Sci 2005;**60**:1083). Glaucoma is not mentioned in the literature for **memantine**.

3.6 HEPATIC IMPAIRMENT

	LOWER RISK	MODERATE RISK	HIGHER RISK
Antipsychotics	Amisulpride[5] Aripiprazole[2] Flupentixol[4] Haloperidol[6] Pimozide[8] Sulpiride[5] Ziprasidone[2] Zuclopenthixol[4]	Clozapine[3] Loxapine[8] Olanzapine[2] Phenothiazines[7] Quetiapine[2] Risperidone[1] Sertindole[2]	Zotepine[2]
Antidepressants	Mianserin[16] Paroxetine[9] Tryptophan[16]	Duloxetine[10] Mirtazapine[11] Moclobemide[16] Reboxetine[14] SSRIs[9] St John's wort[16] Trazodone[13] Tricyclics[12] Venlafaxine[10]	Lofrepramine[12] MAOIs[15]
Anxiolytics and hynpotics	Lorazepam LD[17] Oxazepam LD[17] Temazepam LD[17]	Buspirone[18] Clomethiazole[21] Propranolol LD[20] Zaleplon[19] Zolpidem[19] Zopiclone[19]	Benzodiazepines (esp LA)[17] Chloral[21] Propranolol HD[20]
Anticonvulsants	Carbamazepine[22] Ethosuximide[28] Gabapentin[26] Pregabalin[27] Topiramate?[27] Vigabatrin[27]	Acetazolamide[28] Benzodiazepines[17] Lamotrigine[26] Levetiracetam[27] Oxcarbazepine[22] Paraldehyde[28] Tiagabine[27]	Barbiturates[25] Fosphenytoin[24] Phenytoin[24] Valproate[23]
Others	Buprenorphine[36] Donepezil[29] Lithium[32] Memantine[29]	Acamprosate[31] Anticholinergics[30] Atomoxetine[34] Bupropion[35] Disulfiram[31] Galantamine[29] Methadone[36] Methylphenidate[34] Modafinil[33] Rivastigmine[29]	

LD = low dose   HD = high dose
SA = short-acting   LA = long-acting

GENERAL PRINCIPALS (ADAPTED FROM *MAUDSLEY GUIDELINES*)

1. The greater the degree of hepatic impairment, the greater the degree of impaired drug metabolism, and the greater the risk of drug toxicity, and so the starting and final dose should be lower. People may be more sensitive to common or predictable side-effects.
2. Start low, go slow, and monitor LFTs regularly (eg. weekly).
3. LFTs do not necessarily correlate well with metabolic impairment, although they can give a reasonable indication.
4. Care is needed with drugs with a high first-pass clearance effect.
5. In severe liver disease, avoid drugs with the marked side-effects of sedation and constipation.

3.6.1 ANTIPSYCHOTICS

1. Unbound **risperidone** levels increase in liver impairment and so initial doses and dose increments should be halved, and 4 mg/d not exceeded. Risperidone-induced jaundice has been reported (n = 1, Oyewole *et al*, *Int J Geriatr Psychiatry* 1996;**11**:179), as has rapid onset hepatotoxicity (n = 1, Phillips *et al*, *Ann Pharmacother* 1998;**32**:843).
2. No changes in dose with **aripiprazole** seem necessary with mild, moderate or severe hepatic impairment. A lower **olanzapine** starting dose of 5 mg/d may be appropriate. Transient, asymptomatic elevations in ALT and AST have been noted and monitoring of these in patients with risk factors (eg. hepatic impairment, concomitant hepatotoxic drugs) may be appropriate. A single-dose study with **quetiapine** showed some reduced clearance so the starting dose should be 25 mg/d, with dose increments of 25–50 mg/d (Thyrum *et al*, *Prog Neuropsychopharmacol Biol Psychiatry* 2000;**24**:521–33). Hepatic clearance of **sertindole** is reduced by a half in hepatic impairment, so use slower titration, lower maintenance doses and monitor closely. Sertindole is contraindicated in severe hepatic failure. **Zotepine** levels may be 2–3 times higher with hepatic impairment, so start at 25 mg BD up to a maximum of 75 mg BD and measure LFTs weekly for the first three months. **Ziprasidone** is extensively metabolised

and an extended half-life has been shown in Child-Pugh Class A and B, but dose adjustment is not necessary in mild to moderate impairment (n = 30, open, Everson *et al*, *Br J Clin Pharmacol* 2000;**49**(S3):21–6).
3. Severe hepatic disease is a contraindication for **clozapine**, and so lower doses, regular plasma level monitoring and LFT monitoring would be necessary if used. There are reported cases of toxic hepatitis, with AST levels dramatically raised, eosinophilia developing early and full LFT normalisation within 4–5 weeks of stopping (eg. Thatcher *et al*, *Am J Psychiatry* 1995;**152**:296–7).
4. No dosage adjustments are necessary for **flupentixol** or **zuclopenthixol**, although both undergo hepatic metabolism and so some caution would be wise in significant hepatic impairment.
5. **Sulpiride** and **amisulpride** are virtually un-metabolised with little or no biliary excretion. There is a low incidence of liver toxicity reported, with a transient rise in serum transaminase the only reported effect. Dosage adjustments are thus unnecessary (SPC).
6. There are no apparent problems with **halo-peridol**, although the UK SPC states liver disease to be a caution.
7. **Phenothiazines** (particularly chlorpromazine) may cause hepatocanalicular cholestasis and there have been suggestions of immunological liver damage. Onset is usually during the first month of therapy. Coma may be precipitated due to increased cerebral neuron sensitivity.
8. **Loxapine** is extensively metabolised so use in severe liver disease is likely to be of a higher risk, although no specific problems have been reported. **Pimozide** should be used with caution in hepatic impairment (UK SPC).

3.6.2 ANTIDEPRESSANTS

9. * **Citalopram** and **escitalopram** are metabolised extensively by the liver, with three major meta-bolites. Doses at the lower end of the therapeutic range should be used (n = 1000, Milne and Goa, *Drugs* 1991;**41**:450–77), although no liver enzyme abnormalities were noted in this study. In hepatic impairment, alternate day-dosing of **fluoxetine** is recommended. Patients with cirrhosis show higher plasma levels of fluoxetine and **norfluoxetine** and lengthened half-lives, and a 50% reduction in dose is recommended, especially if a low albumin is

present. **Fluvoxamine** should be started at 50mg/d and monitored carefully, as raised hepatic enzymes have been reported. **Paroxetine** appears to be the safest option, using doses at the lower end of the therapeutic range, although cases of hepatitis (Benbow and Gill, *Br Med J* 1997;**314**:1387) and hepatotoxicity have been reported (n = 3, Azaz-Livshits *et al*, *Pharmacopsychiatry* 2002;**35**:112–5). **Sertraline** is extensively metabolised by the liver and is contraindicated in significant hepatic dysfunction. One study has shown a 2.5–fold increase in half-life and a 1.6–fold increase in sertraline/desmethylsertraline peak levels in 10 patients with stable chronic cirrhosis (cf 10 controls, Demolis *et al*, *Br J Clin Pharmacol* 1996;**42**:394–7; case of hepatotoxicity where rechallenge led to recurrent hepatitis: n = 1, Persky and Reinus, *Dig Dis Sci* 2003;**48**:939–44).

10. * **Venlafaxine** clearance is reduced by about 35% in mild to moderate hepatic impairment, and so doses should be reduced by about 25–50% respectively, although there is much interpatient variability (Anon, *J Clin Psychiatry* 1993;**54**:119–26) and is not recommended in severe hepatic impairment. **Duloxetine** is contraindicated in liver disease causing hepatic impairment (UK SPC). Moderate liver disease (Child-Pugh class B) increases the half-life 2.3-fold and AUC 3.7-fold. The FDA in 2006 noted that duloxetine can cause hepatitis and jaundice, and people with pre-existing liver disease may be at risk of additional problems. There is no data in mild or severe hepatic insufficiency.

11. **Mirtazapine** clearance was reduced by 33% in moderate hepatic impairment in a single dose study (n = 16, Murdoch *et al*, *Br J Clin Pharmacol* 1993;**35**:76P), and so dosage reduction may be necessary. Transient asymptomatic raised liver enzymes (eg. SGTP) have been noted in a few patients in early clinical trials.

12. Most **tricyclics** have a high first-pass clearance by the liver, and so lower starting doses are necessary. Increased sedation with tricyclics is likely to be due to decreased metabolism, eg. amitriptyline has been reported to have doubled or tripled plasma levels in patients with cirrhosis and should be avoided. Increased blood levels may also occur with reduced plasma protein-binding if albumin levels are lower, as with many tricyclics protein-binding is high. Particular care is obviously needed if albumin levels are low. SSRIs such as paroxetine would appear to be easier

to use than tricyclics in liver disease. Cholestatic jaundice has occasionally been noted with tricyclics. **Lofepramine** is contraindicated in severe liver disease.

13. **Trazodone** should be used with care in severe hepatic impairment, as hepatoxicity has been reported (n = 1, Rettman and McClintock, *Ann Pharmacother* 2001;**35**:1559–61).

14. **Reboxetine's** half-life and plasma levels appear to rise in severe hepatic insufficiency and dose adjustment may be necessary. A starting dose of 2 mg BD is recommended (n = 12, Tran *et al*, *Clin Drug Invest* 2000;**19**:473–7).

15. **MAOIs** are hepatotoxic and may precipitate coma. Patients may also be more sensitive to side-effects. If essential, start with a low dose, increase gradually and observe carefully. **Isocarboxazid** is contraindicated with any degree of impaired hepatic function.

16. **Moclobemide's** clearance can be reduced and half-life increased in cirrhosis and so doses should be reduced by a 25–33% to avoid accumulation (Stoeckel *et al*, *Acta Psychiatr Scand* 1990;**360**[Suppl]:94–7). There are no apparent problems with **mianserin** and **tryptophan**. St **John's wort** levels may rise in moderate liver cirrhosis and absorption is decreased in mild cirrhosis (n = 16, Johne *et al*, *Clin Pharmacol Ther* 2002;**71**:P95).

3.6.3 ANXIOLYTICS AND HYPNOTICS

17. The metabolism of **diazepam** and **chlordiazepoxide** is impaired in liver disease. The half-lives of the metabolites desmethylchlordiazepoxide and demoxepam are reported to be prolonged to up to 346 hours and 150 hours respectively (n = 1, Barton *et al*, *Med Tox Adv Drug Exp* 1989;**4**:73–6) which may induce coma, and may be detectable two months after stopping treatment in patients with hepatic encephalopathy (Meier *et al*, *Gastroenterology*, 1991;**101**:274–5). Impaired metabolism has been reported with **alprazolam**, **clobazam** and **midazolam** (significantly impaired in cirrhosis, as it is metabolised by at least three different P450 enzymes, Wandel *et al*, *Br J Anaesthesia* 1994;**73**:658–61). The metabolism of **lorazepam**, **temazepam** and **oxazepam** is unchanged and in low dose these are probably the benzodiazepines of choice (reviewed by Peppers, *Pharmacotherapy* 1996;**16**:49–58).

18. **Buspirone** plasma levels are higher in patients with hepatic failure, with a good correlation between steady-state buspirone levels and serum albumin (open, Barbhaiya et al, Eur J Clin Pharmacol 1994;**46**:41–7). Caution is recommended with a history of hepatic impairment and it should not used in severe hepatic disease.

19. Elimination of **zopiclone** can be reduced with hepatic dysfunction, producing enhanced adverse effects (n = 17, open, Parker and Roberts, Br J Clin Pharmacol 1983;**16**:259). A lower dose of 3.75 mg to 7.5 mg (but no higher) can be used with caution in hepatic disease. Plasma protein binding of **zolpidem** is reduced in hepatic impairment (n = 42, open, Pacifici, Int J Clin Pharmacol Ther Toxicol 1988;**26**:439–43) and it is contraindicated in severe hepatic insufficiency. Reduced doses are recommended in cirrhosis and other hepatic impairment (where half-life may rise to 10 hours). Hepatoxicity has been reported (n = 1, Karsenti et al, Br Med J 1999;**318**:1179). **Zaleplon** is contraindicated in severe hepatic insufficiency and the dose reduced to 5 mg in mild to moderate hepatic impairment.

20. The metabolism of **propranolol** is impaired in decompensated liver disease and by portal systemic shunting. High doses are potentially toxic and so reduced oral doses are needed. Propranolol may increase the risk of developing hepatic encephalopathy.

21.* **Clomethiazole** clearance is reduced by 50% in moderate to severe liver impairment, but with sedation not significantly enhanced in the majority (n = 24, Centerholt et al, Eur J Clin Pharmacol 2003;**59**:1117–22). In severe liver disease a ten-fold increase can occur, so reduced oral doses are needed, eg. a third of normal, and noting that sedation can mask the onset of hepatic coma. **Chloral hydrate** is contraindicated in marked hepatic impairment.

3.6.4 ANTICONVULSANTS

22. Serious problems with **carbamazepine** are rare, but jaundice, hepatitis and liver function disorders have been reported, and so use should be with caution. Although **oxcarbazepine** is rapidly and extensively metabolised, no dose adjustments are generally needed in mild to moderate hepatic impairment. It has not been studied in severe hepatic impairment.

23. * **Valproate** is contraindicated in active liver disease, as it can be hepatotoxic and liver failure can occur in about 1 in 10000 cases. The risk is higher early on in therapy and lessens after a couple of months (review by Eadie et al, Med Tox 1988;**3**:85–106). Electron-microscopy shows lipid droplets and a scarcity of cytoplasmic cells and normal mitochondria (Caparros-Lefebvre et al, Lancet 1993;**341**:1604). Hepatotoxicity occurs mostly in children and presents as worsening epilepsy, drowsiness and with biochemical and/or clinical evidence of liver failure. Some fatal cases have been reported. Care needs to be taken if valproate is used in children, especially if used with other anticonvulsants. Valproate use may be possible in patients with hepatitis C, provided ALT is closely monitored (n=564, Felker et al, Am J Psychiatry 2003;**160**:174–8).

24. **Phenytoin** is highly protein bound and extensively metabolised and so accumulation and toxicity may occur in severe liver disease. Use reduced doses and monitor for toxicity. In uraemia, protein-binding may be reduced but active/free levels remain unchanged so therapeutic control may be possible at plasma levels below the usual range. Severe cardiovascular ADRs have been reported with **fosphenytoin** IV (see 3.2.4), and a reduction in loading dose and/or infusion rate by 10–25% is recommended in hepatic impairment.

25. Increased cerebral sensitivity and the impaired metabolism of **barbiturates** may precipitate coma. Plasma albumin-binding may be reduced but this may have no clinical effect.

26. **Gabapentin** is virtually unmetabolised and so dose adjustments are unnecessary. No adjustment to initial and maintenance doses of **lamotrigine** is necessary for Child-Pugh grade A cirrhosis but should be reduced by 50% in moderate (Child-Pugh grade B) hepatic impairment, and by 75% in severe (Child-Pugh grade C) impairment (n = 36, Marcellin et al, Br J Clin Pharmacol 2001;**51**:410–4).

27. * No dose adjustment of **levetiracetam** is necessary in Child-Pugh classes A and B, but in class C start with half the normal dose as total clearance is reduced by about 57% (n = 16, Brockmoller et al, Clin Pharmacol Ther 2005;**77**:29–41). No dose adjustments are necessary for **pregabalin** in hepatic impairment. **Tiagabine** is metabolised by the liver. Initial doses in mild to moderate hepatic impairment should

be lower. Use in severe hepatic impairment is not recommended (n = 13, open, 8/7, Lau et al, Epilepsia 1997;**38**:445–51). **Topiramate** is not extensively metabolised and about 60% is excreted unchanged via the kidneys. In moderate-to-severe liver disease, clearance is reduced by about 26% although the resultant changes in plasma levels have been considered clinically insignificant by the manufacturers. **Vigabatrin** can cause decreased LFT levels but there is no evidence of hepatic toxicity. **Zonisamide** has not been studied in hepatic impairment so caution is needed.

28. There are no apparent problems with **ethosuximide**. **Acetazolamide** should be used with caution. **Paraldehyde** elimination is slower in hepatic failure and so lower doses may be needed.

3.6.5 OTHERS

29. * **Donepezil** 5 mg/d can be safely given in mild to moderate (Child-Pugh grade A or B) hepatic impairment (n = 35[c = 32], Reyes et al, Br J Clin Pharmacol 2004;**58**[Suppl 1]:9–17, MS), and a 5 mg single-dose study indicated that compromised hepatic function did not significantly alter its kinetics (n = 20, Tiseo et al, Br J Clin Pharmacol 1998;**46**[Suppl 1]:51–5). **Rivastigmine** is contraindicated in severe liver impairment. **Galantamine** is not affected by mild hepatic impairment but clearance is reduced by 23% in moderate impairment and so care is necessary in moderate-to-severe impairment (n = 25, open, Zhao et al, J Clin Pharmacol 2002;**42**:428–36). Start with 4 mg/d, increasing slowly to a maximum of 8 mg BD. In severe impairment (Child-Pugh score > 9), galantamine is contraindicated (due to current lack of safety data). There is no data for the use of **memantine** in hepatic impairment but since it is metabolised only to a minor extent to inactive metabolites, mild to moderate hepatic impairment is unlikely to have a significant effect.

30. The literatures for the **anticholinergics** all urge some caution in hepatic disease.

31. The literature for **disulfiram** recommends caution in liver disease. Although some evidence of further raised LFTs was noted, an open trial showed disulfiram was safe in patients with elevated LFTs and/or evidence of Hepatitis C virus, provided LFTs were monitored regularly (n = 57, Saxon et al, J Clin Psych 1998;**59**:313–6). The literature for **acamprosate** states that use in severe hepatic failure (Child-Pugh grade C) is a contraindication but the pharmacokinetics are not altered in mild to moderate hepatic dysfunction.

32. There are no problems with **lithium** in liver disease.

33. * The maximum **modafinil** dose of 400 mg/d should only be used in the absence of hepatic impairment. The starting dose of **sodium oxybate** should be halved in hepatic impairment as the elimination half-life is increased (UK SPC).

34. * There is no data on **methylphenidate**. The UK SPC recommends possible **atomoxetine** dose modification in hepatic impairment and rare (1 in 50 000 patients) cases have been reported of severe acute hepatitis with markedly elevated hepatic enzymes and bilirubin (MHRA warning).

35. **Bupropion** is extensively metabolised and there are rare reports of abnormal LFTs, liver damage and hepatotoxicity, with some metabolite half-lives prolonged in cirrhosis. Reduced initial doses and close monitoring is required, as a prolonged half-life has been reported in hepatic failure (n = 16, open, DeVane et al, J Clin Psychopharmacol 1990;**10**:328–32).

36. * Cases of QT interval prolongation and torsades de pointes have been reported during treatment with **methadone** (particularly at doses > 100 mg/d) and liver disease (a risk factor for prolonged QTc) is a UK SPC caution. **Buprenorphine** is primarily metabolised by glucuronidation (Tegeder et al, Clin Pharmacokinet 1999;**37**:17–40) and so should have a low risk in mild to moderate hepatic impairment, although it is contraindicated in severe hepatic insufficiency as this may, in itself, possibly be associated with hepatic events (UK SPC).

3.7 OLD AGE

	LOWER RISK	MODERATE RISK	HIGHER RISK
Antipsychotics	Amisulpride[5] Aripiprazole[2] Risperidone[1] Sulpiride[5] Ziprasidone[2]	Butyrophenones[6] Loxapine[8] Olanzapine[2] Phenothiazines[7] Quetiapine[2] Sertindole[2] Thioxanthenes[4]	Clozapine[3] Pimozide[8] Thioridazine[7] Zotepine[2]
Antidepressants	Duloxetine[10] Lofepramine[12] Mirtazapine[11] Moclobemide[16] SSRIs[9] Tryptophan[16] Venlafaxine[10]	Flupentixol[4] MAOIs[15] Mianserin[16] Nortriptyline[12] Reboxetine[14] Trazodone[13]	Tricyclics[12]
Anxiolytics and hypnotics	Alprazolam[17] Buspirone[18] Clobazam[17] Lorazepam[17] Oxazepam[17] Oxprenolol[20] Zaleplon[19] Zopiclone[19]	Clomethiazole[21] Flunitrazepam[17] Flurazepam[17] Propranolol[20] Temazepam[17] Zolpidem[19]	Benzodiazepines, long-acting[17]
Anticonvulsants	Carbamazepine[22] Clobazam[17] Oxcarbazepine[22] Tiagabine[27] Topiramate?[27]	Barbiturates[25] Clonazepam[17] Gabapentin[26] Lamotrigine[26] Levetiracetam[27] Piracetam?[27] Pregabalin[27] Valproate[23]	Acetazolamide[28] Benzodiazepines (most)[17] Fosphenytoin[24] Paraldehyde[28] Phenytoin[24] Vigabatrin[27]
Others	Anticholinesterases[29] Bupropion[35] Memantine[29] Modafinil[33] Sodium oxybate[33]	Anticholinergics[30] Lithium[32]	Acamprosate?[31] Methlyphenidate[34]

In the elderly, drug absorption and distribution are altered, metabolism, cardiac output and renal perfusion are reduced and tissue sensitivity is usually increased.

GENERAL PRINCIPALS (ADAPTED FROM MAUDSLEY GUIDELINES)

1. Increased sensitivity to drugs occurs due to age-related changes in pharmacokinetics (ADME and protein binding) and pharmacodynamics (eg. neuronal changes, and receptor binding). The over 70s have about twice as many ADRs as under 50s, eg. postural hypotension with antipsychotics, longer sedation with hypnotics and increased sensitivity to anticholinergic side-effects of drugs.

2. Hepatic changes (eg. reduced metabolism) and reduced renal clearance will affect many drugs.

3. The lowest effective dose should be used (so 'start low and go slow'), avoid polypharmacy and monitor effects (both positive and negative) regularly and frequently.

4. Avoid drugs with sedative and hypotensive effects, which can increase the under-rated risks of falls. A meta-analysis concluded that psychotropics are associated with a small increase in falls (Leipzig et al, J Am Geriatr Soc 1999;**47**:30–9; reviewed by Shorr, EBMH 1999;**2**:95).

5. Use drugs only when necessary, decide a treatment aim, keep therapy simple, use the smallest effective doses and discontinue gradually if no apparent benefit can be seen, as accumulation of a drug can lead to the subtle and insidious development of side-effects.

6. Most drugs are highly lipophilic and an increased fat to lean body mass ratio, in addition to decreased metabolism and excretion, means that half-lives usually increase.

7. Consider other factors, eg. potential poor compliance due to social or physical reasons, or use of OTC medicines.

Reviews: geriatric psychopharmacology (Turnheim, Exp Gerontol 2003;**38**:843–53; Zubenko and Sunderland, Harvard Rev Psych 2000;**7**:311–33, 202 refs), anticholinergic side-effects (Mintzer and Burns, J Royal Soc Med 2000;**93**:457–62, 37 refs).

3.7.1 ANTIPSYCHOTICS *

Antipsychotics can relieve psychotic symptoms in older adults but pre-treatment assessment, repeated every 3–6 months, is recommended to detect common side-effects such as postural hypotension, anticholinergic effects and Parkinsonism. Single daily doses are usually appropriate once stable (as indeed they are in younger adults). Doses should be reviewed regularly, and a periodic reduction in dose (eg. by 10–25% every four weeks) for some patients may be indicated. recent licensing changes have meant that an association between antipsychotics (especially risperidone and olanzapine) and cerebrovascular events has been highlighted. The evidence for a causal relationship is highly debatable. An enormous Medicaid analysis was unable to show that atypicals (including risperidone) were more likely to

cause CVEs than haloperidol or benzodiazepines (n = 8million, Finkel et al, Int Psychogeriatr 2005;**17**;617–29) and a prospective nursing home study failed to show that antipsychotics increased mortality in dementia (n = 273, 12/12, Suh et al, Int Psychogeriatr 2005;**17**:429–41), nor do risperidone, olanzapine and quetiapine seem to increase the risk of weight gain or diabetes in Alzheimer's patients in nursing homes (n = 36, open, 12/12, Rondanelli et al, Minerva Med 2006;**97**:147–51).

Reviews: general (Sciolla and Jeste, Int J Psychiatr Clin Prac 1998;**2**:S27–34, 55 refs), atypicals in elderly (Yiu-Chung et al, Pharmacotherapy 1999;**19**:811–22; Jeste et al, Am J Geriatr Psychiatry 1999;**7**:70–6; Bouman and Pinner, Adv Psychiatr Treat 2002;**8**:49–58).

1. * **Risperidone** is partially metabolised to an active metabolite and so lower doses may be needed only if hepatic impairment is present (see 3.6.1). Significant age-related differences have been noted, with higher plasma levels in patients over 40 years, and with a 30% increase per decade of life (n = 129, Aichhorn et al, J Psychopharmacol 2005;**19**:395–401). The UK CSM now recommends not using risperidone in elderly demented people with behavioural problems, due to an increased risk of stroke (2.7% vs 1% on placebo), although the absolute risk is low, and the alternatives are not risk-free. The restriction does not apply to elderly demented people without behavioural problems.

2. * No **aripiprazole** dose adjustments are necessary in the elderly. The UK CSM recommends not using **olanzapine** in elderly demented people with behavioural problems, due to an increased risk of stroke (2% vs 1% on placebo), although the absolute risk is low, and the alternatives are far from risk-free. The restriction does not apply to elderly demented people without behavioural problems, where a lower starting dose of 5 mg/d may be appropriate as the mean elimination half-life is 50% longer and clearance slightly reduced in otherwise healthy elderly patients. Periodic blood pressure monitoring is recommended and there may be a slightly higher risk of seizures in people over 65. Transient sedation and somnolence were more marked in the elderly in pre-marketing trials. A naturalistic study showed olanzapine was well-tolerated and superior to haloperidol for acute schizophrenia in elderly patients (n = 20, RCT,

open, Barak et al, Prog Neuropsychopharmacol Biol Psychiatry 2002;**26**:1199–202; review of use in psychosis in old age: Madhusoodanan et al, Ann Clin Psychiatry 2001;**13**:201–13). **Quetiapine** (mean 200 mg/d, range 50–800 mg/d) appears effective and safe in elderly in-patients, but there is a wide and diagnosis-dependent (eg. higher in functional psychosis) dosing range (n = 100 [c = 91], Yang et al, J Psychopharmacol 2005;**19**:661–6). The mean clearance in elderly patients is 30–50% lower than healthy adults so the starting dose should be 25 mg/d, with dose increments of 25–50 mg/d. Quetiapine may be well-tolerated and clinically effective in elderly patients, with somnolence (32%), dizziness (13%) and postural hypotension (13%) the most common side-effects (n = 151, open, 12/52, McManus et al, J Clin Psychiatry 1999;**60**:292–8). It may be a suitable alternative to olanzapine and risperidone, although orthostatic hypotension is more common in the elderly. There is no difference in **sertindole** kinetics in young and elderly adults, but a slower dose titration and perhaps lower final doses may be needed if an increased sensitivity to alpha-blocking activity produces hypotension. **Zotepine** levels may be 2–3 times higher in elderly patients, so start at 25 mg BD up to a maximum of 75 mg BD. Age and gender does not influence the kinetics of **ziprasidone** (n = 35, Wilner et al, Br J Clin Pharmacol 2000;**49**[Suppl 3]:S15–S20).

3. * **Clozapine** may be safe, reasonably well-tolerated (with slower dose titration) and effective in the elderly (n = 133, Barak et al, Compr Psychiatry 1999;**40**:320–5) at doses as low as 50–100 mg, with 6.25–50 mg/d suggested as the optimal dosage (review by Hoeh et al, J Geriatr Psychiatry Neurol 2003;**16**:213–8). There may be an increased incidence of agranulocytosis, so great care should be taken.

4. **Zuclopenthixol** and **flupentixol** should be used with caution in renal disease. Lower doses of flupentixol may be needed due to altered kinetics (review: Jann et al, Clin Pharmacokinet 1985;**10**:315–33), and, as with other antipsychotics, the elderly suffer more side-effects (Balant-Gorgia and Balant, Clin Pharmacokinet 1987;**13**:65–90).

5. Single doses of **amisulpride** are well-tolerated and show a similar pharmacokinetic profile in healthy elderly and young subjects (n = 20, open, Hamon-Vilcot et al, Eur J Clin Pharmacol 1998; **54**:405–9).

6. For the **butyrophenones**, an increased severity of side-effects including EPSE, sedation, hypotension and respiratory depression may occur and so lower starting doses are indicated.

7. It is generally recommended that 33–50% of the adult dose of **phenothiazines** should be used for elderly patients, who are more susceptible to Parkinsonian side-effects (n = 120, open, Caligiuri et al, J Clin Psychopharmacol 1999;**19**:322–8), and which are often then harder to manage. **Thioridazine** should be avoided, as should **chlorpromazine**. **Levomepromazine** is not recommended for use in people over 50 unless the risk of hypotension has been assessed.

8. Doses of **loxapine** of around 40 mg/d have been used (n = 26, open, 12/52, Branchey et al, J Am Geriatr Soc 1978;**26**: 263–7).

3.7.2 ANTIDEPRESSANTS *

Depression increases mortality in the elderly with cardiac disease, so it should not be ignored, especially if long-standing and severe (n = 652, Geerlings et al, Psychol Med 2002;**32**:609–18). Drugs with anticholinergic side-effects may further harm an already compromised cholinergic system. Heart failure is particularly marked in women with depression (n = 2501, 14 years, Williams et al, Psychosom Med 2002;**64**:6–12). A robust trial showed no difference in response between venlafaxine, fluoxetine and placebo in old age depressed out-patients, although the placebo group responded significantly well (n = 300, RCT, p/c, d/b, 8/52, Schatzberg and Roose, Am J Geriatr Psychiatry 2006;**14**:361–70).

9.* **SSRIs** have obvious advantages over other antidepressants in the elderly (fewer anticholinergic effects, a benign cardiovascular profile, ease of use and safety in overdose) but have some unappreciated risks, including hyponatraemia, weight loss, sexual dysfunction, drug interactions (review: Herrmann, Can J Clin Pharmacol 2000;**7**:91–5) and SSRIs may increase the risk of falls and osteoporotic fractures in people aged over 50 (n = 5008, 137 on SSRIs, Richards et al, Arch Int Med 2007;**167**:188–94). A prolonged **citalopram** half-life (up to 3.8 days) and raised steady-state plasma levels may be due to reduced metabolism, with side-effects more prevalent in the elderly, particularly bradycardia, nausea, sweating and headache (n = 1344, > 6/52,

Barak et al, Prog Neuropsychopharmacol Biol Psychiatry 2003;**27**:545–8). Dose reduction (by up to 50%) has been suggested but normal adult doses have been used in some studies with no apparent problem (eg. n = 96, d/b, 6/52, Bouchard et al, Acta Psychiatr Scand 1987;**76**:583–92). In a recent study, however, citalopram 10–40mg/d in people over 75 was no more effective than placebo, although there was huge inter-individual variation (n = 174, RCT, p/c, 8/52, Roose et al, Am J Psychiatry 2004;**161**:2050–9). The manufacturers recommend a starting dose of 20mg/d in all patients. An initial dose of 5mg daily for the first two weeks of treatment is recommended for **escitalopram,** increasing to 10mg/d Depending on individual patient response, the dose may be increased to 10mg/d. The half-life of **fluoxetine** appears not to be significantly different in the elderly (open, 7/7, Lemberger et al, J Clin Psychiatry 1985;**46**:14–9). In an open study of depressed and physically ill hospitalised elderly patients with multiple pathology and polypharmacy, fluoxetine was claimed to be a safe and effective antidepressant in this difficult to treat cohort (n = 20, open, Evans and Lye, J Clin Exp Gerontol 1992;**14**:297–307). No pharmacokinetic differences have been seen with **fluvoxamine** in the elderly and so no dose alterations are necessary (n = 19, open, de Vries et al, Ther Drug Monitor 1992;**14**:493–8) and 200mg/d seems as equally well-tolerated and effective in old age depression as sertraline 150mg/d (n = 93, RCT, d/b, 7/52, Rossini et al, J Clin Psychopharmacol 2005;**25**:471–5). Initially, lower doses of 10mg are recommended for **paroxetine,** as blood levels with 20mg/d in the elderly can be similar to those of 30mg/d in younger people (n = 21, open, 7/52, Lundmark et al, Acta Psychiatr Scand 1989;**80**[Suppl 350]:76–80; review of paroxetine in old age Holliday and Plosker, Drugs Aging 1993;**3**:278–99). **Sertraline** clearance may be slightly reduced and the half-life increased in elderly volunteers, but this does not seem to warrant dosage adjustment (n = 44, open, 30/7, Ronfeld et al, Clin Pharmacokin 1997;**32**[Suppl 1]:S22–S30). It improves depression and is tolerable in elderly even with significant comorbid medical status (n = 752, RCT, d/b, p/c, 8/52, Sheikh et al, J Am Geriatr Soc 2004;**52**:86–92; review by Kurzthaler and Fleischhacker, EBMH 2004;**7**:82).

10. * **Venlafaxine** clearance is reduced by about 15% in the elderly, probably due to reduced renal function, but dosage adjustment is not generally considered necessary (Anon, J Clin Psychiatry 1993;**54**:119–26). However, venlafaxine (up to 150mg/d) may be less well-tolerated and possibly less safe than sertraline (up to 100mg/d) in elderly frail populations (n = 32, RCT, d/b, Oslin et al, J Clin Psychiatry 2003;**64**:875–82; comment by Schneider, EBMH 2004;**7**:47). Postural hypotension may be more common. **Duloxetine's** half-life is about 25% longer in the elderly but no dose adjustment is necessary. It is not recommended in the over 75s, due to lack of safety data rather than the presence of negative information.

11. **Mirtazapine** dosage is the same in the elderly as younger adults, although the manufacturers recommend care with dosage increments, eg. 15–45mg/d has equivalent efficacy to sub-therapeutic amitriptyline 30–90mg/d, but relatively fewer cardiac effects (n = 115, d/b, Hoyberg et al, Acta Psychiatr Scand 1996;**93**:184–90). It appears to be slightly quicker acting and better tolerated than paroxetine in elderly depressed patients (n = 255, RCT, d/b, 8+16/52, Schatzberg et al, Am J Geriatr Psychiatry 2002;**10**:541–50).

12. Reduced initial doses of **tricyclics** are recommended, with perhaps slightly lower final doses, depending upon tolerance, as cognitive and central effects are enhanced in the elderly.

Clomipramine was as well-tolerated in patients 56–70 years old as in younger adults, although postural hypotension and anticholinergic side-effects were more common (n = 150, Stage et al, Acta Psychiatr Scand 2002;**105**:55–9). Single night-time doses of **dosulepin** have been used in the elderly with no increase in side-effects (n = 50, s/b, 4/52, Khan, J Int Med Res 1981;**9**:108–12). Higher serum levels occur with standard doses (reviewed by Hicks et al, J Clin Psychiatry 1981; **42**:374–85) with reduced clearance and doubled half-life shown with **imipramine** (open, Benetello et al, Int J Clin Pharmacol Res 1990;**10**:191–5). Elderly patients may respond to lower doses of **lofepramine** but in depressed elderly in-patients, low dose lofepramine (70mg/d) appears no better than placebo, indicating that full, or at least higher, doses are necessary (n = 63. 4/52, Tan et al, Br J Clin Pharmacol 1994;**37**:321– 4). **Nortriptyline** kinetics appear the same in the elderly as the young (n = 22, mean age 84, open, Katz et al, Neuropsychopharmacology 1989;**2**:229–

36) although individual variation is high and the elderly may respond to lower doses (Kanba et al, Prog Neuropsychopharmacol Biol Psychiatry 1992;16:301–9). ECG changes may occur so care is needed in cardiovascular disease.

It has been noted that when tricyclic non-response has occurred in an elderly person, response to an alternative antidepressant may take up to 5–6 weeks, rather than the 3–4 weeks normally expected (n = 101, open, Flint and Rifat, J Affect Disord 1996;36:95–105), so do not give up too soon.

13. * Single daily dosing of **trazodone** (except when used as a hypnotic) may not be appropriate in the elderly, and reduced doses may be better, eg. one study showed 150 mg/d to be the optimum in the elderly (n = 20, d/b, Mukherjee and Davey, J Int Med Res 1986;14:279–84), as higher plasma levels (n = 97, Prapotnik et al, Int J Clin Pharmacol Ther 2004;42:120–4) and a longer half-life (men only, n = 43, open, Greenblatt et al, Clin Pharmacol Ther 1987;42:193–200) occur in the elderly.

14. The incidence of side-effects with **reboxetine** is no greater in the elderly than in younger people, although the half-life may be doubled (Holm and Spencer, CNS Drugs 1999;12:65–83) and peak plasma levels are also over twice that in younger people (n = 12, Bergmann et al, Eur J Drug Metab Pharmacokinet 2000;25:195–8). The starting dose should probably be 2 mg BD. A delayed lowering of potassium levels and some treatment-emergent tachycardia has been reported. Frail elderly may need dose reductions. The UK SPC does not recommend use in the elderly, due to lack of positive information rather than the presence of negative information.

15. Although **MAOIs** are often considered as more toxic to the elderly, mainly due to postural hypotension and dizziness, they can be highly effective in resistant depression in the elderly (review by Volz and Gleiter, Drugs Aging 1998;13:341–55).

16. **Moclobemide** is considered to be safe, effective and having a seemingly beneficial effect on a range of cognitive functions (use in the elderly reviewed by Nair et al, Acta Psychiatr Scand 1995;91[Suppl 386]:28–35). One trial in elderly depressed and/or demented patients showed it to cause no cognitive impairment, if not a slight improvement (n = 694, d/b, p/c, Roth et al, Br J Psychiatry 1996;168:149–57). **Mianserin**

elimination is highly variable and often prolonged in the elderly (n = 27, open, Begg et al, Br J Clin Pharmacol 1989;27:445–51). Doses may need to be adjusted, although reduced receptor sensitivity may not necessarily lead to increased side-effects. There are no apparent problems with **tryptophan**.

3.7.3 ANXIOLYTICS AND HYPNOTICS

A meta-analysis showed that improvements in sleep with sedative use are significant in the elderly, albeit of small magnitude, but that ADRs and the risk of falls is clinically relevant (s = 24, n = 2417, RCT, Glass et al, Br Med J 2005;331:1169).

Reviews: * management of insomnia in elderly (Bain, Am J Geriatr Pharmacother 2006;4:168–92), sleep in the elderly (Asplund, Drugs Aging 1999;14:91–103).

17. * All **benzodiazepines** should be used with care in the elderly, as side-effects are likely to be enhanced eg. sedation, disturbances in gait, daytime drowsiness, cognitive impairment, hypotension, memory impairment and reduced psychomotor performance. Half-lives are generally lengthened, sometimes only in men, although there is considerable interpatient variability. Prolonged half-lives in the elderly have been reported with **clonazepam** (n = 25, open, Court and Kase, J Neurol Neurosurg Psychiatry 1976;39:297), **clobazam** (n = 29, open, Greenblatt et al, Br J Clin Pharmacol 1981; 12:631–6), **flunitrazepam** (review by Davis and Cook, Clin Pharmacokinet 1986;11:18–35), **nitrazepam**, **flurazepam**, **chlordiazepoxide**, **clorazepate**, **bromazepam** (n = 32, open, Ochs et al, Clin Pharmacol Ther 1987;41:562–70), **diazepam** (n = 24, single dose study, Pomara et al, J Clin Psychiatry 1985;46:185–7) and **midazolam** (n = 18, open, Albrecht et al, Clin Pharmacol Therap 1999;65:630–9). **Temazepam** is relatively safe over 8/52 and CBT may slightly improve the response (n = 60, RCT, 8/52, Morin et al, Hum Psychopharmacol 2003;18:75–82). Normal adult doses of **oxazepam** can be used as there are apparently no clinically significant pharmacokinetic changes in the elderly (Dreyfuss et al, J Clin Psychiatry 1986;47:511–4). If used as a hypnotic, **lorazepam** doses should probably be slightly reduced. **Loprazolam** appears well-tolerated in the elderly, with a half-life similar to young adults, although peak levels are prolonged

(n = 12, Dorling and Hindmarsh, *Drugs Exp Clin Res* 2001;**27**:151–9).

18. There do not appear to be any significant changes in the pharmacokinetics of **buspirone** in the elderly and so dose adjustments are not considered necessary (n = 48, open, Gammans et al, *J Clin Pharmacol* 1989;**29**:72–8).

19.* Normal adult doses of **zopiclone** can be used (Goa and Heel, *Drugs* 1986;**32**:48–65). In elderly people, **zolpidem** at 5 mg is an effective hypnotic dose with no consistent memory or performance effects nor daytime drowsiness (n = 221, Roger and Attali, *Clin Therap* 1993;**15**:127–36), with doses of 10 mg or above reducing REM sleep slightly (n = 30, Scharf et al, *J Clin Psychiatry* 1991;**52**:77–83). In a comparison of zolpidem, zopiclone and lormetazepam in elderly patients, zolpidem caused least cognitive, memory and equilibrium adverse effects and should thus be the preferred hypnotic in the elderly (n = 48, RCT, d/b, p/c, c/o, Allain et al, *Eur J Clin Pharmacol* 2003;**59**:179–88). There appears to be no problem with **zaleplon** in the elderly.

20. Increased **propranolol** side-effects have been reported in the elderly and so reduced initial doses are generally recommended, unlike **oxprenolol** where dose reduction is not considered necessary.

21. **Clomethiazole** doses should be reduced, as the half-life can be at least doubled and plasma levels up to five times normal can occur (Dehlin, *Acta Psychiatr Scand* 1986;**73**[Suppl 329]:112–5).

3.7.4 ANTICONVULSANTS

For anticonvulsants, it is best to avoid renally excreted drugs (eg. **gabapentin**) as the renal excretion of some drugs may be significantly reduced in the elderly compared with younger people. Hepatically metabolised drugs, eg. **carbamazepine** and **lamotrigine** are not influenced by age and are to be preferred.

Reviews: management of epilepsy in old age (Stephen and Brodie, *Lancet* 2000;**355**:1441–6; Bourdet et al, *J Am Pharm Assoc (Wash)* 2001; **41**:421–36; Lackner, *Pharmacotherapy* 2002; **22**: 329–64, 301 refs).

22. * No significant changes have been shown with **carbamazepine** in the elderly (eg. n = 10, Read et al, *Seizure* 1998;**7**:159–62) and so dose

requirements are likely to be the same, although the elderly may be more susceptible to cardiac arrhythmias (Richens, *Pharm J* 1993;**251**:50). Although the AUC with **oxcarbazepine** may be 30–60% higher in the elderly, tolerability is comparable to that in adults (n = 52 cf 1574 adults, Kutluay et al, *Epilepsy Behav* 2003;**4**:175–80). No dose recommendations exist, other than gradual dose titration (n = 48, van Heiningen et al, *Clin Pharmacol Ther* 1991;**50**:410–9), and a lower dose recommended if the patient has compromised renal function.

23. * **Valproate's** half-life may be doubled in the elderly, possibly via reduced metabolism (n = 13, open, Bryson et al, *Br J Clin Pharmacol* 1983;**16**:104–5), but total blood levels are similar to younger adults (n = 12, open, 5/7, Bauer et al, *Clin Pharmacol Ther* 1985;**37**:697–700). A naturalistic retrospective study of valproate in elderly patients showed a 62% response rate, no LFT abnormalities and it was well tolerated (n = 35, retrospective, Kando et al, *J Clin Psychiatry* 1996;**57**:238–40). The proportion of unbound drug may be increased via reduced protein binding but, overall, the effect is likely to be of low significance. However, CNS side effects and nausea are correlated with total and unbound levels, and hence likely to be increased (n = 6, s/b, Felix et al, *J Clin Psychopharmacol* 2003;**23**:471–8). Compared to younger adults, valproate may have a different therapeutic window (65–90mcg/mL) if used for mania in the elderly (n = 59, retrospective, Chen et al, *J Clin Psychiatry* 1999;**60**:181–6).

24. Reduced doses of **phenytoin** may be needed with the elderly. Careful monitoring is necessary, especially in those with hypoalbuminaemia or renal disease, as these individuals may have an increased level of side-effects and risk of toxicity (Hayes et al, *Br J Clin Pharmacol* 1975;**2**:73–9), including cardiac arrhythmias. In people aged from 60 to 80, doses 20% lower will maintain blood levels, compared to younger adults (n = 92, open, Bauer and Blouin, *Clin Pharmacol* 1982;**31**:301–4). It may be that reduced doses are only needed with monotherapy, as opposed to anticonvulsant polypharmacy (review by Bachmann and Belloto, *Drugs Aging* 1999;**15**:235–50). Severe cardiovascular ADRs have been reported with **fosphenytoin** IV (see *3.2*), and a reduction in the loading dose and/or infusion rate by 10–25% in the elderly is recommended.

25. The half-lives of **phenobarbital** and **primidone** are longer in the elderly due to reduced metabolism and so reduced doses should be used (reviewed by Hicks et al, J Clin Psychiatry 1981: **42**:374–85).

26. * **Lamotrigine** is hepatically metabolised and this is influenced by genetic factors rather than age. An increased volume of distribution in the elderly has been shown to increase the half-life of lamotrigine, thus increasing the chance of side-effects, and so reduced doses may be needed. One study, however, showed that the half-life does not appear to be increased in the elderly (Betts, Seizure 1992;**1**:3–6). **Gabapentin** clearance is reduced in old age, probably via reduced renal clearance (Boyd et al, Pharm Res 1990;**7**[Suppl]:S215), although it seems to cause less cognitive impairment than carbamazepine in healthy senior adults (n = 34, RCT, c/o, Martin et al, Epilepsia 2001;**42**:764–71). It has been successful and well-tolerated as add-on therapy for neuroleptics or valproate in geriatric mania (n = 7, open, Sethi et al, J Geriatr Psychiatry Neurol 2003;**16**:117–20).

27. * **Levetiracetam** seems well-tolerated in the elderly, with only headache and tremor occurring more frequently (n = 719 + 1510 + 1023, Cramer et al, Epilepsy Res 2003;**56**:135–45), although reduced doses are recommended in renal impairment (see 3.9.4). No age-related changes in pharmacokinetics have been detected with **topiramate**. The half-life of **piracetam** is extended in the elderly (n = 10, open, Platt et al, Arzneimittel Forschung 1985;**35**:533–5). There is no need to adjust the dose of **tiagabine** on the basis of age, although slightly higher plasma levels may occur in the elderly (n = 24, Snel et al, J Clin Pharmacol 1997;**37**:1015–20). Reduced **pregabalin** doses may be necessary due to decreased renal function (see 3.9.4). **Vigabatrin** is renally excreted and this may be reduced in the elderly to one sixth compared to younger people. Reduced doses have been recommended in people with a creatinine clearance of less than 60ml/min (Grant and Heel, Drugs 1991;**41**:889–926) and it should be avoided in the elderly.

28. Lower **acetazolamide** doses are indicated (n = 12, open, Chapron et al, J Clin Pharmacol 1989;**29**:348–53). Deaths have been reported in debilitated patients given only 8ml **paraldehyde**,

and so use should be with the utmost caution (Baratham and Tinckler, Med J Aust, 1964;**51**:877).

3.7.5 OTHERS

29. There are no specific problems with **donepezil** and **rivastigmine**, provided the dose titration guidelines are followed. **Galantamine** levels are about 30–40% higher in elderly patients than healthy young individuals. **Memantine** has a usual maximum dose of 20mg/d.

30. Confusion can be induced in the elderly by further compromising brain cholinergic activity. An initial low dose is thus usually recommended for **benzhexol/trihexyphenidyl** and **orphenadrine**. Clearance of **procyclidine** may be reduced in the elderly and so BD dosing may be more appropriate than TDS dosing (n = 6, RCT, p/c, Whiteman et al, Eur J Clin Pharmacol 1985;**28**:73–8).

31. The UK SPC for **acamprosate** states that it should not be used in the elderly, due more to lack of data rather than specific reported problems.

32. Reduced **lithium** clearance occurs in the elderly through reduced renal function and increased volume of distribution (review by Sproule et al, Drugs Aging 2000;**16**:165–77), so doses should be reduced by as much as 50%. The elderly may also develop symptoms of lithium toxicity at standard therapeutic blood levels (Nakra and Grossberg, J Geriatr Drug Ther 1987;**2**:47–63). However, lithium can be safely used in the elderly if monitored closely and frequently and, just to prove it, a cross-sectional study in octogenarians showed that lithium can be well-tolerated provided serum levels and renal and thyroid function are monitored regularly (n = 12, Fahy and Lawlor, Int J Geriatr Psychiatry 2001;**16**:1000–3). Hypothyroidism can also occur.

33. * In the elderly, a **modafinil** starting dose of 100mg/d is recommended. **Sodium oxybate** may cause cognitive impairment so care might be needed (SPC).

34. There is no data for **methylphenidate**, but it has been used for depression in the elderly.

35. **Bupropion** appears well-tolerated in the elderly, although some accumulation and greater side-effects might occur (Branconnier et al, J Clin Psychiatry 1983;**44**:130–3). It has been used successfully for depression in the elderly (n = 100, RCT, Weihs et al, J Clin Psychiatry 2000;**61**:196–202).

3.8 PREGNANCY

	LOWER RISK (FDA = A)	MODERATE RISK (FDA = B OR C)	HIGHER RISK (FDA = D OR X)
Antipsychotics		Aripiprazole[2] Butyrophenones[6] Clozapine[3] Loxapine[8] Olanzapine[2] Phenothiazines[7] Quetiapine[2] Risperidone[1] Sertindole[2] Sulpiride[5] Thioxanthenes[4] Ziprasidone[2]	Zotepine[2]
Antidepressants	Flupentixol?[4] Tryptophan?[16]	Duloxetine[10] MAOIs[15] Mianserin[16] Mirtazapine[11] Moclobemide[16] SSRIs (except paroxetine)[9] St John's wort[16] Trazodone[13] Tricyclics[12] Venlafaxine[10]	Paroxetine[9] Reboxetine[14]
Anxiolytics and hynpotics	Chloral[21] Clomethiazole[21]	Beta-blockers[20] Buspirone[18] Chlordiazepoxide[17] Clonazepam[17] Oxazepam[17] Promethazine[21] Zaleplon[19] Zolpidem[19] Zopiclone[19]	Alprazolam[17] Lorazepam[17] Temazepam[17]
Anticonvulsants		Acetazolamide[28] Clonazepam?[17] Gabapentin[26] Lamotrigine[26] Levetiracetam[27] Oxcarbazepine[22] Paraldehyde[28] Pregabalin?[27] Tiagabine[27] Topiramate[27]	Benzodiazepines[17] Carbamazepine[22] Ethosuximide[28] Fosphenytoin[24] Phenobarbital[25] Phenytoin[24] Valproate[23] Vigabatrin[27] Zonisamide[27]

Others		Acamprosate[31]	Lithium[32]
		Anticholinergics[30]	Methadone HD[34]
		Anticholinesterases[29]	
		Atomoxetine[35]	
		Buprenorphine[34]	
		Bupropion[36]	
		Dextroamfetamine[35]	
		Disulfiram[31]	
		Memantine[29]	
		Methylphenidate[35]	
		Modafinil[33]	
		Methadone LD[34]	
		Sodium oxybate[33]	

The **FDA** has established five categories to indicate a drug's potential for teratogenicity, and, where known, these classifications are noted in the text:

A Controlled studies in women fail to show a risk in the first trimester and the risk of fetal harm seems remote.

B Either animal tests do not show a risk but there are no human studies or animal studies show a risk but human studies have failed to show a risk to the fetus.

C Either animal studies show teratogenic or embryocidal effects but there are no controlled studies in humans or there are no studies in either animals or humans.

D Definite evidence of a risk to the fetus exists, but the benefits in certain circumstances (eg. life-threatening situations) may make use acceptable.

X Fetal abnormalities have been shown in animals or humans or both and the risk outweighs any possible benefits.

The **Australian (ADEC) pregnancy category definitions** (in brief) are:

A Drug has been taken by a large number of pregnant women with no proven increase in malformations or other direct or indirect harmful effects on the fetus.

B1 Drug has been taken by a limited number of pregnant women with no proven increase in malformations or other direct or indirect harmful effects on the fetus. Animal studies have not shown evidence of fetal damage.

B2 As B1, but animal studies are inadequate or lacking, but other evidence shows no evidence of fetal damage.

B3 As B1, but animal studies have shown evidence of an increased occurrence of fetal damage of uncertain significance.

C Drugs that have caused or are suspected of causing an increase in fetal malformations or irreversible damage.

X High risk of causing permanent damage so should not be used in pregnancy or where there is a possibility of pregnancy.

Where known, both the FDA and ADEC categories are quoted.

Further information should be sought on individual drugs to balance the risk-benefit ratio in a particular individual patient. The FDA and ADEC risk classification systems may not always be a reliable source of information (Addis *et al*, *Drug Saf* 2000;**23**:245–53).

Reproductive toxicity falls into five domains (Wisner *et al*, *Am J Psychiatry* 2000;**157**:1933–40, 44 refs):

1. Intrauterine fetal death/miscarriage.
2. Physical malformations.
3. Growth impairment.
4. Behavioural toxicity (post-birth).
5. Neonatal toxicity, eg. withdrawal or direct adverse effects.

For the record, spontaneous major or gross malformations (usually defined as incompatible with life or requiring surgical correction) occur in 2–3% of pregnancies and spontaneous abortions in about 10–20% of clinically recognised pregnancies. In the first trimester, teratogenicity is the main drug risk, and growth retardation and neurological damage may occur in the second and third trimesters. After birth, drug withdrawal effects may occur. Although there are a few reports that pregnancy may protect against the risk of, eg. bipolar disorder, other papers show an increased risk (reviewed by Viguera and Cohen, *Psychopharmacol Bull* 1998;**34**:339–46).

Assessing risk: Recent retrospective studies are more useful pointers to risk than the length of time a drug has been on the market or anecdotal case reports.

GENERAL PRINCIPALS (ADAPTED FROM *MAUDSLEY GUIDELINES*)

Planning for possible pregnancy provides time for informed decisions. In bipolar disorder, pregnancy and the postpartum periods can be considered as separate risk periods, and treatment plans may need to be different for each. See also an additional section under anticonvulsants (*3.8.4*).

Pre-conception
1. For planned conception, discuss the risks and benefits of discontinuing or continuing medication, eg. relapse, teratogenicity, etc, the unpredictability of the pre-conceptual duration, and that no decision is risk-free. Avoiding all drugs during the first trimester is the ideal but risks relapse. Other options include continuing at the lowest possible dose (or switch to a drug with the shortest possible half-life) until a positive pregnancy test, or continue throughout pregnancy at the lowest viable dose.
2. Consider the risk of pregnancy even if not currently planned, eg. carry out a pregnancy test before starting teratogenic drugs in a woman of child-bearing age. As up to 50% of pregnancies are unplanned, document the patient's birth control method, document the potential risks for exposure to drug(s) during pregnancy, encourage proper nutrition, exercise and vitamin supplementation, note any other substances taken (eg. excess caffeine, alcohol and natural products) and educate the patient about the potential risks. Inquire about any pregnancy plans and emphasise the need for a pre-pregnancy consultation.

3. For drugs of known significant risk or where there is little data, consider switching to a lower-risk drug before conception.

Pregnancy
1. Avoid all drugs during the first trimester if possible. The maximum teratogenic potential is from days 17–60 (2–9 weeks) after conception, and decisions must balance the relative versus absolute risk.
2. Behavioural teratogenesis and subtle functional disturbances (eg. learning difficulties, neurological deficits and developmental delay), and an effect on labour and delivery may occur in the second and third trimesters.
3. Use the lowest possible (maintenance) dose and monitor effects (adverse and desired) carefully. Maintain a low threshold for reintroduction or dose increase.
4. In many cases, the risk of relapse (and subsequent higher dose drug use) will be higher than the risk of fetal damage.
5. Avoid polypharmacy, as synergistic teratogenicity can occur (up to 16% with multiple AEDs, n = 172, Kaneko *et al*, *Epilepsia* 1988;**29**:459–67).
6. The pharmacokinetics of drugs may change during pregnancy and so doses may need to be adjusted (see eg. lithium, tricyclics).
7. Discontinuation effects have been reported in the newborn (eg. benzodiazepines, antidepressants and opiates) and these psychotropics should, if possible, be gradually reduced or withdrawn over the weeks before delivery is due.

Unexpected pregnancy

If a woman discovers or reports that she is pregnant while taking a drug:
1. Don't panic.
2. If before day 17, consider immediate stopping or temporary discontinuation.
3. If after day 60, the major risk has passed and so decisions are less urgent.
4. Institute immediate nutritional supplements (eg. folic acid).
5. Reduce the dose if possible, at least during the high risk period.

6. Discontinue any non-essential treatments, particularly any that might be at sub-therapeutic doses.

7. Do not stop lithium abruptly (see point 32), and beware of stopping some SSRIs and anticonvulsants.

8. Seek specific specialist advice, and discuss the risk of the possible consequences of relapse versus the published risk to the fetus.

Reviews: * *Drugs in Pregnancy and Lactation: A Reference Guide to Fetal and Neonatal Risk*, by Briggs et al, Williams and Wilkins, Baltimore, MD; general (Craig and Sisodiya, *Prescriber* 2001;**12**:30–6; Pennell, *Neurology* 2003;**61**[6 Suppl 2]:S35–42; Kohen, *Adv Psychiatr Treat* 2004; **10**:59–66, 55 refs), mood stabilisers, atypicals and broad-spectrum psychotropics (Ernst and Goldberg, *J Clin Psychiatry* 2002;**63**[Suppl 4]: S42–S55), pharmacokinetic changes during pregnancy and their clinical relevance to specific drugs (Loebstein et al, *Clin Pharmacokinet* 1997; **33**:328–43), psychotropics in pregnancy in bipolar disorder (Viguera et al, *Can J Psychiatry* 2002;**47**:426–36; Yonkers et al, *Am J Psychiatry* 2004;**161**:608–20).

3.8.1 ANTIPSYCHOTICS *

In recent years, more women taking antipsychotics have been planning to (or have) become pregnant (McKenna et al, *Vet Hum Toxicol* 2004;**46**:44–6), presumably due to the introduction of the atypicals. However, low folate intake and low serum folate levels have been shown in women taking atypicals, increasing the risk of neural tube defects (Koren et al, *Am J Psychiatry* 2002;**159**:136–7) and so dietary advice and folate supplements pre-conception are **essential**. One systematic review suggested that women with schizophrenia have a greater risk of poor pregnancy outcomes than other women, with an increased risk with phenothiazines, although the review omitted two major studies that show no increased risk with phenothiazines (Patton et al, *Can J Psychiatry* 2002;**47**:959–65; comment by Levinson, *EBMH* 2003;**6**:89). More recently, a prospective cohort study of three programmes showed no increase in malformations in women who took atypicals (olanzapine n = 60, risperidone n = 49, quetiapine n = 36, clozapine n = 6), which although relatively underpowered had no bad news (n = 151, McKenna et al, *J Clin Psychiatry* 2005;**66**:444–9; comment by Howard, *EBMH* 2005;**8**:115).

Reviews: * general (Gentile, *Ann Pharmacother* 2004;**38**:126–71; Pinkofsky, *Ann Clin Psychiatry* 1997;**9**:175–9).

1. **Risperidone** (FDA = C; ADEC = B3) has no reported teratogenicity in animal tests.

2. * There is no adequate data on **aripiprazole** (FDA = C), although animal studies have been unremarkable and a healthy child was born to a woman taking aripiprazole 10–15mg/d from 0-8 weeks and then 20 weeks to term. There was, though, a lactation failure, possibly due to aripiprazole-induced regulation of prolactin (n = 1, Mendhekar et al, *Bipolar Disord* 2006;**8**:299– 300). From 23 documented pregnancies with **olanzapine** (FDA = C; ADEC=B3), 5% were premature, spontaneous abortion occurred in 13% and stillbirth in 5%, but with no major malformations. All these were reported as being within normal ranges (n = 23, Goldstein et al, *J Clin Psychopharmacol* 2000;**20**:399–403). Use should only be when the potential benefit outweighs the potential risk. No teratogenic effects have been seen in animal studies nor in anecdotal case reports (eg. n = 2, Malek-Ahmadi, *Ann Pharmacother* 2001;**35**:1294–5; n = 1, Mendhekar et al, *Pharmacopsychiatry* 2002;**35**:122–3). The **quetiapine** (FDA = C) literature recommends using only if the benefits justify the risk. There are cases of 400mg/d (n = 1, Tényi et al, *Am J Psychiatry* 2002;**159**:674) and 200–300mg/d (n = 1, Taylor et al, *Am J Psychiatry* 2003;**160**:587–8) taken throughout pregnancy without complications and with normal development at six months. **Sertindole** is contraindicated in pregnancy, but no teratogenic activity has been shown, although some potential effects on weight gain and delayed development has been suggested. There are no adequate human studies during pregnancy with **ziprasidone** (FDA = C). **Zotepine** crosses the placenta and although there are no indications of teratogenicity (animal study in rats, Fukuhara et al, *Arzneimittel-forschung* 1979;**29**:1600–6), there is insufficient data in humans and the drug is contraindicated in pregnancy.

3. Women are more likely to conceive on **clozapine** (FDA = B; ADEC = C) than most other antipsychotics due to an absence of raised prolactin. In the close study of one patient, there

was clear accumulation of clozapine in the infant, possibly due to higher albumin concentrations (n = 1, Barnas, *Am J Psychiatry* 1994;**151**:945). Of 84 reports of pregnancy with clozapine with known outcomes, there were 51 births, seven miscarriages and 14 elective terminations, of which one was due to known abnormalities (patient taking clozapine 25 mg/d plus lithium). Of the 51 births, 43 were born healthy and normal and eight had abnormalities, ranging from low glucose levels through to malformations. Clozapine is known to pass the placental barrier in animals and is assumed to do so in humans. No clear conclusion can be drawn from this, although combined with animal studies it would appear clozapine is not a major teratogen, but not recommended in pregnancy as such.

4. **Thioxanthenes**:

Flupentixol (ADEC = C) passes across the placenta and fetal levels are about a quarter of the mother's levels (n = 5, open, Kirk and Jorgensen, *Psychopharmacology* 1980;**72**:107–8). There is no positive evidence of teratogenicity although Lundbeck do not recommend its use. Studies in three species have not shown malformations. With **zuclopenthixol**, few birth defects have been recorded at a rate consistent with the spontaneous levels of malformations.

5. **Sulpiride** has been used as an anti-nauseant in pregnancy. There are no published reports of abnormalities in animals or humans (*Int J Res Preg* 1982;**3**:173–7, + MI). **Amisulpride** shows no animal reproductive toxicity but is contraindicated in pregnancy in humans.

6. * **Butyrophenones**: The safety of **haloperidol** (FDA = C; ADEC = C) in pregnancy has not been fully established, but a prospective study showed that of 188 haloperidol pregnancies, there was no significant increase in congenital abnormalities (cf control group) even if taken in the first trimester (although there were two limb defects), but there was a higher incidence of therapeutic termination, preterm birth and low birth weight (n = 188, Diav-Citrin *et al*, *J Clin Psychiatry* 2005;**66**:317–22). There is a case of dyskinesia in a newborn after halo-peridol monotherapy (n = 1, Collins and Comer, *Am J Health Syst Pharm* 2003;**60**:2253–5).

7. **Phenothiazines**: (ADEC: chlorpromazine = C, promazine = C, trifluoperazine = C, flu-phenazine = C, thioridazine = C)

The teratogenicity of phenothiazines has been investigated in some studies, although most of the data is based on low doses and thus not necessarily applicable to higher dose use. The phenothiazines are considered by some as of low risk, although the potential for hypotension, sedation and anticholinergic effects means that any use must be with extreme care. Severe congenital abnormalities were not significantly different in the studies of 543 women taking low-dose phenothiazines, other than **prochlorperazine** (FDA = C) for nausea (Miklovich and van den Berg, *Am J Obstet Gynecol* 1976;**125**:244–8), and in 1309 mothers mostly taking prochlorperazine (prospective, Slone *et al*, *Am J Obstet Gynecol* 1977;**128**:486–8). The largest study, of 315 pregnancies where phenothiazines were taken in the first trimester, showed a statistically significant difference in the malformation rate of 3.5% in the aliphatic (**chlorpromazine** and **promazine**) phenothiazine-treated group (11 malformed infants), compared with 1.6% in the control group. There was no apparent trend in the type of abnormality and the risk is still considered low. There was no difference with the other phenothiazines, which appear to have an incidence of malformations similar to the background incidence (*Teratology* 1977;**15**:57–64). Although **levomepromazine** (methotrimeprazine) is an aliphatic phenothiazine, it has generally been considered safe for both mother and fetus if used occasionally in low dose, later in pregnancy. A follow-up of trifluoperazine pregnancies showed no teratogenic effects (Moriarity, *Can Med Assoc J* 1963;**88**:97). In the neonate, lethargy and extra-pyramidal symptoms have been reported, as has respiratory depression when given in high dose (above 500 mg chlorpromazine equivalents) close to term.

Postnatal development: In the longer term, a lack of impaired mental or physical development has been shown at two and seven years in a follow-up study (n = 16, Ayd, *Int Drug Ther Newsletter* 1976;**11**:5). See also a short comment about 'Is fluphenazine a teratogen?' (Merlob *et al*, *Am J Med Genet* 1994;**52**:231–2).

8. The safety of **loxapine** (FDA = C) in pregnancy is unknown. There are two reports of gastrointestinal malformations in infants whose mothers took loxapine throughout pregnancy, but no similar cases are reported elsewhere.

3.8.2 ANTIDEPRESSANTS *

There is little data on the newer drugs so the lowest risk in the first trimester would appear to be to use either **imipramine**, **amitriptyline** or an **SSRI**, none of which have data suggesting a significant risk. One study (children whose mother took a tricyclic [n = 80], fluoxetine [n = 55] or nothing [n = 84], Nulman et al, NEJM 1997;**336**:258–62) indicates that if women take an antidepressant during their pregnancy, there seems to be no effect on the neurological development or intelligence of their children (see 20 below). Serotonergic drugs may increase the risk of CNS serotonergic adverse effects (tremor, restlessness, rigidity), but these subside quickly without treatment and may be due to serotonergic hyperstimulation rather than withdrawal (prospective, n = 40, p/c, Laine et al, Arch Gen Psychiatry 2003;**60**:720–6).

Review: * general (Gentile, Drug Safety 2005; **28**:137–52; Patkar et al, Ann Clin Psychiatry 2004;**16**:87–100), risks of untreated depression (Bonari et al, Can J Psychiatry 2004;**49**:726–35), depression during pregnancy and postpartum (Cohen et al, CNS Spectr 2004;**9**:209–16).

9.* **SSRIs**: (FDA: citalopram = C, escitalopram = C, fluoxetine = C, fluvoxamine = C, paroxetine = D, sertraline = C, ADEC: citalopam = C, fluoxetine = C, paroxetine = B3, sertraline = B3)

In a prospective, multicentre cohort study of 267 women exposed to an SSRI (fluvoxamine, sertraline or paroxetine) during pregnancy and 267 controls, exposure to SSRIs at recommended doses did not appear to be associated with increased teratogenicity (relative risk 1.06, 95% CI, 0.43–2.62) or higher rates of miscarriage, stillbirth or prematurity. Gestational ages and birth weights were similar among off-spring of both groups of women (prospective, Kulin et al, JAMA 1998;**279**:609–10). A recent review of 138 pregnancies concluded that the rates of congenital anomalies, low birth weight and preterm births were the same as in the general population, although high-dose fluoxetine (40–80 mg/d) may be associated with a risk of lower birth weight (n = 138, Hendrick et al, Am J Obstet Gynaecol 2003;**188**:812–15). Overall, the rate of major birth defects is 1.4%, similar to that seen in the general population.

Postnatal development: In a retrospective study, apparent prenatal SSRI exposure was not associated with malformation or any developmental delay. However, slightly earlier delivery (0.9 week) and decreased birth weight (175 g) were noted and third trimester exposure to SSRIs was associated with a 0.29 decrease in mean Apgar scores at five minutes (n = 185, controls n = 185, Simon et al, Am J Psychiatry 2002;**159**:2055–61). Caution is advised and use should only be if clearly needed.

Withdrawal: Neonatal withdrawal symptoms (irritability, constant crying, shivering, increased tonus, eating and sleeping difficulties and convulsions) have been reported after in utero exposure to paroxetine (n = 3), citalopram (n = 1) and fluoxetine (n = 1), four requiring calming with chlorpromazine (Nordeng et al, Acta Paediatrica 2001;**90**:288–91).

Citalopram (and **escitalopram**):* Of 125 women who took citalopram in the first trimester (including 71 who also took it throughout pregnancy), there were 86% normal live births, 11% spontaneous abortions, 1.5% elective terminations and 1.5% stillbirths, plus one male infant born with major malformations and there was an overall increased risk of admission to a SCBU (n = 125, Sivojelezova et al, Am J Obstet Gynecol 2005;**193**:2004–9). Occasionally, slightly increased doses of citalopram may be needed in pregnancy (n = 11, Heikkinen et al, Clin Pharmacol Ther 2002;**72**:184–91).

Fluoxetine: There is a mass of data on fluoxetine-exposed pregnancies reported in three prospective cohort-controlled studies and four prospective surveys. Based on published studies, use in the first trimester is not associated with increased risk of major malformations (meta-analysis by Addis and Koren, Psychol Med 2000;**30**:89–94; critical review by Gijsman, EBMH 2000;**3**:122). There is an absence of perinatal sequelae and no evidence of an increase in major malformations, spontaneous abortion, poor perinatal state or neurodevelopmental delay. In a prospective study on first-trimester exposure involving 128 women taking fluoxetine, 110 taking no known teratogen and 74 taking a tricyclic, no statistical differences in pregnancy outcome, age or weight were shown, but there was a slight tendency to miscarriage with both drug groups (SSRI 14.8%, TCA 12.2%, no drug 7.8%). The authors concluded that fluoxetine was unlikely to be a major teratogen but further work on miscarriage and any potential developmental effects was needed (n=312, Pastuszak et al, JAMA 1993;**269**:2246–8). Of 544 reported cases in the USA of fluoxetine taken during pregnancy, 91 were electively terminated and there were 72 (15.9%) spontaneous abortions, 13 (3.4%) perinatal major malformations and seven post-perinatal malformations reported. These rates have been concluded as being similar to the unexposed population (Goldstein and Marvel, JAMA, 1993;**270**:2177–8) but this has been disputed, as the previous study (Pastuszak et al, JAMA 1993;**269**:2246–8) showed similar miscarriage rates which were double that in the control group. Chambers et al (NEJM 1996;**335**:1010–5, n=228) could not show increased miscarriage rates, major fetal abnormalities or a consistent pattern of events suggesting teratogenicity, although there was a higher rate of having three or more minor anomalies and no account was taken of the severity of maternal depression (Dwight and Walker, Curr Opin Psychiatry 1998;**11**:85–8).

Postnatal development: A careful prospective study of children (assessed between 18 and 86 months) whose mothers had taken either fluoxetine (n=55) or no drug (n=84) showed fluoxetine to have no effect on global IQ, language development or behavioural development (Nulman et al, NEJM 1997;**336**:258–62). Further data on exposure to fluoxetine throughout pregnancy shows no detectable adverse affect on cognition, language development or temperament, whereas untreated depression was associated with poorer cognitive and language achievement in their children (TCA n=46, fluoxetine n=40, control n=36; open, Nulman et al, Am J Psychiatry 2002;**159**:1889–95). Relatively low plasma fluoxetine levels have been reported in pregnancy, which might lead to therapeutic failure at standard doses, with infant fluoxetine and norfluoxetine plasma levels 65% and 72% respectively at birth (n=11+10 controls, Heikkinen et al, Clin Pharmacol Ther 2003;**73**:330–7).

Paroxetine: * One study has shown an increase in whole and cardiovascular malformations from 3% to 4% and 1% to 2% respectively (cf. general population) and recommends use in pregnancy only when strictly indicated (MHRA December 2005), although previous studies had not provided this signal. The MHRA do not recommend stopping paroxetine abruptly if a women is pregnant as this could precipitate discontinuation symptoms, but to discuss the risks and benefits at the next appointment. When used in the third trimester, paroxetine may cause a high rate of neonatal complications, probably due to a withdrawal syndrome. In a careful prospective study, 22% neonates had complications (9 = respiratory distress, 2 = hypoglycaemia) requiring intensive treatment and hospitalisation, although all symptoms had disappearing within 1–2 weeks (n=55+controls; Costei et al, Arch Pediatr Adolesc Med 2002;**156**:1129–32; more severe case, Morag et al, J Toxicol Clin Toxicol 2004; **42**:97–100).

Sertraline has been included in a number of studies, eg. in a prospective, multicentre cohort study of 267 women exposed to an SSRI (fluvoxamine, sertraline or paroxetine) during pregnancy and 267 controls, exposure to SSRIs at recommended doses did not appear to be associated with increased teratogenicity (relative risk 1.06, 95% CI, 0.43–2.62) or higher rates of miscarriage, stillbirth or prematurity. Gestational ages and birth weights were similar among off-spring of both groups of women (prospective, Kulin et al, JAMA 1998;**279**:609–10).

10. * Data on 150 **venlafaxine** (FDA=C; ADEC=B2) pregnancies showed 125 live births, 18 spontaneous abortions, seven therapeutic abortions and two major malformations, suggesting that the base-rate of malformations does not rise above the spontaneous rate but, as with the SSRIs, the spontaneous abortion rate is slightly higher (n=150, compared to 150 SSRIs exposures and 150 non-teratogenic drug control exposures; Einarson et al, Am J Psychiatry 2001;**158**:1728–30). It is no longer contraindicated in pregnancy in the UK SPC, although there is a warning of the potential for withdrawal symptoms in the neonate (eg. case that resolved with use of low-dose 1 mg/d for 8/7; n=1, de Moor et al, Ned Tijdschr Geneeskd 2003;**147**:1370–2). Animal studies with **duloxetine** (FDA=C) suggest some adverse behavioural effects in one animal species but there is no human data and so caution is recommended.

11.* For **mirtazapine** (FDA=C; ADEC=B3) a recent comprehensive and prospective study has shown no increase in the baseline rate of major malformations but a slight increase in spontaneous abortions (19% vs 17% vs 11%) and preterm births (10% vs 7% vs 2%) (n=104 mirtazapine, vs n=104 other antidepressants vs. control group, Djulus et al, J Clin Psychiatry 2006;**67**:1280-4). Animal tests do not show any teratogenicity or fetal harm. When used for depression, anxiety and *hyperemesis gravidarum* in seven pregnancies, all women improved and all babies were born healthy at term (n=7, Saks, Arch Women's Ment Health 2001;**3**:165–170; see also n=2, Kesim et al, Teratology 2002;**66**:204).

12. **Tricyclic antidepressants:** (FDA: amoxapine=C, clomipramine=C, desipramine=C, doxepin=B, maprotiline=B, trimipramine=C; ADEC: amitriptyline=C, clomipramine=C, dosulepin=C, doxepin=C, imipramine=C, nortriptyline=C, protriptyline= C, trimipramine=C)

In a recent retrospective study, apparent prenatal tricyclic exposure was not associated with malformations, developmental delay or any adverse perinatal outcomes (n=209, controls n=209, Simon et al, Am J Psychiatry 2002;**159**:2055–61). A meta-analysis of the use of tricyclics in pregnancy, reviewing over 300 000 live births (including 414 first trimester exposures), failed to show a significant association between tricyclics and congenital malformations, although withdrawal symptoms were noted (Altshuler et al, Am J Psychiatry 1996;**153**:592–605). The metabolism of tricyclics in the neonate is much slower, so anticholinergic and other side-effects are likely to be more marked.

In pregnancy, mild toxicity in the infant has been seen with **imipramine**, eg. respiratory distress, hypotonia, irritability, tremors, convulsions and jerky movements (eg. n=2, Ware and DeVane, J Clin Psychiatry 1990;**51**:482–4). Phenobarbital can improve these symptoms, which can persist for a total duration of up to two weeks. **Amitriptyline** and **imipramine** are considered the tricyclics of choice, based on cumulative data on their relative safety.

Discontinuation effects have been noted in the neonate, sometimes requiring active treatment, eg. **clomipramine** has caused jittery/twitchy infants which resolves upon introduction of the drug, either via a drip or via breast milk (n=1, Schimmel et al, Clin Toxicol 1991;**29**:479–84), lethargic and cyanotic babies who had

abnormal movements and feeding difficulties where symptomatic treatment was successful (Cowe et al, Br Med J 1982;**284**:1837–8) and fetal seizures unresponsive to phenobarbital and phenytoin, which settled with clomipramine, in a mother who took up to 150mg/d clomipramine and stopped abruptly (child was born prematurely four days later; Bromiker and Kaplan, JAMA 1994;**272**:1722–3).

Postnatal development: A careful study of children (assessed between 18 and 86 months) whose mothers had taken either a tricyclic (n=84) or no drug (n=80) showed tricyclics to have no adverse effect on global IQ, language development or behavioural development compared to no drug (Nulman et al, NEJM 1997;**336**:258–62). Further data shows no adverse affect on cognition, language development or temperament, whereas untreated depression is associated with poorer cognitive and language achievement in their children (tricyclic n=46, fluoxetine n=40, control n=36, open, Nulman et al, Am J Psychiatry 2002;**159**:1889–95).

13. For **trazodone** (FDA=C) at very high doses (15+ times the maximum human dose), there appears to be some fetal resorption and congenital abnormalities in animals but little human data exists to support this.

14. No teratogenic effects have been noted with **reboxetine** in animal studies but little human data exists so the drug should be avoided in pregnancy.

15. **MAOIs:** (FDA: isocarboxazid=C; ADEC: isocarboxazid=B3, phenelzine=B3, tranylcypromine=B2)

There are no reports of human teratogenicity with **phenelzine** or **tranylcypromine**, although it has been suggested that the risk may be roughly doubled if tranylcypromine is taken in the first trimester (AAPCD, Pediatrics 1982;**69**:241–3). Growth retardation and fetal toxicity have been reported. If at all possible, MAOIs should be avoided due to maternal toxicity and lack of published safety data. MAOIs may also interact with drugs used in labour (see also 4.3.4).

16. There is no evidence of teratogenicity with **mianserin** (ADEC=B2) in animals except at toxic doses but little human data is available. No firm data is available on the use of **moclobemide** in pregnancy, but there is a case of 300mg/d taken throughout pregnancy with no problems

and normal development within the first 14 months (n = 1, Rybakowski, *Pharmacopsychiatry* 2001;**34**:82–3). No human data is available for **tryptophan**, but it is a naturally occurring substance in food. Slight *in vitro* uterotonic activity has been reported with **St John's wort** and the lack of safety and toxicity data suggests that it is currently best avoided in pregnancy.

3.8.3 ANXIOLYTICS AND HYPNOTICS

For a review of the treatment of anxiety during pregnancy see McGrath *et al*, (*Drug Saf* 1999;**20**:171–86).
17. * **Benzodiazepines**: (FDA: alprazolam = D, clonazepam = D, lorazepam = D, temazepam = X; ADEC: clonazepam = C, diazepam = C, flunitrazepam = C, lorazepam = C, oxazepam = C, temazepam = C)
Assessment of 104 000 births in the USA has shown a higher incidence of teratogenicity in women taking benzodiazepines, but multiple alcohol and illicit substance exposure could account for this (Bergman *et al*, *Lancet* 1992; **340**:694–6). A population-based case-control study indicated that **nitrazepam**, **medazepam**, **alprazolam** and **clonazepam** taken during pregnancy did not present a detectable teratogenic risk (n = 38,151, Eros *et al*, *Eur J Obstet Gynecol Reprod Biol* 2002;**101**:147–54). With **chlordiazepoxide**, there was slight increase in congenital malformations with use in the 2nd-3rd months, but no specific type or pattern was seen, and so the risk is unlikely to be substantial (n = 469, Czeizel *et al*, *Neurotoxicol Teratol* 2004;**26**:593–8). **Clobazam** is known to cross the placenta and benzodiazepine withdrawal symptoms in the neonate have been suggested. For **diazepam**, studies show a varying risk of oral clefts, with the worst case scenario bringing the risk to seven in 1000. In late pregnancy, doses of 30 mg or more of diazepam IM or IV during the last 15 hours of labour can induce neonatal respiratory depression and feeding problems. 10 mg given IV within 10 minutes of birth has been shown not to affect Apgar scores (n = 23, open, McAllister, *Br J Anaesth* 1980;**52**:423–7). As with other benzodiazepines, withdrawal symptoms in the neonate have been seen (n = 3, Rementeria and Bhatt, *J Pediatr* 1977;**90**:123–6). As **lorazepam** crosses the placenta, the floppy

baby syndrome and respiratory depression can occur, especially if IV doses are used close to birth. Oral use during later pregnancy may show delayed feeding in full-term infants, but premature infants may have lower Apgar scores and respiratory depression (n = 53, open, Whitelaw *et al*, *Br Med J* 1981;**282**:1106–8). **Clorazepate** also passes the placenta. Animal studies have not shown teratogenicity although some cognitive impairment was suggested.

The UK CSM has noted the danger of benzodiazepine use during pregnancy or labour due to the effects on the neonate such as hypothermia, hypotonia, respiratory depression and withdrawal symptoms (*Curr Prob* 1997; **23**:10). Shorter-acting benzodiazepines on a 'when required' basis may be acceptable later in pregnancy, but the first trimester should be avoided if possible. After birth, benzodiazepine withdrawal symptoms have been noticed in the neonate with many benzodiazepines. The 'floppy baby' syndrome, as it is often termed, includes facial features and CNS dysfunction and can occur particularly with higher doses (eg. > 30 mg diazepam equivalent per day) of longer-acting benzodiazepines (n = 8, Laegreid *et al*, *J Pediatrics* 1989;**114**:126–31).
18. There is no evidence of a teratogenic effect from **buspirone** (FDA = B; ADEC = B1) but some effects on survival and weights have been noted in some, but not all, animal tests.
19. **Zopiclone** has not been contraindicated in pregnancy. Animal tests have shown no abnormalities and the limited human data is unremarkable. Little information is currently available on **zolpidem** (FDA = C; ADEC = B3) and **zaleplon** (FDA = C). Until more is known, they should be avoided in pregnancy, especially during the first trimester. None of these three hypnotics are contraindicated in pregnancy.
20. **Beta-blockers**: (FDA: propranolol = C; ADEC = C)
Beta-blockers are not generally considered teratogens but a connection between **propranolol** use in pregnancy and tracheosophageal fistulas (Campbell, *NEJM* 1985;**313**:518) and intrauterine growth retardation has been proposed but not substantiated. Direct effects of beta-blockade on the fetus would also occur, eg. bradycardia (for reviews etc. see Livingstone *et al*, *Clin Exp Hypertens* 1983;**2**:341–50; O'Connor *et al*,

Lancet 1981;**2**:1168). Use in the second and third trimesters may aggravate or produce neonatal hypoglycaemia. Fetal and neonatal bradycardia may occur, especially in pregnancies already complicated by placental insufficiency (eg. severe maternal hypertension). Due to direct cardiac effects, hypoglycaemia and apnoea from beta-blockers, it may be prudent to discontinue treatment 1–2 weeks before delivery.

21. Maternally administered **chloral** (ADEC=A) lowers bilirubin concentrations in the infant (Drew and Kitchen, *J Pediatr* 1976;**89**:657–61). No increase in congenital anomalies was seen in a study of 71 women who took chloral in the first four months of pregnancy or to 358 women who took chloral at some time in pregnancy (Heinonen et al, *Birth Defects and Drugs in Pregnancy,* Publishing Sciences Group 1977:336–7). The UK manufacturers state that **clomethiazole** (ADEC=A) should not be used, particularly in the first and third trimesters, although it has been used widely for pre-eclampsia. Platelet aggregation in the neonate has been reported with **promethazine** (FDA=C;ADEC=C) (Corby and Schulman, *J Pediatr* 1971;**79**:307).

3.8.4 ANTICONVULSANTS

Pregnant women with epilepsy are at increased risk of complications and 25–33% have an increased risk of seizures. One of the main reasons for this increase is the marked alterations in plasma protein-binding of drugs as pregnancy progresses, resulting in declining plasma levels. A number of prospective and retrospective studies have shown that there are a wide range of risks associated with anticonvulsants (some used as mood stabilisers) used throughout pregnancy. Most have an uncomplicated pregnancy and normal healthy offspring (n=151 pregnancies, 124 women, retrospective, Sabers et al, *Acta Neurol Scand* 1998;**97**:164–70), but the risk of abnormal outcomes (10.7%) may be three times that of controls (3.4%), with phenobarbital showing the highest risk (n=211, prospective, Waters et al, *Arch Neurol* 1994;**51**:250–3). There is an association with an increased risk of major congenital abnormalities with most AEDs, in particular, valproate, carbamazepine, benzodiazepines and phenobarbital (n=1411, Samren et al, *Ann Neurol* 1999;**46**:739–44).

Polytherapy carries additional risks, eg. it is associated with a (partly reversible) decline in body dimension (n=963, Swedish survey, Wide et al, *Epilepsia* 2000;**41**:854–61), including the risk of pre-term delivery, lower birthweight, length and head circumference (n=193, controls n=24094, Hvas et al, *Br J Obstet Gynaecol* 2000;**107**:896–902). To place this in perspective, one review of anticonvulsants in pregnancy (Malone and D'Alton, *Semin Perinatol* 1997;**21**:114–23) concluded that the lowest dose of one of the major drugs probably has less risk of teratogenicity than that of recurrent seizures.

Postnatal development: Three recent studies have suggested some specific effects on postnatal development of children exposed to anticonvulsants during pregnancy. One survey suggested a higher frequency of educational needs statements (10.3% drug exposed cf. 5.7% non-drug-exposed). The figures for **valproate** (30%), and possibly also polypharmacy, were much higher, supporting the possibility of a drug-related effect (n=400 school-age children: 150 exposed to monotherapy, 74 to polytherapy and 176 to none; Adab et al, *J Neurol Neurosurg Psychiatry* 2001;**70**:15–21). Another study concluded that while there were no global score differences, phenytoin (n=16, but not CBZ n=35) caused a significant albeit subtle reduction in psychomotor development, which may be more obvious at school age (n=76 exposed, c/w 71 unexposed, Wide et al, *Acta Paediatrica* 2002;**91**:409–14). Finally, in a review of the long-term health and neurodevelopment in children exposed to antiepileptic drugs before birth, developmental delay was seen in 24% of exposed children (cf. 11% non-exposed siblings), childhood medical problems in 31% (cf. 13% of non-exposed siblings) and behaviour disorders in 20% (cf.5% of non-exposed) and concluded that prenatal antiepileptic drug exposure is associated with developmental delay and later childhood morbidity, in addition to congenital malformation (n=129 mothers, 293 children, Dean et al, *J Med Genet* 2002;**39**:251–9).

Summary of the risks of pregnancy in women with epilepsy:

- 25–33% increase in maternal seizure frequency

- 10% risk of vaginal bleeding
- 7% risk of neonatal haemorrhage if no vitamin K is given
- 10% risk of infant facial dysmorphism.
- 4–6% risk of major malformations (30% of which are oral facial defects)
- 1–2% risk of spina bifida with valproate.
- 0.5–1% risk of spina bifida with carbamazepine.

(Yerby, *Epilepsia* 1992;**33**[Suppl 1]:S23–S27.)

UK epilepsy and pregnancy register *

A prospective study (n = 3607, Morrow *et al*, *J Neurol Neurosurg Psychiatry* 2006;**77**:193–8) has shown that only 4.2% of children born to mothers with epilepsy and taking AEDs had major congenital malformations (MCM), subdivided as follows:

- 6% polytherapy exposures had MCMs
- 3.7% monotherapy exposures had MCMs
- more polytherapies with MCM had valproate than those that did not include valproate.

Relative risks with monotherapy:

- 2.2% carbamazepine (least risk)
- 3.2% lamotrigine (> 200 mg/d had higher risk)
- 6% valproate (higher with > 1000 mg/d at 9%).

Summary of risk minimisation strategies:

There is evidence to suggest that recent literature has been slow to positively influence clinical practice and reduce the risks of adverse effects (Wiebe, *Br Med J* 2000;**320**:3–4, editorial).

1. Pre-conception: *

- Education of the patient as to the risks and benefits of continued treatment. This should be documented and supported with written information (n = 300, survey, Fairgrieve *et al*, *Br Med J* 2000;**321**:674–5).
- Adequate oral contraceptive dosage (see individual drugs' interactions, 4.5) until conception is planned, eg. 50 mcg of ethinylestradiol.
- Start regular multivitamins with folate before oral contraceptives are stopped, to reduce the chance of spina bifida. Folic acid antagonists (eg. carbamazepine, phenytoin, phenobarbital) taken during pregnancy increase the risk of cardiovascular birth

defects and oral clefts, and oral folic acid (eg. in multivitamins) may reduce the risks of these defects (n = 6932, Hernandez-Diaz *et al*, *NEJM* 2000;**343**:1608–14), although folic acid is not always successful with valproate (n = 2, Duncan *et al*, *Epilepsia* 2001;**42**:750–3).

- Minimise the exposure to drugs with known associated risks, eg. phenobarbital (n = 211, prospective, Waters *et al*, *Arch Neurol* 1994;**51**:250–3), phenytoin (n = 151, retrospective, Sabers *et al*, *Acta Neurol Scand* 1998;**97**:164–70), valproate, carbamazepine and benzodiazepines (n = 1411, Samren *et al*, *Ann Neurol* 1999;**46**:739–44).
- Seizure control with the lowest dose monotherapy should be targeted.
- Diagnosis should be verified and the need for anticonvulsants confirmed.

2. After conception:

- Education of the patient about risk minimisation eg. vitamins.

3. Seizure control without toxicity during pregnancy:

- Do not change drugs if the patient is stabilised.
- Multivitamins with folate continued.
- Frequent monitoring of free anticonvulsant concentrations and dose adjustment if necessary.
- Monotherapy continued if possible.
- Vitamin K given during last week of pregnancy if possible (Deblay *et al*, *Lancet* 1982;**1**:1247).
- Ultrasound and AFPs carried out.

Facial dysmorphism has been described in patients with uncontrolled seizures, as well as with phenytoin, phenobarbital, primidone, valproate, benzodiazepines and carbamazepine. All appear quite similar, not really drug-specific and some effects, especially digital, appear to resolve with age, although a review and huge multicentered study concluded that the distinctive pattern of physical abnormalities are associated with anticonvulsants rather than epilepsy itself (n = 128 049, Holmes *et al*, *NEJM* 2001;**344**:1132–8).

It is worth noting that one study showed that only 38% of female epileptics were able to recall any pre-pregnancy counselling, only 44% had planned the pregnancy (24% reported contraceptive failure) and only 11% took folate appropriately. Most published advice is directed at neurologists, rather than the GPs caring for many patients. The net result was malformation rates double the background rate and there was an excess of premature deliveries cf. controls (n = 300, survey, Fairgrieve *et al, Br Med J* 2000; **321**:674–5).

Reviews: general (Perucca, *Lancet Neurol* 2005; **4**:781–6; Gagliardo and Krishnan, *Psychopharmacol Bull* 2003; **37**:59–66), advice to patients (Yerby, *Epilepsia* 1997; **38**:957–8), long-term outcomes (Koch *et al, Epilepsia* 1999; **40**:1237–43), kinetics in pregnancy and lactation (Pennell, *Neurology* 2003; **61**[6 Suppl 2]:S35–S42).

22. * **Carbamazepine** (FDA = D; ADEC = D) is now considered to have a higher risk. In a pooled data study of 1255 exposures, carbamazepine was associated with:

- an increased rate of congenital anomalies, mainly neural tube defects (eg. spina bifida, 1% incidence; Rosa, *NEJM* 1991; **324**:674–7), cardiovascular and urinary tract anomalies, and cleft palate (a 'carbamazepine syndrome': Ornoy and Cohen, *Arch Dis Child* 1996; **75**:517)
- some minor abnormalities
- some reduced gestational age at delivery
- increased risk with polytherapy (n = 1255, Matalon *et al, Reprod Toxicol* 2002; **16**:9–17)
- a negative influence on body dimensions (n = 963, Wide *et al, Epilepsia* 2000; **41**: 854–61).

Children exposed to carbamazepine may also have subtle but distinctive facial features (n = 274, Kini *et al, Arch Dis Child Neonatal Ed* 2006; **91**:90–5), although 45% unexposed children also had some facial features too. Other problems include craniofacial defects (11%), fingernail hypoplasia (27%) and developmental delay (20%) (n = 72, retrospective, Jones *et al, NEJM* 1989; **320**:1661–6, + correspondence in *NEJM*, 1989; **321**:1480–1). Population studies indicate a two-fold increase in major congenital malformations and a slight reduction in birth weight (n = 210, 629 controls, Diav-Citrin *et al, Neurology* 2001; **57**:321–4). However, the UK epilepsy and pregnancy register showed that carbamazepine monotherapy may still have a low risk of major malformations (n = 3607, Morrow *et al, J Neurol Neurosurg Psychiatry* 2006; **77**:193-8). The literature recommends the need for counselling and screening for neural tube defects (*Curr Problems* 1993; **19**:8), which can detect 90–95% of neural tube defects if carried out with AFP levels at 16–18 weeks. In late pregnancy, routine vitamin K to mothers and the neonates is usually recommended.

Postnatal development: In a controlled study of *in utero* exposure, 36 children born to mothers taking carbamazepine were compared to matched controls. Allowing for variables, the carbamazepine children had similar IQs and language abilities to those of the controls (n = 36, Scolnik *et al, JAMA* 1994; **271**:767), and a long-term follow-up over up to 10 years showed normal intelligence in children exposed to carbamazepine monotherapy within normal plasma ranges during pregnancy compared to matched controls (n = 323; CBZ n = 86, Gaily *et al, Neurology* 2004; **13**:28–32), suggesting the lack of a clinically important adverse effect on cognitive development.

Oxcarbazepine * (FDA = C) is closely related to carbamazepine. The placenta may contribute to the metabolism of oxcarbazepine (Pienimaki *et al, Epilepsia* 1997; **38**:309–16) and data indicates that oxcarbazepine may cause serious birth defects, and there is significant transfer through the placenta in humans (n = 12, Myllynen *et al, Epilepsia* 2001; **42**:1482–5). However, a study from Argentina suggested that oxcarbazepine had a lower risk of teratogenicity than older AEDs (n = 114, Meischenguiser *et al, Epilepsy Behav* 2004; **5**:163–7). There is a report of an uneventful pregnancy and healthy child with oxcarbazepine taken throughout pregnancy (n = 1, Eisenschenk, *Neurologist* 2006; **12**:249–54). A recent survey showed that there was a higher risk of seizures and higher doses were needed in mothers taking oxcarbazepine and lamotrigine in late pregnancy (n = 1956, EURAP Study Group, *Neurology* 2006; **66**:354–60), because plasma levels of oxcarbazepine and metabolite may decrease markedly during pregnancy and increase several-fold after delivery. Careful monitoring throughout pregnancy and immediately afterwards is essential (n = 5, Mazzucchelli *et al, Epilepsia* 2006; **47**:504–9).

23. * **Valproate** (FDA = D; ADEC = D) crosses the placenta easily and is now well-established as both teratogenic and causing developmental problems and should not be used in women of child-bearing potential.

- **Teratogenicity:** the North American Antiepileptic Drug Pregnancy Registry has shown an increased relative risk of 7.3 of major malformations after first trimester exposure to valproate (10.7% had major malformations cf. 2.9% controls; n = 149, n = 1048 controls, Wyszynski et al, Neurology 2005;**64**:961–5). These include facial dysmorphia, hypospadias, limb malformations and spina bifida. However, dysmorphic features, developmental delay and structural anomalies were found only in children exposed to maternal valproate doses above 1000 mg/d (n = 69, Mawer et al, Seizure 2002;**11**:512–8), an important observation. The literature now states that there have been rare reports of haemorrhagic syndrome in neonates whose mothers took valproate in pregnancy.

- **Postnatal delay:** the Liverpool and Manchester study of children aged 6–16 showed that those exposed to valproate in utero were more likely to have an IQ below 69 and a poorer memory compared to exposure to other AEDs or none. The mother's IQ and number of GTC seizures during pregnancy were significant predictors of verbal IQ in the children (n = 249, Vinten et al, Neurology 2005;**64**:949–54). Exposure to valproate in utero may lead to a higher than expected incidence of education needs statements (n = 400 school-age children: 150 exposed to monotherapy, 74 to polytherapy and 176 to none, Adab et al, J Neurol Neurosurg Psychiatry 2001;**70**:15–21). A long-term follow-up over up to 10 years showed some evidence of reduced verbal intelligence in children exposed to valproate and AED polytherapy during pregnancy compared to matched controls (n = 323; valproate n = 13, polytherapy n = 30, Gaily et al, Neurology 2004;**13**:28–32). These support two previous studies showing an association with a risk of developmental delay (n = 400, Adab et al, J Neurol Neurosurg Psychiatry 2001;**70**:15–21; Dean et al, J Med Genet 2002;**39**:251–9).

- **Polycystic ovary syndrome** (PCOS): There is an association between valproate and PCOS, which may have some effect on reproductive capacity (n = 32, O'Donovan et al, J Clin Psychiatry 2002;**63**:322–30; review by Genton et al, Epilepsia 2001;**42**:295–304) but this may just be because valproate causes weight gain, a risk factor for PCOS.

The UK MHRA noted in September 2003 (Curr Prob Pharmacovig 2003;**29** [Sept]:6) that:

- specialist consultation should be sought for women likely to become pregnant on valproate
- if used in pregnancy, use the lowest effective dose (below 1000 mg/d), monotherapy, divided daily doses and give as an MR prep to reduce peak levels
- 5 mg folic acid should be started as soon as contraception is discontinued.

NICE has recommended (Bipolar Guidelines, 2006) that valproate should not be used in women of child-bearing potential.

Reviews: Valproate disposition in pregnancy (Omtzigt et al, Eur J Clin Pharmacol 1992;**43**:381–8), valproate in women of reproductive age (Piontek and Wisner, J Clin Psychiatry 2000; **61**:161–3).

24. **Phenytoin** (FDA = D; fosphenytoin = D; ADEC: phenytoin = D) crosses the placenta freely and teratogenicity is well-established, particularly the 'fetal hydantoin syndrome'. This syndrome includes growth retardation, microcephaly, mental retardation, facial defects, including cleft lip and/or palate, digit and nail hypoplasia, rib anomalies, hirsuitism, low hairlines and inguinal hernia, plus cardiovascular, gastrointestinal or genitourinary anomalies (n = 2 and review: Ozkinay et al, Turk J Pediatr 1998;**40**:273–8). The full syndrome occurs in about 8–10% of children born to mothers who took phenytoin in the first trimester (Witter et al, Obstet Gynecol 1981;**58**:100S–105S; n = 88, Rodriguez-Palomares et al, Arch Med Res 1995; **26**:371–7) and a part syndrome in a further 30% of children (n = 3, Seeler et al, Pediatrics 1979;**63**:524–7; see also controlled prospective study, n = 34, Nulman et al, Am J Med Genet 1997; **68**:18–24). It appears not to be dose-related (n = 88, Rodriguez-Palomares et al, Arch Med Res 1995;**26**:371–7). Prediction of the teratogenic risk may be possible by measuring microsomal epoxide hydrolase activity (n = 19, Buehler et al, NEJM 1990;**332**:1567–72).

The syndrome may be related to phenytoin-induced reduction in GSH levels, enhancing peroxidative damage to the fetus via the placental circulation (n = 52, controlled, Lui et al, Human Toxicol 1997;**16**:177–81). It has also been noted that epileptic fathers taking phenytoin have increased rates of malformed children (Friis, Acta Neurol Scand 1983;**94**[Suppl]:39–43).

The kinetics of phenytoin change in pregnancy. Elimination increases (single dose study, n = 5, Dickinson et al, Br J Clin Pharmacol 1989;**28**:17– 27) and plasma levels fall steadily as the pregnancy progresses, with a possible change in the seizure frequency (45% increase: Knight and Rhind, Epilepsia 1975;**16**:99–110; no significant change, Tomson et al, Epilepsia 1994;**35**:122–30). Bound levels may be reduced with free (ie. active) levels unchanged in pregnancy and so care with plasma level interpretation is needed (review of phenytoin disposition and metabolism in pregnancy, Eadie et al, Eur J Clin Pharmacol 1992;**43**:389–92; for 'Guidelines for the care of epileptic women of child-bearing age' see CGP+CILAE, Epilepsia 1989;**30**:409–10).

Risk reduction with phenytoin: The general consensus seems to be that where documented seizures are proven to be controlled by phenytoin, the risks of withdrawal are probably greater than with the continued use of phenytoin, with the following precautions:

1. **Use of minimal effective doses.** At least monthly blood level monitoring both during pregnancy, and for up to six months after, are essential to avoid toxicity and an increased teratogenic risk (see above, noting relevance of free levels).

2. **Use of folic acid 5 mg/d** from before conception. One study resulted in no birth defects in the 33 mothers who took folic acid from before conception, or immediately upon becoming pregnant, but there were 10 children with malformations from the 66 born to mothers who did not take folic acid, a **significant** and highly important difference (n = 66 retrospective, n = 22 prospective, Biale and Lewenthal, Eur J Obstet Gynecol Reprod Biol 1984;**18**:211). The neural tube closes around the time of the first missed period and so folic acid supplements need to be started **before** pregnancy is detected.

3. **Vitamin K supplementation**. Phenytoin inhibits the synthesis of vitamin K-dependent clotting factors and neonatal haemorrhage may occur. Vitamin K deficiency may also be the cause of abnormal facial development, via abnormal development of the cartilaginous nasal septum. Early vitamin K supplementation in at-risk pregnancies is thus recommended (n = 10, Howe et al, Am J Med Genet 1995;**58**:238–44) and to the neonate after birth (Yerby, Epilepsia 1987;**28**[Suppl 3]:S29–S36).

After birth, a withdrawal syndrome, including irritability and haemorrhage has been reported (prospective, Hill et al, Am J Dis Child 1974; **127**:645–53).

Postnatal development: One study has indicated a negative neurodevelopmental effect from phenytoin. In a controlled study of in utero exposure, 34 children born to mothers taking phenytoin and 36 children born to mothers taking carbamazepine were compared to matched controls. Allowing for other variables, the phenytoin children had a significantly lower mean IQ and language ability, the carbamazepine children being similar to controls (Scolnik et al, JAMA 1994;**271**:767). This strongly suggests a clinically important adverse effect in the long term. Developmental impairment and reduced growth and head circumference has been reported at seven years (Gal and Sharpless, Drug Intell Clin Pharm 1984;**18**:186–201). Reports of malignancies in the infant have probably been disproven (Koren et al, Teratology 1989;**40**:157–62).

25. **Phenobarbital** (FDA = D) has been implicated as a teratogen, although in many reported cases it has been as part of a combination therapy. Minor digital deformities (finger-like thumbs, rudimentary or missing nails), as well as hip and facial abnormalities have been reported. Withdrawal symptoms, such as seizures and irritability have occurred in the neonate, some delayed by up to two weeks after birth. Neonatal bleeding in the first 24 hours has been reported, as has respiratory depression. However, antenatal phenobarbital exposure does not appear to affect the neurodevelopmental outcome of premature infants at 18–22 months of age (n = 578, Shankaran et al, Am J Obstet Gynecol 2002;**187**:171–7).

Postnatal development: There is some evidence of a direct neurotoxic effect by pheno-barbital on developing fetal neurons, which may be responsible for some cognitive or CNS abnormalities. Prenatal exposure to combined phenobarbital and phenytoin (n = 172) compared to controls (n = 168) produced smaller head size at birth and persistent learning problems (12%) compared to controls (1%) in one study (Dessens et al, Acta Paediatrica 2000;**89**:533–41). In the longer-term, a smaller head circumference and an impaired cognitive development has been suggested in two studies (n = 122, van der Pol et al, Am J Obstet Gynecol 1991;**164**:121–8).

26. * For **lamotrigine** (FDA = C; ADEC = B3), data from the North American Antiepileptic Drug Pregnancy Registry led to the UK MHRA issuing a warning in June 2006 about an increased risk of oral clefts, although they note that now needs confirming by other database analyses. The incidence of major malformations with first-trimester exposure has been reported to be 1.8%, eg. there was one malformation in 51 women taking lamotrigine in an AED study, suggesting a low relative risk (n = 51, Sabers et al, Acta Neurol Scand 2004;**109**:9–13). Use in pregnancy needs additional care to manage seizures, eg. one survey showed that there was a higher risk of seizures, and higher doses were needed, in mothers taking lamotrigine (n = 1956, EURAP Study Group, Neurology 2006;**66**:354–60) because lamotrigine plasma levels can decrease by 65% in trimesters 2 and 3, which reverted rapidly after delivery (n = 11, Petrenaite et al, Epilepsy Res 2005;**65**:185–8; see also n = 12, Tran et al, Neurology 2002;**59**:251–5; n = 1, Tomson et al, Epilepsia 1997;**38**:1039–41). The incidence may be as high as 10% when also taken with valproate. In six mother–baby pairs, fetal **gabapentin** (ADEC = B1) levels were estimated to be 0.2–1.3 mg/kg/d (1.3–3.8% of mother's dose), with no adverse effects detected (n = 6, Ohman et al, Epilepsia 2005;**46**:1621–4) and there were no congenital anomalies in the 11 babies born to mothers taking gabapentin (FDA = C) in the first trimester in the Southampton PMSS (n = 3100, Wilton and Shakir, Epilepsia 2002;**43**:983–92).

27. * Some animal studies show animal reproductive toxicity, and so **levetiracetam** (FDA = C) should not be used unless clearly necessary. Animal studies have shown some animal reproductive toxicity with **pregabalin** (FDA = C) at high dose but the human risk is not known (SPC). No human data is available on **tiagabine** (FDA = C; ADEC = B3) in pregnancy and so use should only be where clearly indicated.

Topiramate (FDA = C; ADEC = B3) appears to pass the placenta easily, with low but detectable levels in children, although no ADRs have been noticed (n = 5 pairs, Ohman et al, Epilepsia 2002;**43**:1157–60). There has been some teratogenicity shown in animals and should not be used in pregnancy unless the benefit clearly outweighs the risk. **Vigabatrin** is contraindicated due to a slight increase in the incidence of cleft palate at high doses in one animal test (n = 2, Tran et al, Br J Clin Pharmacol 1998;**45**:409–11). **Zonisamide** is transferred to the infant via the placenta, the transfer rate being 92% (n = 2, Kawada et al, Brain Dev 2002;**24**:95–7) and adequate contraception in women is necessary during treatment and for one month afterwards.

28. For **acetazolamide** (FDA = C; ADEC = B3), animal tests indicate that it is teratogenic and can increase miscarriages when taken at toxic doses, and two probable human cases exist (Worsham et al, JAMA 1978;**240**:251–2). If use is essential, maternal electrolyte balance should be monitored. There are reported cases of malformations with **ethosuximide** (ADEC = D) alone, and about 35 when combined with other drugs but no cause-effect relationship has been proven. Although animal studies in rats have raised some concerns, no systematic human data is available. Little data is available for **paraldehyde** (FDA = C).

3.8.5 OTHERS

29. Very high doses of **donepezil** (FDA = C; ADEC = B3) may have some minor effects in pregnancy but no teratogenicity has been detected. The safety of **rivastigmine** (FDA = B) in pregnancy has not been established. There is no data on **galantamine** (FDA = B) in pregnancy, although animal studies show a slight delay in fetal and neonatal development. Human data is lacking with **memantine** (FDA = B) but animal data suggests potentially reduced interuterine growth.

30. **Anticholinergics**: (ADEC: benzatropine = B2, procyclidine = A)
There is little data available on these drugs. A 'small left colon syndrome' has been reported in two children born to mothers who took benzatropine and other psychotropic drugs late in pregnancy (Falterman and Richardson, J Paediatr 1980;**92**:308–10) although a cause-effect relationship was not established.

31. For **disulfiram** (ADEC=B2) there have been isolated reports of congenital abnormalities (eg. Gardner and Clarkson, *N Z Med J* 1981;**93**:184–6), although other drugs were often taken and the symptoms were similar to the fetal alcohol syndrome. In animals, disulfiram has been shown to be embryotoxic. The risk-benefit ratio for the risks of alcoholism against disulfiram for the fetus must be assessed carefully. The UK SPC for **acamprosate** (FDA=C) states that use in pregnancy is a contraindication, but animal studies have not shown any evidence of teratogenicity.

32. * **Lithium** (FDA=D; ADEC=D) completely equilibrates across the placenta. Studies show that congenital malformation rates with lithium (2.8%) are similar to control rates (2.4%), and suggest that lithium is not an important human teratogen if used with adequate screening (including level II ultrasound and fetal echo-cardiography) to detect Ebstein's anomaly (n=148, prospective Jacobson *et al*, *Lancet* 1992;**339**:530–3). The malformation risk in the first trimester is in the order of 4–12% and, hence, still greater than the general population. The risk of Ebstein's anomaly (a rare congenital downward displacement of the tricuspid valve into the right ventricle) exists if the drug is taken during weeks two to six post-conception. Ebstein's anomaly is 20 times more common with lithium, but the risk rises from 1 in 20000 to 1 in 1000. However, this risk must be weighed against the 50% chance of relapsing if lithium is stopped abruptly. An important study (n=101, retrospective, Viguera *et al*, *Am J Psychiatry* 2000;**157**:179–84) noted that:

- the heart is formed very early, so stopping lithium when pregnancy is confirmed is too late anyway
- the relapse rates in the 40 weeks after lithium discontinuation are similar for pregnant (52%) and non-pregnant (58%) women, but much higher than the year before discontinuation (21%), so stopping lithium raises the risk of release 2–3-fold but pregnancy itself is relatively 'risk neutral'
- women who remained stable over the first 40 weeks after lithium discontinuation were 2.9 times more likely to relapse than non-pregnant women during weeks 41–62 (70% vs 24%)
- the relapse rates are much higher in rapid rather than gradual lithium discontinuation

- the >50% relapse rate in the first 40 weeks is high, and the risk from consequentially needed drugs is high
- there were no major malformations in the children born to the women (n=9) who continued lithium throughout pregnancy
- an unstudied option might be to stop lithium gradually as soon as pregnancy is known, then reintroduce it in the third trimester.

NICE (Antenatal and postnatal mental health Guideline, 2007) recommends advising a woman to stop lithium if she is planning a pregnancy, is well and not at high risk of relapse. NICE also recommends that if a woman taking lithium becomes pregnant, is well and not at high risk of relapse, lithium should be stopped gradually over four weeks, and then informed that this may not remove the risk of cardiac defects in the fetus (although the author of this book fails to fully comprehend the logic of this). If the woman is not well or at high risk of relapse, NICE recommends switching to an antipsychotic, stopping lithium and restarting in the second trimester or continuing lithium if at high risk of relapse (for which rapid withdrawal would be a risk factor). Renal clearance is increased during pregnancy and so higher doses are needed. However, higher concentrations at delivery are associated with more perinatal complications. Since lithium clearance reduces markedly near the end of term, doses may need to be reduced by up to 30–50% in the last few weeks (or a few doses omitted close to delivery) and plasma levels monitored carefully and frequently (n=10+32, Newport *et al*, *Am J Psychiatry* 2005;**162**:2162–70), eg. NICE recommends monitoring levels every four weeks until the 36th week, then weekly from 36 weeks, then within the first 24 hours after childbirth, with doses adjusted according to those serum levels, and adequate fluid intake maintained.

Postnatal development: A study of 60 healthy children born to mothers who took lithium during the first trimester did not reveal any increased frequency of physical or mental anomalies among the lithium children compared to their non-lithium exposed siblings over 5–10 years (n=60, Schou, *Acta Psychiatr Scand* 1976;**54**:193–7; see also case and review by Pinelli *et al*, *Am J Obstet Gynecol* 2002;**187**:245–9).

Reviews: Llewellyn *et al*, *J Clin Psychiatry* 1998;

59[Suppl 6]:S57–S64; Yonkers et al, CNS Drugs 1998;**9**:261–9.

33. * **Modafinil** (FDA=C) is contraindicated in pregnancy. Pre-clinical studies have shown no teratogenicity but more information is required. There is limited data on **sodium oxybate** (FDA= B) but no evidence of malformations or toxicity after 2nd and 3rd trimester exposure, but there is no data in the 1st trimester and so is not recommended (SPC).

34. * **Methadone** (ADEC=C) at maintenance doses has been used successfully, does not appear to be overtly teratogenic and reduces the risk of poor quality street drugs being used. With potential illicit drug-using mothers, teratogenicity with methadone will obviously be very difficult to ascertain, but there does not appear to be a clear association with malformations (eg. study by Newman et al, Am J Obstet Gynecol 1975;**121**:233–7). Predictably, a fetal withdrawal syndrome, occurring within the first 24 hours has been seen. Symptoms include tremor, irritability, hyperactivity, jitteriness, shrill cry, vomiting, diarrhoea and convulsions. Methadone is associated with longer and more severe neonatal withdrawal than heroin (Malpas et al, Aus NZ J Obstet Gynecol 1995;**35**:175–7) and infant sudden death increased two- to three-fold (Davidson Ward et al, J Pediatrics 1990;**117**:876–87), although in one study, high-dose methadone was not associated with an increased risk of neonatal abstinence syndrome compared to lower doses, but reduced overall maternal drug use (n=81, McCarthy et al, Am J Obstet Gynecol 2005;**193**:606–10; see also breast-feeding, 3.1). Stopping opiates abruptly is dangerous, as withdrawal reactions can damage the fetus more than methadone.

Postnatal development: Long-term developmental outcome seems unaffected by methadone (Kaltenbach and Finnegan, Neurotoxicol Teratol 1987;**9**:311–13. For effect on the child in the first year see Arch Dis Childhood 1989;**64**:235–

45). There have also been numerous reports of sudden death, reduced body weight and head circumference, but these are virtually all in uncontrolled situations and so other effects cannot be excluded. In a study of methadone maintenance in pregnancy, head circumference and birth weight were slightly lower with methadone compared to controls (n=32, Brown et al, Am J Obstet Gynecol 1998;**179**:459–63). Slow-release morphine is no better at reducing neonatal withdrawal symptoms than methadone (n=48, Fischer et al, Addiction 1999;**94**:231–9).

Buprenorphine (FDA=C; ADEC=C) may have some advantages in pregnancy (Nocon, Addiction 2006;**101**:608). In weeks 24–29, buprenorpine had a higher retention rate than methadone, but higher additional opioid use with an earlier onset of NAS in methadone (mean 60 hours) than buprenorphine (72 hours) (n=18[c=14], RCT, d/b, Fischer et al, Addiction 2006;**101**:275–81).

35. No teratogenic effects have been reported in patients who took **dextroamphetamine** (FDA=C) before knowing they were pregnant (Guilleminault, Sleep 1993;**16**:199–201).

36. * There is little information available for **methylphenidate** (FDA=C; ADEC=B2) and the few reported cases are unremarkable, but the literature advises caution. The UK SPC recommends use of **atomoxetine** (FDA=C) only where the benefit justifies the potential risk.

37. * There have been reports of a higher than expected incidence of neonatal malformations with **bupropion** (FDA=C), especially cardiac (n=10, Prescrire Int 2005;**14**:225), but a large US study (1995–2004) showed that exposure to bupropion in the first trimester (n=1213) and 2nd/3rd trimesters (n=1049) was not associated with an increased risk of cardiovascular or other malformations, compared to other antidepressant (n=4743) 1st trimester exposures (Cole et al, Pharmacepidemiol Drug Saf 2007; in press).

3.9 RENAL IMPAIRMENT (SEE ALSO BNF)

	LOWER RISK (FDA=A)	MODERATE RISK (FDA=B OR C)	HIGHER RISK (FDA=D OR X)
Antipsychotics	Loxapine[8] Sertindole[2]	Aripiprazole[2] Butyrophenones[6] Clozapine[3] Olanzapine[2] Phenothiazines[7] Quetiapine[2] Thioxanthenes[4] Ziprasidone[2]	Amisulpride[5] Risperidone[1] Sulpiride[5] Zotepine[2]
Antidepressants	Mianserin[16] Moclobemide[16] Tricyclics[12] Trazodone[13] Tryptophan[16]	Duloxetine[10] MAOIs[15] Mirtazapine[11] Reboxetine[14] SSRIs[9]	Fluoxetine[9] Venlafaxine[10]
Anxiolytics and hynpotics	Benzodiazepines (some)[17] Zaleplon[19] Zopiclone[19]	Benzodiazepines[17] Beta-blockers[20] Clomethiazole[21] Zolpidem[19]	Buspirone[18] Chloral[21]
Anticonvulsants	Phenytoin[24] Tiagabine[27]	Barbiturates[25] Benzodiazepines[17] Carbamazepine[22] Ethosuximide[28] Fosphenytoin[24] Lamotrigine[26] Piracetam[27] Topiramate[27] Zonisamide[27]	Acetazolamide[28] Gabapentin[26] Levetiracetam[27] Midazolam[17] Oxcarbazepine[22] Pregabalin[27] Valproate[23] Vigabatrin[27]
Others	Anticholinesterases[29] Sodium oxybate[33]	Anticholinergics[30] Atomoxetine[34] Bupropion[34] Disulfiram[31] Memantine[29] Modafinil[33]	Acamprosate[31] Lithium[32]

Grade	GFR ml/min	Serum creatinine micromo/L
Mild	20–50	150–300
Moderate	10–20	300–700
Severe	<10	>700

GENERAL PRINCIPALS (ADAPTED FROM *MAUDSLEY GUIDELINES*)

1. The greater the renal impairment, the greater the potential for accumulation of drugs.
2. Serum creatinine may not be raised in the elderly, although renal impairment may be present.
3. Care is needed with drugs or active metabolites predominantly cleared by the kidney, eg. antidepressants and antipsychotics (except substituted benzamides).
4. Start low and go slow, adjusting doses to tolerance.
5. Adverse effects such as postural hypotension, sedation and confusion may be more common.
6. Care is needed with drugs with marked anticholinergic activity, which may cause urinary retention and interfere with U&E measurements.

3.9.1 ANTIPSYCHOTICS

Lower doses of all antipsychotics should be used, due to increased cerebral sensitivity and EPS.

1. * **Risperidone** elimination is reduced in renal disease and so initial doses and dose increments should be halved, up to a maximum of about 4mg/d. Haemodialysis has resulted in reduced risperidone levels, leading to relapse (n = 1, Railton et al, *Ther Drug Monit* 2005;**27**:558–61).
2. Dose adjustment with **aripiprazole** is not necessary even in severe renal impairment. **Olanzapine** is excreted primarily (57%) via the renal pathway and 30% in faeces. A lower olanzapine starting dose of 5mg/d may be appropriate in renal impairment (review: Callaghan et al, *Clin Pharmacokinetics* 1999;**37**:177–93). If creatinine clearance is <10ml/min, there is only a slight (11%) increase in half-life and 17% reduction in clearance. In severe renal impairment, **quetiapine** may have some reduced clearance compared to controls so the starting dose should be 25mg/d, with dose increments of 25–50mg/d (eg. n = 8, Thyrum et al, *Prog Neuropsychopharmacol Biol Psychiatry* 2000;**24**:521–33). Only 4% of an oral dose of **sertindole** is excreted via the kidneys. Clearance is unchanged by deteriorating renal function and in dialysis and usual doses can be used even in patients with severe renal impairment.

A 4mg single dose study showed that no dose adjustment was necessary in varying degrees of impairment (n = 24, Wong et al, *Eur J Clin Pharmacol* 1997;**52**:223–7). 17% of a dose of zotepine is excreted through the kidneys and levels may be 2–3 times higher in patients with renal impairment. Start at 25mg BD up to a maximum of 75mg BD. Only 1% of a **ziprasidone** dose is excreted unchanged via urine (20% excreted as metabolites), so dosage adjustment is not required in renal impairment (n = 39, open, Aweeka et al, *Br J Clin Pharmacol* 2000;**49**[Suppl 3]:27–33).

3. **Clozapine** is contraindicated in severe renal disease. Start at 12.5mg/d and increase slowly in mild to moderate renal failure.
4. **Zuclopenthixol** and **flupentixol** should be used with caution in renal impairment, as some accumulation of metabolites has been reported. No dosage adjustment of flupentixol is usually necessary (review: Jann et al, *Clin Pharmacokinet* 1985;**10**:315–33).
5. **Sulpiride** is mainly cleared by the kidneys and its half-life can range from 6–25 hours, depending upon renal function. Reduce the dose by 35–70% or extend the dosage interval by a factor of 1.5 to 3 if necessary (n = 24, open, Bressolle et al, *Clin Pharmacokinet* 1989;**17**:367–73). **Amisulpride** is principally cleared unchanged through the kidneys, so care is needed in moderate to severe renal insufficiency (GFR 10–30ml/min). It is not appreciably removed during haemodialysis.
6. There are no apparent problems with **haloperidol**. It causes little sedation or postural hypotension. The literature recommends caution as some accumulation might occur.
7. There is little information on **phenothiazines**, but excretion may be slower and accumulation may occur, causing sedation or postural hypotension. **Levomepromazine** (methotrimeprazine) should be used with care in renal disease, and chlorpromazine and thioridazine avoided.
8. **Loxapine** is 70% excreted via the kidneys and 30% via faeces. No specific problems in renal damage are known. The UK SPC for **pimozide** recommends caution in renal impairment.

3.9.2 ANTIDEPRESSANTS

9. * Renal clearance accounts for about 20% of total **citalopram** elimination, and although half-life increases slightly, no reduction of citalopram

dosage is warranted in patients with moderately impaired renal function but slight reduction in severe renal failure may be prudent (RCT, Joffe et al, Eur J Clin Pharmacol 1998;**54**:237–42). Haemodialysis had an insignificant effect on plasma levels (n = 12, open, Spigset et al, Eur J Clin Pharmacol 2000;**56**:699–703). Even severe renal failure did not affect the kinetics of citalopram in a single-dose study. Dosage adjustment with **escitalopram** is not necessary in patients with mild or moderate renal impairment. Caution is advised in patients with severely reduced renal function (CLCR less than 30 ml/min). The UK SPC for **fluoxetine** states that when given 20 mg/day for two months, patients with severe renal failure (GFR < 10 ml/min) requiring dialysis showed no difference in plasma levels of fluoxetine or norfluoxetine compared to controls with normal renal function. **Fluvoxamine** should be used with care, starting at 50 mg/d and increasing only slowly. An unpublished report indicated that fluvoxamine does not accumulate at 100 mg/d in renal impairment. Plasma levels of fluvoxamine are reduced by about 22% by haemodialysis, so higher doses might be needed (n = 7, Kamo et al, Psychiatr Clin Neurosci 2004;**58**:133–7). In moderate renal impairment, reduce the initial dose of **paroxetine** to 10 mg/d and increase only if necessary. Use of **sertraline** is not recommended by the manufacturers, although they have 'data on file' of a single dose study which showed no significant changes in sertraline kinetics in mild, moderate or severe renal failure.

10. About 1–10% of a **venlafaxine** dose is cleared unchanged by the kidney and 30% renally excreted as the major metabolite. Total clearance is reduced by about 35% in mild to moderate renal impairment (GFR 10–30 ml/min) and so doses should be reduced by about 25–50%, although there is much inter-patient variability in renal impairment (Anon, J Clin Psychiatry 1993;**54**:119–26). A study (12 with renal impairment, eight on dialysis and 18 matched controls) showed that clearance was reduced by about 55% in moderate to severe renal disease, and the authors suggested a 50% reduction in venlafaxine dose, given once a day, where GFR was less than 30 ml/min (n = 38, open, Troy et al, Clin Pharmacol Therapeut 1994;**56**:14–21). Daily doses should also be reduced by 50% in dialysis and doses withheld

until after dialysis is complete. Venlafaxine is not recommended in severe renal failure. No dose adjustment is needed for **duloxetine** in mild to moderate renal disease (creatinine clearance 30–80 ml/min), but is contraindicated in severe (< 30 ml/min) renal disease where plasma levels are doubled.

11. **Mirtazapine** clearance is reduced by 33% in moderate and by 50% in severe renal failure, but not in mild renal impairment in a single dose study (n = 40, Bengtsson et al, Hum Psychopharmacol 1998;**13**:357–65). Care with higher doses is recommended.

12. **Tricyclics** should be started at low dose and increased slowly, with divided doses. Avoid lofepramine in severe renal impairment, as 50% is renally excreted.

13. No dosage adjustment is necessary for **trazodone** (Catanese et al, Boll Chim Farm 1978; **117**:424–7).

14. **Reboxetine's** half-life and plasma levels appear to rise (up to two-fold) in severe renal impairment, where dose adjustment may be necessary. In a single-dose study, a reduction in starting dose to 2 mg BD in patients with moderate-to-severe renal dysfunction has been suggested (n = 18, open, Coulomb et al, J Clin Pharmacol 2000;**40**:482–7).

15. No dosage adjustments are usually necessary for the **MAOIs**, although **isocarboxazid** should be used with caution with impaired renal function to prevent accumulation.

16. Dosage adjustments in renal disease are not necessary for **moclobemide** (n = 12, open, Stoeckel et al, Acta Psychiatr Scand 1990;**360**[Suppl]:S94–S97), **mianserin** or **tryptophan**.

3.9.3 ANXIOLYTICS AND HYPNOTICS

17. Low dose anticonvulsant use of **benzo-diazepines** may be acceptable, as higher doses produce an increase in CNS sedative side-effects. **Chlordiazepoxide** can be given in normal doses and is not affected by haemodialysis (review, Bennett et al, Am J Kidney Dis 1983;**3**:155). In severe renal failure, doses of **oxazepam** should be reduced to 75%. In end-stage renal failure and haemodialysis, **clobazam** and metabolite concentrations appear no different to those with normal renal function so there may be no need to change doses in any degree of renal failure or in haemodialysis (n = 1, Roberts and Zoanetti, Ann

Pharmacother 1994;**28**:966–7). Accumulation of metabolites of **midazolam** may be responsible for prolonged sedation, not reversible by flumazenil (n = 5, Bauer *et al*, *Lancet* 1995;**346**:145–7).

18. **Buspirone** plasma levels have been shown to be higher in patients with renal failure, with a good correlation between steady-state levels and serum albumin (n = 54, open, Barbhaiya *et al*, *Eur J Clin Pharmacol* 1994;**46**:41–7). It is contraindicated in moderate or severe renal impairment.

19. Plasma protein-binding of **zolpidem** is reduced in renal failure (n = 54, open, Pacifici, *Int J Clin Pharmacol Ther Toxicol* 1988;**26**:439–43). The half-life may be doubled but no dosage adjustments are recommended in mild renal dysfunction. The pharmacokinetics of **zaleplon** and **zopiclone** are not significantly different in renal insufficiency, and dose alteration is not required.

20. In severe renal disease, plasma levels of **beta-blockers** may be higher and so starting doses should be lower. Beta-blockers may also reduce renal blood flow and adversely affect renal function.

21. Caution is needed with **clomethiazole** in chronic renal disease. **Chloral** is contraindicated in moderate to marked renal impairment.

3.9.4 ANTICONVULSANTS

22. **Carbamazepine** rarely causes renal disturbances although it has been suggested that doses should be reduced by 25% in severe renal failure. The UK SPC has renal impairment as a precaution. For **oxcarbazepine** in renal impairment (creatinine clearance less than 30 ml/min), start at half the usual dose (300 mg/day), increasing no more frequently than at weekly intervals. In patients with pre-existing renal conditions associated with low sodium or in patients treated concomitantly with sodium-lowering drugs (eg. diuretics, desmopressin) as well as NSAIDs, serum sodium levels should be monitored carefully.

23. **Valproate** is eliminated mainly through the kidneys and the literature states that it may be necessary to decrease dosage in renal insufficiency.

24. No specific dose adjustments are required for **phenytoin**, but protein-binding is altered in uraemia which can be problematic in accurately assessing serum levels. Severe cardiovascular ADRs have been reported with **fosphenytoin** IV (see *3.2*) and so a reduced loading dose and/or infusion rate by 10–25% is recommended in renal impairment.

25. **Phenobarbital** causes increased sedation and the dosage interval should be increased to at least 12–16 hours in severe renal failure. Large doses of **primidone** should be avoided. Active metabolites of **amylobarbital** accumulate in severe renal disease.

26. **Gabapentin** is mainly excreted unchanged in the urine (n = 12, open, Hooper *et al*, *Br J Clin Pharmacol* 1991;**31**:171–4). The manufacturer recommends dose reductions as follows:

Creatine clearance	Gabapentin dosage and frequency
60–90 ml/min	400 mg TDS
30–60 ml/min	300 mg BD
15–30 ml/min	300 mg/d
< 15 ml/min	300 mg alternate days

Patients undergoing haemodialysis should receive a gabapentin loading dose of 400 mg, plus 200–300 mg for every four hours of dialysis. Alternatively, a single-dose study of gabapentin 400 mg in adults with varying degrees of renal function (but none on dialysis) showed that clearance correlated well with creatinine clearance, with increased half-life with poorer renal function. The authors of this study suggested normal gabapentin doses for creatinine clearance of 60 ml/min, 600 mg/d for 30–59 ml/min, 300 mg/d for 15–29 ml/min and 150 mg/d for CLcr less than 15 ml/min (n = 60, open, Blum *et al*, *Clin Pharmacol Therapeut* 1994;**56**:154–9). A reduced maintenance dose of **lamotrigine** is usually recommended in severe renal impairment, but the dose probably needs little adjustment in mild to moderate impairment (n = 21, Wootton *et al*, *Br J Clin Pharmacol* 1997;**43**:23–7), and even in end-stage renal failure, although the major glucuronide metabolite levels may increase eight-fold due to reduced renal clearance.

27. * Since 66% of a dose of **levetiracetam** is excreted unchanged in the urine, dose reductions are necessary in impaired renal function as follows:

Renal function	Creatinine clearance	
Normal	80 ml/min	500–1500 mg BD
Mild	50–79 ml/min	500–1000 mg BD
Moderate	30–49 ml/min	250–750 mg BD
Severe	<30 ml/min	250–500 mg BD
End-stage renal disease, undergoing dialysis	–	50–100 mg BD

Following dialysis, a 250–500 mg supplemental dose is recommended.

Piracetam is excreted unchanged via the kidneys and dose adjustments may be needed in renal impairment (review: Tacconi and Wurtman, Adv Neurol 1986;**43**:675–85). **Pregabalin** is mainly excreted unchanged by the kidney, clearance being directly proportional to creatinine clearance (n = 50, Randinitis et al, J Clin Pharmacol 2003;**43**:277–83), so doses in renal impairment must be individually calculated (see SPC). Supplementary doses are necessary after every four-hour haemodialysis (SPC). There are no apparent problems with **tiagabine** (n = 25, Cato et al, Epilepsia 1998;**39**:43–7). About 60–70% of a **topiramate** dose is excreted unchanged via the kidneys. Time to steady state may be 10–15 days in severe renal impairment instead of 4–8 days with normal renal function. Dose titration may thus need to be more careful. Supplemental doses of 50% of the daily dose should be given on haemodialysis days. There is an increased risk of renal stone formation, via its carbonic anhydrase inhibition, carbonic anhydrase being a known inhibitor of renal crystallisation. Care is needed to ensure adequate fluid throughput, especially in patients with known disposition to this problem (Wasserstein et al, Epilepsia 1995;**36**[Suppl 3]:S153). **Vigabatrin** is excreted by the kidneys and so reduced doses are recommended with a creatinine clearance of <60 mL/min. **Zonisamide** and its metabolite are excreted renally and should not be used in acute renal failure or where serum creatinine is significantly raised. Zonisamide AUC is increased by 35% in people

where creatinine clearance is <20 ml/min. It may cause symptomatic renal calculus.
28. **Ethosuximide** doses should be reduced by 25% in severe renal failure.

3.9.5 OTHERS

29. No change in dose is necessary with **donepezil** in mild to moderate renal impairment and a 5 mg single-dose study indicated that even moderate to severe renal impairment did not significantly alter donepezil kinetics (open, n = 22, Tiseo et al, Br J Clin Pharmacol 1998;**46**[Suppl 1]:S56–S60). There are no reported problems with **rivastigmine**. No dosage reduction of **galantamine** is necessary for creatinine clearance greater than 9 ml/min. In severe impairment (<9 ml/min) galantamine is contraindicated (due to a lack of safety data). **Memantine** can be used in renal failure with no dosage adjustments although 5 mg BD is recommended in severe renal failure (n = 32 [c = 31], Periclou et al, Clin Pharmacol Ther 2006;**79**:134–43).
30. The literature recommends some caution in renal disease with the **anticholinergics**.
31. The SPC for **disulfiram** recommends caution in renal disease. The UK SPC for **acamprosate** states that use in renal insufficiency (serum creatinine >120 micromol/L) is a contraindication.
32. **Lithium** is contraindicated in severe renal impairment but if use is unavoidable, use alternate-day dosing, very low doses (25–75% normal) and frequently estimate levels (eg. 125 mg on alternate days in a 78-year-old woman, n=1, Gash et al, J Affect Disord 1995; **34**:51–3). For a review of lithium and the kidney, see Gitlin (Drug Saf 1999;**20**:231–43, 77 refs).
33. * The maximum **modafinil** dose of 400 mg/d should only be used in the absence of renal impairment. **Sodium oxybate** contains a significant dose of sodium (0.75 g in 4.5 g dose) and so dietary restriction of sodium might be considered, but since the kidney is not involved in excretion no dose reduction is thought to be necessary (SPC).
34. **Bupropion** and metabolites are almost exclusively (85%) excreted through the kidneys and so, in renal failure, the initial dose should be reduced and close monitoring for toxicity carried out. For **atomoxetine**, 80% of a dose is excreted in urine and the UK SPC recommends possible dose reduction in renal impairment.

4 DRUG INTERACTIONS

Full reviews, assessments and references for most of these interactions can be found in standard reference books. Resources include *Drug Interactions Facts, Drug Interactions* by Ivan Stockley (Blackwell Scientific, Oxford), or *Drug Interactions in Psychiatry*, edited by Ciraulo, Shader, Greenblatt and Creelman (Williams & Wilkins, Maryland).

Absolute classification of interactions is impossible. Many factors, eg. age, concurrent illness, P450 status, etc. are important. Single case reports merely suggest a possible interaction, and more structured formal studies may show the probable likelihood of an interaction. For completeness, some drugs available worldwide are included and may not be marketed in all countries. To give some guidance, interactions with the drugs in **CAPITAL LETTERS** are those that could be:

- potentially hazardous
- where a dosage adjustment is likely to have to be made
- well-established and documented
- of clinical significance
- rare but important.

How to use this section:
1. Look up the psychiatric drug or group.
2. Look up the drug group of the interacting drug.
3. If no entry there, look up the actual drug.
4. If still no entry, little or nothing has been reported to date.

Review: general psychotropics (Chadwick *et al*, *Adv Psychiatr Treat* 2005;**11**:440–9).

4.1 ANXIOLYTICS AND HYPNOTICS

Reviews: clinically important drug interactions with zopiclone, zaleplon and zolpidem (Hesse *et al*, *CNS Drugs* 2003;**17**:513–32), pharmacokinetics and pharmacodynamics (Drover, *Clin Pharmacokinet* 2004;**43**:227–38).

4.1.1 BENZODIAZEPINES

Benzodiazepines are mainly metabolised by CYP2C and CYP3A3/4.

Review: Tanaka, *J Clin Pharm Therapeut* 1999; **24**:347.

Acamprosate + benzodiazepines
See acamprosate (*4.6.1*).

Alcohol + benzodiazepines
See alcohol (*4.7.1*).

Alosetron + alprazolam
Alosetron, a 5-HT3 receptor antagonist, has no effect on the kinetics of alprazolam (n = 12, RCT, open, D'Souza *et al*, *J Clin Pharmacol* 2001;**41**:452–4).

Amfetamines + benzodiazepines
Amfetamine significantly reverses the sedative and memory-impairing effects of triazolam (n = 20, p/c, d/b, c/o, Mintzer and Griffiths, *J Psychopharmacol* 2003;**17**:17–29, 146).

Amiodarone + clonazepam
Amidarone has been reported to cause clonazepam toxicity at low dose (n = 1, Witt *et al*, *Ann Pharmacother* 1993;**27**:1463–4).

Antacids + benzodiazepines
Benzodiazepine absorption is slightly delayed by antacids, but total absorption remains the same.

Anticholinergics + benzodiazepines
Benzodiazepine absorption may be delayed by anticholinergics, but the amount absorbed remains unchanged.

Anticoagulants + benzodiazepines
Lack of an interaction has been demonstrated and benzodiazepines are a suitable alternative to chloral hydrate. Isolated cases of adverse reactions have been reported.

Antihistamines + benzodiazepines
Enhanced sedation is possible.

Antihypertensives + benzodiazepines
Enhanced hypotension is possible.

Antipsychotics + benzodiazepines
See antipsychotics (*4.2.1*).

Atomoxetine + benzodiazepines
See atomoxetine (*4.6.4*).

Atropine + benzodiazepines
No interaction is thought to occur.

Baclofen + benzodiazepines
Enhanced sedation can occur.

Barbiturates + benzodiazepines
Enhanced sedation and increased benzodiazepine

clearance may occur via CYP3A4 induction. Dose adjustment may be necessary.

Beta-blockers + benzodiazepines

Propranolol and metoprolol produce a small but significant reduction in diazepam clearance, and patients may become more 'accident-prone' on the combination. Propranolol and labetolol have no effect on oxazepam (n=6, Sonne et al, Br J Clin Pharmacol 1990;**29**:33–7), but some effect on reaction times was seen. Metoprolol appears not to interact significantly with lorazepam (n=12, open, Scott et al, Eur J Clin Pharmacol 1991; **40**:405–9).

Buprenorphine + benzodiazepines

Buprenorphine does not inhibit the metabolism of flunitrazepam and so any interaction is likely to be pharmacodynamic rather than metabolic, although deaths have been reported with concomitant buprenorphine and benzodiazepines (n=6, Reynaud et al, Addiction 1998;**93**:1385–92).

Buspirone + benzodiazepines

See buspirone (4.1.2).

CALCIUM-CHANNEL BLOCKERS + BENZODIAZEPINES

Diltiazem significantly increases diazepam levels, probably via CYP3A4 inhibition (n=13, RCT, d/b, c/o, Kosuge et al, Drug Metab Dispos 2001;**29**:1284–9). Both diltiazem and verapamil significantly raise midazolam levels and half-life, via 3A4 induction, increasing sedative side-effects, and so a 50% midazolam dose reduction has been recommended (n=9, RCT, d/b, c/o, 2/7, Backman et al, Br J Clin Pharmacol 1994;**37**:221–5).

Cannabis + benzodiazepines

See cannabis (4.7.2).

Carbamazepine + benzodiazepines

See carbamazepine (4.5.1).

Charcoal, activated + benzodiazepines

25 g of activated charcoal given 30 minutes after diazepam 5 mg reduces diazepam AUC by 27%, but not the peak levels. Concurrent gastric lavage does not provide any additional reductions (n=9, RCT, Lapatto-Reiniluoto et al, Br J Clin Pharmacol 1999;**48**:148–53).

Citalopram + benzodiazepines

See citalopram/escitalopram (4.3.2.1).

Clarithromycin + benzodiazepines

Higher dose clarithromycin (2.5 g/d) may increase the availability of midazolam, probably via CYP3A4 competition (n=16, open, 8/7, Gorski et al, Clin Pharmacol Ther 1998;**64**:133–43).

CLOZAPINE + BENZODIAZEPINES

See clozapine (4.2.3).

Cyclophosphamide + benzodiazepines

Increased cyclophosphamide toxicity has been proposed.

Dehydroepiandrosterone + benzodiazepines

Alprazolam rapidly and significantly increases dehydroepiandrosterone concentrations (n=38, Kroboth et al, J Clin Psychopharmacol 1999;**19**:114–24).

Dextropropoxyphene + alprazolam

Increased sedation can occur with alprazolam.

Digoxin + benzodiazepines

Lack of interaction has been shown.

Diflunisal + benzodiazepines

Diflunisal may reduce the effect of some benzodiazepines (lorazepam, temazepam and oxazepam) by increasing metabolism.

Disulfiram + benzodiazepines

See disulfiram (4.6.8).

Escitalopram + benzodiazepines

See citalopram/escitalopram (4.3.2.1).

Ethambutol + diazepam

Lack of interaction has been shown.

Fluoxetine + benzodiazepines

See fluoxetine (4.3.2.2).

Fluvoxamine + benzodiazepines

See fluvoxamine (4.3.2.3).

Food + benzodiazepines

Food delays the absorption of benzodiazepines; only significant if rapid onset of action is needed.

Gabapentin + benzodiazepines

See gabapentin (4.5.3).

Gingko biloba + benzodiazepines *

GB may increase the AUC for midazolam by 25%, possibly significant (n=10, 4/52, Uchida et al, J Clin Pharmacol 2006;**46**:1290–8).

Grapefruit juice + benzodiazepines

200ml normal-strength grapefruit juice increases plasma triazolam levels, and repeated consumption produces a greater increase (n=12, RCT, Lilja et al, Eur J Clin Pharmacol 2000;**56**:411–5).

H2-blockers + benzodiazepines

Cimetidine inhibits the CYP3A4 metabolism of long-acting benzodiazepines, but not of lorazepam, oxazepam and temazepam. The clinical effect is probably negligible. The other H2-blockers do not interact this way (eg. ranitidine, n=9, RCT, d/b, c/o, 4/7, Klotz et al, J Clin Pharmacol 1987;**27**:210–2), although ranitidine may slightly reduce the absorption of diazepam and increase the absorption of triazolam (n = 30, RCT, open, 3/7, O'Connor-Semmes et al, Clin Pharmacol Ther 2001;**70**:126–31).

Heparin + benzodiazepines
A transient rise in benzodiazepine levels could occur (n = 5, open, Routledge et al, Clin Pharm Ther 1980;**27**:528–32).

Indometacin + diazepam
Increased dizziness may occur (d/b, Nuotto and Saariolho, Pharmacol Toxicol 1988;**62**:293–7).

Isoniazid + benzodiazepines
Isoniazid reduces the clearance of diazepam but not of oxazepam (n = 9, Ochs et al, Clin Pharmacol Ther 1981;**29**:671–8).

Itraconazole/ketoconazole + benzodiazepines
Increased chlordiazepoxide oral bioavailability and midazolam levels/AUC, up to eight-fold higher (n = 9, RCT, d/b, c/o, 3×4/7, Olkkola et al, Clin Pharmacol Ther 1994;**55**:481–5; n = 10, RCT, 12/7, Lam et al, J Clin Pharmacol 2003;**43**:1274–82). Midazolam levels were significantly higher with itraconazole 200mg/d for four days, the effect being detectable up to four days after cessation of treatment (n = 9, open, Backman et al, Eur J Clin Pharmacol 1998;**54**:53–8).

Lamotrigine + benzodiazepines
See lamotrigine (4.5.4).

LEVODOPA + BENZODIAZEPINES
Levodopa can be antagonised by diazepam, nitrazepam and chlordiazepoxide (Yousselson et al, Ann Intern Med 1982;**96**:259–60): observe for worsening of symptoms.

Lithium + benzodiazepines
See lithium (4.4).

MAOIs + benzodiazepines
See MAOIs (4.3.4).

Methadone + benzodiazepines
See methadone (4.6.10).

Metronidazole + benzodiazepines
Lack of interaction has been reported.

Mianserin + benzodiazepines
See mianserin (4.3.3.2).

Mirtazapine + benzodiazepines
See mirtazapine (4.3.3.3).

Moclobemide + benzodiazepines
See moclobemide (4.3.3.3).

Modafinil + benzodiazepines
See modafinil (4.6.12).

Muscle relaxants + benzodiazepines
Variable relatively minor effects have been

reported (n = 113, Driessen et al, Acta Anaesthesiol Scand 1986;**30**:642–6). Diazepam may hasten the onset and prolong the duration of action of vecuronium (n = 20, RCT, Yuan et al, Chung Hua I Hsueh Tsa Chih (Taipei) 1994;**54**:259–64), but midazolam appears not to do this (n = 10, Husby et al, Acta Anaesthesiol Scand 1989;**33**:280–2).

Narcotic analgesics/opioids + benzodiazepines
Synergism (eg. n = 95, RCT, d/b, Kissin et al, Anesth Analg 1990;**71**:65–9) and changes in haemodynamic status (Heikkila et al, Acta Anesthesiol Scand 1984;**28**:683–9) have been reported.

Nimodipine + benzodiazepines
Lack of a clinically significant interaction during chronic oral administration has been reported (n = 24, RCT, c/o, 3×5/7, Heine et al, Br J Clin Pharmacol 1994;**38**:39–43).

Olanzapine + benzodiazepines
See olanzapine (4.2.4).

Ondansetron + benzodiazepines
Lack of interaction has been shown with temazepam (n = 24, RCT, d/b, c/o, 2/7, Preston et al, Anesthesia 1996;**51**:827–30).

Oral contraceptives + benzodiazepines
OCs may increase the effects of longer-acting benzodiazepines, but this is not thought to be of clinical significance.

Oxycodone + benzodiazepines
A fatal interaction has been reported with clonazepam, although the mechanism is unclear (n = 1, Burrows et al, J Forensic Sci 2003; **48**: 683–6).

Paraldehyde + benzodiazepines
Enhanced sedation would be expected.

Paroxetine + benzodiazepines
See paroxetine (4.3.2.4).

Phenytoin + benzodiazepines
See phenytoin (4.5.8).

Physostigmine + benzodiazepines
Physostigmine may reverse diazepam-induced sleep (Speeg et al, J Neurochem 1980;**34**:856–5) and midazolam-induced somnolence (Ho et al, Ma Tsui Hsueh Tsa Chi 1991;**29**:643–7).

Pregabalin + benzodiazepines
See pregabalin (4.5.10).

Progabide + clonazepam
Lack of interaction has been reported.

Propofol + benzodiazepines
Propofol increases the half-life of midazolam by

61%, probably by inhibiting CYP3A4 (n = 24, RCT, Hamaoka et al, Clin Pharmacol Ther 1999;**66**:110–7).

Proton-pump inhibitors + benzodiazepines
Omeprazole, but not pantoprazole (review: Steinijans et al, Int J Clin Pharmacol Ther 1996; **34**:S31–S50), can reduce diazepam clearance by up to 50% (n = 12, 1/52, Andersson et al, Eur J Clin Pharmacol 1990;**39**:51–4), probably by a P450 mechanism (Zomorodi and Houston, Br J Clin Pharmacol 1996;**42**:157–62).

Quetiapine + benzodiazepines
See quetiapine (4.2.5).

Reboxetine + benzodiazepines
See reboxetine (4.3.3.5).

Rifampin + benzodiazepines
CYP3A4 induction by rifampin can lead to increased diazepam clearance (n = 21, 7/7, Ohnhaus, Clin Pharmacol Ther 1987;**42**:148) and reduced midazolam levels (n = 9, 9/7, Backman et al, Eur J Clin Pharmacol 1998;**54**:53–8).

Ritonavir + benzodiazepines
Extensive impairment of triazolam and alprazolam clearance by short-term low-dose ritonavir may occur (editorial: Greenblatt et al, J Clin Psychopharmacol 1999;**19**:293–6).

Rivastigmine + benzodiazepines
See rivastigmine (4.6.3.3).

Sertindole + benzodiazepines
See sertindole (4.2.7).

Sertraline + benzodiazepines
See sertraline (4.3.2.5).

Smoking + benzodiazepines
See smoking (4.7.4).

Sodium oxybate + benzodiazepines*
See sodium oxybate (4.6.13).

St John's wort + benzodiazepines
See St John's wort (4.3.3.9).

Tiagabine + benzodiazepines
See tiagabine (4.5.11).

Tricyclics + benzodiazepines
Enhanced sedation has been reported and would be expected. Reduced hydroxylation of clomipramine has been reported and dose reduction may be necessary (Pharmaceutisch Weekblad 1992;**14**[4] Suppl D:D3).

Valproate + benzodiazepines
Valproate displaces diazepam from plasma protein-binding sites and so doses may need to be reduced. Valproate increases lorazepam levels by up to 40% (n = 16, RCT, Samara et al, J Clin Pharmacol 1997;**37**:442–50) and coma has been reported with the combination, possibly via reduced lorazepam clearance (n = 1, Lee et al, Seizure 2002;**11**:124–5). Concomitant valproate and clonazepam increases clonazepam clearance by 14% and reduces valproate clearance by 18% (n = 317, Yukawa et al, J Clin Pharm Ther 2003;**28**:497–504), probably of minimal significance (n = 4, Wang and Wang, Ther Drug Monit 2002;**24**:532–6).

Venlafaxine + benzodiazepines
See venlafaxine (4.3.3.8).

Warfarin + benzodiazepines
No interaction has been reported but is theoretically possible (mentioned in Sayal et al, Acta Psychiatr Scand 2000;**102**:250–5).

Xanthines + benzodiazepines
Xanthines, eg. theophylline, aminophylline and caffeine antagonise the sedative (and possibly anxiolytic) effects of benzodiazepines (eg. midazolam 12mg is moderately antagonised by 250mg caffeine, n = 114, Mattila et al, Int J Clin Pharmacol Ther 2000;**38**:581–7). This can be useful in the treatment of benzodiazepine overdose, but care must be taken if a patient on a benzodiazepine has theophylline stopped, as respiratory depression can then occur.

Ziprasidone + benzodiazepines
See ziprasidone (4.2.8).

Zotepine + benzodiazepines
See zotepine (4.2.9).

4.1.2 BUSPIRONE

Buspirone may be metabolised by CYP3A4.

Alcohol + buspirone
See alcohol (4.7.1).

Benzodiazepines + buspirone
Two studies with diazepam have shown only a minimal enhanced sedation. Alprazolam appears not to interact with buspirone (n = 24, 7/7, Buch et al, J Clin Pharmacol 1993;**33**:1104–9).

Calcium-channel blockers + buspirone
80mg verapamil or 60mg diltiazem increase buspirone plasma concentrations three-fold and five-fold respectively, peak plasma levels also being raised. This is probably by CYP3A4 inhibition, potentially enhancing the therapeutic and side-effects of buspirone (n = 9, RCT, p/c, c/o, Lamberg et al, Clin Pharmacol Ther 1998;**63**:640–5).

Cimetidine + buspirone
Lack of interaction has been reported (n = 10,

open, Gammans et al, Pharmacotherapy 1987;
7:72–9).

Citalopram + buspirone
See citalopram (4.3.2.1).

Clozapine + buspirone
Near fatal gastrointestinal bleeding and hyper-glycaemia occurring one month after buspirone was added to a stable clozapine regimen has been reported, but no firm explanation found (n = 1, Good, Am J Psychiatry 1997;**154**:1473).

Erythromycin + buspirone
Erythromycin and itraconazole may increase plasma buspirone levels dramatically, probably via CYP3A4 inhibition, with increased side-effects noted (n = 8, Kivisto et al, Clin Pharmacol Ther 1997;**62**:348–54).

Escitalopram + buspirone
See citalopram/escitalopram (4.3.2.1).

Fluvoxamine + buspirone
Fluvoxamine 100mg/d raises buspirone levels, probably via CYP3A4 inhibition, but this is of limited significance (n = 10, RCT, Lamberg et al, Eur J Clin Pharmacol 1998;**54**:761–6).

Fluoxetine + buspirone
Reduced anxiolytic effect, dystonia, akathisia (n = 1, Metz, Can J Psychiatry 1990;**35**:722–3) and anorgasmia (n = 20, open, 8/52, Jenike et al, J Clin Psychiatry 1991;**52**:13–4) have been reported.

Grapefruit juice + buspirone
200ml double-strength grapefruit juice raised peak buspirone plasma levels four-fold, probably via CYP3A4 inhibition or delayed gastric emptying, so avoid buspirone and, at least, large amounts of grapefruit juice, or adjust doses (n = 10, RCT, Lilja et al, Clin Pharmacol Ther 1998;**64**:655–60).

Itraconazole + buspirone
See erythromycin + buspirone.

MAOIs + BUSPIRONE
See MAOIs (4.3.4).

NSAIDs + buspirone
GI side-effects and headache may be slightly more common with the combination (n = 150, Kiev and Domantay, Curr Ther Res 1989;**46**:1086–90).

Phenytoin + buspirone
Buspirone does not appear to displace phenytoin from plasma-binding sites (review: Gammans et al, Am J Med 1986;**80**[Suppl 3B]:41–51).

Propranolol + buspirone
Buspirone appears not to displace propranolol from plasma-binding sites (review: Gammans et al, Am J Med 1986;**80**[Suppl 3B]:41–51).

Rifampin + buspirone
The buspirone UK SPC now states that rifampin decreases buspirone plasma levels, probably via CYP3A4 induction. Significant changes in psychomotor tests have been noted and so dose adjustment may be necessary (n = 10, Lamberg et al, Br J Clin Pharmacol 1998;**45**:381–5).

Ritonavir + buspirone
Severe EPSE have appeared after ritonavir was added to buspirone (n = 1, Clay and Adams, Ann Pharmacother 2003;**37**:202–5).

St John's wort + buspirone
There is a possible case of serotonin syndrome (n = 1, Dannawi, J Psychopharmacol 2002;**16**:401).

Trazodone + buspirone
There are some isolated reports of raised SGPT/ALT levels and a case of serotonin syndrome (n = 1, Goldberg and Huk, Psychosomatics 1992;**3**:235).

Warfarin + buspirone
Buspirone does not appear to displace warfarin from plasma-binding sites (review: Gammans et al, Am J Med 1986;**80**[Suppl 3B]:41–51).

Zidovidine + buspirone
The combination has been used safely (n = 2, Batki, J Clin Psychopharmacol 1990;**10**[Suppl 3]: 111S–5S).

4.1.3 CHLORAL HYDRATE

Chloral is probably metabolised by CYP2E1.

ALCOHOL + CHLORAL HYDRATE
See alcohol (4.7.1)

Fluvoxamine + chloral hydrate
See fluvoxamine (4.3.2.3).

Furosemide + chloral hydrate
Diaphoresis, facial flushing and agitation occurred with chloral hydrate and IV furosemide, which stopped when the chloral hydrate was discontinued (n = 1, Dean et al, Clin Pharm 1991; 10:385–7).

MAOIs + chloral hydrate
See MAOIs (4.3.4).

Methadone + chloral hydrate
See methadone (4.6.10).

Phenytoin + chloral hydrate
See phenytoin (4.5.8).

Nicoumalone + chloral hydrate
An enhanced anticoagulant effect can occur. See also warfarin + chloral hydrate.

Warfarin + chloral hydrate
The anticoagulant effects of warfarin are

increased slightly by chloral hydrate, probably by plasma protein displacement (BCDSP, *N Engl J Med* 1972;**286**:53–5). This can be important if chloral hydrate is given as a PRN hypnotic.

4.1.4 ZALEPLON

Zaleplon is primarily metabolised by aldehyde oxidase, and a small amount by CYP3A4 to inactive metabolites. As with other such drugs, use with other CNS-depressants needs care.

Alcohol + zaleplon
See alcohol (*4.7.1*).

Antipsychotics + zaleplon
Additive psychomotor effects may occur with thioridazine (n = 12, RCT, Hetta *et al*, *Eur J Clin Pharmacol* 2000;**56**:211–7).

Carbamazepine + zaleplon
Co-administration may reduce zaleplon's efficacy through CYP3A4 induction.

Cimetidine + zaleplon
Raised zaleplon levels can occur with cimetidine, via aldehyde oxidase and CYP3A4 inhibition.

Digoxin + zaleplon
Lack of interaction has been shown (n = 20, Sanchez-Garcia *et al*, *Am J Health Syst Pharm* 2000;**57**:2267–70).

Erythromycin + zaleplon
Raised zaleplon levels can occur, via 3A4 inhibition.

Ibuprofen + zaleplon
Lack of significant interaction has been shown (n = 17, open, Sanchez-Garcia *et al*, *Am J Health Syst Pharm* 2000;**57**:1137–41).

Ketoconazole + zaleplon
Raised zaleplon levels can occur, via 3A4 inhibition.

Narcotics + zaleplon
Enhanced euphoria is possible.

Rifampin + zaleplon
A four-fold reduction in zaleplon levels can occur, via CYP3A4 induction.

Phenobarbital + zaleplon
Reduced zaleplon levels can occur, via CYP3A4 induction.

Warfarin + zaleplon
No interaction occurs.

4.1.5 ZOLPIDEM

Zolpidem is mainly metabolised by CYP3A4 but has no effect on 1A2, 2B6, 2C9, 2D6 and 3A4.

Enhanced sedation would be expected with concurrent use with any CNS depressant.

Alcohol + zolpidem
See alcohol (*4.7.1*).

Antipsychotics + zolpidem
Excessive sedation has been reported with chlorpromazine (n = 6, d/b, single-dose, Desager *et al*, *Psychopharmacol* 1988;**96**:63–6).

Bupropion + zolpidem
See bupropion (*4.6.6*).

Caffeine + zolpidem
In a parallel group study, 300 mg caffeine did not antagonise the sedative effects of zolpidem given during the day (n = 45+, d/b, p/c, Mattila *et al*, *Eur J Clin Pharmacol* 1998;**54**:421–5).

Fluconazole + zolpidem
See itraconazole + zolpidem.

Food + zolpidem
The rate of absorption of zolpidem is slowed significantly by food.

H2-blockers + zolpidem
Lack of a significant interaction has been shown with both cimetidine and ranitidine (n = 6, c/o, 18/7, Hulhoven *et al*, *Int J Clin Pharmacol Res* 1988;**8**:471–6).

Itraconazole + zolpidem
Single doses of itraconazole or fluconazole slightly lengthen the half-life of zolpidem (n = 12, RCT, Greenblatt *et al*, *Clin Pharmacol Ther* 1998;**64**:661–71). However, itraconazole 200 mg/d for four days had no marked effect on the pharmacokinetics of zolpidem, although central effects were slightly increased (n = 10, Luurila *et al*, *Eur J Clin Pharmacol* 1998;**54**:163–6).

Ketoconazole + zolpidem
See itraconazole + zolpidem.

Oral Contraceptives + zolpidem
Zolpidem clearance is slightly higher and half-life slightly shorter in women using OCs (n = 16, Olubodun *et al*, *J Clin Pharmacol* 2002;**42**:1142–6).

Rifampin + zolpidem
Rifampin significantly reduces zolpidem's plasma levels and therapeutic effect, via CYP3A4 induction (n = 8, RCT, Villikka *et al*, *Br J Clin Pharmacol* 1997;**43**:629–34).

Smoking + zolpidem
Zolpidem's half-life may be 30% shorter in smokers than non-smokers, probably of low clinical significance and due to minor CYP1A2 induction (n = 16, Olubodun *et al*, *J Clin Pharmacol* 2002;**42**:1142–6).

Sodium oxybate + zolpidem *
See sodium oxybate (4.6.13).

SSRIs + zolpidem *
SSRIs may enhance zolpidem-associated hallucinations (n = 5, Elko et al, J Toxicol Clin Toxicol 1998;**36**:195–203; n = 1 Coleman and Ota, J Forensic Sci 2004;**49**:392–3). One study showed a minimal pharmacokinetic interaction between **fluoxetine** and regular zolpidem in healthy women, with no significant psychomotor function changes, although zolpidem's half-life increased slightly (n = 29, 5/52, Allard et al, Drug Metab Dispos 1998;**26**:617–22). Visual hallucinations and amnesia triggered by **fluvoxamine** have been reported (n = 1, Kito and Koga, Int Psychogeriatr 2006;**18**:749–51). The combination with **sertraline** may lead to a shorter onset of action and an increased effect from zolpidem (n = 28, RCT, Allard et al, J Clin Pharmacol 1999;**39**;184–91).

Valproate + zolpidem
Somnambulism has been reported with the combination in a 47-year-old male (n = 1, Sattar et al, Ann Pharmacother 2003;**37**:1429–33).

4.1.6 ZOPICLONE

Zopiclone is mainly metabolised by CYP3A4.

Alcohol + zopiclone
See alcohol (4.7.1).

Aspirin + zopiclone
Lack of interaction has been shown.

Atropine + zopiclone
See metoclopramide + zopiclone below.

Caffeine + zopiclone
Caffeine may moderately antagonise the psychomotor impairment caused by zopiclone (d/b, Mattila et al, Pharmacol Toxicol 1992;**70**:286–9).

Erythromycin + zopiclone
Erythromycin accelerates zopiclone absorption, leading to a more rapid onset, which could be clinically significant in the elderly (n = 10, Aranko et al, Br J Clin Pharmacol 1994;**38**:363–7).

Itraconazole + zopiclone
Itraconazole significantly increased zopiclone plasma levels by 28% and half-life by 40%, but had no clinically significant effect in the young volunteers (n = 10, d/b, p/c, c/o, Jalava et al, Eur J Clin Pharmacol 1996;**51**:331–4).

Ranitidine + zopiclone
Lack of interaction has been shown.

Rifampin + zopiclone
Rifampin significantly reduces zopiclone plasma levels and therapeutic effect, via CYP3A4 induction (n = 8, RCT, Villikka et al, Br J Clin Pharmacol 1997;**43**:471–4).

Tricyclics + zopiclone
One study showed decreased levels of trimipramine and zopiclone, but this is of doubtful significance (n = 10, RCT, Caille et al, Biopharm Drug Dispos 1984;**5**:117–25).

4.2 ANTIPSYCHOTICS
Aripiprazole (4.2.2), clozapine (4.2.3), olanzapine (4.2.4), quetiapine (4.2.5), risperidone (4.2.6), sertindole (4.2.7), ziprasidone (4.2.8) and zotepine (4.2.9) also have their own sections

4.2.1 ANTIPSYCHOTICS — GENERAL

There are few specific interactions reported for some antipsychotics, other than additive sedation. Sulpiride has no significant effect on 1A2, 2C9, 2C19, 2D6 2E1 or 3A4 enzymes (Niwa et al, Biol Pharm Bull 2005;**28**:188–91).

ACE inhibitors + antipsychotics
An enhanced hypotensive effect can occur, with severe postural hypotension with chlorpromazine and other antipsychotics, eg. captopril plus chlorpromazine (White, Arch Int Med 1986;**146**:1833–4).

Activated charcoal + phenothiazines
Decreased antipsychotic absorption is likely.

ALCOHOL + ANTIPSYCHOTICS
See alcohol (4.7.1).

Amfetamines + antipsychotics
The antipsychotic effects of phenothiazines can be antagonised by amfetamines, although haloperidol and other antipsychotics can be used to treat amfetamine-induced psychosis.

Amiodarone + phenothiazines
The literature notes an increased risk of ventricular arrhythmias with phenothiazines.

Antacids + antipsychotics
Antacids may reduce chlorpromazine and possibly haloperidol serum levels. Sulpiride absorption may be reduced by sucralfate or aluminium-containing antacids. Any problem can be minimised by separating doses by a couple of hours.

Anticholinergics + antipsychotics
Anticholinergics may reduce the improvement in

positive symptoms produced by antipsychotics, probably by lowering the serum levels of oral and depot antipsychotics (n = 25, Bamrah et al, Br J Psychiatry 1986;**149**:726–33), but not by increased clearance (n = 31, open, Chetty et al, Eur J Clin Pharmacol 1994;**46**:523–6). Additive anticholinergic effects may also occur, eg. acute intestinal pseudo-obstruction has been reported with benzatropine and haloperidol (n = 1, Sheikh et al, Am J Gastroenterol 2001;**96**:934–5).

ANTICONVULSANTS + ANTIPSYCHOTICS

Antipsychotics lower the seizure threshold and may thus antagonise anticonvulsant actions. See also individual anticonvulsants (4.5).

ANTIHISTAMINES + ANTIPSYCHOTICS

Loratadine and fexofenadine are currently considered suitable, although there are three unproven reports of arrhythmia with loratadine. Loratadine is metabolised by CYP2D6 and CYP3A4, allowing alternate pathways to be used if one is inhibited.

Antihypertensives + phenothiazines

Combined hypotensive effect may occur.

Antimalarials + chlorpromazine

One study showed markedly increased chlorpromazine levels with anti-malarials, eg. chloroquine and 'Fansidar' (open, Makanjuola et al, Trop Geogr Med 1988;**40**:31–3).

Aripiprazole + antipsychotics

See aripiprazole (4.2.2).

Ascorbic acid + fluphenazine

An isolated case exists of reduced fluphenazine levels (Dysken et al, JAMA 1979;**241**:2008) with 1 g/d of ascorbic acid.

BARBITURATES+ANTIPSYCHOTICS

Additive sedative effects can occur acutely with this combination, and death has been reported (n = 1, Hino et al, Leg Med (Tokyo) 1999;**1**:48–51). Barbiturates may induce the metabolism of many antipsychotics, eg. haloperidol levels reduced by 40–75%. Antagonism of the anticonvulsant effects may also occur.

Benzodiazepines + antipsychotics

Enhanced sedation and impaired psychomotor function can occur (see 1.1).

Beta-blockers + antipsychotics

Generally, raised antipsychotic plasma levels occur, of possible clinical significance, eg. chlorpromazine levels may rise by up to 100–500% with propranolol (Peet et al, Lancet 1980;**ii**:978), although pindolol has no significant effect on haloperidol levels (n = 26, open, Greendyke and Gulya, J Clin Psychiatry 1988;**49**:105–7). Thioridazine is contraindicated with propranolol due to QTc prolongation (see general review by Markowitz et al, Ann Pharmacother 1995;**29**:603–9).

Betel nut + antipsychotics

Betel nut (Areca catechu), which contains the cholinergic alkaloid arecoline, has been reported to cause EPSE, bradykinesia, stiffness and akathisia with flupentixol and fluphenazine (n = 1, Deahl, Mov Disord 1998;**4**:330–3).

Bromocriptine + antipsychotics

A predictable reversal of the antipsychotic effect may occur. Antipsychotics may also antagonise the hypoprolactinaemic and anti-parkinsonian effects of bromocriptine.

Calcium-channel blockers + antipsychotics

Increased antipsychotic plasma levels or enhanced hypotension could be predicted (review by Markowitz et al, Ann Pharmacother 1995;**29**:603–9).

Cannabis + antipsychotics

See cannabis (4.7.2).

CARBAMAZEPINE + ANTIPSYCHOTICS

See carbamazepine (4.5.1).

Citalopram + antipsychotics

See citalopram/escitalopram (4.3.2.1).

CLARITHROMYCIN + ANTIPSYCHOTICS

References report an increased risk of arrhythmias with phenothiazines and recommend avoiding the combination. Death has been reported when clarithromycin was added to pimozide in a man with a documented prolonged QT interval (n = 1, Flockhart et al, J Clin Psychopharmacol 2000;**20**:317–24).

Clonidine + antipsychotics

Animal studies have shown phenothiazines and haloperidol (but not pimozide) to antagonise the hypotensive effect of clonidine. Case reports exist of severe hypotension (Fruncillo et al, Am J Psychiatry 1985;**142**:274) and of delirium (review by Markowitz et al, Ann Pharmacother 1995; **29**:603–9).

Clozapine + antipsychotics

See clozapine (4.2.3).

Cocaine + antipsychotics

See cocaine (4.7.3).

Desferrioxamine + prochlorperazine

Prolonged unconsciousness may occur.

Diazoxide + chlorpromazine

Enhanced hypoglycaemia has been reported (n = 1,

Aynsley-Green and Illig, *Lancet* 1975;**2**:658).

Disopyramine + antipsychotics

Increased anticholinergic effects may occur.

Disulfiram + antipsychotics

See disulfiram (*4.6.8*).

Domperidone + antipsychotics

There is an enhanced risk of EPSE.

Donepezil + antipsychotics

See donepezil (*4.6.3.1*).

Erythromycin + antipsychotics

See clarithromycin + antipsychotics.

Escitalopram + antipsychotics

See citalopram/escitalopram (*4.3.2.1*).

FLUOXETINE + ANTIPSYCHOTICS

Severe EPSE have been reported with fluoxetine and **haloperidol** (n = 1, Tate, *Am J Psychiatry* 1989;**146**:399–400), dystonia with **fluphenazine** 2.5 mg (n = 1, Katai, *Am J Psychiatry* 1993;**150**:836–7), and stupor and confusion (n = 1, Hansen-Grant et al, *Am J Psychiatry* 1993;**150**:1750–1) and severe bradycardia and drowsiness (n = 1, Friedman, *Can J Psychiatry* 1994;**39**:634) with **pimozide**. The probable mechanism is CYP2D6 inhibition leading to raised levels. The combination should thus be avoided if possible (Ahmed et al, *Can J Psychiatry* 1993;**38**:62–3). Citalopram, escitalopram and sertraline would be suitable alternatives.

Fluvoxamine + antipsychotics

See fluvoxamine (*4.3.2.3*).

Ginseng + haloperidol

Ginseng may potentiate the general effects of haloperidol (Mitra et al, *Indian J Exp Biol* 1996; **34**:41–7).

H2-blockers + antipsychotics

Chlorpromazine levels may be reduced by 30% by cimetidine (Howes et al, *Eur J Clin Pharmacol* 1983;**24**:99–102). Ranitidine is a suitable alternative.

Haloperidol + chlorpromazine

Chlorpromazine may significantly increase haloperidol levels, probably via CYP2D6 inhibition (n = 43, Suzuki et al, *Ther Drug Monit* 2001;**23**:363–8).

Hydroxyzine + phenothiazines

The antipsychotic effect of phenothiazines may be decreased (Ross and Priest, *Dis Nerv Syst* 1970;**31**:412).

Hypoglycaemics + chlorpromazine

Chlorpromazine 100 mg or more can induce hyperglycaemia and upset the control of diabetes with oral hypoglycaemics (Schwarz and Munoz, *Am J Psychiatry* 1968;**125**:253).

Indometacin + haloperidol

One study showed profound drowsiness and confusion on the combination (Bird et al, *Lancet* 1983;i:830–1).

Itraconazole + haloperidol

Itraconazole 200 mg/d for seven days significantly increases haloperidol and metabolite levels, leading to increased side-effects, presumably due to CYP3A4 inhibition (n = 13, Yasui et al, *J Clin Psychopharmacol* 1999;**19**:149–54).

LEVODOPA + ANTIPSYCHOTICS

The therapeutic effect of levodopa is antagonised by antipsychotics and vice versa. Levodopa may worsen antipsychotic-induced EPSE.

Lithium + antipsychotics

See lithium (*4.4*).

MAOIs + antipsychotics

See MAOIs (*4.3.4*).

Memantine + antipsychotics

See memantine (*4.6.9*).

Methyldopa + haloperidol

Pseudo-dementia with haloperidol and methyl-dopa has been reported (n = 3, Nadel and Wallach, *Br J Psychiatry* 1979;**135**:484). There is also an enhanced risk of EPSE and postural hypotension.

Metirosine + antipsychotics

An enhanced risk of EPSE exists.

Metoclopramide + antipsychotics

An enhanced risk of EPSE exists.

Minocycline + phenothiazines

There is a case of pigmented galactorrhoea with the combination (n = 1, Basler and Lynch, *Arch Dermatol* 1985;**121**:417).

Naltrexone + phenothiazines

Severe drowsiness may occur with thioridazine (Maany et al, *Am J Psychiatry* 1987;**144**:966) or chlorpromazine.

Olanzapine + antipsychotics (other)

See olanzapine (*4.2.4*).

Oral contraceptives + chlorpromazine

There is a report of a combined oral contraceptive raising chlorpromazine levels six-fold (n = 1, Chetty and Miller, *Ther Drug Monit* 2001; **23**:556–8).

Orlistat + haloperidol

A small trial suggested a lack of interaction (n = 8, open, 8/52, Hilger et al, *J Clin Psychopharmacol* 2002;**22**:68–70).

Oxcarbazepine + antipsychotics

See oxcarbazepine (4.5.6).

Paroxetine + antipsychotics

See paroxetine (4.3.2.4).

Pethidine + phenothiazines

Increased CNS toxicity and hypotension can occur (n = 10, open, c/o, Stambaugh and Wainer, *J Clin Pharmacol* 1981;**21**:140–6).

Phenylpropanolamine + thioridazine

A single fatal case of ventricular arrhythmia exists (n = 2841, Chouinard et al, *Can Med Assoc J* 1978;**119**:729).

PHENYTOIN + ANTIPSYCHOTICS

Phenytoin may reduce haloperidol levels by 40–75%, probably via enzyme induction (n = 30, open, Linnoila et al, *Am J Psychiatry* 1980;**137**:819). Chlorpromazine may increase phenytoin levels by up to 50% (n = 27, open, Sands et al, *Drug Intell Clin Pharm* 1987;**21**:267–72), although other studies show a nil or opposite effect. Antipsychotics lower the seizure threshold and may antagonise the anticonvulsant effect of phenytoin.

Piperazine + chlorpromazine

The validity of a single case of convulsions with the combination has been queried by a small study (Sturman, *Br J Pharmacol* 1974;**50**:153–5).

Polymyxin + phenothiazines

The neuromuscular blocking effects of polypeptide antibiotics may be increased by phenothiazines with prolonged respiratory depression possible (Pohlmann, *JAMA* 1966; **196**: 181).

Procarbazine + antipsychotics

Enhanced sedation is possible.

Quetiapine + antipsychotics (other)

See quetiapine (4.2.5).

Reboxetine + antipsychotics

See reboxetine (4.3.3.5)

RIFAMPIN + HALOPERIDOL

Rifampin may reduce haloperidol serum levels by a third (n = 17, Kim et al, *J Clin Psychopharmacol* 1996;**16**:247–52), a clinically significant effect. Care would also be needed if rifampin were stopped.

Sertindole + antipsychotics (other)

See sertindole (4.2.7).

Sertraline + pimozide *

Sertraline (up to 200 mg/d) may cause pimozide levels to rise by 35%, but with no prolonged QTc (n = 15, Alderman, *Clin Ther* 2005;**27**:1050–63).

Smoking + antipsychotics

See smoking (4.7.4).

Suxamethonium + promazine

Prolonged apnoea has been reported (n = 1, Regan and Aldrete, *Anesth Analg* 1967;**46**:315–8).

Sucralfate + antipsychotics

See antacids + antipsychotics.

Tea or coffee + antipsychotics

Typical antipsychotics precipitate out of solution to form a tannin complex with tea and coffee (Kulhanek et al, *Lancet* 1979;ii:1130–1). The clinical significance is thought to be minimal (Bowen et al, *Lancet* 1981;i:1217–8).

Tetrabenazine + antipsychotics

Only a single case exists of enhanced EPSE in a Huntington's patient (Moss and Stewart, *Can J Psychiatry* 1986;**31**:865–6), although it would be a predictable outcome of this combination.

Thiazide diuretics + antipsychotics

Although no case reports exist, enhanced thioridazine cardiotoxicity has been suggested (Thornton and Pray, *Am J Nurs* 1976;**76**:245–6).

Trazodone + antipsychotics

See trazodone (4.3.3.6).

Tricyclics + antipsychotics

See tricyclics (4.3.1).

Valproate + antipsychotics

Chlorpromazine may inhibit the metabolism of valproate and so monitoring of valproate levels may be appropriate (open, Ishizaki et al, *J Clin Psychopharmacol* 1984;**4**:254–61). Valproate has no significant effect on the plasma levels of **haloperidol** (n = 27, 4/52, Hesslinger et al, *J Clin Psychopharmacol* 1999;**19**:310–5) nor **risperidone** and 9-hydroxyrisperidone (n = 33, Spina et al, *Ther Drug Monit* 2000;**22**:481–5; n = 22, s/b, p/c, 28/7, Ravindran et al, *Clin Pharmacokinet* 2004;**43**:733–40). Valproate has no significant effect on the plasma levels of **haloperidol** (n = 27, 4/52, Hesslinger et al, *J Clin Psychopharmacol* 1999;**19**:310–5) but there are cases of dose-related generalised oedema with **risperidone** and valproate (n = 2, Sanders and Lehrer, *J Clin Psychiatry* 1998;**59**:689–90). Two studies have shown that valproate produces a non-clinically significant rise in **clozapine**, but lower norclozapine levels (n = 37 + 6, Facciola et al, *Ther Drug Monit* 1999;**21**:341–5). No interaction occurs with **aripiprazole** (Citrome et al, *Int J Neuropsychopharmacol* 2002;**5**[Suppl 1]:S187). Antipsychotics lower the seizure threshold and may antagonise the anticonvulsant effect of valproate.

Venlafaxine + antipsychotics
See venlafaxine (4.3.3.8).

Warfarin + antipsychotics
An interaction is theoretically possible (mentioned in Sayal et al, Acta Psychiatr Scand 2000; 102:250–5).

Zaleplon + antipsychotics
See zaleplon (4.1.4).

Zolpidem + antipsychotics
See zolpidem (4.1.5).

Zotepine + antipsychotics (other)
See zotepine (4.2.9).

4.2.2 ANTIPSYCHOTICS — ARIPIPRAZOLE *

Aripiprazole is metabolised by several enzyme systems, eg. mainly CYP2D6 and 3A4, but not CYP1A1, 1A2 or 2C9/19. It has no effect on CYP 2C9, 2C19, 2D6 and 3A4.

Alcohol + aripiprazole
See alcohol (4.7.1).

Antipsychotics + aripiprazole
There is a theoretical interaction with potent D2 antagonists such as older neuroleptics and risperidone with aripiprazole. Aripiprazole apparently has a very high affinity for D2 receptors and would displace almost any other antipsychotic from these receptors.

Carbamazepine + aripiprazole
See antipsychotics + carbamazepine (4.5.1).

Dextromethorphan + aripiprazole
Lack of interaction has been shown.

H2-blockers + aripiprazole
Lack of significant interaction has been shown with famotidine.

Itraconazole + aripiprazole
Although itraconazole is a potent CYP3A4 inhibitor, it made no clinically significant difference to aripiprazole levels in one study (n = 24, Kubo et al, Drug Metab Pharmacokinet 2005;20:55–64).

Ketoconazole + aripiprazole
Ketoconazole decreases aripiprazole metabolism and so an aripiprazole dose should be decreased by a half during co-administration.

Lithium + aripiprazole
See lithium (4.4).

Omeprazole + aripiprazole
Lack of interaction has been shown.

Quinidine + aripiprazole
Quinidine decreases aripiprazole metabolism and so aripiprazole doses should be halved.

Smoking + aripiprazole
See smoking (4.7.4)

Valproate + aripiprazole
See valproate + antipsychotics (4.2.1)

Warfarin + aripiprazole
Lack of interaction has been shown.

4.2.3 ANTIPSYCHOTICS — CLOZAPINE
See 4.2.1 for other, more general interactions

The major metabolic route of clozapine is to norclozapine, which is more stable but more toxic to stem cells (Gerson et al, Br J Haematology 1994;86:555–61). CYP1A2 is the major metabolising enzyme, with 2D6 and 3A4 possibly having an effect, as well as many other P450 and FMO enzymes being involved.

Reviews: general (Linnet et al, Drug Metab Dispos 1997;25:1379–82; Chang et al, Prog Neuropsychopharmacol Biol Psychiatry 1998; 22:723–9).

ACE inhibitors + clozapine
Clozapine plus diltiazem or enalapril (Aronowitz et al, J Clin Psychopharmacol 1994;14:429–30) has been reported to produce additional hypotension. There is also a well-documented case of a clinically important rise in clozapine and norclozapine levels with lisinopril, via an unknown mechanism (n = 1, Abraham et al, Am J Psychiatry 2001;158:969).

Alcohol + clozapine
See antipsychotics + alcohol (4.7.1).

ANTIBIOTICS + CLOZAPINE *
Antibiotics reported to cause leucopenia/ neutropenia may enhance the likelihood of clozapine-induced neutropenia and should, if possible, be avoided. It should be noted, however, that respiratory infections can themselves inhibit CYP1A2, raising clozapine levels, and so antibiotics may not always be the cause of apparent interactions (Leon, J Clin Psychiatry 2004;65:1144–5).

1. Antibiotics LESS likely to cause neutropenia (safer to use): penicillins (all except benzylpenicillin G), all tetracyclines, aminoglycosides, macrolides, clarithromycin, some anti-TBs (ethambutol, pyrazinamide, streptomycin), clofazimide, hexamine, sodium fusidate, spectinomycin, colistin, polymixin B and cicloserin.

2. Antibiotics MORE likely/CAN cause leucopenia and/or neutropenia (less safe to use):

cephalosporins and cephamycins, clindamycin, lincomycin, sulphonamides and trimethoprim, some anti-TBs (capreomycin, isoniazid, rifampin), dapsone, metronidazole, tinidazole, nitrofurantoin, chloramphenicol, vancomycin, teicoplanin and the 4-quinolones (ciprofloxacin, nalidixic acid, etc), eg. there is a case of clozapine levels falling by nearly 50% when ciprofloxacin was stopped, probably due to CYP1A2 inhibition (Markowitz et al, Am J Psychiatry 1997;**153**:881). Where possible, choose antibiotics from the first list as first choice and be aware of the potential for problems if drugs from the second list must be used. See also individual drugs for other interactions.

Anticholinergics + clozapine
See antipsychotics (4.2.1).

Antihypertensives + clozapine
Potentiation of the antihypertensive effects may occur. This can be particularly important during the upward dose titration period.

ANTIPSYCHOTICS (other) + CLOZAPINE *
There is an enhanced risk of agranulocytosis, which would additionally be complicated by the long-term nature of any antipsychotic given as a depot, eg. a case of thrombocytopenia associated with **fluphenazine** and clozapine has been reported (n = 1, Mihaljevic-Peles et al, Nord J Psychiatry 2001;**55**:449–50). **Amisulpride** has no apparent effect on plasma clozapine concentrations (Bergemann et al, J Clin Psychopharmacol 2005; **25**:494–7). Elevated **haloperidol** levels have been reported in combination with clozapine (n = 1, Allen, J Clin Pharmacol 2000;**40**:1296–7), as have myoclonic and GTC seizures (n = 1, Haberfellner, Eur Psychiatry 2002;**17**:55–6). Although **risperidone** 2–4mg/d may not affect serum clozapine (250–650mg/d) levels to any significant degree (n = 18, Raaska et al, Eur J Clin Pharmacol 2002;**58**:587–91), there are cases of raised clozapine levels with this combination, eg. 73% higher with risperidone 2mg/d (Tyson et al, Am J Psychiatry 1995;**152**:1401–2), agranulocytosis six weeks after risperidone 6mg/d was added to a stable clozapine regimen (n = 1, Godleski and Sernyak, Am J Psychiatry 1996;**153**:735), and a neurotoxic reaction or mild NMS (n = 1, Kontaxakis et al, Prog Neuropsychopharmacol Biol Psychiatry 2002;**26**:407–9). The mechanism cannot be explained by inhibition of CYP1A2, 2D6 or 2C19 (n = 8, Eap et al, Ther Drug Monit 2001;**23**:228–31).

BENZODIAZEPINES + CLOZAPINE
There are rare cases of severe hypotension and respiratory depression (eg. n = 3, Finkel et al, N Engl J Med 1991;**325**:518), sudden death after IV lorazepam (n = 1, Klimke and Klieser, Am J Psychiatry 1994;**151**:780), sedation (n = 2, Cobb et al, Am J Psychiatry 1991;**148**:1606–7) and delirium with lorazepam (n = 3, Jackson et al, Ann Clin Psychiatry 1995;**7**:139–41). Monitor for enhanced sedation and take particular care when a clozapine dose is being increased.

Buspirone + clozapine
See buspirone (4.1.2).

Caffeine + clozapine*
Caffeine and clozapine are both metabolised by CYP1A2 and so some competitive inhibition of metabolism may occur. Caffeine, in doses of 400–1000mg, inhibits the metabolism of clozapine to an extent that might be significant in some people (n = 12, RCT, open, Hagg et al, Br J Clin Pharmacol 2000;**49**:59–63), eg. mean serum trough levels of clozapine increased by about 26% have been reported, probably of minor clinical significance in most patients (n = 12[c = 6], RCT, d/b, Raaska et al, Basic Clin Pharmacol Toxicol 2004;**94**:13–8). Drowsiness and sialorrhoea have occurred with the combination, with clozapine levels halving when caffeine was stopped (n = 1, Odom-White and de Leon, J Clin Psychiatry 1996;**57**:175–6).

CARBAMAZEPINE + CLOZAPINE
See antipsychotics + carbamazepine (4.5.1).

Chloramphenicol + clozapine
There is an enhanced risk of agranulocytosis.

Citalopram + clozapine *
See antipsychotics + citalopram/escitalopram (4.3.2.1).

Clonidine + clozapine
See clonidine + antipsychotics (4.2.1).

Cocaine + clozapine
See antipsychotics + cocaine (4.7.3).

Co-trimoxazole + clozapine
There is an enhanced risk of agranulocytosis.

Cytotoxic agents + clozapine
There is an enhanced risk of agranulocytosis.

Digoxin + clozapine
The SPC for clozapine advises caution with highly bound drugs, which would include digoxin. Monitor for adverse effects and adjust doses as necessary.

Erythromycin + clozapine
Raised clozapine levels have been reported, with

seizures seven days after erythromycin 250 mg/d was added to clozapine 800 mg/d, with levels falling by 50% when the erythromycin was stopped (Funderburg et al, Am J Psychiatry 1994;**151**:1840) and increased toxicity, eg. somnolence and leukocytosis (n = 1, Cohen et al, Arch Intern Med 1996;**156**:675–7). Reduced clozapine metabolism via CYP1A2 is the probable mechanism

Escitalopram + clozapine *

See antipsychotics + citalopram/escitalopram (4.3.2.1).

FLUOXETINE + CLOZAPINE

Fluoxetine produces significant increases in plasma clozapine and norclozapine levels, with some inter-individual variation (n = 80, open, Centorrino et al, Am J Psychiatry 1996;**153**:820–2). There are several case reports (eg. n = 6, Centorrino et al, Am J Psychiatry 1994;**151**:123–5), including death (n = 1, Ferslew et al, J Forensic Sci 1998;**43**:1082–5) and uncontrollable myoclonic jerks (n = 1, Kingsbury and Puckett, Am J Psychiatry 1995;**152**:473–2). The mechanism is possibly CYP2D6 inhibition. The risk of clozapine toxicity must be considered and measuring clozapine levels may be useful.

FLUVOXAMINE + CLOZAPINE *

Fluvoxamine increases clozapine AUC by 40% and increases the half-life by 370% (sic) by 1A2 inhibition, although peak levels may remain unchanged (n = 9, Wang et al, J Clin Pharmacol 2004;**44**:785–92). There are other reports of clozapine plasma levels rising by up to 900% with fluvoxamine 100–200 mg/d (eg. n = 2, Dequardo and Roberts, Am J Psychiatry 1996;**153**:840–1; n = 1, Armstrong and Stephans, J Clin Psychiatry 1997;**58**:499). So predictable is the effect, that fluvoxamine has been used to counteract 1A2 induction by smoking which can lead to clozapine non-response (n = 3, Bender and Eap, Arch Gen Psychiatry 1998;**55**:1048–50) in 1A2 rapid metabolisers. In a study in Chinese male in-patients, 50 mg/d fluvoxamine increased clozapine levels by a mean of 130% (137 to 327 ng/ml), and norclozapine levels by 78% (from 65 to 116 ng/ml) within two weeks. Clozapine levels rose further (to 440–480 ng/ml) with 100 mg/d (n = 12, Lu et al, J Clin Psychopharmacol 2002;**22**:626–8). Close pharmacokinetic monitoring is thus necessary, as the effect can be dramatic over a few days in some patients even with very low doses, eg. 10–20 mg/d fluvoxamine.

Grapefruit juice + clozapine

Grapefruit juice has no effect on clozapine levels (n = 15, open, 12/52, Lane et al, Drug Metabol Drug Interact 2001;**18**:263–78).

H2-blockers + clozapine

Clozapine levels may rise by over 50% with cimetidine (n = 1, Czymanski et al, J Clin Psychiatry 1991;**52**:21). Ranitidine is a safer alternative.

Influenza vaccine + clozapine

Influenza vaccine has no effect on clozapine levels (n = 14, Raaska et al, Eur J Clin Pharmacol 2001;**57**:705–8).

Itraconazole/ketoconazole + clozapine

Itraconazole 200 mg/d over seven days had no effect on plasma clozapine and norclozapine levels (RCT, n = 7, Raaska and Neuvonen, Eur J Clin Pharmacol 1998;**54**:167–70), and ketoconazole also has no effect on clozapine (Lane et al, Drug Metabol Drug Interact 2001;**18**:263–78).

Lamotrigine + clozapine

An unexplained three-fold increase in clozapine levels was seen two weeks after lamotrigine 100 mg/d was added to a stable clozapine 400 mg/d regimen (n = 1, Kossen et al, Am J Psychiatry 2001;**158**:1930).

Lithium + clozapine

See antipsychotics + lithium (4.4).

MAOIs + clozapine

See antipsychotics + MAOIs (4.3.4).

Oral contraceptives + clozapine

Elevated plasma clozapine levels have been reported with norethindrone, resolving on OC discontinuation (n = 1, Gabbay et al, J Clin Psychopharmacol 2002;**22**:621–2).

Orlistat + clozapine

A small trial suggested lack of interaction (8/52, Hilger et al, J Clin Psychopharmacol 2002;**22**:68–70).

PAROXETINE + CLOZAPINE *

Paroxetine produces significant increases in plasma clozapine and norclozapine levels (n = 60, open, Centorrino et al, Am J Psychiatry 1996;**153**:820–2), and so the risk of clozapine toxicity must be considered carefully. NMS with no leukocytosis and normal CPK has also been reported with the combinaton (n = 1, Gambassi et al, Aging Clin Exp Res 2006;**18**:266–70).

Penicillamine + clozapine

There is an enhanced risk of agranulocytosis (mandatory precaution in SPC).

Phenobarbital + clozapine

Elevated plasma clozapine levels (requiring

dose reduction) have been reported after discontinuation of phenobarbital, presumably from removal of CYP1A2 induction (n = 1, Lane et al, J Clin Psychiatry 1998;**59**:131–3).

Phenylbutazone + clozapine

There is an enhanced risk of agranulocytosis (mandatory precaution in SPC).

PHENYTOIN + CLOZAPINE

Serum concentrations of clozapine may be markedly reduced by phenytoin (n = 2, Miller et al, J Clin Psychiatry 1991;**52**:23) via CYP1A2 induction, so monitor for reduced effect.

Proton Pump Inhibitors + clozapine

A switch from omeprazole to pantoprazole does not alter average clozapine plasma levels, although some individual increases may be seen (n = 13, Mookhoek and Loonen, Br J Clin Pharmacol 2002;**53**:545P).

Pyrazolone analgesics + clozapine

There is an enhanced risk of agranulocytosis (mandatory precaution in SPC).

Reboxetine + clozapine

See reboxetine (4.3.3.5).

Rifampin + clozapine

There is a case of a 600% reduction in clozapine levels 2–3 weeks after rifampin was started, probably via 1A2 and 3A4 induction (n = 1, Joos et al, J Clin Psychopharmacol 1998;**18**:83–5).

Sertraline + clozapine

Sertraline may produce significant increases in plasma clozapine and norclozapine levels, with some inter-individual variations (n = 80, Centorrino et al, Am J Psychiatry 1996;**153**:820–2). There is a case of sudden death with the combination, probably as a result of cardiac arrhythmia (n = 1, Hoehns et al, Ann Pharmacother 2001;**35**:826–6). The risk of clozapine toxicity must be considered carefully.

Smoking + clozapine

See antipsychotics + smoking (4.7.4).

Sulphonamides + clozapine

There is an enhanced risk of agranulocytosis (mandatory precaution in SPC).

Tricyclics + clozapine

See antipsychotics + tricyclics (4.3.1).

Valproate + clozapine

Although valproate is often used as anticonvulsant cover for higher doses of clozapine, a careful study showed valproate to produce a 15% drop in clozapine levels and a 65% drop in norclozapine levels (n = 7, Longo and Salzman, Am J Psychiatry 1995;**152**:650), although raised clozapine levels have been reported (n = 1, Costello and Suppes, J Clin Psychopharmacol 1995;**15**:139–41). Since norclozapine is more toxic than clozapine, this may be a useful effect with careful manipulation of the dose. Clozapine may, of course, also lower the seizure threshold and antagonise the anticonvulsant effect of valproate.

Venlafaxine + clozapine

See venlafaxine (4.3.3.8).

Warfarin + clozapine

The SPC for clozapine advises caution with highly bound drugs, which would include warfarin. There are no case reports, although caution is still needed (mentioned in Sayal et al, Acta Psychiatr Scand 2000;**102**:250–5). Monitor carefully for an enhanced warfarin effect and adjust doses as necessary.

4.2.4 ANTIPSYCHOTICS — OLANZAPINE

See 4.2.1 for other, more general, interactions

Olanzapine is metabolised by CYP1A2 and 2D6, with little or no effect on 1A2, 2D6, 2C19, 2C9 and 3A4 at normal doses. It is highly bound to albumin (90%) and alpha 1-acid glycoprotein (77%), and interactions may be possible through this mechanism. The metabolic pathways of olanzapine also include N-glucuronidation, reducing its overall sensitivity to drugs that might induce or inhibit its own metabolism via CYP or flavin-containing mono-oxygenase (FMO) systems. Olanzapine is approximately 60% excreted in urine and 30% in faeces. Fixed doses appear to give higher levels in women.

Review: extensive, of pharmacokinetics and pharmacodynamics (Callaghan et al, Clin Pharmacokinetics 1999;**37**:177–93, 56 refs).

Alcohol + olanzapine

See antipsychotics + alcohol (4.7.1).

Antacids + olanzapine

Antacids have no effect on olanzapine bio-availability.

Antipsychotics (other) + olanzapine

An interaction has been suggested with **halo-peridol** and olanzapine (Gomberg, J Clin Psychopharmacol 1999;**19**:272–3) and NMS has been reported (n = 1, Mujica and Weiden, Am J Psychiatry 2001;**158**:650–1). Seizures have been reported with **quetiapine** and olanzapine (n = 1, Hedges and Jeppson, Ann Pharmacother

2002;**36**:437–9). Unchanged olanzapine levels with **flupentixol** were mentioned in one study (Bergemann et al, Pharmacopsychiatry 2004; **37**:63–8).

Benzodiazepines + olanzapine *

Single dose studies show no effect of olanzapine on the metabolism of **diazepam**. Mild increases in heart rate, sedation and dry mouth were noted, but no dose adjustment considered necessary. Unchanged olanzapine levels with **lorazepam** were mentioned in one study (Bergemann et al, Pharmacopsychiatry 2004;**37**:63–8). Concommitant IM olanzapine and IM BDZs are contraindicated (UK SPC) and must be separated by at least one hour. There is one case report of significant hypotension (down to 66/30 within four hours) lasting 12 hours in a patient given olanzapine IM with lorazepam 2 mg IM 30 minutes later (n = 1, Zacher and Roche-Desilets, J Clin Psychiatry 2005;**66**:1614–5).

Biperiden + olanzapine

Lack of interaction has been reported.

Carbamazepine + olanzapine

See carbamazepine (4.5.1).

Charcoal (activated) + olanzapine

Activated charcoal reduces olanzapine bioavailability by 50–60%.

Cimetidine + olanzapine

There is no effect on olanzapine bioavailability.

Ciprofloxacin + olanzapine

Raised olanzapine levels have been reported, possibly caused by ciprofloxacin (n = 1, Markowitz and DeVane, J Clin Psychophamacol 1999; **19**:289–91).

Lithium + olanzapine

See antipsychotics + lithium (4.4).

Opioids + olanzapine *

Opioid-induced delirium has been reported with the combination (n = 2, Estfan et al, J Pain Symptom Manage 2005;**29**:330–2)

Oxcarbazepine + olanzapine *

See oxcarbazepine (4.5.6).

Probenecid + olanzapine

Probenecid appears to decrease olanzapine glucuronidation (n = 12, RCT, d/b, c/o, Markowitz et al, Clin Pharmacol Ther 2002;**71**:30–8).

Smoking + olanzapine

See antipsychotics + smoking (4.7.4).

SSRIs + olanzapine *

Fluvoxamine (but not **sertraline**) inhibits the metabolism of olanzapine, probably via CYP1A2 (n = 165, Weigmann et al, Ther Drug Monit 2001;**23**:410–13; Bergemann et al, Pharmacopsychiatry 2004;**37**:63–8), with 100 mg/d raising peak levels by 49%, AUC by 70%, half-life by 40% and steady-state olanzapine levels by 12–112% and so care is needed (n = 8, open, Hiemke et al, J Clin Psychopharmacol 2002;**22**:502–6; n = 10, Chiu et al, J Clin Pharmacol 2004;**44**:1385–90, n = 12, Wang et al, J Clin Pharmacol 2004;**44**:785–92). Use of fluvoxamine 25 mg/d has allowed a 26% reduction in olanzapine dose for the same plasma level, or would have increased OLZ levels by 25% without increasing the dose (n = 10, 6/52, open, Albers et al, J Clin Psychopharmacol 2005;**25**:170–4). This could be a useful trick for keeping olanzapine doses within BNF limits with the MHA commissioners around. Higher doses of **fluoxetine** may slightly increase olanzapine levels, probably via CYP2D6 inhibition (n = 15, Gossen et al, AAPS PharmSci 2002;**4**:E11). Melancholic depression has been reported with fluoxetine and olanzapine (n = 1, Nelson and Swartz, Ann Clin Psychiatry 2000;**12**:167–70), although the combination has been licensed in USA for psychotic depression.

Tricyclics + olanzapine

Single dose studies show no effect of olanzapine on the metabolism of imipramine (n = 9, open, Callaghan et al, J Clin Pharmacol 1997;**37**:971–8) and desipramine. Seizures have been reported with olanzapine and clomipramine (Deshauer et al, J Clin Psychopharmacol 2000;**20**:283–4). Lower olanzapine levels with trimipramine but unchanged levels with amitriptyline were mentioned in one study (Bergemann et al, Pharmacopsychiatry 2004;**37**:63–8).

Valproate + olanzapine *

Valproate lowers the plasma levels of olanzapine (Bergemann et al, J Clin Psychopharmacol 2006; **26**:432–4).

Warfarin + olanzapine

Single dose studies show no effect of olanzapine on the metabolism of warfarin, although it could be possible (mentioned in Sayal et al, Acta Psychiatr Scand 2000;**102**:250–5).

Xanthines + olanzapine

Lack of interaction has been shown with aminophylline and theophylline (n = 19, RCT, Macias et al, Pharmacotherapy 1998;**18**:1237–48).

4.2.5 ANTIPSYCHOTICS — QUETIAPINE
See *4.2.1* for other, more general, interactions

Quetiapine is metabolised primarily by CYP3A4.
Alcohol + quetiapine
See alcohol (*4.7.1*).
Antipsychotics (other) + quetiapine
Thioridazine 400mg/d significantly decreased quetiapine 600mg/d plasma levels by up to 68%, but haloperidol 15mg/d and risperidone 6mg/d had no effect (n=36, RCT, 9/7, Potkin *et al, J Clin Psychopharmacol* 2002;**22**:121–30). See also olanzapine (*4.2.4*).
Barbiturates + quetiapine
Lower levels of quetiapine would be expected, due to CYP3A4 induction by barbiturates.
Benzodiazepines + quetiapine
Single doses of lorazepam and diazepam are unaffected by quetiapine.
Carbamazepine + quetiapine
See antipsychotics + carbamazepine (*4.5.1*).
Cimetidine + quetiapine
No interaction occurs (n=13, open, Strakowski *et al, J Clin Psychopharmacol* 2002;**22**:201–5).
Erythromycin + quetiapine
Raised quetiapine levels are likely via CYP3A4 inhibition.
KETOCONAZOLE + QUETIAPINE *
Ketoconazole 200mg/d increases quetiapine plasma levels 3.5-fold, presumably by CYP3A4 inhibition, potentially clinically significant (n=12, Grimm *et al, Br J Clin Pharmacol* 2006; **61**:58–69).
Lovastatin + quetiapine
A prolonged QTc interval has been reported with the combination (n=1, Furst *et al, Biol Psychiatry* 2002;**51**:264–5).
Lithium + quetiapine
Slightly increased lithium levels may occur.
Phenytoin + quetiapine
Lower levels of quetiapine would be expected, due to CYP3A4 induction by phenytoin.
Rifampin + quetiapine
Lower levels of quetiapine would be expected, due to CYP3A4 induction by rifampin.
SSRIs + quetiapine
Fluoxetine 60mg/d has no significant effect on quetiapine kinetics (n=26, RCT, Potkin *et al, J Clin Psychopharmacol* 2002;**22**:174–82).
Tricyclics + quetiapine
Imipramine 150mg/d has no significant effect

on quetiapine (n=26, RCT, Potkin *et al, J Clin Psychopharmacol* 2002;**22**:174–82) but quetiapine has caused a falsely elevated estimation of nortriptyline levels (n=1, Schussler *et al, Am J Psychiatry* 2003;**160**:589).
Warfarin + quetiapine
No interaction is likely to occur routinely (mentioned in Sayal *et al, Acta Psychiatr Scand* 2000;**102**:250–5), but an isolated case has been reported (n=1, Rogers *et al, J Clin Psychopharmacol* 1999;**19**:382–3).

4.2.6 ANTIPSYCHOTICS — RISPERIDONE
See *4.2.1* for other, more general, interactions

Reviews: general (DeVane and Nemeroff, *J Clin Psychopharmacol* 2001;**21**:408–16), P450 metabolism (Berecz *et al, Curr Drug Targets* 2004; **5**:573–9).
Caffeine + risperidone *
Caffeine appears to have no effect on plasma risperidone levels (n=136, Kakihara *et al, Int Clin Psychopharmacol* 2005;**20**:71–8).
CARBAMAZEPINE + RISPERIDONE
See antipsychotics + carbamazepine (*4.5.1*).
CLOZAPINE + RISPERIDONE
See antipsychotics + clozapine (*4.2.3*).
Donepezil + risperidone
See antipsychotics + donepezil (*4.6.3.1*).
FLUOXETINE + RISPERIDONE
Fluoxetine 20mg/d has caused a 75% increase in risperidone levels over four weeks, resulting in side-effects in 30% (n=10, Spina *et al, J Clin Psychopharmacol* 2002;**22**:419–23), and severe EPSE and urinary retention has been reported (n=1, Bozikas *et al, J Psychopharmacol* 2001;**15**:142–3).
Fluvoxamine + risperidone
Neurotoxicity (eg. confusion, diaphoresis and myoclonus) has been reported within two days when fluvoxamine was added to risperidone (n=1, Reeves *et al, Ann Pharmacother* 2002; **36**:440–3).
Galantamine + risperidone
See antipsychotics + galantamine (*4.6.3.2*).
Itraconazole + risperidone *
One week of itraconazole 200mg/d raised risperidone and metabolite levels by around 70–75%, presumably via 3A4 inhibition, returning to normal over the next week (n=19, 2/52, Jung *et al, Clin Pharmacol Ther* 2005;**78**:520–8).

Lamotrigine + risperidone *

Increasing lamotrigine from 175 mg/d to 225 mg/d produced a rise in risperidone levels from 70 ng/ml to 412 ng/ml in one patient also on clozapine, although the mechanism was unknown (n = 1, Bienentreu and Kronmüller, *Am J Psychiatry* 2005;**162**:811–2) and others have disputed this (n = 15 + 211 controls, Castberg and Spigset, *J Clin Psychiatry* 2006;**67**:1159).

Lithium + risperidone

See antipsychotics + lithium (*4.4*).

Methadone + risperidone

See methadone (*4.6.10*).

Mirtazapine + risperidone

See mirtazapine (*4.3.3.3*).

Oxcarbazepine + risperidone *

See oxcarbazepine (*4.5.6*).

Paroxetine + risperidone *

Paroxetine causes a dose-dependent rise in risperidone and metabolite levels (up to double with paroxetine 40 mg/d), and so risperidone dose reduction might be needed should side-effects occur (n = 12, open, 12/52, Saito et al, *J Clin Psychopharmacol* 2005;**25**:527–32; n = 10, open, 4/52, Spina et al, *Ther Drug Monit* 2001;**23**:223–7; n = 1, Barnhill et al, *Pharmacopsychiatry* 2005; **38**:223–5).

Phenothiazines + risperidone *

Leveomepromazine had no effect on risperidone plasma levels when used as an adjuvant (n = 20, 2/52, Yoshimura et al, *Pharmacopsychiatry* 2005; **38**:98–100).

Phenytoin + risperidone

Severe EPSE have been reported (n = 1, Sanderson, *J Clin Psychiatry* 1996;**57**:177).

Probenecid + risperidone

Probenecid has no effect on risperidone kinetics (n = 12, RCT, d/b, c/o, Markowitz et al, *Clin Pharmacol Ther* 2002;**71**:30–8).

Reboxetine + risperidone

See reboxetine (*4.3.3.5*).

Ritonavir/indinavir + risperidone

Addition of ritonavir/indinavir to risperidone has led to severe EPSE, dystonia (n = 1, Kelly et al, *Ann Pharmacother* 2002;**36**:827–30) and reversible coma (n = 1, Jover et al, *Clin Neuropharmacol* 2002;**25**:251–3), probably due to risperidone toxicity.

Sertraline + risperidone

High doses of sertraline (150 mg/d) can elevate risperidone levels by about 40%, presumably via

2D6 inhibition (n = 11, open, Spina et al, *Ther Drug Monit* 2004;**26**:386–90).

Thioridazine + risperidone *

Thioridazine may significantly inhibit the metabolism of risperidone (Nakagami et al, *J Clin Psychopharmacol* 2005;**25**:89–91).

Tricyclics + risperidone

See antipsychotics + tricyclics (*4.3.1*).

Valproate + risperidone

See antipsychotics (*4.2.1*).

Venlafaxine + risperidone

Steady-state venlafaxine had no significant effect on the kinetics of a single 1 mg dose of risperidone, although some enzyme inhibition led to slightly raised risperidone plasma levels (n = 30, open, Amchin et al, *J Clin Pharmacol* 1999;**39**:297–309).

4.2.7 ANTIPSYCHOTICS — SERTINDOLE

See *4.2.1* for other, more general, interactions

Sertindole is extensively metabolised by CYP2D6 and 3A4 and is a weak 2D6 and 3A4 inhibitor. It is contraindicated in patients also receiving drugs known to prolong the QT interval.

Aluminium-magnesium antacids + sertindole

There is no effect on sertindole absorption.

ANTIPSYCHOTICS (other) + SERTINDOLE

The UK SPC for sertindole states that it is contraindicated with drugs known to prolong the QT interval, eg. thioridazine, ziprasidone and antihistamines.

ANTI-ARRHYTHMICS + SERTINDOLE

The UK SPC for sertindole states that it is contraindicated with drugs known to prolong the QT interval, eg. class Ia and III antiarrhythmics, eg. quinidine, amiodarone, sotalol, dofetilide, etc.

Benzodiazepines + sertindole

Sertindole has no significant effect on alprazolam (n = 14, open, Wong et al, *Psychopharmacol* [Berl] 1998;**135**:236–41).

Calcium-channel blockers + sertindole

Minor, non-significant increases in sertindole levels have been detected with calcium-channel antagonists via CYP3A4 inhibition.

CARBAMAZEPINE + SERTINDOLE

Carbamazepine can reduce sertindole levels 2–3-fold by CYP3A4 induction, so higher maintenance doses might be needed.

CIMETIDINE + SERTINDOLE

The UK SPC for sertindole states that it is contraindicated for use with cimetidine due to CYP3A4 inhibition. Ranitidine would be a suitable alternative.

Citalopram + sertindole
No interaction via CYP2D6 appears to occur.

Escitalopram + sertindole
See citalopram above.

MACROLIDES + SERTINDOLE
QT prolongation potential makes this combination a contraindication. Minor, non-significant increases in sertindole levels have been detected with **erythromycin** and other macrolides, via CYP3A4 inhibition.

FLUOXETINE + SERTINDOLE
Plasma levels of sertindole are increased 2–3-fold via CYP2D6 inhibition, so lower maintenance doses might be needed or use of a non-2D6 inhibiting antidepressant.

HIV PROTEASE INIBITORS + SERTINDOLE
The UK SPC for sertindole states that it is contraindicated with drugs such as indinavir due to 3A4 inhibition.

ITRACONAZOLE/KETOCONAZOLE + SERTINDOLE
The UK SPC for sertindole states that it is contraindicated for use with systemic itraconazole and ketoconazole due to CYP3A4 inhibition.

LITHIUM + SERTINDOLE
The QT prolongation potential makes this combination a contraindication.

PAROXETINE + SERTINDOLE
Plasma levels of sertindole are increased 2–3-fold via CYP2D6 inhibition, so lower maintenance doses might be needed or use of a non-2D6 inhibiting antidepressant. There is a case of sertindole enhancing paroxetine withdrawal symptoms (Walker-Kinnear and McNaughton, *Br J Psychiatry* 1997;**170**:389).

PHENYTOIN + SERTINDOLE
Phenytoin can reduce sertindole levels 2–3-fold by 3A4 induction, so higher maintenance doses might be needed.

Propranolol + sertindole
No interaction via 2D6 seems to occur.

QUINIDINE + SERTINDOLE
Plasma levels of sertindole are thought to be increased 2–3-fold via 2D6 inhibition, so use is contraindicated. The UK SPC for sertindole also states that it is contraindicated with drugs known to prolong the QT interval, eg. quinidine.

QUINOLONE ANTIBIOTICS + SERTINDOLE
The QT prolongation potential makes the combination with, eg. gatifloxacin a contraindication.

Sertraline + sertindole
No interaction via CYP2D6 appears to occur.

TRICYCLICS + SERTINDOLE
The UK SPC for sertindole states that it is contraindicated with drugs known to prolong the QT interval, eg. some tricyclics. No interaction via CYP2D6 appears to occur with the tricyclics.

4.2.8 ANTIPSYCHOTICS — ZIPRASIDONE

Ziprasidone is partly metabolised by CYP3A4 (with a minor amount from 1A2), plus around 65% via aldehyde reductase. It has no effect on CYP1A2, 2C9/19, 2D6 nor 3A4. It is 99% plasma bound. Due to the QTc prolonging effect, ziprasidone should not be used with drugs also likely to prolong the QTc interval, eg. sotalol, quinidine, other Class Ia and III anti-arrhythmics, phenothiazines, tricyclics, pimozide, mefloquine and dolasetron (see SPC).

Antacids + ziprasidone
Lack of interaction has been shown with 30ml Maalox (n=11, RCT, Wilner *et al*, *Br J Clin Pharmacol* 2000;**49**[S3]:57–60).

Anticholinergics + ziprasidone
Lack of interaction has been shown with benzatropine.

Benzodiazepines + ziprasidone
Lack of interaction with lorazepam has been shown.

Beta-blockers + ziprasidone
Lack of interaction has been shown with propranolol.

Carbamazepine + ziprasidone
Carbamazepine decreases ziprasidone AUC by about 35%, which may require slightly raised doses (n=25, RCT, 4/52, Miceli *et al*, *Br J Clin Pharmacol* 2000;**49**[S3]:65–70).

Cimetidine + ziprasidone
Lack of interaction has been shown (n=11, RCT, Wilner *et al*, *Br J Clin Pharmacol* 2000;**49**[S3]: 57–60).

Dextromethorphan + ziprasidone
Lack of interaction has been shown (Wilner *et al*, *Br J Clin Pharmacol* 2000;**49**(S3):43–8).

Ketoconazole + ziprasidone
Ketoconazole decreases ziprasidone AUC by about 35%, which may require slightly raised doses.

Levodopa + ziprasidone
Ziprasidone may antagonise the effects of

levodopa and other dopaminergic agents.

Lithium + ziprasidone *

Lack of interaction has been shown (n = 25, RCT, Apseloff et al, Br J Clin Pharmacol 2000; **49**[S3]:61–4), although lithium toxicity (n = 2, Miodownik et al, Clin Neuropharmacol 2005; **28**:295–7) and NMS (n = 1, Borovicka et al, Ann Pharmacother 2006;**40**:139–42) have been reported with the combination.

Oral contraceptive + ziprasidone

Lack of interaction has been shown with a combined oral contraceptive (n = 19, d/b, p/c, c/o, Muirhead et al, Br J Clin Pharmacol 2000;**49**[S3]:49–56).

QT-prolonging drugs + ziprasidone

See introduction.

Smoking + ziprasidone

See antipsychotics + smoking (4.7.4) .

Warfarin + ziprasidone

Lack of interaction has been shown.

4.2.9 ANTIPSYCHOTICS — ZOTEPINE

See 4.2.1 for other, more general, interactions

Zotepine is metabolised by CYP1A2 and 3A4 to norzotepine and both have a plasma protein binding of 97%, making protein-displacement interactions unlikely. Zotepine has no significant effect on CYP2D6.

Alcohol + zotepine

Zotepine should not be used in people with alcohol intoxication.

Anticonvulsants + zotepine

Zotepine lowers the seizure threshold, particularly at doses above 300 mg/d.

Anticholinergics + zotepine

Biperiden had no effect on zotepine kinetics, side-effects or efficacy in one study (n = 21, Otani et al, Br J Psychiatry 1990;**157**:128–30).

Anticoagulants + zotepine

The Japanese SPC notes that zotepine has been reported to enhance the risk of bleeding when given with anticoagulants, eg. with nicoumalone, dicoumarol and warfarin, possibly via a change in protein binding.

Antipsychotics (other) + zotepine

Co-prescribing other antipsychotics with zotepine can raise the incidence of seizures.

Benzodiazepines + zotepine

Diazepam increases zotepine levels by 10% (higher in Japanese patients) and doubles

norzotepine levels (n = 17, open, Kondo et al, Psychopharmacol [Berl] 1996;**127**:311–4), possibly via CYP3A4 inhibition.

Carbamazepine + zotepine

See antipsychotics + carbamazepine (4.5.1).

Clonidine + zotepine

The Japanese SPC notes that zotepine has alpha-1-adrenergic antagonistic properties, which may decrease the hypotensive actions of clonidine and other hypotensive agents.

Hypotensive drugs + zotepine

See clonidine.

Phenytoin + zotepine

The Japanese SPC notes that zotepine may increase phenytoin plasma levels, so more frequent monitoring is required.

Smoking + zotepine

See antipsychotics + smoking (4.7.4).

SSRIs + zotepine

Fluoxetine increases zotepine levels by 10% and doubles norzotepine levels. Deep vein thrombosis, possibly linked to concurrent **paroxetine** and zotepine, has been reported (n = 2, Pantel et al, Pharmacopsychiatry 1997;**30**:109–11).

Tricyclics + zotepine

Desipramine does not seem to affect zotepine levels.

4.3 ANTIDEPRESSANTS

Reviews: significant drug interactions with antidepressants in the elderly (Spina and Scordo, Drugs Aging 2002;**19**:299–320, 95 refs).

4.3.1 TRICYCLIC ANTIDEPRESSANTS

Tricyclics are metabolised by a range of P450 enzymes, eg. CYP1A2, 2D6 and 3A3/4. Some tricyclics have several metabolic routes, which may vary with concentration and where another might take over should one be inhibited.

Acamprosate + tricyclics

See acamprosate (4.6.1).

Acetazolamide + tricyclics

An interaction is unlikely to occur.

ALCOHOL + TRICYCLICS

See alcohol (4.7.1).

Amiodarone + tricyclics

The literature notes an increased risk of ventricular arrhythmias with tricyclics.

Anaesthetics + tricyclics

Halothane, pancuronium or gallamine should

be used with care with tricyclics with strong anticholinergic actions. Enflurane may be a safer alternative.

Anticholinergics + tricyclics
Enhanced anticholinergic effects may occur, especially in the elderly.

Antihistamines + tricyclics
Enhanced sedation and anticholinergic effects are possible.

Antipsychotics + tricyclics
Tricyclic levels may be up to twice as high if haloperidol is taken concurrently, eg. with desipramine (n=30, open, Nelson et al, Am J Psychiatry 1980;**137**:1232–4), nortriptyline and imipramine. Tricyclic levels may also rise with phenothiazines (eg. Siris et al, Am J Psychiatry 1982;**143**:104–6) giving enhanced side-effects, eg. perphenazine increases nortriptyline levels by about 25%, probably by CYP2D6 inhibition (n=25, Mulsant et al, J Clin Psychopharmacol 1997;**17**:318–21). Thioridazine may increase imipramine levels (n=1, Maynard and Soni, Ther Drug Monit 1996;**18**:728–31). No significant interaction has been reported with the thioxanthenes, although raised imipramine levels with flupentixol have occurred (n=1, Cook et al, Can J Psychiatry 1986;**31**:235–7). Up to 100mg/d amitriptyline may have no effect on risperidone (n=12, open, Sommers et al, Int Clin Psychopharmacol 1997;**12**:141–5) but risperidone may raise maprotiline levels, not a thing you'd want to do accidentally (Normann et al, J Clin Psychopharmacol 2002;**22**:92–4).

Aspirin + imipramine
Imipramine plasma levels may rise and ADRs increase when aspirin is added to imipramine (n=20, Juarez-Olguin et al, Clin Neuropharmacol 2002;**25**:32–6).

Atomoxetine + tricyclics
See atomoxetine (4.6.4).

Baclofen + tricyclics
A patient with multiple sclerosis lost muscle tone when nortriptyline and imipramine were added to baclofen (n=1, Silverglat, JAMA 1981;**246**:1659).

BARBITURATES + TRICYCLICS
Barbiturates can reduce the serum levels of amitriptyline, protriptyline (n=30, Moody et al, Eur J Clin Pharmacol 1977;**11**:51–6) and nortriptyline by 14–60%, via CYP3A4 induction. Pentobarbital may affect nortriptyline metabolism within two days, both when starting (induction) and on discontinuation (n=6, von Bahr et al, Clin Pharmacol Ther 1998;**64**:18–26). Use an alternative to barbiturates or monitor tricyclic levels.

Benzodiazepines + tricyclics
See benzodiazepines (4.1.1).

Beta-blockers + tricyclics
Enhanced maprotiline toxicity has been reported, labetolol increases imipramine plasma levels by 28% (n=12, RCT, p/c, c/o, Hermann et al, J Clin Pharmacol 1992;**32**:176–83) and there are two uncertain cases of propranolol possibly raising imipramine levels in children (n=2, Gillette and Tannery, J Am Acad Child Adolesc Psychiatry 1994;**33**:223–4), possibly via 2D6 inhibition. This would appear to be a rare but possible interaction.

Buprenorphine + amitriptyline
No enhanced CNS depressant or respiratory effects have been seen (n=12, d/b, p/c, c/o, Saarialho-Kere et al, Eur J Clin Pharmacol 1987; **33**:139–46).

Bupropion + tricyclics
See bupropion (4.6.6).

Cannabis + tricyclics
See antidepressants + cannabis (4.7.2).

Calcium-channel blockers + tricyclics
Amitriptyline clearance was reduced by diltiazem and verapamil in one study, with adverse effects increased (n=32, Hermann et al, J Clin Pharmacol 1992;**32**:176–83). Diltiazem may increase nortriptyline concentrations (n=1, Krahenbuhl et al, Eur J Clin Pharmacol 1996;**49**:417–9). Enhanced cardiac side-effects are also possible.

CARBAMAZEPINE + TRICYCLICS
See carbamazepine (4.5.1).

Charcoal, activated + tricyclics
5–10g may reduce the absorption of tricyclics by up to 75% if given within 30 minutes and may be an effective treatment for overdose, even up to two hours after the overdose is taken (open, Dawling et al, Eur J Clin Pharmacol 1978;**14**:445–7).

Cholestyramine + doxepin
Plasma levels of doxepin may be reduced to a third by cholestyramine (n=1, Geeze et al, Psychosomatics 1988; **29**:233–5).

CLONIDINE + TRICYCLICS
Tricyclics can be expected to antagonise the hypotensive effects of clonidine (eg. Hui, J Am Geriatr Soc 1983;**31**:164–5).

Cocaine + tricyclics
See antidepressants + cocaine (4.7.3).

Co-trimoxazole + tricyclics
Five cases of relapse have been reported when co-trimoxazole was added to antidepressant therapy (L'Encephale 1987;**8**:123–6).

Dextropropoxyphene + doxepin
There are reports of doxepin plasma levels raised by up to 150% with dextropropoxyphene, via 2D6 inhibition.

Dicoumarol + tricyclics
An enhanced dicoumarol half-life is possible (Veseil et al, N Engl J Med 1970;**283**:1484–8), shown with amitriptyline and nortriptyline (Pond et al, Clin Pharmacol Ther 1975;**18**:191).

Disopyramide + tricyclics
Increased anticholinergic effects may be seen (Hartel et al, Clin Pharmacol Ther 1974;**15**:551–5) and the BNF notes an increased risk of ventricular arrhythmias.

Disulfiram + tricyclics
Amitriptyline may enhance the effects of disulfiram (MacCallum, Lancet 1969;i:313) and tricyclic levels may be increased by about 30% by enzyme inhibition (n=2, Ciraulo et al, Am J Psychiatry 1985;**142**:1373–4).

Duloxetine + tricyclics
See duloxetine (4.3.3.1).

Fibre + tricyclics
There are several cases of a high fibre diet reducing tricyclic levels by up to a third (and hence to inactive levels), eg. with doxepin. This might explain non-response in some patients.

Fluconazole + tricyclics
Inhibition of CYP3A4 by fluconazole has resulted in cases of elevated, toxic nortriptyline levels (n=1, Gannon, Ann Pharmacother 1992; **26**:1456–7) and syncope (Robinson et al, Ann Pharmacother 2000;**34**:1406–9). Delirium (Duggal, Gen Hosp Psychiatry 2003;**25**:297–8) has been associated with concurrent amitriptyline and fluconazole therapy.

Glyceryl trinitrate + tricyclics
See nitrates + tricyclics.

H2-blockers + tricyclics
CYP1A2 inhibition by **cimetidine** may decrease the metabolism and increase the half-life and plasma levels of tricyclics, eg. amitriptyline (by 37–80%, Curry et al, Eur J Clin Pharmacol 1985; **29**:429–33), doxepin (by 30%, n=10, RCT, Abernethy and Todd, J Clin Psychopharmacol 1986;**6**:8–12), imipramine (by over 100%, n=12, RCT, d/b, p/c, c/o, Wells et al, Eur J Clin Pharmacol 1986;**31**:285–90) and nortriptyline (by 20%, Henauer and Hollister, Clin Pharmacol Ther 1984;**35**:183–7). Other H2-blockers, eg. **ranitidine**, do not appear to interact this way (n=6, open, Sutherland et al, Eur J Clin Pharmacol 1987;**32**:159–64).

Hypoglycaemics + tricyclics
There are two isolated cases of enhanced hypoglycaemia with doxepin and nortriptyline (n=2, True et al, Am J Psychiatry 1987;**144**:1220–1), so monitor blood glucose regularly.

Levodopa + tricyclics
A small reduction in the effect of levodopa may be seen (open, Morgan et al, Neurology 1975;**25**:1029), but this is of low clinical significance.

Levothyroxine + tricyclics
This is usually a synergistic interaction (see 1.14) but a few isolated cases of tachycardia and hypothyroidism have been reported.

Lithium + tricyclics
The combination is well used (see depression, 1.14) but some adverse reactions have been reported, eg. myoclonus (Devanand et al, J Clin Psychopharmacol 1988;**8**:446) and neurotoxicity with motor symptoms and seizures (eg. Austin et al, J Clin Psychiatry 1990;**51**:344). NMS has been reported with amoxapine and lithium (n=1, Gupta and Racaniello, Ann Clin Psychiatry 2000; **12**:107–9).

MAOIs + TRICYCLICS
See MAOIs (4.3.4).

Methadone + tricyclics
See methadone (4.6.10).

Methyldopa + desipramine
The hypotensive effect of methyldopa may be decreased, with possible tachycardia and CNS stimulation (Van Spanning et al, Int J Clin Pharmacol Biopharm 1975;**11**:65–7).

Methylphenidate + tricyclics
See methylphenidate (4.6.11).

Mirtazapine + tricyclics
See mirtazapine (4.3.3.3).

Moclobemide + tricyclics
See moclobemide (4.3.3.4).

Modafinil + tricyclics
See modafinil (4.6.12).

Morphine + tricyclics
Tricyclics such as amitriptyline and clomipramine increase the bioavailability of morphine and

potentiate the analgesic effect, so this is usually a beneficial combination (Ventafridda *et al*, *Lancet* 1987;**i**:1204).

Nitrates (sublingual) + tricyclics

Dry mouth may reduce the dissolution of sublingual nitrates.

Olanzapine + tricyclics

See olanzapine (*4.2.4*).

Oral Contraceptives/estrogens + tricyclics

Akathisia (n=3, Krishnan *et al*, *Am J Psychiatry* 1984;**141**:696–7), reduced tricyclic effectiveness and enhanced tricyclic toxicity have been reported. Best to monitor the tricyclic closely.

Orlistat + tricyclics

A small trial suggested lack of interaction with clomipramine (n=8, 8/52, Hilger *et al*, *J Clin Psychopharmacol* 2002;**22**:68–70).

Phenindione + tricyclics

An enhanced risk of bleeding may occur with this combination.

Phenylbutazone + tricyclics

Tricyclic absorption may get delayed or reduced by phenylbutazone (Consolo *et al*, *Eur J Pharmacol* 1970;**10**:239–42).

PHENYTOIN + TRICYCLICS

See phenytoin (*4.5.8*).

Quetiapine + tricyclics

See quetiapine (*4.2.5*).

Quinine/quinidine + tricyclics

Studies have shown a much reduced clearance of nortriptyline with quinidine and quinine (n=10, Steiner *et al*, *Clin Pharmacol Ther* 1988; **43**:577–81), via 2D6 inhibition. Best to monitor tricyclic levels.

Reboxetine + tricyclics

See reboxetine (*4.3.3.5*).

SERTINDOLE + TRICYCLICS

See sertindole (*4.2.7*).

Smoking + tricyclics

See smoking (*4.7.4*).

Sodium oxybate + tricyclics *

See sodium oxybate (*4.6.13*).

SSRIs + TRICYCLICS

Tricyclics are metabolised by CYP2D6 and SSRIs produce a dose-related inhibition of this enzyme. **Fluoxetine**, **paroxetine** and **fluvoxamine** all cause significant inhibition at therapeutic doses, whereas citalopram/escitalopram and sertraline cause little clinically significant 2D6 inhibition at standard doses. **Citalopram** (and presumably escitalopram) has no effect on some tricyclic levels (n=5, Baettig

et al, *Eur J Clin Pharmacol* 1993;**44**:403–5), although desipramine (but not imipramine) levels may rise slightly (Gram *et al*, *Ther Drug Monit* 1993;**15**:18–24; n=1, Ashton, *J Clin Psychiatry* 2000;**61**:144). **Fluoxetine** may double or triple tricyclic levels, eg. with amitriptyline (eg. fatality reported by Preskorn and Baker, *JAMA* 1997;**277**:1682; n=29, open, Vandel *et al*, *Pharmacol Res* 1995; **31**:347–53), clomipramine (n=4, Vandel *et al*, *Neuropsychobiology* 1992;**25**:202–7), imipramine (Leroj and Walentynowicz, *Can J Psychiatry* 1996; **41**:318–9) and nortriptyline (eg. n=5, case series, Aranow *et al*, *Am J Psychiatry* 1989;**146**:911–3). Potentiation may occur even if the tricyclic is used after an extended interval (Extein, *Am J Psychiatry* 1991;**148**:1601–2). It has been suggested that tricyclic dosage should be reduced by 75% when fluoxetine is added (n=3, Wester-Meyer, *J Clin Pharmacol* 1991;**31**:388–92). **Fluvoxamine** has been shown to increase amitriptyline, clomipramine (n=1, Bertschy *et al*, *Eur J Clin Pharmacol* 1991;**40**:119–20) and imipramine levels (Maskall and Lam, *Am J Psychiatry* 1993; **50**:1566). Fluvoxamine may inhibit both hydroxylation and N-demethylation, indicating a dual effect on tricyclic metabolism (Hartter *et al*, *Psychopharmacology* 1993;**110**: 302–8). **Paroxetine** significantly reduces the metabolism of amitriptyline and imipramine (eg. Skjelbo and Brosen, *Br J Clin Pharmacol* 1992;**34**:256–61), resulting in enhanced tricyclic toxicity. **Sertraline** 50mg/d may produce a 31–60% increase in desipramine levels (Lydiard *et al*, *Am J Psychiatry* 1993;**150**:1125–6; n=18, RCT, 7/52, Preskorn *et al*, *J Clin Psychopharmacol* 1994;**14**:90–8). However, sertraline 150mg/d increased desipramine levels by 70%, with a 200–300% increase in four patients (Zussman *et al*, *Br J Clin Pharmacol* 1995;**39**:S530–S551; See also n=12, RCT, open, Kurtz *et al*, *Clin Pharmacol Ther* 1997;**62**:145–56) so the potential for interaction is present. A serotonin syndrome has been reported with many SSRI-tricyclic combinations (see *5.14*).

St John's wort + tricyclics

See St John's wort (*4.3.3.9*).

Sucralfate + amitriptyline

One small study showed a marked reduction in amitriptyline absorption (*Fed Proc* 1986;**45**:205).

Tea or coffee + tricyclics

Studies have shown that some tricyclics (eg. amitriptyline and imipramine) precipitate out of solution to form a tannin complex with tea and coffee (*J Pharm Sci* 1984;**73**:1056–8). The clinical significance is thought to be minimal (Bowen *et al*, *Lancet* 1981;**i**:1217–8).

Terbinafine + tricyclics *

Terbinafine, a potent 2D6 inhibitor, may triple desipramine plasma levels (n = 1, O'Reardon *et al*, *Am J Psychiatry* 2002;**159**:492) and induce imipramine (eg. n = 1, Teitelbaum and Pearson, *Am J Psychiatry* 2001;**158**:2086) and nortriptyline toxicity (n = 1, van der Kuy *et al*, *Ann Pharmacother* 2002;**36**:1712–4), and a significant rise may occur in amitriptyline levels, an effect that may, extraordinarily, last for up to three to six months after stopping terbinafine (n = 1, Castberg *et al*, *Ther Drug Monit* 2005;**27**:680–2).

Valproate + tricyclics

See antidepressants + valproate (*4.5.12*).

VASOCONSTRICTOR SYMPATHOMIMETICS + TRICYCLICS

A greatly enhanced response, eg. hypertension and arrhythmias, to norepinephrine and phenylephrine in patients taking tricyclics has been shown in many reports. Doxepin and maprotiline may have a lesser effect. Local anaesthetics with epinephrine appear safe. Moderate doses of cold cures containing sympathomimetics should present little risk in healthy patients.

Venlafaxine + tricyclics

Venlafaxine increases imipramine levels, showing a consistent but probably clinically modest effect (n = 8, Albers *et al*, *Psychiatr Res* 2000;**6**:35–43). Serotonin syndrome has been reported with venlafaxine and amitriptyline (n = 1, *Postgrad Med J* 2000;**76**:254–6) and a GTC fit with venlafaxine 150 mg/d and trimipramine 100 mg/d (n = 1, Schlienger *et al*, *Ann Pharmacother* 2000;**34**: 1402–5).

Warfarin + tricyclics *

Normally there is no problem, but occasional control problems have been reported with lofepramine (mentioned in Sayal *et al*, *Acta Psychiatr Scand* 2000;**102**:250–55 and Duncan *et al*, *Int Clin Psychopharmacol* 1998;**13**:87–94).

Yohimbine + tricyclics

Tricyclics can potentiate the blood pressure changes caused by yohimbine, especially if blood pressure is already raised (mentioned in Fugh-Berman, *Lancet* 2000;**355**:134–8).

Zopiclone + tricyclics

See zopiclone (*4.1.6*).

Zotepine + tricyclics

See zotepine (*4.2.9*).

4.3.2 SSRIs (SELECTIVE SEROTONIN REUPTAKE INHIBITORS)

Drug interactions involving the P450 system have been described for all SSRIs, but there are significant differences in the isoenzymes inhibited and the degree of inhibition.

The *in vitro* inhibition of 2D6 on a molar basis is: paroxetine (most potent), norfluoxetine, fluoxetine, sertraline, fluvoxamine and citalopram (least potent). *In vivo* is probably broadly similar. Fluoxetine and paroxetine are probably broadly similar in 2D6 inhibition, but with some variation (n = 31, RCT, using multiple-dose fluoxetine 60 mg/d, fluvoxamine 100 mg/d, paroxetine 20 mg/d, or sertraline 100 mg/d; Alfaro *et al*, *J Clin Psychopharmacol* 1999;**19**:155–63).

Reviews: overview and review of SSRI interactions and P450 effects (Hemeryck and Belpaire, *Curr Drug Metab* 2002;**3**:13–37) and clinically significant SSRI-CNS interactions (Sproule *et al*, *Clin Pharmacokinet* 1997;**33**:454–71, 106 refs).

4.3.2.1 CITALOPRAM AND ESCITALOPRAM

Citalopram is a weak inhibitor of CYP2D6 (Baetig *et al*, *Eur J Clin Pharmacol* 1993;**44**:403–5) and is metabolised by 3A4. A review (Brosen and Naranjo, *Eur Neuropsychopharmacol* 2001; **11**:275–83) concludes that citalopram is neither a source nor a cause of clinically important drug–drug interactions. Escitalopram would be expected to have similar characteristics.

Alcohol + citalopram/escitalopram

See alcohol (*4.7.1*).

Alimemazine (trimeprazine) + citalopram/escitalopram

See antipsychotics + citalopram/escitalopram in this section.

Acenocoumarol + citalopram/escitalopram

There is a reported case of interaction (n = 1, Borras-Blasco *et al*, *Ann Pharmacother* 2002; **36**:345).

Antipsychotics + citalopram/escitalopram *

Levomepromazine and alimemazine may both increase plasma levels of citalopram by about a third (Milne and Goa, *Drugs* 1991;**41**:450–77), possibly via enzyme inhibition and of minimal clinical significance. There has been no detectable effect from citalopram on the plasma levels of other antipsychotics (n=90, d/b, Syvalahti et al, J Intern Med Res 1997;**25**:24–32), eg. citalopram 40mg/d had no effect over eight weeks on the plasma levels of **clozapine** (n=8, 200–400mg/d), **risperidone** (n=7, 4–6mg/d) and their active metabolites in patients with chronic schizophrenia (Avenoso et al, Clin Drug Investigation 1998;**16**:393–8). Despite this, the FDA issued a warning in December 2005 about citalopram raising clozapine levels by clinically significant levels.

Atomoxetine + citalopram/escitalopram
See SSRIs + atomoxetine (4.6.4).

Benzodiazepines + citalopram/escitalopram
No pharmacokinetic interaction could be demonstrated between citalopram and the CYP3A4 substrate triazolam (n=18, open, Nolting and Abramowitz, Pharmacother 2000; **20**:750–5) and citalopram does not prolong the half-life of alprazolam (Hall et al, J Clin Psychopharmacol 2003;**23**:349–57).

Buspirone + citalopram/escitalopram
Hyponatraemia and serotonin syndrome has been reported with this combination (Spigset and Adielsson, Int Clin Psychopharmacol 1997;**12**:61–3).

Carbamazepine + citalopram/escitalopram
Carbamazepine may reduce the proportion and concentration of the escitalopram isomer (n=6, Steinacher et al, Eur Neuropsychopharmacol 2002;**12**:255–60). Citalopram had no effect on carbamazepine kinetics in another study (n=12, open, Moller et al, J Clin Psychophamacol 2001; **21**:493–9).

Charcoal, activated + citalopram/ escitalopram
25g activated charcoal given 30 minutes after citalopram reduced citalopram AUC by 51%, and peak levels by over 50%. Concurrent gastric lavage did not provide any additional reductions (n=9, RCT, Lapatto-Reiniluoto et al, Br J Clin Pharmacol 1999;**48**:148–53).

Ciclosporin + citalopram/escitalopram
Citalopram had no effect on ciclosporin kinetics in one report (Liston et al, Psychosomatics 2001; **42**:370–2).

Cimetidine + citalopram/escitalpram *
Cimetidine increases escitalopram levels but this is unlikely to be clinically significant (n=16, RCT, p/c, Malling et al, Br J Clin Pharmacol 2005;**60**: 287–90).

Digoxin + citalopram/escitalopram
Steady state citalopram 40mg/d had no effect on the kinetics of single doses of digoxin 1mg (n=11, open, c/o, 50/7, Larsen et al, J Clin Pharmacol 2001;**41**:340).

Donepezil + citalopram/escitalopram
See SSRIs + donepezil (4.6.3.1).

Duloxetine+citalopram/escitalopram
See SSRIs + duloxetine (4.3.3.1).

Fluvoxamine + citalopram/escitalopram
Fluvoxamine may increase the ratio of escitalopram to R-citalopram, enhancing its action (n=7, open, Bondolfi et al, Psychopharmacol [Berl] 1996;**128**:421–5).

Ketoconazole + citalopram/escitalopram
Single doses of ketoconazole have no effect on the kinetics of citalopram (n=18, RCT, d/b, c/o, Gutierrez and Abramowitz, Pharmacotherapy 2001;**21**:163–8).

Lamotrigine + citalopram/escitalopram *
Myoclonus has been reported with the combination (n=1, Rosenhagen et al, J Clin Psychopharmacol 2006;**26**:346–7).

Linezolid + citalopram/escitalopram *
In people taking SSRIs, serotonin syndrome may occur about nine days after the introduction of linezolid (longer the older you are); symptoms may resolve in three days or longer (n=12, Morales-Molina et al, J Antimicrob Chemother 2005;**56**:1176–8; n=1, Tahir, J Am Med Dir Assoc 2004;**5**:111–3; n=1, Ann Pharmacother 2005; **39**:956–61).

Lithium + citalopram/escitalopram
No pharmacokinetic interaction was noted in one study (n=24, open, Gram et al, Ther Drug Monit 1993;**15**:18–24).

MAOIs + citalopram/escitalopram
See MAOIs (4.3.4).

Melatonin + citalopram/escitalopram *
Citalopram may slow the metabolism of exogenous melatonin (n=15, RCT, d/b, p/c, 21/7, Huuhka et al, Methods Find Exp Clin Pharmacol 2006;**28**:447–50).

Moclobemide + citalopram/escitalopram
See SSRIs + moclobemide (4.3.3.4).

NSAIDs + citalopram/escitalopram
See NSAIDs + fluoxetine (4.3.2.2).

Omeprazole + citalopram/escitalopram *
Omeprazole increases escitalopram levels but this is unlikely to be clinically significant (n=16, RCT, p/c, Malling et al, Br J Clin Pharmacol 2005;**60**:287–90).

Oxcarbazepine + citalopram/escitalopram
See oxcarbazepine (4.5.6).

Perhexiline + citalopram/escitalopram
Perhexiline toxicity with citalopram has been reported (n = 1, Nyfort-Hansen, Med J Aust 2002; **176**:560–1).

Ritonavir + citalopram/escitalopram
No pharmacokinetic interaction occurs (n = 21 [c = 18], RCT, open, c/o, Gutierrez et al, Clin Ther 2003;**25**:1200–10).

Selegiline + citalopram/escitalopram
One study showed the lack of a clinically significant interaction (n = 18, RCT, Laine et al, Clin Neuropharmacol 1997;**20**:419–33).

Sertindole + citalopram/escitalopram
See sertindole (4.2.7).

Silbutramine + citalopram/escitalopram
A case of hypomania has been reported with this combination (n = 1, Benazzi, J Clin Psychiatry 2002;**63**:165).

St John's wort + citalopram/escitalopram
See SSRIs + St John's wort (4.3.3.9).

Sympathomimetics + citalopram/escitalopram
Augmentation of amfetamines is theoretically possible (see sympathomimetics + fluoxetine).

Tramadol + citalopram/escitalopram
Serotonin syndrome has been reported with tramadol 50 mg/d and citalopram 10 mg/d in a patient with slow metabolising 2D6 and 2C19 enzymes (n = 1, Mahlberg et al, Am J Psychiatry 2004;**161**:1129).

Trazodone + citalopram/escitalopram
No pharmacokinetic interaction occurs (n=41, Prapotnik et al, Int J Clin Pharmacol Ther 2004; **42**:120–4).

Tricyclics + citalopram/escitalopram
See SSRIs + tricyclics (4.3.1).

Triptans + citalopram/escitalopram
The literature notes an increased risk of CNS toxicity with sumatriptan and recommends avoiding the combination. See also triptans + fluoxetine (4.3.2.2).

Warfarin + citalopram/escitalopram
Citalopram 40 mg/d may produce a small increase in prothrombin time (n = 12, Preskorn et al, Br J Clin Pharmacol 1997;**44**:199–202), but this is probably clinically insignificant (Sayal et al, Acta Psychiatr Scand 2000;**102**:250–5).

Zolpidem + citalopram/escitalopram
See SSRIs + zolpidem (4.1.5).

4.3.2.2 FLUOXETINE

Fluoxetine substantially inhibits CYP2D6 and probably 2C9/10, moderately inhibits 2C19 and weakly inhibits 3A3/4 and may have a higher incidence of interactions with drugs metabolised by these enzymes. Norfluoxetine is a potent CYP3A4 inhibitor and appears a moderately potent inhibitor of 2D6.

Alcohol + fluoxetine
See alcohol (4.7.1).

Alosetron + fluoxetine
There is no significant effect from the 5-HT3 antagonist alosetron on fluoxetine kinetics (n = 12, D'Souza et al, J Clin Pharmacol 2001;**41**:455–8).

Amfetamines + fluoxetine
See sympathomimetics + fluoxetine.

ANTIPSYCHOTICS + FLUOXETINE
See antipsychotics (4.2.1), clozapine (4.2.3), olanzapine (4.2.4), quetiapine (4.2.5) and risperidone (4.2.6).

Atomoxetine + fluoxetine
See SSRIs + atomoxetine (4.6.4).

Beta-blockers + fluoxetine
Bradycardia may occur in people taking fluoxetine and metoprolol, possibly due to CYP2D6 inhibition. Atenolol or sotalol may be suitable alternatives (n = 2, Proudlove, Lancet 1993;**341**:967). Fluoxetine may inhibit the metabolism of R-carvedilol (rather than S-carvedilol), but this appears to have little clinical significance (n = 10, RCT, d/b, c/o, 28/7, Graff et al, J Clin Pharmacol 2001;**41**:97–106).

Benzodiazepines + fluoxetine
Fluoxetine may slightly increase the plasma levels of some benzodiazepines (eg. **diazepam**: n = 10, Lemberger et al, Clin Pharmacol Ther 1988;**43**:412–9) although probably not **midazolam** (n = 10, RCT, 12/7, Lam et al, J Clin Pharmacol 2003;**43**:1274–82). Desmethyldiazepam levels may be lower, which may explain the lack of additive psychomotor impairment (review: Ciraulo and Shader, J Clin Psychopharmacol 1990;**10**:213–7). Fluoxetine increases **alprazolam's** half-life by 16% (Hall et al, J Clin Psychopharmacol 2003;**23**:349–57) due to decreased clearance (RCT, p/c, Greenblatt et al, Clin Pharmacol Ther 1992;**52**:479–86). The clinical significance is minor.

Bupropion + fluoxetine
See bupropion (4.6.6).

Buspirone + fluoxetine
See buspirone (4.1.2).

Calcium-channel blockers + fluoxetine

Oedema, weight gain and headache have occurred with verapamil and fluoxetine (n=2, Sternbach, *J Clin Psychopharmacol* 1991;**11**:390). Lowering doses is recommended if an interaction is suspected.

Cannabis + fluoxetine

See antidepressants + cannabis (4.7.2).

Carbamazepine + fluoxetine

Two studies have shown that fluoxetine and norfluoxetine inhibit carbamazepine metabolism, increasing levels by up to 25% (n=14, Gidal *et al*, *Ther Drug Monit* 1993;**15**:405–9). One small study however, showed fluoxetine 20mg/d to have no effect on carbamazepine levels (n=8, open, Spina *et al*, *Ther Drug Monit* 1993;**15**:247–50). A toxic serotonin syndrome has been reported (n=1, Dursun *et al*, *Lancet* 1993;**342**:442–3).

Ciclosporin + fluoxetine

Ciclosporin plasma concentrations were nearly doubled by fluoxetine 20mg/d in one report, probably by CYP3A4 inhibition (n=1, Holton and Bonser, *Br Med J* 1995;**311**:422).

Clarithromycin + fluoxetine

Acute delirium has been reported when clarith-romycin was added to fluoxetine (eg. n=1, Tracy and Johns Cupp, *Ann Pharmacother* 1996;**30**:1199–200), probably via CYP3A4 inhibition.

Cocaine + fluoxetine

See antidepressants + cocaine (4.7.3).

Cyproheptadine + fluoxetine

Patients treated with cyproheptadine for fluoxetine-induced anorgasmia may relapse (n=3, Feder, *J Clin Psychiatry* 1991;**52**:163–4), and interaction has been reported in a bulimic patient (n=2, Goldbloom and Kennedy, *J Clin Psychiatry* 1991;**52**:261–2).

Dextromethorphan + fluoxetine *

Visual hallucinations lasting 6–8 hours occurred in a patient taking fluoxetine 20mg/d who also took a cough mixture containing dextromethorphan (Achamallah, *Am J Psychiatry* 1992;**149**:1406). and a serotonin syndrome has been reported in a patient also taking lithium (n=1, Navarro *et al*, *Gen Hosp Psychiatry* 2006;**28**:78–80).

Digoxin + fluoxetine *

In a nested case-control study, there was no apparent increased risk of digoxin toxicity after initiation of paroxetine, fluoxetine, sertraline and fluvoxamine compared to tricyclics and benzodiazepines (n=3144, Juurlink *et al*, *Br J Clin Pharmacol* 2005;**59**:102–7).

Donepezil + fluoxetine

See SSRIs + donepezil (4.6.3.1).

Duloxetine + fluoxetine

See SSRIs + duloxetine (4.3.3.1).

Lithium + fluoxetine

See lithium (4.4).

LSD + fluoxetine

GTC convulsions occurred in one patient who took a double dose of LSD while on fluoxetine 20mg/d, having previously taken single doses of LSD uneventfully (n=1, Achamallah, *Am J Psychiatry* 1992;**149**:843–4).

MAOIs + FLUOXETINE

See MAOIs (4.3.4)

Methadone + fluoxetine

See methadone (4.6.10).

Metoclopramide + fluoxetine *

Fluoxetine increases metoclopramide plasma levels, increasing Cmax by 42% and half-life by 53% (n=24, c/o,Viase *et al*, *Biopharm Drug Dispos* 2006;**27**:285–9).

Mirtazapine + fluoxetine

See mirtazapine (4.3.3.3).

Moclobemide + fluoxetine

See SSRIs + moclobemide (4.3.3.4).

Morphine + fluoxetine

Fluoxetine may mildly enhance the analgesic effects of morphine and reduce its side-effects (n=15, d/b, Erjavec *et al*, *J Clin Pharmacol* 2000; **40**:1286–95).

NSAIDs + SSRIs

Use NSAIDs and SSRIs together with caution in the over 80s, in those with a history of GI bleeding and in those taking aspirin or other NSAIDs (*Drug Ther Bull* 2004;**42**:17–8).There is a three-fold increase in upper GI bleeding, although the absolute risk remains low (three admissions per 1000 patient years).

Olanzapine + fluoxetine

See SSRIs + olanzapine (4.2.4).

Oral contraceptives + fluoxetine

Lack of interaction has been shown (n=1698, Koke *et al*, *Am J Obstet Gynecol* 2002;**187**:551–5).

Pentazocine + fluoxetine

Rapid toxicity has been reported, although an interaction was not proven (n=1, Hansen *et al*, *Am J Psychiatry* 1990;**147**:949–50).

PHENYTOIN + FLUOXETINE

See phenytoin (4.5.8).

Quetiapine + fluoxetine
See SSRIs + quetiapine (4.2.5).
Reboxetine + fluoxetine
See reboxetine (4.3.3.5).
RISPERIDONE + FLUOXETINE
See risperidone (4.2.6).
Rivastigmine + fluoxetine
See rivastigmine (4.6.3.3).
Selegiline + fluoxetine
There are isolated cases of toxic reactions, eg. hypomania, hypertension and shivering (Suchowersky and de Vries, Can J Neurol Sci 1990;**17**:352), ataxia in a complex regimen (n = 1, Jermain et al, Ann Pharmacother 1992;**26**:1300) and hypertension (Montastruc et al, Lancet 1993; **341**:555).
SERTINDOLE + FLUOXETINE
See sertindole (4.2.7).
Sertraline + fluoxetine
See sertraline (4.3.2.5).
St John's wort + fluoxetine
See SSRIs + St John's wort (4.3.3.9).
Sympathomimetics + fluoxetine
An interaction has been suggested by reports of extreme restlessness, agitation and psychotic symptoms apparently caused by fluoxetine-augmentation of amfetamines (n = 2, Barrett et al, Br J Psychiatry 1996;**168**:253).
Tolterodine + fluoxetine
Fluoxetine has been shown to inhibit the metabolism of tolterodine (n = 13, open, Brynne et al, Br J Clin Pharmacology 1999;**48**:553–63), probably via 2D6.
Tramadol + fluoxetine
Serotonin syndrome and mania has been reported with this combination (n = 1, Kesavan and Sobala, J Roy Soc Med 1999;**92**:474–5; n = 1, Gonzalez-Pinto et al, Am J Psychiatry 2001; **158**:964–5).
Trazodone + fluoxetine
No pharmacokinetic interaction occurs (n = 16, Prapotnik et al, Int J Clin Pharmacol Ther 2004; **42**:120–4), although trazodone toxicity (eg. Neirenberg et al, J Clin Psychiatry 1992;**53**:83) and myoclonus have been reported (n = 1, Darko et al, Vet Hum Toxicol 2001;**43**:214–5).
TRICYCLICS + FLUOXETINE
See SSRIs + tricyclics (4.3.1).
Triptans + fluoxetine
Lack of significant interaction has been reported with sumatriptan (n = 14, open, Blier and Bergeron, J Clin Psychopharmacol 1995;**15**:106–9),

although post-marketing surveillance in Canada indicated that a serotonin-like syndrome may occur rarely with the combination (n = 22, Joffe and Sokolov, Acta Psychiatr Scand 1997;**95**:551–2). The literature notes an increased risk of CNS toxicity and recommends avoiding the combination. Fluoxetine 60 mg/d has only a modest effect on alotriptan peak levels, with no clinically significant side-effects or changes in vital signs or ECGs (n = 14, RCT, c/o, 8/7, Fleishaker et al, J Clin Pharmacol 2001;**41**:217–23).
Tryptophan + fluoxetine
Central toxicity has been reported (n = 5, Steiner and Fontaine, Biol Psychiatry 1986;**21**:1067–71).
Valproate + fluoxetine
Valproate levels may rise by up to 50% if fluoxetine is added, although the mechanism is not established (eg. Lucena et al, Am J Psychiatry 1998;**155**:575) and reduced valproate levels have been reported (Droulers et al, J Clin Psychopharmacol 1997;**17**:139–40).
Venlafaxine + fluoxetine
Serotonin syndrome has been reported when venlafaxine was started immediately after fluoxetine was discontinued (n = 1, Bhatara et al, Ann Pharmacother 1998;**32**:432–6), as have severe anticholinergic side-effects (n = 4, Benazzi, J Clin Psychopharmacol 1999;**19**:96–8, letter).
WARFARIN + FLUOXETINE
An in vitro study indicated fluoxetine has a potentially potent effect on warfarin (Schmider et al, Br J Clin Pharmacol 1997;**44**:495–8). Raised INR has been reported within ten days of starting fluoxetine (n = 2, Woolfrey et al, Br Med J 1993;**307**:241) and two patients on warfarin with stable INRs experienced dramatic increases in INR when fluoxetine 20 mg/d was added (n = 2, Hanger and Thomas, N Z Med J 1995;**108**:157). There is also a case report of an elderly man prescribed warfarin, diazepam and fluoxetine who developed an elevated INR and died from a cerebral haemorrhage (n = 1, Dent and Orrock, Pharmacotherapy 1997;**17**:170–2).
Zolpidem + fluoxetine
See SSRIs + zolpidem (4.1.5).
Zotepine + fluoxetine
See SSRIs + zotepine (4.2.9).

4.3.2.2 FLUVOXAMINE *
Fluvoxamine strongly inhibits CYP1A2, 2D6, 3A4 and 2C19 (and possibly 2C8 weakly) and

may have a high incidence of interactions with drugs metabolised by these enzymes (n = 20, *Clin Pharmacol Ther* 1998;**64**:257–68).

Alcohol + fluvoxamine
See alcohol (4.7.1).

Antipsychotics + fluvoxamine *
Seizures have been reported with **levomepro-mazine** and fluvoxamine (n = 1, Grinshpoon et al, *Int Clin Psychopharmacol* 1993;**8**:61–2), although levomepromazine does not appear to increase fluvoxamine levels (n = 15, Yoshimura et al, *Int Clin Psychopharmacol* 2000;**15**:233–5). Fluvoxamine 100 mg/d had no effect on plasma levels of **risperidone** 3–6 mg/d but 200 mg/d increased concentrations by 26% (n = 11, open, 8/52, D'Arrigo et al, *Pharmacol Res* 2005;**52**:497–501). **Thioridazine** is contraindicated with fluvoxamine due to QTc prolongation. Fluvoxamine produces a dose-dependent increase in **haloperidol** levels, 150 mg/d raising levels by 60%, although this was without additional side-effects at 6 mg/d (n = 12, Yasui-Furukori et al, *Psychopharmacol* [Berl] 2003; **171**:223–7). See also clozapine (4.2.3).

Benzodiazepines + fluvoxamine
Plasma concentrations of **bromazepam** are doubled by fluvoxamine, but **lorazepam** is unaffected (van Harten et al, mentioned in *Clin Pharmacokinet* 1993;**24**:203–20). A study showed that fluvoxamine 100 mg/d increased **alprazolam** plasma levels by 100%, and so, reduced doses of alprazolam should be used (n = 60, Fleishaker and Hulst, *Eur J Clin Pharmacol* 1994;**46**:35–9). A slight increase (66%) in **midazolam** (n = 10, RCT, 12/7, Lam et al, *J Clin Pharmacol* 2003;**43**:1274–82) and **quazepam** levels (n = 12, RCT, d/b, c/o, p/c, 14/7, Kanda et al, *J Clin Pharmacol* 2003;**43**:1392–7) has been reported.

Beta-blockers + fluvoxamine
Lack of significant interaction has been shown with atenolol. Propranolol plasma levels can be raised by fluvoxamine by up to 500%, but apparently without major clinical effect (reviewed by Benfield and Ward, *Drugs* 1988;**32**:313–34).

Buspirone + fluvoxamine
See buspirone (4.1.2).

Caffeine + fluvoxamine *
Even low-dose fluvoxamine (10–20 mg/d) inhibits the metabolism of caffeine, presumably via 1A2 inhibition (n = 10, Christensen et al, *Clin Pharmacol Ther* 2002;**71**:141–52), and half-life may rise from five hours to 22 hours (Slaughter and Edwards,

Ann Pharmacother 1995;**29**:619–24). An enhanced effect is possible but one study indicated that the effect was likely to be minimal (n = 10, Spigset, *Eur J Clin Pharmacol* 1998;**54**:665–6). Caffeine decreases plasma levels of fluvoxamine but not its pharmacodynamic effects (n = 12, RCT, 11/7, d/b, p/c, c/o, Fukasawa et al, *Ther Drug Monit* 2006; **28**:308–11).

Carbamazepine + fluvoxamine
One small study showed fluvoxamine 100 mg/d to have no effect on carbamazepine levels (n = 15, RCT, Spina et al, *Ther Drug Monit* 1993;**15**:247–50), although several cases exist of fluvoxamine apparently increasing carbamazepine levels and toxicity (eg. Martinelli et al, *Br J Clin Pharmacol* 1993;**36**:615–6).

Ciclosporin + fluvoxamine
There is a case report of ciclosporin levels elevated by the introduction of fluvoxamine to a ciclosporin-treated allograft recipient, probably via CYP3A4 inhibition. Intensive monitoring of the serum creatinine and ciclosporin level was recommended, along with appropriate dose reductions (Vella and Sayegh, *Am J Kidney Dis* 1998;**31**:320–3).

Chloral + fluvoxamine
Lack of interaction has been reported (Wagner et al, *Adv Pharmacother* 1986;**2**:34–56).

CLOZAPINE + FLUVOXAMINE
See clozapine (4.2.3).

Digoxin + fluvoxamine *
See digoxin + fluoxetine (4.3.2.2).

Donepezil + fluvoxamine
See SSRIs + donepezil (4.6.3.1).

DULOXETINE + FLUVOXAMINE
See duloxetine (4.3.3.1).

Enoxacin + fluvoxamine *
Enoxacin appears to increase the sleepiness caused by fluvoxamine (n = 10, RCT, d/b, c/o, 11/7, Kunii et al, *Ther Drug Monit* 2005;**27**:349–53).

Glimepiride + fluvoxamine
Fluvoxamine may produce a modest increase in glimepiride plasma concentrations (n = 12, RCT, d/b, c/o, 4/7, Niemi et al, *Clin Pharmacol Ther* 2001;**69**:194–200).

Lansoprazole + fluvoxamine *
Fluvoxamine increases lansoprazole levels 2–3-fold in extensive (but not poor) metabolisers, probably by 2C19 inhibition (n = 18, RCT, p/c, Yasui-Furukori et al, *J Clin Pharmacol* 2004;**44**:1223–9; n = 18, Muira et al, *Br J Clin*

Pharmacol 2005;**60**:61–8).

Lidocaine + fluvoxamine *

Lidocaine metabolism is reduced by fluvoxamine, leading to potential toxicity (n=8, RCT, d/b, p/c, c/o, Isohanni *et al, Basic Clin Pharmacol Toxicol* 2006;**99**:168–72), although the effect of the interaction lessens as liver function worsens (n= 30, RCT, d/b, c/o, Orlando *et al, Clin Pharmacol Ther* 2004;**75**:80–8).

Lithium + fluvoxamine *

Although lack of interaction has been reported (Hendrickx and Floris, *Curr Ther Res* 1991;**49**:106–10), case reports exist of serotonin syndrome (n=1, Ohman and Spigset, *Pharmacopsychiatry* 1993;**26**:263–4), irresistible somnolence (n=1, Evans and Marwick, *Br J Psychiatry* 1990;**156**:286) and diurnal somnolence (n=1, Marchesi *et al, Pharmacopsychiatry* 2005;**38**:145–6).

MAOIs + FLUVOXAMINE

See MAOIs (*4.3.4*).

Melatonin + fluvoxamine

Fluvoxamine 50 mg inhibits the metabolism of oral melatonin 5 mg, increasing plasma levels (n=5, open, Hartter *et al, Clin Pharmacol Ther* 2000;**67**:1–6), supported by a further case, where combining the treatments improved sleep (n=1, Grozinger *et al, Arch Gen Psychiatry* 2000; **57**:812–3).

Methadone + fluvoxamine

See methadone (*4.6.10*).

Metoclopramide + fluvoxamine

Acute dystonia has been associated with the combination (n=1, Palop *et al, Ann Pharmacother* 1999;**33**:382).

Mirtazapine + fluvoxamine

See mirtazapine (*4.3.3.3*).

Moclobemide + fluvoxamine

See SSRIs + moclobemide (*4.3.3.4*).

NICOUMALONE + FLUVOXAMINE

The anticoagulant effects may be enhanced by fluvoxamine.

NSAIDs + FLUVOXAMINE

See NSAIDs + fluoxetine (*4.3.2.2*).

Olanzapine + fluvoxamine

See olanzapine (*4.2.4*).

Oxycodone + fluvoxamine *

Serotonin syndrome has been reported with oxycodone 80 mg/d and fluvoxamine 200 mg/d (n=1, Karunatilake and Buckley, *Ann Pharmacother* 2006;**40**:155–7).

PHENYTOIN + FLUVOXAMINE

See phenytoin (*4.5.8*).

Pipamperone + fluvoxamine

ECG changes have occurred as a result of acute overdose with this combination (Gallerani *et al, Clin Drug Invest* 1998;**15**:64–8).

Quinidine + fluvoxamine

Fluvoxamine significantly inhibits the clearance of quinidine, probably by 3A4 inhibition (n=6, open, Damkier *et al, Eur J Clin Pharmacol* 1999;**55**:451–6).

Reboxetine + fluvoxamine

See reboxetine (*4.3.3.5*).

Risperidone + fluvoxamine

See risperidone (*4.2.6*).

Rosiglitazone + fluvoxamine*

There appears no significant interaction, although rosiglitazone levels may rise in some people (n=23, open, c/o, Pedersen *et al, Br J Clin Pharmacol* 2006;**62**:682–9).

Sildenafil + fluvoxamine *

Fluvoxamine increases sildenafil AUC by 40% and half-life by 19%, probably via CYP3A4 inhibition (n=12, Hesse *et al, J Clin Psychopharmacol* 2005; **25**:589–92).

Smoking + fluvoxamine

See smoking (*4.7.4*).

St John's wort + fluvoxamine

See SSRIs + St John's wort (*4.3.3.9*).

Sympathomimetics + fluvoxamine

Augmentation of amfetamines is theoretically possible (see also fluoxetine, *4.3.2.2*).

Tacrine + fluvoxamine

Fluvoxamine is a potent inhibitor of tacrine metabolism *in vivo* (n=18, RCT, open, Teilmann-Larsen *et al, Eur J Clin Pharmacol* 1999;**55**:375–82).

THEOPHYLLINE + FLUVOXAMINE

Several cases of theophylline toxicity have been reported (eg. Devane *et al, Am J Psychiatry* 1997;**154**:1317–18), probably via CYP1A2 inhibition. The literature recommends avoiding the combination (*Curr Prob* 1994;**20**:12).

TIZANIDINE + FLUVOXAMINE

Fluvoxamine increases tizanidine's AUC 33-fold and peak levels 12-fold, a dramatic and important interaction (n=10, RCT, d/b, c/o, 4/7, Granfors *et al, Clin Pharmacol Ther* 2004;**75**:331–41).

Tolbutamide + fluvoxamine

Fluvoxamine 150 mg/d may increase tolbutamide levels by about 20% (n=14, RCT, Madsen *et al, Clin Pharmacol Ther* 2001;**69**:41–7).

TRICYCLICS + FLUVOXAMINE

See SSRIs + tricyclics (*4.3.1*).

Triptans + fluvoxamine

The literature notes an increased risk of CNS toxicity with sumatriptan and recommends avoiding the combination. See also fluoxetine (4.3.2.2).

Tryptophan + fluvoxamine

Central toxicity has been suggested with fluvoxamine (n=5, Steiner and Fontaine, *Biol Psychiatry* 1986;**21**:1067–71).

Valproate + fluvoxamine

Augmentation of fluvoxamine has been seen with valproate (Corrigan, *Biol Psychiatry* 1992;**31**:1178–9).

WARFARIN + FLUVOXAMINE

An *in vitro* study indicated fluvoxamine has the most potent effect on warfarin of the SSRIs (Schmider *et al*, *Br J Clin Pharmacol* 1997;**44**:495–8). Fluvoxamine can increase warfarin levels by up to 65%, increasing prothrombin time (Benfield and Ward, *Drugs* 1986;**32**:313–34; n=1, Limke *et al*, *Ann Pharmacother* 2002;**36**:1890–2), and elevated INR has occurred up to two weeks after fluvoxamine was stopped, a prolonged effect (n=1, Yap and Low, *Singapore Med J* 1999; **40**:480–2).

Zolpidem + fluvoxamine

See zolpidem (4.1.5).

Zotepine + fluvoxamine

See SSRIs + zotepine (4.2.9).

4.3.2.4 PAROXETINE

Paroxetine is probably the most potent SSRI inhibitor of CYP2D6 but does not appear to inhibit any other P450 enzyme. It may thus have a higher incidence of interactions with drugs metabolised by this enzyme. The main metabolite has approximately one third the CYP2D6 inhibition potency of paroxetine.

Alcohol + paroxetine

See alcohol (4.7.1).

Anticholinergics + paroxetine

See SSRIs + anticholinergics (4.6.2).

Antipsychotics + paroxetine (see also clozapine)

Lack of interaction between haloperidol and paroxetine has been shown (Cooper *et al*, *Acta Psychiatr Scand* 1989;**80**[Suppl 350]:53–5). Paroxetine (three-day course) had no detectable effect on thiothixene (a thioxanthene) pharmacokinetics in a small study (n=10, Guthrie *et al*, *J Clin Pharm Ther* 1997;**22**:221–6).

Atomoxetine + paroxetine

See SSRIs + atomoxetine (4.6.4).

Benzodiazepines + paroxetine *

Lack of interaction has been shown (Boyer and Blumhardt, *J Clin Psychiatry* 1992;**53**[Suppl 2]:132–24), eg. with oxazepam (Cooper *et al*, *Acta Psychiatr Scand* 1989;**80**[Suppl 350]: 53–5) and alprazolam (n=25, d/b, p/c, c/o, 4×15/7, Calvo *et al*, *J Clin Psychopharmacol* 2004; **24**:268–76), but NMS has been reported with paroxetine 20mg/d and alprazolam 1.2mg/d (n=1, Naranjo=6, *Prog Neuropsychopharmacol Biol Psychiatry* 2006;**30**:1176–8). Serotonin syndrome has been reported in a person taking maintenance paroxetine after a single dose clonazepam (Rella and Hoffman, *J Toxicol Clin Toxicol* 1998;**36**:257–8).

Beta-blockers + paroxetine

CYP2D6 inhibition by paroxetine 20mg/d leads to an accumulation of S-metoprolol, and so reduced metoprolol levels might be needed (n=8, open, Hemeryck *et al*, *Clin Pharmacol Ther* 2000;**67**:283–91). Raised paroxetine levels after the addition of pindolol has been reported, probably via 2D6 inhibition (n=1, Olver and Burrows, *Int J Psych Clin Pract* 1998;**2**:225–7).

Bupropion + paroxetine

See bupropion (4.6.6).

Carbamazepine + paroxetine

Lack of significant interaction has been shown (n=20, s/b, p/c, c/o, 23/7, Andersen *et al*, *Epilepsy Res* 1991;**10**:201–4), although hyponatraemia has been reported (n=1, Sempere I Verdu *et al*, *Aten Primaria* 2004;**33**:473–4).

Cimetidine + paroxetine

Cimetidine may inhibit the first-pass metabolism of paroxetine, increasing bioavailability by up to 50% (Bannister *et al*, *Acta Psychiatr Scand* 1989; **80**[Suppl 350]:102–6), so use ranitidine instead.

CLOZAPINE + PAROXETINE *

See clozapine (4.2.3).

Dextromethorphan + paroxetine

Paroxetine would be expected to increase dextromethorphan levels by CYP2D6 inhibition (see reported case with fluoxetine, 4.3.2.2).

Digitalis + paroxetine *

Paroxetine has been reported to cause digitalis intoxication (n=1, Yasui-Furukori and Kaneko, *Lancet* 2006;**367**:788).

Digoxin + paroxetine *

See digoxin + fluoxetine (4.3.2.2).

Donepezil + paroxetine

See SSRIs + donepezil (4.6.3.1).

Duloxetine + paroxetine

See SSRIs + duloxetine (4.3.3.1).

Galantamine + paroxetine

See galantamine (4.6.3.2).

Interferon alpha + paroxetine

A previous good response to paroxetine and trazodone was reversed by interferon alpha, which has anti-serotonergic actions (n = 1, McAllister-Williams et al, Br J Psychiatry 2000;**176**:93).

Lithium + paroxetine

There are some cases (n = 4) of a possible serotonin syndrome (n = 17, Fagiolini et al, J Clin Psychopharmacol 2001;**21**:474–8).

Methadone + paroxetine

Steady-state plasma methadone levels may rise with paroxetine, but only in poor 2D6 metabolisers (n = 10, 12/7, Begre et al, J Clin Psychopharmacol 2002;**22**:211–5).

Mirtazapine + paroxetine

See mirtazapine (4.3.3.3).

Moclobemide + paroxetine

See SSRIs + moclobemide (4.3.3.4).

MAOIs + PAROXETINE

See MAOIs (4.3.4).

NSAIDs + SSRIs

See NSAIDs + fluoxetine (4.3.2.2).

Oral contraceptives + paroxetine

Lack of interaction has been shown (Boyer and Blumhardt, J Clin Psychiatry 1992;**53**[Suppl 2]: 132–4).

Phenytoin + paroxetine

Paroxetine bioavailability may be decreased slightly (Andersen et al, Epilepsy Res 1991: **10**:201–4).

Phenobarbital + paroxetine

Paroxetine bioavailability may be decreased slightly, resulting in a 25% decrease in plasma concentrations (Bannister et al, Acta Psychiatr Scand 1989;**80**[Suppl 350]:102–6). No interaction occurs with amylobarbital (Cooper et al, Acta Psychiatr Scand 1989;**80**[Suppl 350]:53–5).

Risperidone + paroxetine

See risperidone (4.2.6).

SERTINDOLE + PAROXETINE

See sertindole (4.2.7).

St John's wort + paroxetine

See SSRIs + St John's wort (4.3.3.10).

Sympathomimetics + paroxetine

Augmentation of amfetamines is theoretically possible (see sympathomimetics + fluoxetine 4.3.2.2).

TRICYCLICS + PAROXETINE

See SSRIs + tricyclics (4.3.1).

Triptans + paroxetine

The literature notes an increased risk of CNS toxicity and recommends avoiding sumatriptan and paroxetine, although almost complete lack of interaction has been shown with rizatriptan and paroxetine (n = 12, RCT, 14/7, Goldberg et al, J Clin Pharmacol 1999;**39**:192–9). See also fluoxetine (4.3.2.2).

Valproate + paroxetine

No significant interaction occurs (n = 20, s/b, p/c, c/o, 23/7, Andersen et al, Epilepsy Res 1991; **10**:201–4).

Warfarin + paroxetine

An in vitro study indicated that all SSRIs have an effect on warfarin (Schmider et al, Br J Clin Pharmacol 1997;**44**:495–8), eg. up to a three-point rise in INR has been reported in several patients (mentioned by Askinazi, Am J Psychiatry 1996;**153**:135–6).

Zolpidem + paroxetine

See SSRIs + zolpidem (4.1.5).

Zotepine + paroxetine

See SSRIs + zotepine (4.2.9).

4.3.2.5 SERTRALINE *

Sertraline produces a dose-related inhibition of CYP2D6 but has little, if any, effect on CYP1A2, 2C9/10, 2C19 or 3A3/4. It appears a less potent inhibitor of CYP2D6 than most other SSRIs (Baettig et al, Eur J Clin Pharmacol 1993;**44**:403–5) and has, at 50–100 mg/d, a low incidence of interactions with drugs metabolised by 2D6. It is metabolised by a wide range of P450 enzymes, plus monoamine oxidase and UGT2B7 (Obach et al, Drug Metab Disp 2005;**33**:262–70).

Alcohol + sertraline

See alcohol (4.7.1).

Anticholinergics + sertraline

See SSRIs + anticholinergics (4.6.2).

Atomoxetine + sertraline

See SSRIs + atomoxetine (4.6.4).

Benzodiazepines + sertraline

A study in male volunteers showed no effect of sertraline on diazepam and suggested no effect on the CYP2C and CYP3A4 enzymes (n = 20, RCT, d/b, p/c, c/o, Gardner et al, Clin

Pharmacokinetics 1997; **31**[Suppl 1]:43–9), but a slight decrease in plasma levels by 13% may occur (review: Warrington, *Int Clin Psychopharmacol* 1991;**6**[Suppl 2]:11–21).

Beta-blockers + sertraline

No pharmacodynamic interaction has been found with atenolol (eg. n = 10, RCT, Ziegler and Wilner, *J Clin Psychiatry* 1996;**57**[Suppl 1]:12–15).

Bupropion + sertraline *

See bupropion (4.6.6).

Carbamazepine + sertraline

Lack of significant interaction has been reported, but there are cases where sertraline 100 mg/d increased carbamazepine (600 mg/d) plasma levels, probably via 3A4 inhibition (d/b, p/c, Joblin, *N Z Med J* 1994;**107**:43; Lane, *N Z Med J* 1994; **107**:209). Non-response to sertraline has been due to low plasma levels associated with carbamazepine use, possibly via CYP3A4 induction (n = 2, Khan et al, *J Clin Psychiatry* 2000; **61**:526–7).

Clozapine + sertraline

See clozapine (4.2.3).

Digoxin + sertraline *

See digoxin + fluoxetine (4.3.2.2).

Dolasetron + sertraline

A serotonin syndrome has been reported with the combination (n = 1, Sorscher, *J Psychopharmacol* 2002;**16**:191).

Donepezil + sertraline

See SSRIs + donepezil (4.6.3.1).

Duloxetine + sertraline

See SSRIs + duloxetine (4.3.3.1).

Erythromycin + sertraline

Serotonin syndrome has been reported with the combination, possibly via CYP3A4 inhibition (n = 1, Lee and Lee, *Pharmacother* 1999;**19**:894–6).

Fluoxetine + sertraline

A possible serotonin syndrome has been reported (see switching antidepressants, 2.2.5).

Lamotrigine + sertraline

See lamotrigine (4.5.4).

Linezolid + sertraline *

A single case of serotonin syndrome has been reported (n = 1, Clark et al, *Pharmacotherapy* 2006;**26**:269–76).

Lithium + sertraline

See SSRIs + lithium (4.4).

MAOIs + SERTRALINE

See MAOIs (4.3.4).

Mirtazapine + sertraline

See SSRIs + mirtazapine (4.3.3.3).

Moclobemide + sertraline

See SSRIs + moclobemide (4.3.3.4).

NSAIDs + SSRIs

See NSAIDs + fluoxetine (4.3.2.2).

Olanzapine + sertraline

See SSRIs + olanzapine (4.2.4).

Oxycodone + sertraline

Visual hallucinations and tremor induced by sertraline and oxycodone in a bone marrow transplant patient have been reported (n = 1, Rosebraugh et al, *J Clin Pharmacol* 2001;**41**:224).

Phenytoin + sertraline

Lack of significant interaction has been shown (n = 30, RCT, Rapeport et al, *J Clin Psychiatry* 1996;**57**[Suppl 1]:24–8), but dramatically raised phenytoin levels have been reported after the addition of sertraline (n = 2, Haselberger et al, *J Clin Psychopharmacol* 1997;**17**:107–9), as has a significant reduction in sertraline levels by phenytoin (Pihlsgard and Eliasson, *Eur J Clin Pharmacol* 2002;**57**:915–6). Monitoring levels would seem sensible.

Pimozide + sertraline

The use of sertraline with pimozide is not advised since increased pimozide levels have been shown.

Risperidone + sertraline

See risperidone (4.2.6).

Sertindole + sertraline

See sertindole (4.2.7).

St John's wort + sertraline

See SSRIs + St John's wort (4.3.3.10).

Sumatriptan + sertraline

The literature notes an increased risk of CNS toxicity and recommends avoiding the combination. See also fluoxetine (4.3.2.2).

Sympathomimetics + sertraline

Augmentation of amfetamines is theoretically possible (see sympathomimetics + fluoxetine, 4.3.2.2).

Tolbutamide + sertraline

In a parallel-group study, 200 mg/d sertraline produced a 16% decrease in tolbutamide clearance, possibly via inhibition of CYP2C9 (n = 25, RCT, Tremaine et al, *Clin Pharmacokinet* 1997; **31** [Suppl 1]:31–6; n = 25, RCT, Warrington, *Int Clin Psychopharmacol* 1991;**6**[Suppl 2]:11–21).

Tramadol + sertraline

Serotonin syndrome has been reported when a tramadol dose was increased with concomitant sertraline (n=1, Mason and Blackburn, *Ann Pharmacother* 1997;**31**:175–7).

Tricyclics + sertraline
See SSRIs + tricyclics (*4.3.1*).

Venlafaxine + sertraline
Acute liver damage possibly related to sertraline and venlafaxine ingestion has been reported (Kim et al, *Ann Pharmacother* 1999;**33**:381–2, letter).

Warfarin + sertraline
An *in vitro* study indicated that, of the SSRIs, sertraline had the least potent effect on warfarin (Schmider et al, *Br J Clin Pharmacol* 1997;**44**:495–8). It may produce only a modest increase in prothrombin time, considered clinically insignificant (n=12, RCT, 22/7, Apseloff et al, *Clin Pharmacokinet* 1997;**32**[Suppl 1]:37–42). However, prothrombin time can be increased by 9% (Wilner et al, *Biol Psychiatry* 1991;**29**:354S–355S) and up to a three-point rise in INR has been reported in several patients (mentioned by Askinazi, *Am J Psychiatry* 1996;**153**:135–6).

Zolpidem + sertraline
See SSRIs + zolpidem (*4.1.5*).

Zotepine + sertraline
See zotepine (*4.2.9*).

4.3.3 OTHER ANTIDEPRESSANTS

4.3.3.1 DULOXETINE *
Duloxetine is metabolised by 1A2 (but probably does not inhibit it) and 2D6, is a minor inhibitor of 2D6 but has no effect on 3A4. Data on interactions is limited but caution is recommended with sedative drugs, eg. alcohol, benzodiazepines, antipsychotics and sedative antihistamines. Elimination is primarily via urine, after extensive metabolism by multiple oxidative pathways, methylation and conjugation (review of kinetics, Wernicke et al, *Expert Opin Drug Saf* 2005;**4**:987–93).

Antacids + duloxetine
Lack of interaction has been shown with a single 40 mg dose of duloxetine (UK SPC).

CIPROFLOXACIN + DULOXETINE
This combination is a UK SPC contraindication due to the potential for raised duloxetine levels from 1A2 inhibition by ciprofloxacin (UK SPC).

ENOXACINE + DULOXETINE
This combination is a UK SPC contraindication due to the potential for raised duloxetine levels from 1A2 inhibition by enoxacine (UK SPC).

FLUVOXAMINE + DULOXETINE
Fluvoxamine may decrease duloxetine's clearance by 77% and increase AUC six-fold, and this combination is a UK SPC contraindication because of the potential for raised duloxetine levels.

H2-blockers + duloxetine
Lack of interaction has been shown with a single 40 mg dose of duloxetine (UK SPC).

MAOIs + DULOXETINE
This combination is a UK SPC contraindication, due to the risk of serotonin syndrome. Do not use duloxetine within 14 days of stopping an MAOI, or use an MAOI until five days after stopping duloxetine.

Moclobemide + duloxetine
The UK SPC recommends caution when duloxetine is used with moclobemide, due to the risk of serotonin syndrome.

Oral contraceptives + duloxetine
There is no reason to suspect an interaction would occur, but there are no formal studies.

Pethidine + duloxetine
Due to the risk of serotonin syndrome, duloxetine should only be used with care with pethidine.

SMOKING + DULOXETINE
Smokers may have duloxetine plasma levels 50% lower than non-smokers (UK SPC).

SSRIs + duloxetine
Due to the risk of serotonin syndrome, duloxetine should only be used with care with SSRIs (see also fluvoxamine, where the risk is higher).

St John's wort + duloxetine
The UK SPC recommends caution when duloxetine is used with St John's wort.

Theophylline + duloxetine
Duloxetine had no effect on theophylline in a study in male patients (UK SPC).

Tolterodine + duloxetine *
There is no significant interaction between tolterodine and duloxetine (n=16, RCT, d/b, c/o, 2×5/7, Hua et al, *Br J Clin Pharmacol* 2004;**57**:652–6).

Tramadol + duloxetine
Due to the risk of serotonin syndrome, duloxetine should only be used with care with tramadol.

Tricyclics + duloxetine
Due to the risk of serotonin syndrome, duloxetine should only be used with care with tricyclics.

Triptans + duloxetine
Due to the risk of serotonin syndrome, duloxetine should only be used with care with triptans.

Tryptophan + duloxetine
Due to the risk of serotonin syndrome, duloxetine should only be used with care with tryptophan.

Venlafaxine + duloxetine
Due to the risk of serotonin syndrome, duloxetine should only be used with care with venlafaxine.

Warfarin + duloxetine *
There are cases of duloxetine causing severe elevation of INR when combined with warfarin (n = 3, Glueck et al, JAMA 2006;**295**:1517–8).

4.3.3.2 MIANSERIN
ALCOHOL + MIANSERIN
See alcohol (4.7.1).

Benzodiazepines + mianserin
Enhanced sedation may occur.

Carbamazepine + mianserin
Plasma levels of mianserin and enantiomers may be halved by carbamazepine, probably via 3A4 induction (n = 12, Eap et al, Ther Drug Monit 1999;**21**:166–70).

Warfarin + mianserin
There is normally no problem but occasional control difficulties have been reported (Warwick and Mindham, Br J Psychiatry 1983;**143**:308).

4.3.3.3 MIRTAZAPINE
Mirtazapine does not inhibit CYP2D6, 1A2 and 3A and so interactions via these enzymes are unlikely. Mirtazapine is mainly metabolised by CYP2D6 and 1A2 (Montgomery, Int Clin Psychopharmacol 1995;**10**[Suppl 4]:37–45) and if one enzyme is inhibited, the other takes over, so mirtazapine appears less susceptible to P450 interactions. It has linear kinetics from 15–75 mg/d, with 100% excreted via the urine and faeces.
Review: Clinical pharmacokinetics (Timmer et al, Clin Pharmacokinet 2000;**38**:461–74).

Alcohol + mirtazapine
See alcohol (4.7.1).

Atomoxetine + mirtazapine
See atomoxetine (4.6.4).

Benzodiazepines + mirtazapine
The combination of diazepam and mirtazapine, not surprisingly, produces an additive sedative effect (n = 12, RCT, d/b, c/o, Mattila et al, Pharmacol Toxicol 1989;**65**:81–8) and so anyone on the combination should be warned about driving and other activities.

Carbamazepine + mirtazapine
Mirtazapine does not significantly effect carba-

mazepine levels but carbamazepine produces a 60% decrease in mirtazapine levels, probably by CYP3A4 induction, and mirtazapine doses may need to be increased (RCT, 4/52, Sitsen et al, Eur J Drug Metab Pharmacokinet 2001;**26**:109–21).

Cimetidine + mirtazapine
Mirtazapine has no effect on cimetidine but mirtazapine levels may be higher (probably by CYP3A4 inhibition by cimetidine), but not enough to require dose reduction (n = 12, d/b, p/c, c/o, Sitsen et al, Eur J Clin Pharmacol 2000; **56**:389–94).

Clozapine + mirtazapine
Lack of significant interaction has been shown (n = 9, 6/52, Zoccali et al, Pharmacol Res 2003; **48**:411–4).

Fluoxetine + mirtazapine
Fluoxetine 20–40 mg/d caused a clinically in-significant 32% increase in mirtazapine (15 mg/d) plasma levels after an abrupt switch (n = 40, Preskorn et al, Biol Psychiatry 1997;**41**:96S), although mania associated with mirtazapine augmentation of fluoxetine has been reported (n = 1, Ng, Depress Anxiety 2002;**15**:46–7).

Fluvoxamine + mirtazapine
Fluvoxamine 50–100 mg/d may increase mirta-zapine serum levels 3–4-fold, a significant effect (n = 2, Anttila et al, Ann Pharmacother 2001;**35**:1221–3) and a serotonin syndrome has been reported with the combination (n = 1, Demers and Malone, Ann Pharmacother 2001;**35**:1217–20).

Levodopa + mirtazapine
Psychosis has been reported when mirtazapine was added to a stable levodopa regimen (n = 1, Normann et al, Pharmacopsychiatry 1997;**30**:263–5).

Lithium + mirtazapine
No pharmacokinetic interaction has been detected between lithium 600 mg/d and mirtazapine 30 mg (n = 12, 10/7, Sitsen et al, J Clin Psychopharmacol 2000;**14**:172–6).

MAOIs + mirtazapine
The manufacturers cautiously recommend a two-week gap between stopping an MAOI and starting mirtazapine.

Olanzapine + mirtazapine
Lack of significant interaction has been shown (n = 7, 6/52, Zoccali et al, Pharmacol Res 2003; **48**:411–4).

Paroxetine + mirtazapine

Mirtazapine had no effect on the kinetics of paroxetine and the combination was better tolerated than either alone, suggesting a lack of clinically relevant interaction (n = 24, RCT, c/o, 6/7 per arm, Ruwe et al, Hum Psychopharmacol 2001;16:449–59).

Phenytoin + mirtazapine

A multiple dose study showed that mirtazapine had no effect on the steady-state kinetics of phenytoin, but that phenytoin reduced mirtazapine levels by a mean of 46%, probably clinically significant (n = 17, RCT, open, Spaans et al, Eur J Clin Pharmacol 2002;58:423–9).

Risperidone + mirtazapine

Mirtazapine 30 mg/d had no effect on risperidone 2–6 mg/d in one trial (n = 6, open, 8/52, Loonen et al, Eur Neuropsychopharmacol 1999;10:51–7) and lack of significant interaction has been shown (n = 8, 6/52, Zoccali et al, Pharmacol Res 2003;48:411–4).

Sertraline + mirtazapine

Hypomania has been reported when mirtazapine 15 mg/d was used as augmentation of sertraline 250 mg/d, which had been only partially effective (n = 1, Soutullo et al, J Clin Psychiatry 1998;59:320).

Tricyclics + mirtazapine

Amitriptyline causes clinically insignificant increases in mirtazapine plasma levels and vice versa (n = 24, Sennef et al, Hum Psychopharmacol 2003;38:91–101).

Venlafaxine + mirtazapine

Serotonin syndrome has been reported during a cross-over (n = 1, Dimellis, World J Biol Psychiatry 2002;3:167), and when both were also combined with tramadol (n = 1, Houlihan, Ann Pharmacother 2004;38:411–3). See also 1.14 for rational use of this combination.

Warfarin + mirtazapine

No interaction is known or suspected, but there is insufficient information to confirm this at present (Sayal et al, Acta Psychiatr Scand 2000;102:250–5).

4.3.3.4 MOCLOBEMIDE

Moclobemide is metabolised by CYP2C19, and inhibits 2D6, 2C19 and 1A2.

Review: general (Berlin and Lecrubier, CNS Drugs 1996;5:403–13).

Alcohol + moclobemide

See alcohol (4.7.1).

Benzodiazepines + moclobemide

No significant interaction occurs (Zimmer et al, Acta Psychiatr Scand 1990;360:84–6).

Bupropion + moclobemide

See MAOIs + bupropion (4.6.6).

CIMETIDINE + MOCLOBEMIDE

Cimetidine may reduce the clearance and prolong the half-life of moclobemide, so start with lower doses and monitor closely (n = 8, open, Schoerlin et al, Clin Pharmacol Ther 1991;49:32–8)

Digoxin + moclobemide

Lack of interaction has been reported (Berlin and Lecrubier, CNS Drugs 1996;5:403–13).

Duloxetine + moclobemide

See duloxetine (4.3.3.1).

Ecstasy/MDMA + moclobemide

Deaths have been reported, with the victims apparently taking moclobemide in an attempt to enhance the effects of MDMA (n = 4, Vuori et al, Addiction 2003;98:365–8).

Ibuprofen + moclobemide

Moclobemide is alleged to potentiate the effect of ibuprofen, but lack of interaction has been reported (Berlin and Lecrubier, CNS Drugs 1996;5:403–13).

Metoprolol + moclobemide

Concurrent metoprolol and moclobemide results in further lowering of blood pressure, although postural hypotension was not reported (Zimmer et al, Acta Psychiatr Scand 1990;360:84–6).

Nifedipine + moclobemide

No significant interaction occurs, apart from some slight reduction in blood pressure (Zimmer et al, Acta Psychiatr Scand 1990;360:84–6).

Opiates + moclobemide

Moclobemide is alleged to potentiate the effect of opiates, and dose reductions of morphine and fentanyl may be considered necessary.

Oral contraceptives + moclobemide

No significant interaction has been detected (Zimmer et al, Acta Psychiatr Scand 1990;360:84–6).

SELEGILINE + MOCLOBEMIDE

Selegiline is an MAO-B inhibitor and if combined with an MAO-A inhibitor, such as moclobemide, could produce full MAO inhibition (albeit reversible). The combination is not recommended but, if the two need to be used together, then full MAOI dietary precautions might be required.

SSRIs + moclobemide

A fatal serotonin syndrome has been reported with moclobemide and **citalopram** (n = 1, Dams et al, J Anal Toxicol 2001;**25**:147–51) and disputed (Isbister et al, J Anal Toxicol 2001;**25**:716–7). Excitation, insomnia and dysphoria have been reported with **fluvoxamine** and moclobemide in refractory depression (n = 36, open, 6/52, Ebert, Psychopharmacology 1995;**119**:342–4), as have headaches and fatigue (review, Dingemanse, Int Clin Psychopharmacol 1993;**7**:167–80). In a study where up to 600 mg/d moclobemide was added to established **fluoxetine** therapy, there was no change in the number, intensity or type of adverse events. Fluoxetine markedly inhibited the metabolism of moclobemide but did not lead to excessive accumulation or any indication of development of a serotonin syndrome (n = 18, RCT, open, Dingemanse et al, Clin Pharmacol Ther 1998;**63**:403–13). A serotonin syndrome would also be a possibility with the combination and the UK SPC for moclobemide contraindicates the combination. A fatal case, following overdose of **paroxetine** and moclobemide and subsequent serotonin syndrome, has been reported (Singer and Jones, J Anal Toxicol 1997;**21**:518–20). A case of serotonin syndrome has been reported with **sertraline** and metoclopramide (n = 1, Ann Pharmacother 2002;**36**:67–71).

Sympathomimetics + moclobemide

The UK SPC recommends avoiding this combination. Phenylephrine may slightly raise blood pressure in people taking high dose (600 mg/d) moclobemide (Amrein et al, Psychopharmacology 1992;**106**:S24–S31) but ephedrine produces a greater rise in bp (Dingemanse, Int Clin Psychopharmacol 1993;**7**:167–80). Another study noted no clinically significant interaction, although the pressor effect may be slightly enhanced (review: Zimmer et al, Acta Psychiatr Scand 1990; **360**:84–6).

Tricyclics + moclobemide

A rapid and fatal serotonin syndrome has been caused by moclobemide-clomipramine overdose (n = 1, Ferrer-Dufol et al, J Toxicol Clin Toxicol 1998;**36**:31–2).

Triptans + moclobemide

The literature notes an increased risk of CNS toxicity with sumatriptan or zolmitriptan and moclobemide (review by Rolan, Cephalalgia 1997;**17**[Suppl 18]:21–7; Morales Asin, Neuro-

logia 1998;**13**[Suppl 2]:25–30), and that lower doses should be used, although a small study suggested combined use with sumatriptan was safe with care (n = 14, open, Blier and Bergeron, J Clin Psychopharmacol 1995;**15**:106–9). Moclobemide may significantly potentiate the effects of rizatriptan and the combination is not recommended (n = 12, RCT, Van Haarst et al, Br J Clin Pharmacol 1999;**48**:190–6). Moclobemide increases the plasma concentration of almotriptan but the combination appears well-tolerated (n = 12, RCT, open, c/o, Fleishaker et al, Br J Clin Pharmacol 2001;**51**:437–41) and it may be the triptan of choice. Well, it does the trick for me.

Tyramine + moclobemide

Moclobemide does not appear significantly to potentiate the pressor effects of tyramine. Dietary restrictions are generally not required, but patients should avoid eating excessive amounts of tyramine-containing foods, especially if they have pre-existing hypertension. Minor pressor effects are not seen until about 100 mg tyramine (Zimmer et al, Acta Psychiatr Scand 1990;**360**:84–6). Even 150 mg tyramine is suggested by some as being safe (Acta Psychiatr Scand 1990;**360**[Suppl]:78–80). The use of this combination has, however, been used to treat severe postural hypotension (eg. n = 1, Karet et al, Lancet 1994;**344**:1263–5) and in counteracting clozapine-induced hypotension, allowing dose increases to an active therapeutic level (n = 1, Taylor et al, Br J Psychiatry 1995;**167**:409–10).

Tricyclics + moclobemide

The UK SPC contraindicates the combination if the tricyclic (or metabolite) is a serotonin reuptake inhibitor, eg. clomipramine or imipramine. Serotonin syndrome has been reported with moclobemide and clomipramine, imipramine (Brodribb et al, Lancet 1994;**343**:475–6) or an SSRI (eg. Spigest et al, Br Med J 1993;**306**:248), and after moclobemide plus either citalopram or clomipramine overdoses (n = 5, fatal, Neuvonen et al, Lancet 1993;**342**:1419), where aggressive therapy may be needed. Lack of interaction has been noted with desipramine (review: Zimmer et al, Acta Psychiatr Scand 1990;**360**:84–6) and amitriptyline 150 mg/d (eg. n = 21, Amrein et al, Psychopharmacology 1992;**106**:S24–S31).

Venlafaxine + moclobemide

See venlafaxine (4.3.3.8).

Warfarin + moclobemide

No interaction has been reported, but moclobemide inhibits CYP1A2 and 2C19 and so the potential for warfarin potentiation exists (Sayal et al, Acta Psychiatr Scand 2000;**102**:250–5).

4.3.3.5 REBOXETINE

Reboxetine is extensively (97%) bound to plasma proteins (particularly the alpha-1 acid glycoprotein fraction) and may interact with drugs with a high affinity for this fraction, eg. dipyridamole, propranolol, methadone, imipramine, chlorpromazine (see antipsychotics below) and local anaesthetics. Concomitant tricyclics, SSRIs, MAOIs and lithium have not been assessed. The UK SPC states that in high doses reboxetine inhibits CYP3A4 and 2D6 in vitro and is metabolised by 3A4, but there is a wide safety margin.

Alcohol + reboxetine

See alcohol (4.7.1).

Antipsychotics + reboxetine

An interaction is possible (see above). Reboxetine has no effect on clozapine or risperidone plasma levels (n = 7, Spina et al, Ther Drug Monit 2001;**23**:675–8).

Benzodiazepines + reboxetine

Lack of interaction has been reported, although some mild-to-moderate drowsiness and transient increases in heart rate have been noted.

Dipyridamole + reboxetine

An interaction is possible (see above).

Disopyramide + reboxetine

The literature advises caution with combination.

Diuretics + reboxetine

There may be an increased risk of hypokalaemia with loop diuretics or thiazides (BNF).

Erythromycin + reboxetine

The literature advises caution with combination.

Flecainide + reboxetine

The literature advises caution with combination.

Fluoxetine + reboxetine

There are no statistically significant effects of reboxetine on fluoxetine or norfluoxetine pharmacokinetics, and a minimal clinical impact is suggested (n = 30, RCT, d/b, p/c, 8/7, Fleishaker et al, Clin Drug Investigat 1999;**18**:141–50), although urinary retention has been reported with the combination (n = 1, Benazzi, Can J Psychiatry 2000;**45**:936).

Fluvoxamine + reboxetine

The literature advises caution with combination.

Ketoconazole + reboxetine

Ketoconazole decreases the clearance of the two enantiomers of reboxetine, with no adverse effects, but some caution may be advisable (n = 11, open, Herman et al, Clin Pharmacol Therapeut 1999;**66**:374–9)

Lidocaine + reboxetine

An interaction is possible (see introduction to 4.3.3.4), and with other local anaesthetics. The literature advises caution with the combination.

MAOIs + reboxetine

This has not been evaluated so avoid until further notice, and leave a two-week gap after an MAOI and one week after reboxetine before switching to the other.

Methadone + reboxetine

An interaction is possible (see introduction to 4.3.3.4).

Potassium-losing diuretics + reboxetine

See diuretics (introduction to 4.3.3.4).

Propafenone + reboxetine

The literature advises caution with combination.

Propranolol + reboxetine

An interaction is possible (see introduction to 4.3.3.4).

Tricyclics + reboxetine

An interaction is possible (see introduction to 4.3.3.4).

Warfarin + reboxetine

No interaction is known or suspected, but there is insufficient information to confirm this at present (Sayal et al, Acta Psychiatr Scand 2000;**102**:250–5).

4.3.3.6 TRAZODONE

Trazodone is metabolised by CYP2D6 and inhibits 3A4.

ALCOHOL + TRAZODONE

See alcohol (4.7.1).

Antipsychotics + trazodone

Enhanced hypotension may occur when trazodone was added to either chlorpromazine or trifluoperazine (n = 2, Asayesh, Can J Psychiatry 1986;**31**:857–8). Thioridazine may raise trazodone levels by about 25% (n = 11, Yasui et al, Ther Drug Monit 1995;**17**:333–5).

Buspirone + trazodone

See buspirone (4.1.2).

Carbamazepine + trazodone
See carbamazepine (4.5.1).

Citalopram + trazodone
See citalopram (4.3.2.1).

Cocaine + trazodone
See antidepressants + cocaine (4.7.3).

Digoxin + trazodone
Cases of digoxin toxicity exist with trazodone (n = 2, Rauch and Jenike, *Psychosomatics* 1984; **25**: 334–5).

Fluoxetine + trazodone
See fluoxetine (4.3.2.2).

Gingko biloba + trazodone
Coma has been reported with concomitant use in an Alzheimer's patient (n = 1, Galluzzi et al, *J Neurol Neurosurg Psychiatry* 2000;**68**:679–80).

Interferon alpha + trazodone
See interferon alpha + paroxetine (4.3.2.4).

MAOIs + trazodone
See MAOIs (4.3.4).

Phenytoin + trazodone
See phenytoin (4.5.8).

Venlafaxine + trazodone
See venlafaxine (4.3.3.8).

Warfarin + trazodone
INR and PT fell when trazodone was added to warfarin, and rose when trazodone was stopped, and so caution is necessary (adjust doses and/or monitor) if trazodone is used, especially if used as a PRN hypnotic (eg, n = 1, Small and Giamonna, *Ann Pharmacother* 2000;**34**:734–6).

4.3.3.7 TRYPTOPHAN

Duloxetine + tryptophan
See duloxetine (4.3.3.1).

Fluoxetine + tryptophan
See fluoxetine (4.3.2.2).

Fluvoxamine + tryptophan
See fluvoxamine (4.3.2.3).

MAOIs + tryptophan
See MAOIs (4.3.4).

4.3.3.8 VENLAFAXINE *
Venlafaxine is metabolised by CYP2D6 to O-desmethylvenlafaxine, a major active metabolite and by CYP3A4 to N-desmethylvenlafaxine. Other, minor, metabolic pathways exist. Venlafaxine has a low potential for CYP2D6 and 3A4 inhibition (Ball et al, *Br J Clin Pharmacol* 1997;**43**:619–26) and does not appear to have a significant effect on other P450 enzymes.

In 2006, the UK MHRA revised their SPC guidance:
- Use of venlafaxine with potent CYP3A4 inhibitors (eg. ketoconazole, erythromycin) or combinations that inhibit both CYP3A4 and CYP2D6 should be avoided if possible.
- Bizarrely, the new advice also states that 'specialist supervision is recommended for use of concomitant SSRIs', although it is unclear if this is for the patient or the prescriber.

Alcohol + venlafaxine
See alcohol (4.7.1).

Antipsychotics + venlafaxine *
Urinary retention has been reported with **haloperidol** (Benazzi, *Pharmacopsychiatry* 1997; **30**:27) and the UK SPC notes that venlafaxine causes a 70% increase in haloperidol AUC and 88% increase in peak levels, so care is needed. Increased **clozapine** levels and adverse effects have also been reported, although one study showed that even moderate doses of venlafaxine had no significant effect on clozapine plasma levels (n = 11, Repo-Tiihonen et al, *Neuropsychobiol* 2005;**51**:173–6).

Atomoxetine + venlafaxine
See atomoxetine (4.6.4).

Benzodiazepines + venlafaxine
A study showed that diazepam 10mg had no significant effect on venlafaxine or metabolite kinetics, but venlafaxine slightly increased diazepam clearance. No clinically significant interaction thus seems likely (n = 17, Troy et al, *J Clin Pharmacol* 1995;**35**:410–9).

Bupropion + venlafaxine
See bupropion (4.6.6).

Carbamazepine + venlafaxine *
Carbamazepine 200–400mg does not appear to effect venlafaxine plasma levels (mean 200mg/d) and metabolite (n = 10, open, 8/52, Ciusani et al, *J Psychopharmacol* 2004;**18**:559–66).

Cimetidine + venlafaxine
A 45% reduction in venlafaxine clearance via reduced first-pass metabolism can result in increased venlafaxine levels and patients should be monitored for dose-related side-effects, eg. nausea and bp changes. The major metabolite, O-desmethylvenlafaxine, is unaffected.

Co-amoxiclav + venlafaxine
Serotonin syndrome has been reported after single doses of co-amoxiclav during

venlafaxine therapy (n = 1, Connor, *J R Soc Med* 2003;**96**:233–4).

Duloxetine + venlafaxine
See duloxetine (*4.3.3.1*).

Fluoxetine + venlafaxine
See fluoxetine (*4.3.2.2*).

Indinavir + venlafaxine
A study has shown that venlafaxine reduced indinavir's peak plasma levels by 36% and AUC by 28%, a potentially clinically significant effect (n = 9, Levin et al, *Psychopharmacol Bull* 2001;**35**:62–71).

Ketoconazole + venlafaxine *
Ketoconazole increases venlafaxine's AUC and Cmax by about 30% in CYP3A4 extensive metabolisers, but the effect appears erratic in poor metabolisers, variably increasing AUC (0–206%) and Cmax (0–119%), so it's a good job they're relatively rare (n = 21, open, Lindh et al, *Eur J Clin Pharmacol* 2003;**59**:401–6).

Linezolid + venlafaxine *
Serotonin syndrome has been reported with the combination (n = 1, Jones et al, *J Antimicrob Chemother* 2004;**54**:289–90; n = 1, Bergeron et al, *Ann Pharmacother* 2005;**39**:956–61).

Lithium + venlafaxine *
Venlafaxine has been shown to have no significant effect on lithium kinetics in a single dose study (open, Troy et al, *J Clin Pharmacol* 1996;**36**:175–81), but there are cases of raised lithium levels and of serotonin syndrome (eg. Mekler and Woggon, *Pharmacopsychiatry* 1997; **30**:272–3; n = 1, Naranjo = probable, *J Clin Pharm Ther* 2006;**31**:397–400). Lithium reduces the renal clearance of venlafaxine but without apparent clinical significance.

MAOIs + VENLAFAXINE
Wyeth state that venlafaxine and MAOIs should not be used together and recommend a 14-day gap after stopping an MAOI before starting venlafaxine, and a seven-day gap after venlafaxine before starting an MAOI. There are many reported cases of severe reactions, eg. extreme agitation, diaphoresis, rapid respiration and raised CPK levels (n = 1, Phillips and Ringo, *Am J Psychiatry* 1995;**152**:1400–1), hypomania, heavy perspiration, shivering and dilated pupils (n = 1, Klysner et al, *Lancet* 1995;**346**:1298–9), and several of serotonin syndrome (eg. n = 1, Weiner et al, *Pharmacother* 1998;**18**:399–403). Follow manufacturer's recommendations carefully.

Mirtazapine + venlafaxine
See mirtazapine (*4.3.3.3*).

Moclobemide + venlafaxine
The UK SPC for venlafaxine states very cautiously that venlafaxine and moclobemide should not be used together and that serious adverse reactions may occur. It recommends a 14-day gap after stopping moclobemide before starting venlafaxine, and a seven-day gap after venlafaxine before moclobemide is used. This seems overcautious, although a serotonin syndrome has been reported (n = 1, *Ann Pharmacother* 2002; **36**:67–71).

Propafenone + venlafaxine
An organic psychosis has been reported, with raised venlafaxine levels (n = 1, Pfeffer and Grube, *Int J Psychiatr Med* 2001;**31**:427–32).

Risperidone + venlafaxine
See risperidone (*4.2.6*).

Selegiline + venlafaxine
The SPC for venlafaxine states that the combination should not be used and that serious adverse reactions may occur. It recommends a 14-day gap after stopping selegiline before starting venlafaxine, and a seven-day gap after venlafaxine before selegiline is used.

Sertraline + venlafaxine
See sertraline (*4.2.5*).

Sour date nut + venlafaxine
A severe serotonin syndrome with anaphylactic features has been reported with combined sour date nut (jujube) and venlafaxine 37.5 mg/d (n = 1, Stewart, *Am J Psychiatry* 2004;**161**:1129–30).

Trazodone + venlafaxine
A serotonin syndrome has been reported (n = 1, McCue and Joseph, *Am J Psychiatry* 2001; **158**:2088–9).

Tricyclics + venlafaxine
See tricyclics (*4.3.1*).

Verapamil + venlafaxine
A fatality has been reported (n = 1, Kusman et al, *J Forensic Sci* 2000;**45**:926–8).

Warfarin + venlafaxine
Potentiation of the anticoagulant effects of warfarin has been reported, including increased PT or INR.

4.3.3.9 ST JOHN'S WORT
Although not approved for depression in the UK, this section has been included because concerns about its interactions are frequently

raised. Minor serotonin, norepinephrine and dopamine reuptake inhibition activity has been detected from St John's wort (SJW) and might thus potentiate any antidepressants, and so any combinations should in theory be avoided, particularly at high dose. SJW, when taken at recommended doses for depression, is unlikely to inhibit CYP2D6 or 3A4 activity (n = 7, open, Markowitz et al, Life Sci 2000;**66**:133–9), but is probably a CYP3A4 and 2C9 inducer (n = 2, Ruschitzka et al, Lancet 2000;**355**:548–9). SJW increases the expression of P-glycoprotein (a liver enzyme), which may have implications for drug interactions (n = 22, Hennessy et al, Br J Clin Pharmacol 2002;**53**:75–82). There are reports of serotonin syndrome with SJW and antidepressants in elderly patients (n = 5, Lantz et al, J Geriatr Psychiatry Neurol 1999;**12**:7–10). SJW is widely used as self-medication so remember to ask about it (up to 15% have used it recently, and 7% may be taking it at any one time; n = 101, Redvers et al, Psychiatr Bull 2001;**25**:254–6).

Reviews: * herbal medicine interactions (Cupp, Am Fam Physician 1999;**59**:1239–45), general interactions (Zhou et al, J Psychopharmacol 2004; **18**:262–76; Hammerness et al, Psychosomatics 2003;**44**:271–82; Izzo, Int J Clin Pharmacol Ther 2004;**42**:139–48; s = 22, Mills et al, Br Med J 2004; **329**:27–30).

Androgens + St John's wort ***
Short-term administration of SJW does not significantly alter circulating androgen levels in men and women, although 5-alpha-reduced-androgen levels may drop (n = 12, 14/7, Donovan et al, Phytother Res 2005;**19**:901–6).

Anti-HIV drugs + St John's wort
SJW may induce the metabolism of anti-HIV drugs, reducing efficacy, and so should not be taken together (CSM warning, 2000). Suddenly stopping SJW may require dose adjustment of any anti-HIV drug.

Benzodiazepines + St John's wort ***
SJW halves **alprazolam's** half-life (n = 12, open, Markowitz et al, JAMA 2003;**290**:1519–20) but there was no significant interaction between stat doses of alprazolam 1 mg and the Esbericum brand of SJW (n = 28, RCT, p/c, Arold et al, Planta Med 2005;**71**:31–7). SJW significantly reduces **quazepam** plasma levels (n = 13, RCT, p/c, c/o, 14/7, Kawaguchi et al, Br J Clin Pharmacol 2004;**58**:403–10).

Buspirone + St John's wort
See buspirone (4.1.2).

Caffeine + St. John's wort ***
There was no significant interaction between stat doses of caffeine 100 mg and the Esbericum brand of SJW (n = 28, RCT, p/c, Arold et al, Planta Med 2005;**71**:331–7).

Carbamazepine + St John's wort ***
Carbamazepine reduces hypericum levels by 30%, probably clinically insignificant (n = 33, RCT, p/c, 7/7, Johne et al, Eur J Clin Pharmacol 2004;**60**:617–22). SJW may have no effect on carbamazepine clearance (n = 8, 5/52, Burstein et al, Clin Pharmacol Ther 2000;**68**:605–12), but the CSM has warned that SJW may induce the metabolism of carbamazepine, increasing the risk of seizures, and so should not be taken together (CSM warning, 2000). Suddenly stopping SJW may require dose adjustment of carbamazepine so check levels before and after stopping SJW.

Ciclosporin + St John's wort
SJW causes rapid (within three days) and significant (60%) reduction in ciclosporin plasma levels and may alter the metabolite ratio as well (n = 11, open, 14/7, Bauer et al, Br J Clin Pharmacol 2003;**55**:203–11), so these should not be taken together (CSM warning, 2000; n = 1, Barone et al, Ann Pharmacother 2000;**34**:1013–6; Moschella and Jaber, Am J Kidney Dis 2001;**38**:1105–7). Heart transplant rejection due to SJW has been reported (n = 2, Ruschitzka et al, Lancet 2000;**355**:548).

Cimetidine + St. John's wort ***
Cimetidine produces a 25% increase in hypericum levels, probably clinically insignificant (n = 33, RCT, p/c, 7/7, Johne et al, Eur J Clin Pharmacol 2004;**60**:617–22).

Digoxin + St John's wort ***
SJW may induce the metabolism of digoxin, reducing AUC by up to 25%, and so these should not be taken together (n = 25, 10/7, s/b, p/c, Johne et al, Clin Pharmacol Ther 1999;**66**:338–45; Cheng, Arch Intern Med 2000;**160**:2548). Suddenly stopping SJW may also require dose adjustment of digoxin. There was no significant interaction between stat doses of digoxin and the Esbericum brand of SJW (n = 28, RCT, p/c, Arold et al, Planta Med 2005;**71**:331–7).

Duloxetine + St John's wort
See duloxetine (4.3.3.1).

Fexofenadine + St John's wort

SJW may inhibit the metabolism of fexofenadine (open, c/o, Wang et al, Clin Pharmacol Therapeutics 2002;**71**:414–20).

Indinavir + St John's wort

SJW may reduce the levels of indinavir (AUC reduced by 57%), reducing efficacy, and so these should not be taken together (n = 8, Piscitelli et al, Lancet 2000;**355**:547). The same would probably be true for other protease inhibitors, eg. ritonavir and saquinavir.

MAOIs + St John's wort

Minor MAOI activity has been detected from SJW, which might potentiate existing MAOI therapy, and should be avoided, particularly at high dose.

Methadone + St John's wort

SJW induces methadone metabolism, decreasing levels by up to 47% and may precipitate withdrawal symptoms (n = 4, Eich-Hochli et al, Pharmacopsychiatry 2003;**36**:35–7).

Omeprazole + St John's wort

SJW may produce 'enormously' decreased omeprazole levels (n = 12, RCT, c/o, Wang et al, Clin Pharmacol Ther 2004;**75**:191–7).

Oral contraceptives + St John's wort

The UK CSM has recommended that, since SJW reduces the effectiveness of oral contraceptives, the two should not be taken together (two cases of pregnancy mentioned in Pharm J 2002;**268**:198) and reduced efficacy has been shown (n = 12, open, Hall et al, Clin Pharmacol Ther 2003;**74**:525–35).

Phenytoin + St John's wort

The CSM has warned that SJW may induce the metabolism of phenytoin, increasing the risk of seizures, and so should not be taken together (CSM warning, 2000). Suddenly stopping SJW may require dose adjustment of phenytoin so check levels before and after stopping SJW.

Phenobarbital + St John's wort

The CSM has warned that SJW may induce the metabolism of phenobarbital, increasing the risk of seizures, and so should not be taken together (CSM warning, 2000). Suddenly stopping SJW may require dose adjustment of phenobarbital so check levels before and after stopping SJW.

SSRIs + St John's wort

Minor serotonin reuptake inhibition activity has been detected from SJW which might potentiate existing SSRI therapy and so should, in theory, be avoided, particularly at high dose.

Statins + St John's wort

SJW may decrease simvastatin (but not pravastatin) plasma levels (n = 16, d/b, c/o, 14/7, Fujimura et al, Clin Pharmacol Ther 2002;**71**:63).

Tacrolimus + St John's wort

SJW induces tacrolimus metabolism via 3A4, which may lead to organ rejection (n = 10, Hebert et al, J Clin Pharmacol 2004;**44**:89–94).

Theophylline + St John's wort

SJW may induce the metabolism of theophylline, reducing efficacy, and so these should not be taken together (CSM warning, 2000), although suddenly stopping SJW may require dose adjustment of theophylline (Nebel et al, Ann Pharmacother 1999;**33**:502, letter). Check theophylline levels before and after stopping SJW. One study showed no significant changes from 14 days SJW and a single dose of theophylline (n = 12, open, RCT, c/o, 15/7, Morimoto et al, J Clin Pharmacol 2004;**44**:95–101), so there may be interindividual variation.

Tolbutamide + St. John's wort *

There was no significant interaction between stat doses of tolbutamide 500 mg and Esbericum brand SJW (n = 28, RCT, p/c, Arold et al, Planta Med 2005;**71**:331–7).

Tricyclics + St John's wort

Minor serotonin and norepinephrine reuptake inhibition activity has been detected from SJW, which might thus potentiate existing tricyclic therapy, and so should, in theory, be avoided, particularly at high dose. Amitriptyline and nortriptyline levels reduced by 22% have been reported (n = 12, Johne et al, J Clin Psychopharmacol 2002;**22**:46–54).

Triptans + St John's wort

The CSM has warned that SJW may increase the serotonergic effects of sumatriptan, naratriptan, rizatriptan and zolmitriptan, with increased adverse effects so avoid the combination.

Tyramine + St John's wort

There is not thought to be an interaction (mentioned by Cupp, Am Fam Physician 1999; **59**:1239–45).

Verapamil + St John's wort

SJW significantly reduces verapamil bioavailability (AUC 50–60% decreased) via increased first-pass gut metabolism (n = 8, open, Tannergren et al, Clin Pharmacol Ther 2004;**75**:298–309).

Warfarin + St John's wort

SJW may induce the metabolism of warfarin,

reducing efficacy, and so these should not be taken together (CSM warning, 2000). Suddenly stopping SJW may require dose adjustment of warfarin so check INR before and after stopping SJW and adjust doses as necessary.

4.3.4 MONO-AMINE OXIDASE INHIBITORS (MAOIs)

Review of MAOI interactions; Berlin and Lecrubier, *CNS Drugs* 1996;**5**:403–13.

Adrenaline + MAOIs
See norepinephrine+ MAOIs.

ALCOHOL + MAOIs
See alcohol (4.7.1).

Amantadine + MAOIs
Hypertension occurred in one patient taking amantadine, 48 hours after starting phenelzine (Jack and Daniel, *Arch Gen Psychiatry* 1984;**41**:726), with one reported case of safe use of both (Greenberg and Meyers, *Am J Psychiatry* 1985;**142**:273).

AMFETAMINE + MAOIs
See dexamfetamine + MAOIs.

Anaesthetics + MAOIs
With proper monitoring, general and local anaesthesia can be given safely with MAOIs (n = 27, el-Ganzouri *et al*, *Anesth Analg* 1985;**64**:592–6) although occasional cases of reactions have been reported (eg. *Anesthesia* 1987;**42**:633–5). This is generally considered safe although care with analgesics and sympathomimetics is needed.

Anticholinergics + MAOIs
Enhanced anticholinergic effects have been postulated.

Anticoagulants + MAOIs
An enhanced anticoagulant effect has been shown in animals.

Antipsychotics + MAOIs
Unexplained deaths with levomepromazine exist, but are probably not related to a drug interaction. The combination is a risk factor for NMS and may enhance anticholinergic and EPSEs. Enhanced sedation could occur.

Aspartane + MAOIs
Recurrent headaches following aspartane ingestion have been reported (n = 1, Ferguson, *Am J Psychiatry* 1985;**142**:271).

Atomoxetine + MAOIs
See atomoxetine (4.6.4).

Atracurium + MAOIs
A single case report exists of atracurium-induced hypertension (n = 1, Sides, *Anesthesia* 1987;**42**:633).

Barbiturates + MAOIs
Barbiturate sedation may be prolonged. Although little human data exists, be aware of the potential toxicity as one fatality has been reported.

Benzodiazepines + MAOIs
Although there are isolated cases of MAOI toxicity, oedema and hepatotoxicity (eg. Young and Walpole, *Med J Aust* 1986;**144**:166–7), this is normally considered a safe combination.

Beta-blockers + MAOIs
Propranolol used with MAOIs has caused severe hypertension (Risch *et al*, *J Clin Psychiatry* 1982;**43**:16) and slight bradycardia (*Psychosomatics* 1989;**30**:106–8), although not invariably so (review: Davidson *et al*, *J Clin Psychiatry* 1984;**45**:81–4). Best to monitor bp carefully, especially in the elderly.

Bretylium + MAOIs
Bretylium may increase the heart rate with MAOIs but it is only dangerous if other sympathomimetics are present. There are no case reports.

Bupropion + MAOIs
See bupropion (4.6.6).

BUSPIRONE + MAOIs
There are four unpublished reports of increased bp and possible CVA, although the combination has been used safely.

Caffeine + MAOIs
Case reports exist of increased jitteriness with caffeine taken while on MAOIs (Berkowitz *et al*, *Eur J Pharmacol* 1971;**16**:315).

Carbamazepine + MAOIs
Carbamazepine is structurally related to the tricyclics and so an interaction has been postulated. There have been case reports of raised carbamazepine levels but a lack of inter-action with **tranylcypromine** (Lydiard *et al*, *J Clin Psychopharmacol* 1987;**7**:360) and **phenelzine** (Yatham *et al*, *Am J Psychiatry* 1990;**147**:367).

Chloral hydrate + MAOIs
There are two poorly documented case reports of fatal hyperpyrexia and hypertension with chloral hydrate and **phenelzine**. This is not thought to be an important interaction.

Citalopram + MAOIs
There are many reported cases of serotonin syndrome (see 1.32) with other SSRIs and MAOIs and so care is needed if this combination

is used (review: Graber et al, Ann Pharmacother 1994;**28**:732–5).

Clozapine + MAOIs

See clozapine (4.2.3).

Cyproheptadine + MAOIs

An isolated case of hallucinations with cyproheptadine and phenelzine exists (Hahn, Am J Psychiatry 1987;**144**:1242–3).

DEXAMFETAMINE + MAOIs

There is a case report of a death with phenelzine and dexamfetamine (Lloyd and Walker, Br Med J 1965;ii:168-9) and one with amfetamine.

Dextromethorphan + MAOIs

Although this is mainly extrapolation from pethidine, case reports exist with cough mixtures containing dextromethorphan, but, since all also contained sympathomimetics, these are questionable. Two were fatal so care is advised. Dizziness and muscle spasms with dextromethorphan have been reported (Harrison et al, J Clin Psychiatry 1989;**50**:64–5), as has a serotonin syndrome (Nierenberg et al, Clin Pharmacol Ther 1993;**53**:84–8).

Dextropropoxyphene + MAOIs

Dextropropoxyphene plus **phenelzine** has been reported to produce sedation (n=1, Garbutt, Am J Psychiatry 1987;**144**:251–2), severe hypotension, ataxia and impaired coordination (n=1, Zornberg and Hegarty, Am J Psychiatry 1993;**150**:1270).

Disulfiram + MAOIs

See disulfiram (4.6.8).

DOPAMINE/DOXAPRAM + MAOIs

Animal studies show a clear interaction, with side-effects enhanced by MAOIs. The manufacturers recommend that dopamine or doxapram can be used if their initial dose is reduced to one tenth the normal dose and great care is taken.

DULOXETINE + MAOIs

See duloxetine (4.3.3.1).

Ecstasy/MDMA + MAOIs

There is a case of a hypertensive crisis with MDMA/ecstasy and phenelzine (n=1, Smilkstein et al, J Toxicol Clin Toxicol 1987;**25**:149–59) and two of muscle tension, coma and delirium with raised blood pressure (Kaskey, Am J Psychiatry 1992;**192**:411–2).

Escitalopram + MAOIs

See citalopram + MAOIs above.

FLUOXETINE + MAOIs

There are several reported interactions (eg.

Sternbach, Lancet 1988;ii:850–1), including four deaths. A gap must be also be left when switching from one to the other (see 2.2.5).

FLUVOXAMINE + MAOIs

There is an SPC recommendation to allow a two-week gap between therapies. There are many reported cases of serotonin syndrome with other SSRIs and MAOIs and so care is needed with this combination.

Ginseng + MAOIs

There are cases of headache, tremor (Shader and Greenblatt, J Clin Psychopharmacol 1985;**5**:65) and mania (Jones and Runikis, J Clin Psychopharmacol 1987;**7**:201–2) with ginseng and phenelzine.

Hypoglycaemics + MAOIs

An enhanced hypoglycaemic effect with insulin and sulphonylureas has been noted.

Indoramin + MAOIs

The SPC for indoramin states this to be a contraindication, as indoramin antagonises alpha-receptors, thus competing with norepinephrine for post-synaptic alpha-receptors, which could cause vasoconstriction and raised blood pressure. No case reports are known.

Isoprenaline + MAOIs

This is a postulated interaction with some evidence that no interaction occurs. No case reports exist.

LEVODOPA + MAOIs

Low dose levodopa with carbidopa or benserazide seems safe but higher doses should be avoided, as should levodopa on its own (Clin Pharmacol Ther 1975;**18**:273).

Lithium + MAOIs

Lack of an interaction has been reported (Am J Psychiatry 1988;**145**:249–50).

MAOIs + MAOIs

There is some evidence that different MAOIs may interact with each other, especially if abruptly changed, eg. isocarboxazid to tranylcypromine (n=1, Bazire, Drug Intell Clin Pharm 1986;**20**: 54–5) and phenelzine to isocarboxazid (Safferman and Masiar, Ann Pharmacother 1992;**26**:337–8). Tranyl-cypromine is metabolised to an amfetamine and an internal autoreaction (ie. interacts with itself) has been postulated (Br Med J 1989;**298**:964).

Methadone + MAOIs

Lack of an interaction has been reported (Med J Aust 1979;**1**:400).

METHOXAMINE + MAOIs

There is evidence of enhanced bp with

methoxamine and MAOIs (*J Lab Clin Med* 1960;**56**:747).

Methyldopa + MAOIs

There is a single case report of hallucinations with methyldopa and pargyline.

METHYLPHENIDATE + MAOIs

A less severe interaction than with amfetamines would be expected. A single case of headaches and hyperventilation has been reported.

Mirtazapine + MAOIs

See mirtazapine (4.3.3.3).

Modafinil + tranylcypromine *

There is a report of successful use of tranylcypromine and modafinil for refractory narcolepsy (n = 1, Clemons et al, *Sleep Med* 2004; **5**:509–11).

Morphine + MAOIs

This is mainly extrapolation from pethidine. Two cases exist of hypotension and loss of consciousness with IV morphine (Barry, *Anaesth Intens Care* 1979;**7**:194), responsive to naloxone. Low dose morphine and other narcotics, eg. codeine and fentanyl are probably safe. Methadone may be a suitable alternative. If opiates are used, it is best to start at a third or half the normal dose of opiate and titrate carefully, noting blood pressure and levels of consciousness. See also pethidine.

NEFOPAM + MAOIs

The manufacturers of nefopam recommend avoiding this combination.

Norepinephrine + MAOIs

Norepinephrine is potentially dangerous by injection and/or if other sympathomimetics are present, but is unlikely to cause problems if used with care.

Orciprenaline + MAOIs

The manufacturers recommend caution if the two are used together.

Oxcarbazepine + MAOIs

See oxcarbazepine (4.5.6).

Oxymetazoline/xylometazoline + MAOIs

There is thought to be little systemic effect when these drugs are used nasally, but use in nose drops and sprays has not been studied.

Paraldehyde + MAOIs

Enhanced CNS sedation and respiratory depression have been suggested.

Paroxetine + MAOIs

Nothing has been reported but see other SSRIs in this MAOI section.

PETHIDINE + MAOIs

This is a well-documented, rapid, severe and potentially fatal interaction, although not inevitable (Evans-Prosser, *Br J Anaest* 1968;**40**:279-82).

Reboxetine + MAOIs

See reboxetine (4.3.3.5).

Salbutamol + MAOIs

No interaction occurs.

SERTRALINE + MAOIs

The manufacturers suggest a one-week washout period after sertraline before an MAOI is used. Several cases of suspected serotonergic syndrome have been reported, so care is essential (eg. cases and review, Graber et al, *Ann Pharmacother* 1994;**28**:732–5).

St John's wort + MAOIs

See St John's wort (4.3.3.9).

Sulphonamides + MAOIs

An isolated case exists of adverse effects with sulphafurazole and phenelzine (Boyer and Lake, *Am J Psychiatry* 1983;**140**:264–5).

Suxamethonium + MAOIs

There are three cases of enhancement of suxamethonium by phenelzine (Bodley et al, *Br Med J* 1969;**3**:510–2).

SYMPATHOMIMETICS + MAOIs

Hypertension has been reported with many indirectly acting sympathomimetic amines, eg. ephedrine, metaraminol, pseudoephedrine and phenylpropanolamine. Phenylephrine is found in many OTC cough and cold remedies and can cause a massive rise in blood pressure with MAOIs. Use in nasal sprays and drops is not recommended, although there are no case reports.

Tetrabenazine + MAOIs

Reports exist of a central excitation and hypertension with tetrabenazine.

Trazodone + MAOIs

There are many reported cases of serotonin syndrome with SSRIs and MAOIs and so care may be needed if this combination is used (n = 1, Graber et al, *Ann Pharmacother* 1994;**28**:732–5).

TRICYCLICS + MAOIs

The combination of tranylcypromine and **clomipramine** has caused four deaths and one fatality between tranylcypromine and a single dose of **imipramine** (n = 1, Birkenhager and van den Broek, *Eur Psychiatry* 2003;**18**:264–5). There are cases of excitation, seizures and hyperpyrexia and a serotonin syndrome after a clomipramine overdose (325–750 mg) with phenelzine (Nierenberg et al, Clin Pharmacol Ther 1993;**53**:84–8). Other MAOI/tricyclic combinations have been used with extreme care (Graham et al, Lancet 1982;**ii**:440). The dangers could have been exaggerated and the combination may be relatively event-free if the following precautions are taken:

- avoid imipramine, desipramine, clomipramine and tranylcypromine
- prefer amitriptyline
- use oral doses only
- monitor patient closely
- start both drugs simultaneously at low dose and increase slowly.

See also combinations in depression (1.14) for a review of the potentially beneficial effects.

TRIPTANS + MAOIs

The SPCs recommend sumatriptan is not used with MAOIs, or for two weeks after an MAOI has stopped. The UK SPC contraindicates MAOIs with rizatriptan.

Tryptophan + MAOIs *

There are cases of hypomania (n = 2, Goff, Am J Psychiatry 1985;**142**:1487–8), behavioural and neurological toxicity with high doses of tryptophan, mostly with tranylcypromine (n = 8, Pope et al, Am J Psychiatry 1985;**142**:491–2), which may respond to propranolol (Guze and Baxter, J Clin Psychopharmacol 1986;**6**:119–20). Potentiation of the therapeutic effect is well known so monitor carefully.

Patient information: warning signs of a reaction

If a patient experiences any of the following symptoms, expecially after eating, taking drugs of any type or if unexpected or severe, a reaction should be suspected and appropriate medical attention sought immediately: headache (especially at the back of the head), lightheadedness or dizziness, flushing of the face, pounding of the heart, numbness or stiffness in the neck, photophobia, chest pain or nausea and vomiting. It usually occurs about two hours after the ingestion of the compound.

TYRAMINE + MAOIs

Ingestion of dietary tyramine, levodopa or a sympathomimetic drug by a patient on an MAOI can produce a hypertensive crisis, eg. headache, rapid and prolonged rise in blood pressure, intracranial haemorrhage, acute cardiac failure and death. The effect is probably only seen with slow acetylators, as fast acetylators seem able to handle tyramine and other monoamines better. The effect is hugely variable, but 8 mg tyramine can produce a 30 mm Hg rise in bp in 50% people, and 25 mg and above is potentially dangerous (Blackwell and Mabbitt, Lancet 1965;**1**:938–40). 20–50 mg tyramine produces hypertension with tranylcypromine (Berlin et al, Clin Pharmacol Ther 1989;**46**:344–51). In a normal person, bp rises within 10–20 minutes (range 0–60) of tyramine ingestion, peaking at 20–110 minutes, prolonged if an MAOI is taken. For advice on dietary tyramine, see the following section.

Treatment for MAOI hypertensive crisis:

- Phenotamine 2–10 mg by slow IV infusion (adults), repeated if necessary.
- If not phentolamine, chlorpromazine 50–100 mg IM can be used, as can diazoxide (50–100 mg by IV injection). Repeat after 10 minutes if necessary.
- Alternative advice might be to bite open a 10 mg capsule of nifedipine, swallow the contents with water (Am J Psychiatry 1991;148:1616) then go immediately to a hospital casualty department. This produces a consistent and prompt fall in arterial blood pressure but due to serious adverse events (stroke, hypotension etc), s/l nifedipine should only be used with care (Marwick, (JAMA 1996;**275**:423–4; Grossman et al, JAMA 1996;**276**:1328–31). NB: nifedipine is light-sensitive and should not be left in bright light. Safer alternatives include sublingual captopril, clonidine and labetolol (review Matuschka, J Pharm Tech 1999;**15**:199–203).
- Cool any fever with external cooling.

Blood pressure should be monitored frequently.

VENLAFAXINE + MAOIs
See venlafaxine (4.3.3.8).

Warfarin + MAOIs
No interaction is known, although tranylcypromine is known to inhibit CYP2C19 and so some potential exists (Sayal et al, Acta Psychiatr Scand 2000;**102**:250–5).

Xylometazoline + MAOIs
See oxymetazoline + MAOIs.

FOOD
Compliance with the MAOI diet is often very poor.

Reviews: Cheese and drink tyramine contents (Berlin and Lecrubier, CNS Drugs 1996;**5**:403–13), 'The making of a user-friendly MAOI diet' (Gardner et al, J Clin Psychiatry 1996;**57**:99–104).

1. General principles
Freshness of food is vital. If there is any sign of spoilage then avoid. Avoid foods that are matured or might be 'spoiling'. Avoid tyramine-containing foods. Generally, the more 'convenience' the food, the safer it is, eg. packet soups are generally safe. Although many foods have only small amounts of tyramine, it is possible to have local concentrations, which might give a reaction.

2. Tyramine-containing foods to avoid
The following may be of use as general guidelines:

- Dairy products

Hard cheeses and soft cheeses must be avoided. Special care is needed with salty, bitter tasting, refrigerated cheese. Foods containing cheese (eg. pizzas and pies, see below) must also be avoided and are a known cause of inadvertent ingestion and death. However, cottage cheese, cream cheeses (eg. Philadelphia), Ricotta and processed cheese contain only minute amounts of tyramine and large quantities would be needed to produce a reaction.

- Fruit and vegetables

Broad bean pods (but not the beans) and banana skins (occasionally cooked as part of whole unripe bananas in a stew) must be avoided. Avocado has been reported to produce a reaction and should be avoided if possible.

- Game, meat and fish

Pickled or salted dried herrings and any hung or badly stored game, poultry or other meat

that might be 'spoiling' must be avoided. NB. the original reports with pickled herrings may have been due to spoilage in the brine surrounding the fish, and are probably safe.

- Meat products

Avoid chicken liver pâté, liver pâté and any other liver that is not fresh. Avoid aged and cured meats (eg. salami, mortadella, pastrami). Fresh chicken liver, fresh beef liver and fresh pâté should be safe.

- Pizzas

Commercially available pizzas from large chain outlets seem safe (analysis by Shulman and Walker, J Clin Psychiatry 1999;**60**:191–3; comment by Feinberg and Holzer, reply by Shulman and Walker, J Clin Psychiatry 2000;**61**:145–6), and even those with double orders of cheese appear safe. Gourmet pizzas from smaller outlets have higher tyramine contents, especially if mature cheeses are used.

- Soy and soybean

Some samples of Soy sauce and soybean preparations may have very high tyramine levels. Either avoid entirely or a 10ml maximum is recommended.

> **Soy sauce** (Pearl River, etc) — some have high quantities, ie. up to 3.4mg/15ml, and so double or triple helpings could be well above the threshold for a reaction (Shulman and Walker, J Clin Psychiatry 1999;**60**:191–3)
>
> **Soybean curd** (eg. Tofu) — some have high quantities, especially if kept refrigerated for seven days or longer, ie. up to 5mg per 300mg helping, and so double or triple helpings could well be above the threshold for a reaction (Shulman and Walker, J Clin Psychiatry 1999;**60**:191–3).

- Yeast and meat extracts

'Oxo', 'Marmite', 'Bovril' and other meat or yeast extracts must be avoided. Gravy made with 'Bisto' is safe (all contain less than 0.0022mg/g tyramine and a full, half-pint of gravy would contain less than 0.05mg tyramine). Gravy made from juices of the roast or fresh meat should be safe. Brewers yeast (Shulman et al, J Clin Psychopharmacol 1989;**9**:397–402) and bread are safe.

3. Foods known to contain some tyramine where excessive consumption is not advisable, albeit unlikely
Plums, matured pork, sauerkraut, spinach.

4. Foods thought to contain only minute amounts of tyramine

Banana pulp (skins unsafe), chocolate (one anecdotal report of headache), cottage cheese, cream cheese, eggplant, fruit juices, octopus, peanuts, raspberries (minor reports of raised tyramine), sausages, soy milk, tomato, vinegar, yoghurt (commercial), Worcester sauce, eg. Lee and Perrins and others (very low, Shulman and Walker, J Clin Psychiatry 1999;**60**:191–3).

5. Other foods with isolated reports

Chicken nuggets, chapatti, protein dietary supplement, sea kale.

6. Alcoholic drinks

Patient instructions usually state that all alcoholic and some non-alcoholic drinks must be avoided. Real ales may contain up to 110mg/L, with reports of hypertensive crisis after 0.6 pint (79 brand study, Tailor et al, J Clin Psychopharmacol 1994;**14**:5–14). There is some evidence that low or non-alcoholic beers contain significant amounts of tyramine (Murray et al, Lancet 1988;**i**,167–8), shown by three reactions to less than two-thirds of a pint of alcohol-free and 'de-alcoholised' beer (n = 3, Thakore et al, Int Clin Psychopharmacol 1992;**7**:59–60). There is a large variation in other beers, so take in moderation (ie. 1–2 bottles a day maximum), prefer canned beers from major brewers and take care with de-alcoholised beers. The maximum reported level in Chianti wine is 12mg/L, likely to be dangerous only in overdose. The following may, however, be of use where a particular patient wishes to drink:

> **Avoid:**
> - Chianti
> - Home-made beers and wines
> - Real ales
> - Red wines
>
> **True moderation (eg. one unit):**
> - White wines
> - Non-alcoholic beers and lagers
>
> **Safest:**
> - Gin, vodka, other clear spirits

Red wines contain phenolic flavanoids, which inhibit the enzymes which metabolise catecholamines, including tyramine (Br Med J 1990;**301**:544).

Over-the-counter medicines

Each patient should be warned about the possibility of interactions with over-the-counter medicines. The general advice for patients is:

1. **Only buy medicines from a pharmacy**
Do not use medicines from supermarket shelves, drug stores or newsagents. Do not take medicines given to you by friends or relatives. Do not take medicines taken before the MAOI was prescribed until advice has been sought.

2. **Carry an MAOI card and show it to any doctor, dentist or pharmacist who may treat you.**

3. **Take special care over any medicines for coughs, colds, 'flu, hay fever, asthma and catarrh.**

4.4 LITHIUM

Lithium may interact with other drugs, particularly via changes in renal excretion.

Reviews: clinical relevance of lithium interactions (Finley et al, Clin Pharmacokinetics 1995;**29**:172–91, 147 refs), interactions with serotonergic agents (may increase prevalence of lithium-induced polyuria; n = 75, 4/12, open, Movig et al, Br J Psychiatry 2003;**182**:319–23).

ACE INHIBITORS + LITHIUM *

There are many cases of lithium toxicity with ACE inhibitors (n = 9, open, DasGupta et al, J Clin Psychiatry 1992;**53**:398–400), especially in the elderly (n = 20, Finley et al, J Clin Psychopharmacol 1996;**16**:68–71), so either monitor very carefully (review: Lehmann and Ritz, Am J Kidney Dis 1995;**25**:82–7) or use an alternative, eg. beta-blockers. In a case control study, ACE inhibitors were most likely to increase lithium toxicity within a month of starting (Juurlink et al, J Am Geriatr Soc 2004;**52**:794–8; review by Jacoby, EBMH 2004;**7**:120) and there is a case of a five-fold increase in lithium levels after switching from fosinopril to lisinopril, the authors recommending monitoring carefully for four to six weeks after any such change (n = 1, Meyer et al, Int Clin Psychopharmacol 2005;**20**:115–8).

Acetazolamide + lithium

Lithium excretion may be increased or, less likely, possibly decreased by acetazolamide (n = 2, Gay et al, Encephale 1985;**11**:261–2). This is inadequately studied and probably of minimal importance.

Alcohol + lithium

See alcohol (4.7.1).

AMINOPHYLLINE + LITHIUM

See theophylline + lithium.

Amiodarone + lithium

The literature notes an increased risk of hypothyroidism with the combination.

Amfetamines + lithium

Lithium may suppress amfetamine 'highs' (n = 3, Flemenbaum, Am J Psychiatry 1974;**131**:820–1).

Antacids + lithium

See sodium + lithium.

Antibiotics + lithium *

Antibiotics may lead to raised lithium levels (cases within n = 102, Wilting et al, Bipolar Disord 2005;**7**:274–80).

Antipsychotics + lithium *

Although generally considered a potentially useful combination, cases of mostly reversible neurotoxicity were reported in the 1980s, particularly with haloperidol (although these may have been undiagnosed NMS), encephalopathy, enhanced EPSE, neurotoxicity or irreversible brain damage. One review suggested that all these symptoms are consistent with lithium toxicity alone, the antipsychotic affecting fluid balance mechanisms and lithium intracellular concentrations (Knorring, Hum Psychopharmacol 1990;**5**:287–92). The main risk factors seem to be if high doses of both drugs are used and signs of impending toxicity are ignored.

There are a number of reports for individual drugs. **Chlorpromazine** levels may be lowered by up to 40% by lithium, with enhanced EPSE and rarely neurotoxicity. Reports with **risperidone** include delirium (n = 1, Chen and Cardasis, Am J Psychiatry 1996;**153**:1233–4), possible NMS (n = 1, Swanson et al, Am J Psychiatry 1995;**152**:1096; Bourgeois and Kahn, J Clin Psychopharmacol 2003;**23**:315–7), diabetic ketoacidosis, rabbit syndrome (n = 1, Mendhekar, Can J Psychiatry 2005;**50**:369) and myocardial infarction (n = 1, Ananth et al, J Clin Psychiatry 2004;**65**:724). Lower **olanzapine** levels were mentioned in one study (Bergemann et al, Pharmacopsychiatry 2004;**37**:63–8), NMS is possible (n = 1, Berry et al, Pharmacother 2003;**23**:55–9) and severe delirium and EPSE have occurred in an elderly patient (n = 1, Tuglu et al, J Korean Med Sci 2005; **20**:691–4). Combined lithium and **clozapine** appears safe within moderate dose limits and without co-prescription of serotonergic or 1A2-inhibiting drugs (n = 44, Bender et al, Int J

Neuropsychopharmacol 2004;**7**:59–63), although there are reports of increased risk of NMS and reversible neurotoxicity (n = 1, Blake et al, J Clin Psychopharmacol 1992;**12**:297–9), including one where lithium levels were below 0.5 mEq/L (n = 1, Lee and Yang, Chung Hua I Hsueh Tsa Chih (Taipei) 1999;**62**:184–7). Cases of diabetic ketoacidosis have also been reported (eg. n = 1, Peterson and Byrd, Am J Psychiatry 1996;**153**:737–8), and so glucose monitoring might be indicated with this particular combination. **Amisulpride** 200 mg/d (n = 24, RCT, d/b, p/c, Canal et al, Int J Neuropsychopharmacol 2003;**6**:103–9), **aripiprazole** (n = 22, 2/52, Citrome et al, J Clin Pharmacol 2005;**45**:89–93) and **quetiapine** have no significant effect on lithium kinetics (n = 10, open, 4/52, Potkin et al, Clin Ther 2002;**24**:1809–23).

Baclofen + lithium

Cases of aggravation of movement disorder in Huntington's disease exist (n = 2, Anden et al, Lancet 1973;**ii**:93).

Beta-blockers + lithium

A case of bradycardia with propranolol and lithium has been reported (Becker, J Clin Psychiatry 1989;**50**:473), although propranolol and nadolol (n = 1, Dave and Langbart, Ann Clin Psychiatry 1994;**6**:51–2) have been used uneventfully for lithium-induced tremor.

Benzodiazepines + lithium

There have been several anecdotal reports of reactions, eg. hypothermia (Naylor et al, Br Med J 1977;**2**:22) and, although a neurotoxic syndrome in combination with lithium has been reported (n = 5, Koczerginski et al, Int Clin Psychopharm 1989;**4**:195–9), extensive use of this usually beneficial combination suggests it to be safe.

Bumetanide + lithium

Although studies have shown a minimal effect, bumetanide may cause lithium toxicity (Kerry et al, Br Med J 1980;**281**:371).

Calcium-channel blockers + lithium

Cases of enhanced effect and toxicity with unchanged plasma levels have been reported with verapamil (Price and Giannini, J Clin Pharmacol 1986;**26**:717–9), as have reduced lithium levels (Weinrauch et al, Am Heart J 1984;**108**:1378–80). Acute EPSE and bradycardia have been reported with diltiazem (n = 1, Binder et al, Arch Intern Med 1991;**151**:373–4).

Candesartan + lithium

There is a case of a patient prescribed 16 mg/d

candesartan (an Angiotensin II antagonist) who developed severe lithium toxicity eight weeks later (n = 1, Zwanzger et al, J Clin Psychiatry 2001; **62**:208–9).

Cannabis + lithium
See cannabis (4.7.2).

Carbamazepine + lithium
See carbamazepine (4.5.1), plus 'combinations' in bipolar disorder (1.10) for a review of some beneficial effects.

Cisplatin + lithium
Reports exist of lithium levels decreased by up to 64% (eg. Vincent et al, Cancer Chemother Pharmacol 1995;**35**:533–4).

Citalopram + lithium
See citalopram (4.3.2.1).

Clonidine + lithium
Lithium may reduce the hypotensive effect of clonidine (Goodnick and Meltzer, Biol Psychiatry 1984;**19**:883–9), so monitor carefully.

Cocaine + lithium
See cocaine (4.7.3).

Corticosteroids + lithium
An isolated case exists of lithium reducing the effect of corticosteroids on the kidneys (Stewart et al, Clin Endocrinol 1987;**27**:63).

Co-trimoxazole + lithium
Two cases exist of enhanced toxicity with reduced levels (N Z Med J 1984;**97**:729–32).

COX-2 inhibitors + lithium
See NSAIDs + lithium.

Dextromethorphan + lithium *
Serotonin syndrome has been reported with the combination in a patient also taking fluoxetine (n = 1, Navarro et al, Gen Hosp Psychiatry 2006; **28**:78–80).

Digoxin + lithium
Lack of interaction has been shown (n = 6, open, Cooper et al, Br J Clin Pharmacol 1984;**18**:21–5).

Dipyridamole + lithium
Lack of interaction has been shown (Wood et al, Br J Clin Pharmacol 1989;**27**:749–56).

Disulfiram + lithium
See disulfiram (4.6.8).

Domperidone + lithium
An enhanced risk of EPSE exists.

Escitalopram + lithium
See citalopram/escitalopram (4.3.2.1).

Fluoxetine + lithium
The incidence of problems may be low (n = 110, open, Bauer et al, J Clin Psychopharmacol 1996;

16:130–4) and lack of significant pharma-cokinetic interaction has been shown (n = 10, open, Breuel et al, Int J Clin Pharmacol Ther 1995;**33**:415–9). The combination may, however, be poorly tolerated (n = 14, open, Hawley et al, Int Clin Psychopharmacol 1994;**9**:31–3), with reports of serotonin syndrome (n = 1, Muly et al, Am J Psychiatry 1993;**150**:1565), absence seizures (Sacristan et al, Am J Psychiatry 1991;**148**:146–7) and acute confusion or lithium toxicity (Int J Geriatr Psychiatry 1992;**7**:687–8; review by Levinson et al, DICP Ann Pharmacother 1991;**25**:657–61).

Fluvoxamine + lithium
See fluvoxamine (4.3.2.3).

Furosemide + lithium
Studies have shown a minimal effect and furosemide to be the safest diuretic with lithium (eg. n = 13, RCT, Crabtree et al, Am J Psychiatry 1991;**148**:1060–3). In a case control study, loop diuretics most likely to increase lithium toxicity within a month of starting (Juurlink et al, J Am Geriatr Soc 2004;**52**:794–8; review by Jacoby, EBMH 2004;**7**:120).

Gabapentin + lithium
Although both are exclusively eliminated by renal excretion, a single-dose study showed that the pharmacokinetics of lithium are not altered by gabapentin (n = 13, Frye et al, J Clin Psychopharmacol 1998;**18**:461–4).

Herbal diuretics + lithium
A clear case of life-threatening lithium toxicity (4.5 mmol/L) induced by a herbal diuretic preparation has been reported (n = 1, Pyevich and Bogenschutz, Am J Psychiatry 2001;**158**:1329).

Hypoglycaemics + lithium
Lithium has been used to improve glucose metabolism and assist the effects of oral hypoglycaemics and insulin (n = 38, Hu et al, Biol Trace Elem Res 1997;**60**:131–7).

Iodides + lithium
Enhanced antithyroid and goiter effects of lithium have been reported.

Ispaghula husk + lithium
A single case exists of reduced lithium levels (Perlman, Lancet 1990;**335**:416).

Lamotrigine + lithium
Lamotrigine does not cause a significant change in the pharmacokinetics of lithium (n = 20, RCT, 6/7, Chen et al, Br J Clin Pharmacol 2000;**50**:193–6).

Levodopa + lithium
Lithium has been used to treat levodopa-induced

psychiatric side-effects, eg. psychosis and mania (n = 1, Braden, *Am J Psychiatry* 1977;**134**:808). Reversible Creutzfeldt-Jakob-like syndrome has also been reported (n = 1, Broussolle *et al*, *J Neurol Neurosurg Psychiatry* 1989;**52**:686–7).

Levofloxacin + lithium

A case has been reported of severe lithium toxicity (with plasma levels more than doubled) two days after starting levofloxacin in a stable bipolar patient (n = 1, Takahashi *et al*, *J Clin Psychiatry* 2000;**61**:949–50).

Losartan + lithium

A case has been reported of marked lithium toxicity five weeks after losartan 50 mg/d was added to stable therapy (n = 1, Blanche *et al*, *Eur J Clin Pharmacol* 1999;**52**:501).

MAOIs + lithium

See MAOIs (*4.3.4*).

METHYLDOPA + LITHIUM

Many cases of rapidly appearing lithium toxicity with normal plasma levels have been reported (eg. Yassa, *CSAJ* 1986;**134**:141–2).

Metoclopramide + lithium

An enhanced risk of EPSE and of neurotoxicity exists.

Metronidazole + lithium

Cases of toxic lithium levels induced by metronidazole exist (Teicher *et al*, *JAMA* 1987; **257**:3365–6).

Mirtazapine + lithium

See mirtazapine (*4.3.3.3*).

Neuromuscular blocking agents + lithium

A few cases of enhanced blockade have been reported with neostigmine (eg. Martin and Kramer, *Am J Psychiatry* 1982;**139**:1326–8). Animal studies indicate the possibility of an interaction and so the last dose or two of lithium could be omitted before the use of an NMBA.

NON-STEROIDAL ANTI-INFLAMMATORY DRUGS/COX-2 INHIBITORS + LITHIUM

This is a well-known interaction, probably due to inhibition of renal prostaglandin PGE2 and reduced blood flow. Lithium levels should be monitored frequently if the combination is to be used.

Reviews: NSAIDs (Brouwers and de Smet, *Clin Pharmacokinet* 1994;**27**:462–85), COX-2 (Phelan *et al*, *J Clin Psychiatry* 2003;**64**:1328–34).

Avoid:

- **Indometacin:** lithium levels increased by 61% have been reported (eg. n = 10,

open, Reimann *et al*, *Arch Gen Psychiatry* 1983;**40**:283–6).

Extra care:

- **Ibuprofen:** studies show a variable effect, with a 25% increase in lithium levels possible (eg. n = 9, open, Ragheb, *J Clin Psychiatry* 1987;**48**:161–3; Bailey *et al*, *South Med J* 1989;**82**:1197). As ibuprofen is available over-the-counter, this interaction should be considered carefully.

- **Diclofenac:** lithium levels may rise by up to 23% (n = 5, Reimann and Frolich, *Clin Pharmacol Ther* 1981;**30**:348–52).

- **Piroxicam:** several cases exist of a slow-onset (eg. several months) lithium toxicity (eg. n = 1, Walbridge and Bazire, *Br J Psychiatry* 1985;**147**:206–7).

Care:

- **Azapropazone:** the literature notes the possibility of raised lithium levels.

- **Celecoxib:** several interactions have been reported (eg. Gunja *et al*, *Intern Med J* 2002;**32**:494) including one life-threatening (Slordal *et al*, *Br J Clin Pharmacol* 2003;**55**:413–4).

- **Ketoprofen:** raised lithium levels have been reported (n = 1, Singer *et al*, *Therapie* 1981;**36**:323–6).

- **Ketorolac:** lithium levels nearly doubled by ketorolac have been reported (n = 1, Langlois and Paquette, *Can Med Assoc J* 1994;**150**:1455–6; n = 5, Cold *et al*, *J Clin Psychopharmacol* 1998;**18**:33–7).

- **Mefenamic acid:** acute lithium toxicity, possibly with renal damage, has been reported (n = 2, MacDonald and Neale, *Br Med J* 1988;**297**:1339).

- **Meloxicam:** meloxicam 15 mg moderately increases plasma lithium, so plasma levels should be closely monitored (n = 16, Turck *et al*, *Br J Clin Pharmacol* 2000;**50**:197–204).

- **Naproxen:** short-term naproxen has little effect on lithium levels (n = 12, Levin *et al*, *J Clin Psychopharmacol* 1998;**18**:237–40), although one study showed some increased lithium levels (n = 7, Ragheb and Powell, *J Clin Psychopharmacol* 1986;**6**:150–4).

- **Phenylbutazone:** doubled lithium levels have been reported (n = 1, Singer *et al*, *L'Encephale* 1978;**4**:33–40; see also Ragheb, *J Clin Psychopharmacol* 1990;**10**:49–50).

- **Rofecoxib:** 50 mg/d can increase lithium levels, particularly with higher starting lithium levels (n = 10, Sajbel et al, *Pharmacotherapy* 2001;**21**:380; abstract; n = 1, Lundmark et al, *Br J Clin Pharmacol* 2002;**53**:403–4), with a life-threatening lithium intoxication reported (n = 1, Bravo et al, *Ann Pharmacother* 2004;**38**:1189–93).
- **Tiaprofenic acid:** increased serum lithium levels (requiring a dose reduction) occurred in a woman taking fosinopril and lithium to which tiaprofenic acid was added (n = 1, Alderman and Lindsay, *Ann Pharmacother* 1996;**30**:1411–3).

Least risk:

- **Aspirin:** 4 g/d for seven days had no effect on lithium levels in one study (n = 10, open, Reimann et al, *Arch Gen Psychiatry* 1983; **40**:283–6), and other studies have only shown a mildly variable effect (eg. Ragheb, *J Clin Psychiatry* 1987;**48**:425; Bendz and Feinberg, *Arch Gen Psychiatry* 1984;**41**:310–11).
- **Sulindac:** Reports show either a slightly reduced level of lithium (n = 2, Furnell and Davies, *Drug Intell Clin Pharm* 1986;**19**:374–6), no effect (n = 4, Ragheb and Powell, *J Clin Psychiatry* 1986;**47**:33–4) or raised levels (n = 2, Jones and Stoner, *J Clin Psychiatry* 2000;**61**:527–8).

Oxcarbazepine + lithium
See oxcarbazepine (4.5.6).

Phenytoin + lithium
There are several reports of lithium neurotoxicity, without increased lithium levels (eg. Raskin, *J Clin Psychopharmacol* 1984;**4**:120).

Potassium iodide + lithium
An additive effect may cause hypothyroidism.

Psyllium + lithium
See Ispaghula husk + lithium.

Quetiapine + lithium
See quetiapine (4.2.5).

SERTINDOLE + LITHIUM
See sertindole (4.2.7).

Smoking + lithium
See smoking (4.7.4).

Sodium + lithium
Excess sodium (eg. as bicarbonate in antacids) can reduce lithium levels (eg. McSwiggan, *Med J Aust* 1978;**1**:38–9) and sodium restriction can lead to lithium intoxication (eg. Baer et al, *J Psychiatr Res* 1971;**8**:91–105).

Spironolactone + lithium
A rise in lithium levels has been reported (Baer et al, *J Psychiatr Res* 1971;**8**:91–105), as has synergism (see combinations, 1.10).

SSRIs + lithium
See citalopram/escitalopram (4.3.2.1), fluoxetine (4.3.2.2), fluvoxamine (4.3.2.3) and paroxetine (4.3.2.4). No interaction has been seen yet with sertraline.

Tetracyclines + lithium
Cases of lithium intoxication (eg. McGennis, *Br Med J* 1978;**2**:1183) have been reported so monitor lithium regularly.

THEOPHYLLINE + LITHIUM
Theophylline may reduce lithium levels by 20–30% (Cook et al, *J Clin Psychiatry* 1985; **46**:278–9) as may aminophylline, probably by increased excretion. An increased lithium dose can counteract this so monitoring of levels is essential, especially if theophylline is then stopped. The interaction has been made use of to treat lithium toxicity.

THIAZIDE DIURETICS + LITHIUM
Thiazides reduce the renal clearance of lithium and levels can rise within a few days. Thiazides should only be used where unavoidable and where strict monitoring is used, although it is possible that the effect on lithium is not always dramatic. The combination has occasionally been used in patients where large doses of lithium do not produce therapeutic levels.

- **Chlorothiazide:** A 50% rise in lithium levels has been reported (Levy et al, *Am J Psychiatry* 1973;**130**:1014–8).
- **Bendroflumethiazide** (bendrofluazide): a 24% reduction in lithium excretion has been shown, (Petersen et al, *Br Med J* 1974;**2**:143–5), as has lithium toxicity (n = 1, Vipond et al, *Anesthesia* 1996;**51**:1156–8).
- **Co-amilozide:** Single case report (Dorevitch and Baruch, *Am J Psychiatry* 1986;**143**:257–8).
- **Hydroflumethiazide:** One study showed a 24% reduction in lithium excretion (Petersen et al, *Br Med J* 1974;**2**:143–5).
- **Hydrochlorthiazide:** The effect may only be minor (n = 13, RCT, Crabtree et al, *Am J Psychiatry* 1991;**148**:1060–3).
- **Triamterene:** increased lithium clearance may occur (n = 8, open, Wetzels et al, *Nephrol Dial Transplant* 1989;**4**:939–42).

Topiramate + lithium *
Elevated and toxic lithium levels have been reported with higher (800mg/d) doses of topiramate, but not with 500mg/d (Pinninti and Zelinski, *J Clin Psychopharmacol* 2002;**22**:340; Abraham and Owen, *J Clin Psychopharmacol* 2004;**24**:565–7).

Tricyclics + lithium
See tricyclics (*4.3.1*).

Trimethoprim + lithium
Lithium toxicity has been reported following addition of trimethoprim (n=1, de Vries, *Ned Tijdschr Geneeskd* 2001;**145**:539–40).

Triptans + lithium
The literature notes an increased risk of CNS toxicity with sumatriptan.

Venlafaxine + lithium
See venlafaxine (*4.3.3.8*).

Warfarin + lithium
No interaction is suspected nor reported (mentioned in Sayal *et al*, *Acta Psychiatr Scand* 2000;**102**:250–5).

Ziprasidone + lithium
See ziprasidone (*4.2.8*).

4.5 ANTICONVULSANTS

Combining anticonvulsants is a common and essential strategy and so knowledge of interactions is vital, both when adding drugs (or increasing doses) or stopping drugs (or decreasing doses).

Reviews: detailed reviews of pharmacokinetic interactions between anticonvulsants (Tanaka, *J Clin Pharm Ther* 1999;**24**:87; Hachad *et al*, *Ther Drug Monit* 2002;**24**:91–103), anticonvulsant-OC interactions (Crawford, *CNS Drugs* 2002;**16**:263–72, which concludes that a woman taking carbamazepine, oxcarbazepine, phenobarbital, phenytoin or topiramate, would need an OC with at least 50mcg ethinylestradiol, or Depot Provera given every 10 weeks rather than 12), and anticonvulsants with other drugs (Patsalos and Perucca, *Lancet Neurol* 2003;**2**:473–81).

4.5.1 CARBAMAZEPINE *

Carbamazepine is principally metabolised by CYP3A4 (also CYP2C8), but is also a potent inducer of CYP3A4 and other oxidative mechanisms in the liver. This auto-induction takes up to four weeks to occur, although it is virtually complete after a week. Carbamazepine (CBZ) is metabolised to carbamazepine epoxide (CBZ-E), which may be more toxic than carbamazepine itself and so alteration of the CBZ:CBZ-E ratio by another drug would alter toxicity. Carbamazepine is extensively plasma protein-bound. Major diurnal variations in plasma levels occur, which can be as much as 90% during polytherapy compared to monotherapy (Hoppener *et al*, *Epilepsia* 1980;**21**:341–50).
Review: significant interactions (Spina *et al*, *Clin Pharmacokinet* 1996;**31**:198–214).

Acetazolamide + carbamazepine
CYP3A4 inhibition may raise carbamazepine levels (mentioned in Spina *et al*, *Clin Pharmacokinet* 1996;**31**:198–214).

Alcohol + carbamazepine
See alcohol (*4.7.1*).

Atorvastatin + carbamazepine *
Transient carbamazepine toxicity has been reported after combination with atorvastatin and roxithromycin (n=1, Corbin *et al*, *Therapie* 2004;**59**:267–9).

ANTIPSYCHOTICS + CARBAMAZEPINE *

Antipsychotics lower the seizure threshold, antagonising the anticonvulsant effects and there are also a variety of other well-documented interactions. Carbamazepine reduces haloperidol levels, with 240mg/d halving haloperidol levels (n=11, Yasui-Furukori *et al*, *J Clin Psychopharmacol* 2003;**23**:435–40), in a dose-dependent manner, resulting in worsening symptoms and outcome (eg. n=27, 4/52, Hesslinger *et al*, *J Clin Psychopharmacol* 1999;**19**:310–5). More importantly, a significantly extended QT interval has been shown, probably by increased haloperidol metabolite concentrations. Care is thus needed (n=2, Iwahashi *et al*, *Am J Psychiatry* 1996;**153**:135). Loxapine may raise CBZ-E levels, which may enhance toxicity, even with normal carbamazepine levels (n=1, Collins *et al*, *Ann Pharmacother* 1993;**27**:1180–3). There are cases of clozapine levels increasing by up to 100% after carbamazepine was stopped (Raitasuo *et al*, *Am J Psychiatry* 1993;**150**:169) and of neurotoxicity (n=1, Yerevanian and Hodgman, *Am J Psychiatry* 1985;**142**:785–6). There is also the very real enhanced risk of agranulocytosis (mandatory precaution in SPC), so carbamazepine and clozapine should not be used together (n=1, Gerson, *Lancet* 1991;**338**:262–3). Carbamazepine may halve plasma levels of risperidone and 9-hydroxyrisperidone, probably via 2D6 and 3A4 induction (n=34, Spina *et al*, *Ther Drug Monit* 2000;**22**:481–5; n=11, Ono *et al*, *Psychopharmacol (Berl)* 2002;**162**:50–4), and there are cases of EPSE after carbamazepine was discontinued from a combination with risperidone (n=2, Takahashi *et al*, *Clin Neuropharmacol* 2001;**24**:358–60). Alternatively, risperidone 1mg/d may increase steady-state carbamazepine levels by 10% over 24 hours and 20% over two weeks (n=8, Mula and Monaco, *Clin Neuropharmacol* 2002;**25**:97–100). Carbamazepine increases olanzapine clearance by 44% and reduces half-life by 20% (n=31+16, Linnet and Olesen, *Ther Drug Monit* 2002;**24**:512–7), probably by CYP1A2 induction, but dose adjustment is not needed as olanzapine has a wide therapeutic index (n=11, Lucas *et al*, *Eur J Clin Pharmacol* 1998;**54**:639–43). Toxic levels of CBZ-E (the toxic CBZ metabolite) raised 3–4-fold have been reported with concurrent quetiapine (n=2, Fitzgerald and Okos, *Pharmacother* 2002; **22**:1500–3). Carbamazepine 600–800mg/d decreases quetiapine plasma levels by 80%, presumably by CYP3A4 induction, a potentially clinically significant (n=18, Grimm *et al*, *Br J Clin Pharmacol* 2006;**61**:58–69; n=2, Hasselstrom and Linnet, *Ther Drug Monit* 2004;**26**:486–91). The Japanese SPC notes that carbamazepine may reduce zotepine levels, via CYP3A4 induction. Increased aripiprazole metabolism occurs through 3A4 induction and the aripiprazole dose should be doubled.

Benzodiazepines + carbamazepine
A large study concluded that concomitant clonazepam and carbamazepine results in a 22% increase in clonazepam clearance and a 20% decrease in carbamazepine clearance (n=183, Yukawa *et al*, *J Clin Psychopharmacol* 2001;**21**:588–93), so slightly higher benzodiazepine doses may be needed (Baba *et al*, *Br J Clin Pharmacol* 1990;**29**:766–9). Carbamazepine toxicity has occurred after the addition of clobazam (Genton *et al*, *Epilepsia* 1998;**39**:1115–8), probably related to progressive increases in norclobazam.

Bupropion + carbamazepine
See bupropion (4.6.6).

Caffeine + carbamazepine
Carbamazepine induces the CYP1A2 metabolism of caffeine (n=5, Parker *et al*, *Br J Clin Pharmacol* 1998;**45**:176–8).

CALCIUM-CHANNEL BLOCKERS + CARBAMAZEPINE
One study showed that **verapamil** increases carbamazepine plasma levels by 50%, via CYP3A4 inhibition (n=6, open, McPhee *et al*, *Lancet* 1986;i:700–3; n=43, open, Bahls *et al*, *Neurology* 1991;**41**:740–2). Other evidence, eg. with **diltiazem** (postoperative ophthalmoplegia and ataxia, n=1, Wijdicks *et al*, *J Neuroophthalmol* 2004;**24**:95) and verapamil suggests a substantial risk of toxicity. The antihypertensive effect of **nilvadipine** (n=1, Yasui-Furukori and Tateishi, *J Clin Pharmacol* 2002;**42**:100–3) and isradipine may be reduced. Since no interaction occurs with **nifedipine** (n=43, open, Bahls *et al*, *Neurology* 1991;**41**:740–2; n=1, Brodie and MacPhee, *Br Med J* 1986;**292**:1170–1), it is the calcium-channel blocker of choice with carbamazepine, although the BNF notes the efficacy of **nifedipine** may be reduced, so care is needed.

Charcoal, activated + carbamazepine
Carbamazepine absorption may be almost completely stopped if activated charcoal is given five minutes after ingestion, with a lesser effect if given after an hour (Neuvonen and Elonen, *Eur J Clin Pharmacol* 1980;**17**:51–7).

Chinese medicines + carbamazepine
Paeoniae Radix, a traditional Chinese medicine, may increase carbamazepine absorption (in rats, Chen *et al*, *Biol Pharm Bull* 2002;**25**:532–5).

CICLOSPORIN + CARBAMAZEPINE
Ciclosporin metabolism is accelerated by carbamazepine, to give reduced plasma levels.

Citalopram + carbamazepine
See citalopram/escitalopram (4.3.2.1).

Cocaine + carbamazepine
See cocaine (4.7.3).

CORTICOSTEROIDS + CARBAMAZEPINE
Corticosteroid CYP3A4 metabolism is accelerated by carbamazepine, giving a reduced effect (n=15, open, Bartoszek *et al*, *Clin Pharmacol Ther* 1987;**42**:424–32).

Clarithromycin + carbamazepine
See erythromycin + carbamazepine.

DANAZOL + CARBAMAZEPINE
Danazol inhibits carbamazepine metabolism to give an increased effect (n=6, open, Zielinski

et al, Ther Drug Monit 1987;**9**:24–7) so monitor levels and observe for side-effects.

Dantrolene + carbamazepine *

Carbamazepine toxicity has been reported when dantrolene and oxybutinin were added to a stable carbamazepine dose (n = 1, Vander *et al, Spinal Cord* 2005;**43**:252–5).

DEXTROPROPOXYPHENE + CARBAMAZEPINE

Dextropropoxyphene enhances carbamazepine toxicity via CYP3A4 inhibition (eg. *Neurology* 1987;**37**[Suppl 1]:87) and levels may rise by 44–77%. In one case, carbamazepine levels increased four-fold over 24 hours and led to cerebellar dysfunction, which resolved over 48 hours (n = 1, Allen, *Postgrad Med J* 1994;**70**:764). Monitor closely if used together, especially in the elderly (n = 84, open, Bergendal *et al, Eur J Clin Pharmacol* 1997;**53**:103–6).

Digoxin + carbamazepine

An isolated case exists of bradycardia with digitalis and carbamazepine but not with digoxin.

Disulfiram + carbamazepine

See disulfiram (4.6.8).

Diuretics + carbamazepine

Hyponatraemia may uncommonly occur with furosemide or thiazides (n = 2, Yassa *et al, J Clin Psychiatry* 1987;**48**:81–3; n = 1, Ranta and Wooten, *Epilepsia* 2004;**45**:879).

DOXYCYCLINE + CARBAMAZEPINE

Doxycycline metabolism is accelerated by carbamazepine, reducing efficacy and halving half-life (Penttila *et al, Br Med J* 1974;**2**:470–2). Other tetracyclines appear not to interact.

Enteral feeds + carbamazepine

Carbamazepine suspension absorption has been shown to be slightly slowed and reduced during nasogastric feeding (n = 8, RCT, c/o, Bass *et al, Epilepsia* 1989;**30**:364–9), so take care with dosing after enteral feeding is stopped.

Escitalopram + carbamazepine

See citalopram/escitalopram (4.3.2.1).

Ethosuximide + carbamazepine

See ethosuximide (4.5.2).

Etretinate + carbamazepine

One girl treated with the combination only responded to etretinate when her carbamazepine was withdrawn (n = 1, Mohammed, *Dermatology* 1992;**185**:79).

ERYTHROMYCIN + CARBAMAZEPINE

A rapid 100–200% rise in carbamazepine levels has been reported (n = 4, Wroblewski

et al, JAMA 1986;**255**:165–7; n = 1, Tatum and Gonzalez, *Hosp Pharm* 1994;**29**:45) and with IV erythromycin use (Mitsch, *Drug Intell Clin Pharm* 1989;**23**:878–9), probably via CYP3A4 inhibition. Monitor levels or use an alternative antibiotic. A review of the interaction concluded that the greatest risk is with high doses of both drugs, and least with clarithromycin (Pauwels, *Pharmacol Res* 2002;**45**:291–8).

Fluconazole + carbamazepine

Fluconazole-induced carbamazepine toxicity has been reported (n = 1, Nair and Morris, *Ann Pharmacother* 1999;**33**:790–2), with elevated CBZ levels (n = 1, Finch *et al, South Med J* 2002;**95**:1099–2000; Ulivelli *et al, J Neurol* 2004; **251**:622–3).

Gestrinone + carbamazepine

The UK SPC states that carbamazepine may reduce the activity of gestrinone.

Grapefruit juice + carbamazepine

300 ml grapefruit juice increased carbamazepine levels by 40% and AUC by 41%, probably by CYP3A4 inhibition in the gut wall and liver (n = 10, RCT, Garg *et al, Clin Pharmacol Ther* 1998; **64**:286–8).

Griseofulvin + carbamazepine

A reduced griseofulvin level by enzyme induction (*Am J Hosp Pharm* 1986;**16**:52) has been postulated.

H2-BLOCKERS + CARBAMAZEPINE

Studies have shown a transient 20% rise in carbamazepine levels with **cimetidine** (n = 8, open, 7/7, Dalton *et al, Epilepsia* 1986;**27**:553–8), reduced clearance, prolonged half-life (n = 12, open, 8/52, Webster *et al, Eur J Clin Pharmacol* 1984;**27**:341–3) and inhibition of non-renal elimination (n = 8, RCT, c/o, Dalton *et al, Epilepsia* 1985;**26**:127–30) via CYP3A4 inhibition. Studies show no interaction with **ranitidine** (eg. n = 8, RCT, Dalton *et al, Drug Intell Clin Pharm* 1985; **19**:941–4), which would thus appear a safer option.

Herbal tea + carbamazepine

For completeness, I thought you'd like to know that rats drinking herbal tea may have raised carbamazepine levels (Thabrew *et al, Drug Metabol Drug Interact* 2003;**19**:177–87).

Honey + carbamazepine

Yes, I was surprised when I saw this too, but you'll be relieved to find there is no interaction (n = 10, RCT, c/o, 1/52, Malhotra *et al, Methods Find Exp Clin Pharmacol* 2003;**25**:537–40).

Indinavir + carbamazepine

See protease inhibitors + carbamazepine.

Influenza vaccine + carbamazepine

A transient 10% increase in carbamazepine levels occurred in one study (n = 55, open, Jann and Fidone, *Clin Pharm* 1986;**5**:817–20) and there is a report of carbamazepine toxicity after influenza vaccination (Robertson, *Pediatr Neurol* 2002;**26**:61–3).

ISONIAZID + CARBAMAZEPINE

Rapid carbamazepine toxicity may occur via 3A4 inhibition by isoniazid in this potentially serious interaction (Valsalan and Cooper, *Br Med J* 1982;**285**:261–2). It may be potentiated by cimetidine (n = 1, Garcia *et al*, *Ann Pharmacother* 1992;**26**:841–2). Monitor carefully for toxicity.

Isotretinoin + carbamazepine

Isotretinoin may slightly reduce carbamazepine plasma levels and alter the CBZ:CBZ-E ratio (n = 1, Marsden *et al*, *Br J Dermatol* 1988;**119**: 403).

Itraconazole + carbamazepine

Sub-therapeutic itraconazole levels may occur with carbamazepine, so monitor for lack of efficacy (n = 12, open, Tucker *et al*, *Clin Infect Dis* 1992;**14**:165–74).

Lamotrigine + carbamazepine

See lamotrigine (4.5.4).

Levetiracetam + carbamazepine

See levetiracetam (4.5.5).

Levothyroxine (thyroxine) + carbamazepine

Levothyroxine metabolism is accelerated by carbamazepine, increasing the thyroxine requirements in hypothyroidism.

Lithium + carbamazepine

Although the combination is often used in rapid-cycling bipolar disorder, neurotoxicity may rarely occur without increased plasma levels (Marcoux, *Ann Pharmacother* 1996;**30**:547), and while this is mostly in patients with pre-existing brain damage (n = 5, Shukla *et al*, *Am J Psychiatry* 1984;**141**:1604–6), there is some evidence of minor cognitive impairment with the combination (*Hum Psychopharmacol* 1990;**5**:41–5). An additive anti-thyroid effect can occur, lowering T4 and free T4 levels (n = 23, open, Post *et al*, *Am J Psychiatry* 1990;**147**:615–20) and there is a case of lithium intoxication due to carbamazepine-induced renal failure (n = 1, Mayan *et al*, *Ann Pharmacother* 2001;**35**:560–2). Monitor carefully and regularly for signs of toxicity.

MAOIs + carbamazepine

See MAOIs (4.3.4).

Mefloquine + carbamazepine

The SPC states that mefloquine may antagonise the anticonvulsant effect of carbamazepine.

Methadone + carbamazepine

See methadone (4.6.10).

Methylphenidate + carbamazepine

See methylphenidate (4.6.11).

Metoclopramide + carbamazepine

There is a report of apparent carbamazepine neurotoxicity occurring after metoclopramide 30 mg/d was added, which resolved when metoclopramide was stopped (n = 1, Sandyk, *Br Med J* 1984;**288**:830).

Metronidazole + carbamazepine

Plasma carbamazepine levels rose by 60% in one case when metronidazole was added, resulting in symptoms of toxicity (n = 1, Patterson, *Ann Pharmacother* 1994;**28**:1304).

Mianserin + carbamazepine

See mianserin (4.3.3.2).

Miconazole + carbamazepine

An isolated case report of an adverse response has appeared (n = 1, *Therapie* 1982;**37**:437–41).

Mirtazapine + carbamazepine

See mirtazapine (4.3.3.3).

Modafinil + carbamazepine

See modafinil (4.6.12).

Neuromuscular blocking agents + carbamazepine

Studies show reduced responses and recovery times to NMBAs (*Anaesthesiology* 1989;**71**:A784), eg. vecuronium doses need to be significantly higher in patients on maintenance carbamazepine (n = 8, open, Whalley and Ebrahim, *Br J Anaesth* 1994;**72**:125–6) and recovery times can be 40–60% faster with atracurium and pancuronium (n = 53, open, Tempelhoff *et al*, *Anesth Analg* 1990;**71**:665–9).

NICOUMALONE + CARBAMAZEPINE

The metabolism of nicoumalone is accelerated by carbamazepine to give a reduced effect.

ORAL CONTRACEPTIVES + CARBAMAZEPINE

The CYP3A4 metabolism of OCs is accelerated by carbamazepine to give a **reduced contra-ceptive effect** (n = 10, open, Crawford *et al*, *Br J Clin Pharmacol* 1990;**30**:892–6). Any OC needs to contain at least 50 mcg ethinylestradiol or Depot Provera given every 10 rather than 12 weeks (review by Crawford, *CNS Drugs* 2002;

16:263–72) or alternative methods used. In the UK, one tablet each of Marvelon® and Mercilon® (Organon), or two tablets of Ovranette® (Wyeth) are often recommended as daily oral contraception.

Orlistat + carbamazepine
A small trial suggested lack of interaction (n = 8, open, 8/52, Hilger et al, J Clin Psychopharmacol 2002;**22**:68–70).

Oxcarbazepine + carbamazepine
See oxcarbazepine (4.5.6).

Oxybutynin + carbamazepine *
See dantrolene + carbamazepine.

Paracetamol + carbamazepine *
Co-administration with carbamazepine may reduce the bioavailability of paracetamol (UK SPC) and hepatotoxicity has been reported (n = 1, Parikh et al, Intern Med J 2004;**34**:441–2).

Paroxetine + carbamazepine
See paroxetine (4.3.2.4).

Phenobarbital + carbamazepine
Phenobarbital induces carbamazepine CYP3A4 metabolism, slightly reducing plasma levels (Christiansson and Dam, Acta Neurol Scand 1973;**49**:543–6). Carbamazepine may raise phenobarbital levels but not by a clinically significant amount (d/b, c/o, 4×21/7, Cereghino et al, Clin Pharmacol Ther 1975;**18**:733–41).

PHENYTOIN + CARBAMAZEPINE
Phenytoin induces carbamazepine CYP3A4 metabolism, reducing levels, often dramatically (eg. n = 2, Chapron et al, Drug Intell Clin Pharm 1993;**27**:708–11) but with some evidence of increased carbamazepine metabolites in the CSF (discussion by Morris et al, Neurology 1987;**37**:1111–8). Monitoring of CBZ levels is useful, although seizure control may not be affected. Raised carbamazepine levels may result from withdrawal of phenytoin via removal of enzyme induction (n = 2, Chapron et al, Ann Pharmacother 1993;**27**:708–11), so carbamazepine levels must be monitored during the de-induction stage to prevent toxicity developing. Raised phenytoin concentrations may occur due to CYP2C19 inhibition (Lakehal et al, Epilepsy Res 2002;**52**:79–83) and mean serum levels increase by 35% (some studies by up to 100%), producing neurotoxicity (Browne et al, Neurology 1988;**38**:1146–50). The clinical effect may be limited but best to monitor the levels of both drugs.

Pregabalin + carbamazepine
See pregabalin (4.5.10).

Probenecid + carbamazepine *
Probenecid has a minimal effect on carbamazepine kinetics, but can increase the proportion of CBZ-E via enzyme induction (n = 10, RCT, open, Kim et al, Eur J Clin Pharmacol 2005;**61**:275–80).

Progabide + carbamazepine
Progabide has no effect on carbamazepine levels (n = 24, open, Bianchett et al, Epilepsia 1987;**28**:68–73), but may slightly increase CBZ-E levels.

Protease inhibitors + carbamazepine *
The UK SPC notes the possibility of reduced plasma **indinavir**, **rotinavir** and **saquinavir** levels, probably by 3A4 inhibition. Carbamazepine toxicity has been reported when **lopinavir/ ritonavir** and then **nelfinavir** were added separately to carbamazepine, both increasing CBZ plasma levels by 53%, where reducing CBZ dose by 33% solved the problem (n = 1, Bates and Herman, Ann Pharmacother 2006;**40**:1190-5). Raised carbamazepine levels and toxicity (including hepatic) have been reported with ritonavir (n = 1, Kato et al, Pharmacother 2000; **20**:851–4; Antonio et al, Ann Pharmacother 2001;**35**:125–6).

PROTON-PUMP INHIBITORS + CARBAMAZEPINE
Carbamazepine induces the CYP3A4 metabolism of **omeprazole**, but has little or no effect on hydroxylation via CYP2C19 (n = 5, open, Bertilsson et al, Br J Clin Pharmacol 1997;**44**:186–9). Multiple dose omeprazole may decrease carbamazepine clearance by 40% and thus increase levels (Naidu et al, Drug Invest 1994;**7**:8–12). **Pantoprazole** appears to have no effect on carbamazepine (n = 20, RCT, Huber et al, Int J Clin Pharmacol Ther 1998;**36**:521–4).

RIFAMPIN + CARBAMAZEPINE
Rapid CYP3A4 induction may lower carbamazepine levels (n = 1, Zolezzi, Am J Psychiatry 2002;**159**:874).

Ritonavir + carbamazepine
See protease inhibitors + phenytoin.

Roxithromycin + carbamazepine *
See atorvastatin + carbamazepine.

Saquinavir + carbamazepine
See protease inhibitors + phenytoin.

SERTINDOLE + CARBAMAZEPINE
See sertindole (4.2.7).

Sertraline + carbamazepine
See sertraline (4.3.2.5).

Simvastatin + carbamazepine
Carbamazepine reduces the AUC for simvastatin by 75% and the peak by 68%, so increased simvastatin doses would be needed (n = 12, RCT, c/o, Ucar et al, Eur J Clin Pharmacol 2004;**59**:879–82).

Smoking + carbamazepine
See smoking (4.7.4).

St John's wort + carbamazepine
See St John's wort (4.3.3.9).

Stiripentol + carbamazepine
Stiripentol appears to be a potent inhibitor of CBZ-E formation (n = 14, Tran et al, Clin Pharmacol Ther 2002;**71**:33; Cazali et al, Br J Clin Pharmacol 2003;**56**:526–36).

Terfenadine + carbamazepine *
There is a case of raised CBZ levels leading to toxicity after starting terfenadine (n = 1, Naranjo = 6, Baath et al, Can J Clin Pharmacol 2006;**13**:228-31).

Theophylline + carbamazepine
Theophylline metabolism is accelerated by carbamazepine to give a reduced effect (Mitchell et al, N Z Med J 1986;**99**:69–70).

Thiazides + carbamazepine *
Hyponatremia has been reported with the combination (n = 1, Ranta and Wooten, Epilepsia 2004;**45**:879).

Tiagabine + carbamazepine
See tiagabine (4.5.11).

Tibolone + carbamazepine
The SPC states that carbamazepine may reduce the activity of tibolone.

Topiramate + carbamazepine
See topiramate (4.5.12).

Tramadol + carbamazepine
Carbamazepine may reduce the activity of tramadol.

Trazodone + carbamazepine
Raised carbamazepine levels have been reported with 100mg/d trazodone (n = 1, Romero et al, Ann Pharmacother 1999;**33**:1370).

TRICYCLICS + CARBAMAZEPINE
The CYP3A4 metabolism of imipramine, doxepin and amitriptyline may be accelerated by carbamazepine to give plasma levels reduced by 42–50% (eg. n = 29 + 22, Leinonen et al, J Clin Psychopharmacol 1991;**11**:313–8). This is a common combination and other evidence supports this to be a clinically significant, but

not well recognised, interaction. However, one study concluded that while the total blood concentration of imipramine drops with carbamazepine, the free fraction remains unchanged, so dose increases may not be necessary (n = 13, Szymura-Oleksiak et al, Psychopharmacology [Berl] 2001;**154**:38–42).

VALPROATE + CARBAMAZEPINE
Valproate seems to inhibit several carbamazepine metabolic pathways, resulting in raised CBZ-E concentrations (which has led to CBZ-E-induced psychosis, n = 1, McKee et al, Lancet 1989;i:167, and so watch closely for toxicity) but sometimes with unchanged carbamazepine levels (n = 27, Bernus et al, Br J Clin Pharmacol 1997;**44**:21). In one study, carbamazepine levels fell by about 25% when valproate was added (n = 7, open, Levy et al, Epilepsia 1984;**25**:338–45). Valproate may also displace carbamazepine from binding sites on plasma proteins (n = 8, open, Macphee, Br J Clin Pharmacol 1988;**25**:59–66). Conversely, carbamazepine induces valproate metabolism, reducing plasma levels by about 20% (n = 8, RCT, d/b, c/o, Larkin et al, Br J Clin Pharmacol 1989;**27**:313–22). This is probably minor but a mean 59% increase in valproate levels can occur on carbamazepine withdrawal (n = 6, open, Jann et al, Epilepsia 1988;**29**:578–81). Overall, no adjustments in carbamazepine doses are generally necessary, but, beware of the altered metabolite ratio and monitor if clinical symptoms change.

Venlafaxine + carbamazepine
See venlafaxine (4.3.3.8).

Vigabatrin + carbamazepine
See vigabatrin (4.5.14).

Vincristine + carbamazepine
Carbamazepine significantly increases the clearance of vincristine, probably by CYP3A4 induction (n = 15, open, Villikka et al, Clin Pharmacol Therapeut 1999;**66**:589–93).

WARFARIN + CARBAMAZEPINE *
The metabolism of warfarin is accelerated by carbamazepine, reducing efficacy. Warfarin doses may need to be doubled (n = 5 + 54, Herman et al, Eur J Clin Pharmacol 2006;**62**:291–6), monitored frequently and reduced carefully if carbamazepine is discontinued (n = 1, Denbow and Fraser, South Med J 1990;**83**:981).

Zaleplon + carbamazepine
See zaleplon (4.1.4).

Ziprasidone + carbamazepine
See ziprasidone (4.2.8).

Zonisamide + carbamazepine *
See zonisamide (4.5.15).

4.5.2 ETHOSUXIMIDE

Barbiturates + ethosuximide
See phenobarbital (4.5.7).

Carbamazepine + ethosuximide
Carbamazepine induces ethosuximide metabolism, reducing plasma levels by about 17% (n = 6, open, 55/7, Warren et al, Clin Pharmacol Ther 1980;**28**:646–51), although this is probably of minor significance.

Phenytoin + ethosuximide
Phenytoin may reduce ethosuximide plasma levels (n = 198, retrospective, Battion et al, Clin Pharmacokinet 1982;**7**:176–80).

Sodium oxybate + ethosuximide
See sodium oxybate (4.6.13).

Valproate + ethosuximide
Valproate may increase ethosuximide plasma levels by up to 50% via enzyme inhibition, although this may only be a transient effect (n = 6, Pisani et al, Epilepsia 1984;**25**:229–33), and standard regular monitoring will probably suffice. Adding ethosuximide to valproate may reduce valproate levels by 28% (n = 4) and stopping ethosuximide from an ethosuximide/valproate combination has led to valproate levels rising by 36% (n = 9). The mechanism is unknown (open, Salke-Kellermann et al, Epilepsy Res 1997;**26**:345–9).

Zotepine + ethosuximide
See anticonvulsants + zotepine (4.2.9).

4.5.3 GABAPENTIN

Gabapentin is not protein-bound so there is little chance of an interaction via this mechanism. Excretion is almost completely via the kidney.

Antacids + gabapentin
The antacid 'Maalox' reduces gabapentin levels by 20% when given concurrently. Separating the doses by two hours resulted in only a 5% reduction in levels (Busch et al, Epilepsia 1993;**34**[Suppl 2]:158), although nothing has been reported with other antacids.

Benzodiazepines + gabapentin
No significant interaction has been noted with

clonazepam (n = 127, d/b, p/c, UKGSG, Lancet 1990;**335**:1114–7).

Carbamazepine + gabapentin
No significant interaction has been noted (eg. n = 26, open, Radulovic et al, Epilepsia 1994; **35**:155–61).

Cimetidine + gabapentin
Cimetidine 1200 mg/d reduces gabapentin clearance by about 10%, which requires no dosage adjustment (Busch et al, Epilepsia 1993; **34**[Suppl 2]:158).

Levetiracetam + gabapentin
See levetiracetam (4.5.5).

Lithium + gabapentin
See lithium (4.4).

Oral contraceptives + gabapentin
No change in the kinetics of norethisterone and ethinylestradiol were seen with gabapentin (Busch et al, Epilepsia 1993;**34**[Suppl 2]:158).

Phenobarbital + gabapentin
One study showed no significant interaction (n = 12, open, 52/7, Hooper et al, Br J Clin Pharmacol 1991;**31**:171–4).

Phenytoin + gabapentin
Only a slight trend towards an increase in phenytoin levels has been observed (eg. Graves et al, Pharmacotherapy 1989;**9**:196) although toxic phenytoin levels have occurred with gabapentin 600 mg/d (eg. n = 1, Sanchez-Romero et al, Rev Neurol 2002;**34**:52–3).

Pregabalin + gabapentin
See pregabalin (4.5.10).

Valproate + gabapentin
No significant interaction has been noted (n = 127, d/b, p/c, UKGSG, Lancet 1990; **335**:1114–7).

Zotepine + gabapentin
See anticonvulsants + zotepine (4.2.7).

4.5.4 LAMOTRIGINE *

A large naturalistic study showed that lamotrigine levels are lower with co-medication with carbamazepine, ethinylestradiol, fluoxetine, lithium, phenytoin, phenobarbital and topiramate. No other antidepressants or any antipsychotics lowered levels (n = 829, Reimers et al, J Clin Psychopharmacol 2005;**25**:342–8).

Barbiturates + lamotrigine
Lamotrigine has no significant effect on primidone and phenobarbital (Epilepsia 1991;**32** [Suppl 1]:96).

Benzodiazepines + lamotrigine

Lamotrigine has no significant effect on clonazepam (*Epilepsia* 1991;**32**[Suppl 1]:96).

Bupropion + lamotrigine

In a small study, steady-state bupropion 300mg/d had no effect on a single 10mg dose of lamotrigine (n = 12, RCT, Odishaw and Chen, *Pharmacotherapy* 2000;**20**:1448–53).

Carbamazepine + lamotrigine *

A higher incidence of CNS side-effects has been noted with the combination (Gilman, *Ann Pharmacother* 1995;**29**:144–51). Toxicity appears more likely to occur when lamotrigine is added to CBZ if the initial CBZ level is high, eg. greater than 8mg/L, probably via a pharmacodynamic interaction (n = 47, open, Besag et al, *Epilepsia* 1998;**39**:183–7). However, lamotrigine does not seem to raise the levels of CBZ-E and, in fact, may reduce the levels of this active but toxic metabolite (n = 14, open, Eriksson and Boreus, *Ther Drug Monit* 1997;**19**:499–501). Carbamazepine reduces the half-life of lamotrigine from 29 hours to about 15 hours via enzyme induction (n = 23, open, 4/52, Jawad et al, *Epilepsia Res* 1987;**1**:194–201) with clinically important reductions in lamotrigine plasma concentrations reported with carbamazepine (Koch et al, *Eur Psychiatry* 2003;**18**:42). A case of serious lamotrigine rash has been reported after carbamazepine was stopped presumably as lamotrigine levels increased (n = 1, Surja et al, *J Clin Psychiatry* 2005;**66**:400–1) and there is a case of toxic epidermal necrolysis associated with concomitant use of these two drugs (n = 1, Mansouri et al, *Arch Dermatol* 2005;**141**:788–9).

Citalopram/escitalopram + lamotrigine *

See citalopram/escitalopram (*4.3.2.1*).

Clozapine + lamotrigine

See clozapine (*4.2.3*).

Fosphenytoin + lamotrigine

See phenytoin + lamotrigine.

Levetiracetam + lamotrigine

See levetiracetam (*4.5.5*).

Lithium + lamotrigine

See lithium (*4.4*).

LOPINAVIR/RITONAVIR (Kaletra®, Abbott) **+ LAMOTRIGINE ***

Kaletra® (Abbott) reduced lamotrigine levels by 55%, with a doubling of lamotrigine dose needed to compensate (n = 24, 31/7, van der Lee et al, *Clin Pharmacol Ther* 2006;**80**:159–68).

Oral contraceptives + lamotrigine *

The UK SPC was changed in June 2005 to include advice that lamotrigine reduces the effectiveness of hormonal contraceptives, and OCs may reduce lamotrigine serum levels (52% in AUC and 39% decrease in Cmax for Microgynon 30® (Schering Health); n = 7, Sabers et al, *Epilepsy Res* 2001;**47**:151–4). In women starting lamotrigine while on OCs, the normal dose escalation should be used. In women starting OCs while on lamotrigine, the maintenance dose of lamotrigine may need to be increased two-fold (unless also taking any drug inducing lamotrigine glucuronidation). In women stopping OCs, lamotrigine doses may need to be halved (unless also taking any drug inducing lamotrigine glucuronidation). In a controlled study, only the ethinylestradiol component of OCs reduced lamotrigine serum levels, but progestogens did not alter the levels (n = 45, Reimers et al, *Epilepsia* 2005;**46**:1414–7).

Oxcarbazepine + lamotrigine

See oxcarbazepine (*4.5.6*).

Phenytoin + lamotrigine *

Lamotrigine has no effect on phenytoin but phenytoin reduces the half-life of lamotrigine from 29 hours to about 15 hours via enzyme induction (n = 23, open, 4/52, Jawad et al, *Epilepsia Res* 1987;**1**:194–201) by increasing lamotrigine's clearance by 125% (n = 570, chart analysis, Weintraub et al, *Arch Neurol* 2005;**62**:1432–6).

Pregabalin + lamotrigine

See pregabalin (*4.5.10*).

Risperidone + lamotrigine *

See risperidone (*4.2.6*).

Sertraline + lamotrigine

Sertraline may increase lamotrigine levels, eg. sertraline 25mg/d doubled lamotrigine levels in one case and, in another, a 25mg/d dose reduction halved lamotrigine levels, despite a 33% lamotrigine dose increase (n = 2, Kaufman and Gerner, *Seizure* 1998;**7**:163–5).

Topiramate + lamotrigine

Topiramate does not cause a significant change in lamotrigine levels (n = 24, Berry et al, *Epilepsia* 2002;**43**:818–23) at standard doses (n = 13, open, 22/52, Doose et al, *Epilepsia* 2003; **44**:917–22).

VALPROATE + LAMOTRIGINE *

Lamotrigine generally has no significant effect on valproate levels (n = 372, open, Mataringa et al, *Ther Drug Monit* 2002;**24**:631–6). Valproate inhibits lamotrigine glucuronidation resulting in reduced clearance (by 21%), and half-life lengthening from 29 hours to about 59 hours (eg. Panay et al, Lancet 1993;**341**:445; n = 570, chart analysis, Weintraub et al, Arch Neurol 2005; **62**:1432–6), probably a dose-dependent (n = 28, open, Kanner and Frey, Neurology 2000;**55**:588–91) rather than concentration-dependent effect (n = 62, open, Gidal et al, Epilepsy Res 2000;**42**:23–31). Lamotrigine should thus start at half the usual dose when used with valproate. The interaction has been used to enhance the effect of both drugs with striking responses in adults and children with intractable epilepsy (Pisani et al, Lancet 1993;**341**:1224). Enhanced ADRs have been reported, eg. rash (n = 112, open, Faught et al, Epilepsia 1999;**40**:1135–40), disabling postural and action tremor (n = 3, Reutens et al, Lancet 1993;**342**:185–6), lupus (n = 1, Echaniz-Laguna et al, Epilepsia 1999;**40**:1661–3), delirium (n = 1, Mueller and Beeber, Am J Psychiatry 2004;**161**:1128–9) and toxic epidermal necrolysis (n = 1, Chang et al, Prog Neuropsychopharmacol Biol Psychiatry 2006;**30**:147–50).

Zotepine + lamotrigine

See anticonvulsants + zotepine (4.2.9).

4.5.5 LEVETIRACETAM

Levetiracetam has, as yet, no demonstrable drug interactions. It is not bound to plasma proteins, is not extensively metabolised and does not inhibit or induce CYP1A2, 2A6, 2C8/9/10, 2C19, 2D6, 2E1 and 3A4, nor UGT enzymes. A review concluding that there was no need to adjust levetiracetam doses if prescribed with any other AED (n = 590, Perucca et al, Epilepsy Res 2003;**53**:47–56).

Review: * Levetiracetam, serum levels and influence of dose and other drugs (n = 297, May et al, Ther Drug Monit 2003;**25**:690–9).

Alcohol + levetiracetam

No data is available.

Carbamazepine + levetiracetam

Lack of pharmacokinetic interaction has been shown, although disabling symptoms consistent with carbamazepine toxicity (but with unchanged levels) have been reported (n = 4, Sisodiya et al, Epilepsy Res 2002;**48**:217–9).

Digoxin + levetiracetam

Lack of pharmacokinetic interaction has been

demonstrated (n = 11, RCT, Levy et al, Epilepsy Res 2001;**46**:93–9).

Food + levetiracetam

Levetiracetam absorption is slightly slowed by food, but total absorption remains unchanged.

Gabapentin + levetiracetam

Lack of pharmacokinetic interaction has been demonstrated.

Lamotrigine + levetiracetam

Lack of pharmacokinetic interaction has been demonstrated.

Oral contraceptives + levetiracetam

Lack of pharmacokinetic interaction has been demonstrated (n = 18, RCT, d/b, c/o, Ragueneau et al, Epilepsia 2002;**43**:697–702).

Phenobarbital + levetiracetam

Lack of pharmacokinetic interaction has been demonstrated.

Phenytoin + levetiracetam

Levetiracetam has no effect on the kinetics of phenytoin (n = 6, open, Browne et al, J Clin Pharmacol 2000;**40**:590–5).

Probenecid + levetiracetam

Probenecid may inhibit the clearance of the primary (inactive) metabolite of levetiracetam, but not of the parent drug.

Valproate + levetiracetam

Lack of pharmacokinetic interaction has been demonstrated (n = 16, open, c/o, Coupez et al, Epilepsia 2003;**44**:171–8).

Warfarin + levetiracetam

Lack of pharmacokinetic interaction has been demonstrated (n = 42, RCT, Ragueneau-Majlessi et al, Epilepsy Res 2001;**47**:55–63).

Zotepine + levetiracetam

See anticonvulsants + zotepine (4.2.6).

4.5.6 OXCARBAZEPINE

Oxcarbazepine and its metabolite MHD inhibit CYP2C19 and induce 3A4 and 3A5 at higher doses (n = 4, open, Patsalos et al, Eur J Clin Pharmacol 1990;**39**:187–8), but probably not at lower doses (n = 8, Larkin et al, Br J Clin Pharmacol 1991;**31**:65–71).

Alcohol + oxcarbazepine

Caution should be exercised if alcohol is taken, as additive sedation can occur.

Antipsychotics + oxcarbazepine *

It should be well known that carbamazepine reduces the plasma levels of many antipsychotics.

However, as oxcarbazepine seems to have little enzyme-inducing activity, when substituted for carbamazepine, it can lead to plasma levels of some antipsychotics (eg. haloperidol, chlorpromazine and clozapine) increasing by 50–200% over 2–4 weeks (n = 6, Raitasuo et al, Psychopharmacology [Berl] 1994;**16**:115–6). Oxcarbazepine (up to 1200mg/d), however, may have no effect on olanzapine (n = 13) nor risperidone (n = 12) levels (5/52, Rosaria Muscatello et al, Epilepsia 2005;**46**:771–4).

Carbamazepine + oxcarbazepine
Addition of oxcarbazepine to carbamazepine has resulted in a 0–22% decrease in carbamazepine levels and a 40% reduction in MHD levels (UK SPC).

Ciclosporin + oxcarbazepine
Trough ciclosporin levels may fall slightly with oxcarbazepine (n = 1, Rosche et al, Clin Neuropharmacol 2001;**24**:113–6).

Cimetidine + oxcarbazepine
Cimetidine has no effect on the kinetics of oxcarbazepine (n = 8, c/o, Keranen et al, Acta Neurol Scand 1992;**85**:239–42).

Citalopram + oxcarbazepine
Carbamazepine may induce the plasma levels of citalopram, and when oxcarbazepine is substituted, citalopram plasma levels may rise (n = 2, Leinonen et al, Pharmacopsychiatry 1996; **29**:156–8).

Erythromycin + oxcarbazepine
Erythromycin has no effect on the kinetics of oxcarbazepine (n = 8, c/o, Keranen et al, Acta Neurol Scand 1992;**86**:120–3).

Escitalopram + oxcarbazepine
See citalopram above.

Felodipine + oxcarbazepine
Repeated doses of oxcarbazepine reduce felodipine AUC and plasma levels by 28% and 34% respectively, which might slightly reduce its clinical effect (n = 8, open, Zaccara et al, Ther Drug Monit 1993;**15**:39–42).

Fosphenytoin + oxcarbazepine
See phenytoin + oxcarbazepine.

Furosemide + oxcarbazepine
There is a case of acute encephalopathy with this combination (n = 1, Siniscalchi et al, Ann Pharmacother 2004;**38**:509–10).

Lamotrigine + oxcarbazepine *
There appears to be no significant interaction (n = 47, RCT, s/b, Theis et al, Neuropsychopharmacol

2005;**30**:2269–74), although ADRs may be more common and a retrospective review suggested that lamotrigine plasma levels may fall by 29% and that reduced lamotrigine doses may be necessary if oxcarbazepine is discontinued (n = 222, May et al, Therap Drug Monit 1999;**21**:175–81).

Lithium + oxcarbazepine
The combination of lithium and oxcarbazepine might theoretically cause enhanced neurotoxicity.

MAOIs + oxcarbazepine
A theoretical risk of interaction exists.

ORAL CONTRACEPTIVES + OXCARBAZEPINE
Oxcarbazepine can produce significant reductions in some OC plasma levels, with some breakthrough bleeding (n = 13, Klosterskov-Jensen et al, Epilepsia 1992;**33**:1149–52; n = 16, RCT, Fattore et al, Epilepsia 1999;**40**:783–7). Any OC needs to contain at least 50mcg ethinylestradiol, Depot Provera given every 10 rather than 12 weeks (review by Crawford, CNS Drugs 2002;**16**:263–72), or alternative methods used. In the UK, one tablet each of Marvelon® and Mercilon® (Organon), or two tablets of Ovranette® (Wyeth) are often recommended as daily oral contraception.

Phenobarbital + oxcarbazepine
Phenobarbital levels raised by 14% and reduced oxcarbazepine/MHD levels by 30% have been observed with the combination. The clinical significance has not been quantified.

Phenytoin + oxcarbazepine
Doses of oxcarbazepine above 1200mg/d have been reported to increase phenytoin levels by up to 40% (less than 10% for doses below 1200mg/d), probably due to CYP2C19 inhibition (microsomes, Lakehal et al, Epilepsy Res 2002;**52**:79–83) and so close monitoring of phenytoin is essential, especially at higher doses (n = 4, Patsalos et al, Eur J Clin Pharmacol 1990;**39**:187–8).

Propoxyphene + oxcarbazepine
Unlike carbamazepine, propoxyphene has no significant effect on oxcarbazepine kinetics (n = 8, open, Mogensen et al, Acta Neurol Scand 1992;**85**:14–7).

Valproate + oxcarbazepine
Valproate levels may rise if oxcarbazepine replaces carbamazepine (n = 4, Patsalos et al, Eur J Clin Pharmacol 1990;**39**:187–8). There is also a theoretical increase in the risk of teratogenicity, due to the presence of increased levels of metabolites.

Verapamil + oxcarbazepine

Verapamil can produce a 20% reduction in MHD levels, which could be clinically significant (UK SPC).

Warfarin + oxcarbazepine

Oxcarbazepine does not appear to affect the anticoagulant activity of warfarin (n = 10, 1/52, Kramer et al, Epilepsia 1992;**33**:1145–8).

Zotepine + oxcarbazepine

See anticonvulsants + zotepine (4.2.9).

4.5.7 PHENOBARBITAL AND PRIMIDONE

Alcohol + barbiturates

See alcohol (4.7.1).

ANTICOAGULANTS + BARBITURATES

A well-documented and clinically significant reduction in anticoagulant levels and effects occur with concurrent barbiturates. Doses of the anticoagulant may need to be raised by up to 60% if a barbiturate is started.

ANTIPSYCHOTICS + BARBITURATES

See antipsychotics (4.2.1) and quetiapine (4.2.5).

Benzodiazepines + barbiturates

See benzodiazepines (4.1.1).

Beta-blockers + barbiturates

Blood levels of metoprolol and propranolol are reduced by barbiturates (open, Seideman et al, Br J Clin Pharmacol 1987;**23**:267–71), but timolol (n = 12, RCT, c/o, Mantyla et al, Eur J Clin Pharmacol 1983;**24**:227–30), atenolol and nadolol do not appear to be affected.

Bupropion + phenobarbital

See bupropion (4.6.6).

CALCIUM-CHANNEL BLOCKERS + BARBITURATES

Phenobarbital may induce the CYP3A4 metabolism of verapamil (open, Rutledge et al, J Pharmacol Exp Therap 1988;**246**:7–13), diltiazem, isradipine, nicardipine and nifedipine, reducing efficacy and so some care may be needed.

Carbamazepine + phenobarbital

See carbamazepine (4.5.1).

Charcoal, activated + barbiturates

If given within five minutes, activated charcoal can almost completely prevent barbiturate absorption and can be an effective adjunct in overdose treatment (Neuvonen and Elonen, Eur J Clin Pharmacol 1980;**17**:51–7).

Chloramphenicol + barbiturates

Chloramphenicol metabolism is accelerated by barbiturates to reduce oral chloramphenicol efficacy (n = 1, Koup et al, Clin Pharmacol Ther 1978;**24**:571–5).

CICLOSPORIN + PHENOBARBITAL

Even low dose phenobarbital induces the CYP3A4 metabolism of ciclosporin (Carstensen, et al, Br J Clin Pharmacol 1986;**21**:550–1).

Cimetidine + phenobarbital

Reduced actions of both can occur but this is of very limited significance (n = 8, open, 6/52, Somogyi et al, Eur J Clin Pharmacol 1981;**19**:343).

Clozapine + phenobarbital

See clozapine (4.2.3).

CORTICOSTEROIDS + PHENOBARBITAL

CYP3A4 induction reduces the effect of some corticosteroids (Brooks et al, NEJM 1972; **286**:1125–8).

Digoxin + phenobarbital

Digitoxin (but not digoxin) levels can be reduced by up to 50% by phenobarbital, probably via enzyme induction and of little significance (Kaldor et al, Int J Clin Pharmacol Biopharm 1975; **12**:403–7).

Disopyramide + phenobarbital

Barbiturates induce the CYP3A4 metabolism of disopyramide, reducing plasma levels (n = 14, open, Kapil et al, Br J Clin Pharmacol 1987;**24**: 781–91).

Doxorubicin + phenobarbital

Indirect results from one study showed that doxorubicin clearance may be increased by barbiturates and so doses may need to be increased (Riggs et al, Clin Pharmacol Ther 1982; **31**:263).

Doxycycline + phenobarbital

Doxycycline levels are reduced via CYP3A4 induction, reducing its effect, with a halved half-life (Neuvonen and Penttila, Br Med J 1974;**2**:535–6). Other tetracyclines appear not to interact.

Ethosuximide + phenobarbital

A possible interaction may lead to reduced phenobarbital effectiveness. A study showed that ethosuximide levels may fall if primidone is used (n = 198, Battino et al, Clin Pharmacokinet 1982;**7**:176–80).

Fenoprofen + phenobarbital

Phenobarbital may slightly increase fenoprofen metabolism and reduce its efficacy (Helleberg et al, Br J Clin Pharmacol 1974;**1**:371).

Furosemide + phenobarbital

One study showed no effect of barbiturates on furosemide diuresis (n = 10, open, Lambert et al,

Clin Pharmacol Ther 1983;**34**:170–5).

Gabapentin + phenobarbital
See gabapentin (*4.5.3*).

Glyceryl trinitrate + phenobarbital
A reduced nitrate effect via enzyme induction may occur.

Griseofulvin + phenobarbital
Cases have been reported of griseofulvin levels reduced by up to 45% by phenobarbital, either by enzyme induction (eg. *Am J Hosp Pharm* 1986;**16**:52) or reduced absorption.

Indinavir + barbiturates
The plasma levels of indinavir may be reduced by barbiturates via CYP3A4 induction.

Influenza vaccine + phenobarbital
A transient 20% rise in barbiturate levels has been reported (n = 35, open, Jann and Fidone, *Clin Pharm* 1986;**5**:817–20).

Isoniazid + primidone
Steady state primidone levels rose by 80% in a patient given isoniazid 300 mg/d (n = 1, Sutton and Kupferberg, *Neurology* 1975;**25**:1179–81). Blood levels should be monitored.

Ketoconazole + phenobarbital
A case exists of reduced ketoconazole levels in a man taking phenobarbital (n = 1, *Antimicrob Ag Chemother* 1982;**21**:151–8).

Lamotrigine + barbiturates
See lamotrigine (*4.5.4*).

Levetiracetam + phenobarbital
See levetiracetam (*4.5.5*).

Levonorgestrel + phenobarbital
There is a case of a levonorgestrel implant (Norplant) failing twice in a woman also taking phenobarbital (Shane-McWhorter et al, *Pharmacotherapy* 1998;**18**:1360–4).

Levothyroxine (thyroxine) + barbiturates
Levothyroxine metabolism is accelerated by barbiturates to give a reduced effect and this may increase requirements in hypothyroidism.

Lidocaine + barbiturates
Serum lidocaine levels may be lower in people taking barbiturates than in those not (LeLorier, *Toxicol Appl Pharmacol* 1978;**44**:657), via CYP3A4 induction.

MAOIs + barbiturates
See MAOIs (*4.3.4*).

Memantine + barbiturates
See memantine (*4.6.9*).

Methadone + barbiturates
See methadone (*4.6.10*).

Methyldopa + phenobarbital
Methyldopa levels are not reduced by phenobarbital (Kristensen et al, *Br Med J* 1973;**1**:49).

Metronidazole + phenobarbital
One study showed metronidazole metabolism to be accelerated by barbiturates, reducing levels by a third (*Clin Pharmacol Ther* 1987;**41**:235).

Modafinil + phenobarbital
See modafinil (*4.6.12*).

Nicotinamide + primidone
There are reports of reduced conversion from primidone to phenobarbital (n = 1, Bourgeois et al, *Neurology* 1982;**32**:1122).

NICOUMALONE + BARBITURATES
Nicoumalone metabolism is accelerated by barbiturates, giving a reduced anticoagulant effect.

ORAL CONTRACEPTIVES + PHENOBARBITAL
Contraceptive failure via CYP3A4 induction is well-established (eg. n = 5, Back et al, *Contraception* 1980;**22**:495–503). Use higher dose OC (equivalent to at least 50 mcg ethinylestradiol), Depot Provera given every 10 rather than 12 weeks (Crawford, *CNS Drugs* 2002;**16**:263–72) and adjust the dose if necessary, or use alternative contraceptive methods. See also levonorgestrel. In the UK, one tablet each of Marvelon® and Mercilon® (Organon) or two tablets of Ovranette® (Abbott) are often recommended as daily oral contraception.

Oxcarbazepine + phenobarbital
See oxcarbazepine (*4.5.6*).

Paracetamol + phenobarbital
An isolated case of enhanced hepatotoxicity exists (Pirotte, *Ann Int Med* 1984;**101**:403).

Paroxetine + phenobarbital
See paroxetine (*4.3.2.4*).

Pethidine + phenobarbital
Severe CNS sedation with the combination has been reported (n = 12, open, c/o, Stambaugh et al, *J Clin Pharmacol* 1978;**18**:482–90).

Phenylbutazone + phenobarbital
Reduced levels of phenylbutazone may occur (Levi et al, *Lancet* 1968;i:1275).

Phenytoin + phenobarbital
See barbiturates + phenytoin (*4.5.8*).

Pregabalin + phenobarbital
See pregabalin (*4.5.10*).

Pyridoxine + phenobarbital
Large doses of pyridoxine (eg. 200 mg/d) can reduce phenobarbital levels by up to 40–50% (Hansson and Sillanpaa, *Lancet* 1976;i:256).

Quetiapine + barbiturates
See quetiapine (4.2.5).

Quinidine + phenobarbital
CYP3A4 induction may reduce quinidine levels by up to 50% (Rogers and Blackman, *Drug Intell Clin Pharm* 1983;**17**:819–20).

Rifampin + barbiturates
Rifampin can induce barbiturate metabolism, so a decreased efficacy might be predicted (for effect on hexobarbital: n = 40, open, See Richter *et al*, *Eur J Clin Pharmacol* 1980;**17**:197–202).

Smoking + phenobarbital
See smoking (4.7.3).

St John's wort + phenobarbital
See St John's wort (4.3.3.9).

Testosterone + phenobarbital
A reduced steroid effect can occur via CYP3A4 induction.

THEOPHYLLINE + BARBITURATES
Theophylline metabolism is accelerated by barbiturates in premature neonates, giving a reduced effect (n = 24, Kandrokas *et al*, *Ther Drug Monit* 1990;**12**:139–43).

Tiagabine + phenobarbital
See tiagabine (4.5.11).

Topiramate + phenobarbital
See topiramate (4.5.12).

TRICYCLICS + BARBITURATES
See tricyclics (4.3.1).

Tropisetron + barbiturates
Phenobarbital reduces the plasma levels of tropisetron (BNF).

WARFARIN + PHENOBARBITAL
See anticoagulants + barbiturates in this section.

VALPROATE + PHENOBARBITAL
Valproate may reduce glucuronidation and increase phenobarbital plasma concentrations by up to 25% (mean of 5.87 mg/L, n = 20, Bernus *et al*, *Br J Clin Pharmacol* 1994;**38**:411–6), increasing sedation and other side-effects (eg. Kapetanovic *et al*, *Clin Pharmacol Ther* 1981;**99**:314), although this may only be transient (review by Keys, *Drug Intell Clin Pharm* 1982;**16**:737–9). Reduce phenobarbital dosage if sedation occurs, and monitor blood levels regularly.

Vigabatrin + phenobarbital
See vigabatrin (4.5.14).

Zaleplon + phenobarbital
See zaleplon (4.1.4).

Zotepine + phenobarbital
See anticonvulsants + zotepine (4.2.9).

4.5.8 PHENYTOIN *

Phenytoin has a narrow therapeutic index and is prone to drug-drug interactions via several mechanisms. It is primarily metabolised by 2C9, secondary is 2C19, with genetic polymorphism affecting levels. It is extensively bound to plasma proteins, induces CYP3A4 and has a saturable metabolism. It can be displaced, giving an increased proportion of free active phenytoin, significant where TDM just measures total phenytoin rather than the proportion of free (hence active) phenytoin. Measuring free phenytoin levels may be more appropriate in certain circumstances, eg. interactions with drugs displacing it from binding sites, as well as hypoalbuminaemia and renal failure, eg. total plasma levels may be within the alleged therapeutic range. Decreased protein binding produces a decline in total concentration, but no change in free levels (Wilkinson, *Pharmacol Rev* 1987;**39**:1–47).

Thus, low concentrations may appear below the normal therapeutic range, but free (active) levels are appropriate, prompting inappropriately increased doses or discontinuation. More usual concentrations could have toxic (seizure-inducing) free levels, which might then provoke an increase in dosage to bring it into the 'optimum' range (see Toler, *Ann Pharmacother* 1994;**28**:808–9).

Review: pharmacokinetic interactions (Nation *et al*, *Clin Pharmacokinet* 1990;**18**:37–60).

Acetazolamide + phenytoin
Case reports indicate that acetazolamide may enhance the osteomalacia secondary to phenytoin use in a few patients (n = 2, Mallette, *Arch Intern Med* 1977;**137**:1013).

ALCOHOL + PHENYTOIN
See alcohol (4.7.1).

Allopurinol + phenytoin
Phenytoin toxicity may occur with repeated high-dose allopurinol (Ogiso *et al*, *J Pharmacobiodyn* 1990;**13**:36–43).

AMIODARONE + PHENYTOIN
Amiodarone reduces phenytoin metabolism, toxicity developing over two weeks (n = 7, open, 8/52, Nolan *et al*, *Am J Cardiol* 1990;**65**:1252–7), so reduce the phenytoin dose by at least 25%.

Anaesthetics + phenytoin
Documentation of an interaction is limited but case reports exist of phenytoin toxicity following

halothane (Karlin and Kutt, *J Pediatr* 1970;**76**:941–4) and so caution is needed.

Antacids + phenytoin

Antacids probably reduce phenytoin levels, shown in several studies (eg. n=6, McElnay *et al*, *Br J Clin Pharmacol* 1982;**13**:501) and seizure control could be impaired. It is thus best to separate doses by about three hours or use ranitidine (see also cimetidine).

ANTIPSYCHOTICS + PHENYTOIN

See antipsychotics *(4.2.1)*, clozapine *(4.2.3)*, quetiapine *(4.2.5)*, risperidone *(4.2.6)* and zotepine *(4.2.9)*.

Atomoxetine + phenytoin

See atomoxetine *(4.6.4)*.

Ayurvedic herbal mixtures + phenytoin

See shankhapushpi + phenytoin.

Barbiturates + phenytoin

At normal doses it is thought that phenobarbital induces the metabolism of phenytoin, reducing plasma levels, but the clinical effect is probably minimal (n=6, open, Browne *et al*, *Neurology* 1988;**38**:639–42). Phenytoin serum levels are increased by very high dose barbiturates and the effect may be dose-dependent with a curvilinear relationship (n=1, Kuranari *et al*, *Ann Pharmacother* 1995;**29**:83–4). Care is also needed if phenobarbital is stopped, as phenytoin levels may change. Phenytoin may raise phenobarbital levels by up to 100%, resulting in increased sedation, probably of minor clinical significance (n=1, Porro *et al*, *Br J Clin Pharmacol* 1982;**14**:294–7) but regular monitoring should still be done, especially as a case of fatal agranulocytosis has been reported with the combination (n=1, Laurenson *et al*, *Lancet* 1994;**344**:32–3).

Benzodiazepines + phenytoin

Diazepam, clonazepam and chlordiazepoxide have been reported to potentiate phenytoin leading to possible intoxication (eg. n=1, Murphy and Wilbur, *Ann Pharmacother* 2003;**37**:659–63), although some studies have not shown this effect. It is best to monitor phenytoin plasma levels regularly. Conversely, phenytoin induces the metabolism of clonazepam, reducing levels by up to 50% (n=27, open, Sjo *et al*, *Eur J Clin Pharmacol* 1975;**8**:249–54).

Bupropion + phenytoin

See bupropion *(4.6.6)*.

Buspirone + phenytoin

See buspirone *(4.1.2)*.

Calcium-channel blockers + phenytoin

High dose **diltiazem** (240 mg TDS) increases phenytoin levels and toxicity, and in one patient a 40% reduction in phenytoin dose was needed to stabilise levels (n=2, Clarke *et al*, *Pharmacotherapy* 1993;**13**:402–5; n=43, Bahls *et al*, *Neurology* 1991;**41**:740–2). **Isradipine** can raise phenytoin levels, producing toxicity probably by P450 inhibition (n=1, Cachat and Tufro, *Ann Pharmacother* 2002;**36**:1399–402). Lack of interaction between **nifedipine** and phenytoin has been noted in several studies (eg. n=8, open, Schellens *et al*, *Br J Clin Pharmacol* 1991;**31**:175–8), although tremor, headache and restlessness with phenytoin levels tripled has been reported, falling to normal after nifedipine was discontinued (n=1, Ahmad *et al*, *J Am Coll Cardiol* 1984;**3**:1581). Verapamil may inhibit phenytoin metabolism (*Neurology* 1991;**41**:740–2). Almost complete lack of **verapamil** absorption (at up to 400 mg/d) has been reported (n=1, Woodcock *et al*, *N Engl J Med* 1991;**325**:1179). The effects of isradipine and nicardipine may be reduced by phenytoin.

CARBAMAZEPINE + PHENYTOIN

See carbamazepine *(4.5.1)*.

Charcoal, activated + phenytoin

Phenytoin absorption is almost completely (98%) prevented if activated charcoal is taken within five minutes and reduced by about 80% if given after one hour (n=6, open, c/o, Neuvonen *et al*, *Eur J Clin Pharmacol* 1978;**13**:213–8). Multiple-dose activated charcoal has been used successfully over several days for phenytoin toxicity secondary to hepatitis and, extraordinarily, may have some use even up to a week after phenytoin ingestion (n=1, Howard *et al*, *Ann Pharmacother* 1994;**28**:201–3).

Chinese medicines + phenytoin

Phenytoin poisoning after using Chinese proprietary medicines has been reported (n=1, Lau *et al*, *Hum Experimental Toxicol* 2000;**19**:385–6).

Chloral + phenytoin

Dichloralphenazone has been shown to decrease phenytoin levels (n=5, Riddell *et al*, *Br J Clin Pharmacol* 1980;**9**:118P), although whether the chloral part of the molecule was responsible for this is not known.

CHLORAMPHENICOL + PHENYTOIN

Phenytoin toxicity may occur with oral chloramphenicol via enzyme inhibition (*Aust J Hosp Pharm* 1987;**17**:51–3). This is an uncommon combination but a well-documented and serious interaction. Monitor very carefully if the combination has to be used.

Chlorphenamine + phenytoin

Two isolated cases exist of phenytoin intoxication (Pugh et al, Br J Clin Pharmacol 1975;**2**:173–5) and so care may be needed.

CICLOSPORIN + PHENYTOIN

Ciclosporin levels can be reduced by 80% by phenytoin, via increased metabolism (n = 6, Freeman et al, Br J Clin Pharmacol 1984;**18**:887–93).

Ciprofloxacin + phenytoin

Phenytoin toxicity would be expected to occur via P450 enzyme inhibition. Raised phenytoin levels from oral ciprofloxacin have been reported (n = 1, Hull, Ann Pharmacother 1993;**27**:1283). However, IV ciprofloxacin has led to halved phenytoin levels (n = 1, Int Pharm J 1992;**6**:109), and resulted in sub-therapeutic levels, seizures and increased phenytoin dose requirements (Dillard et al, Ann Pharmacother 1992;**26**:263; n = 1, Brouwers and de Boer, Ann Pharmacother 1997;**31**:498). There is a case of a phenytoin dose increased during ciprofloxacin therapy, only for toxic levels to appear when the antibiotic course was completed (n = 1, Pollak and Slayter, Ann Pharmacother 1997;**31**:61–4). More frequent phenytoin plasma level monitoring would be wise.

Clinafloxacin + phenytoin

Higher steady state phenytoin levels have been reported with clinafloxacin (Randinitis et al, Drugs 1999;**58**[Suppl 2]:254–5).

CLOZAPINE + PHENYTOIN

See clozapine (4.2.3).

CORTICOSTEROIDS + PHENYTOIN

Steroid metabolism is accelerated by phenytoin to give a reduced effect (McLelland and Jack, Lancet 1978;i:1096–7) and so higher doses may be needed. Hydrocortisone may be less affected than other steroids. Phenytoin levels may also be changed.

Co-trimoxazole + phenytoin

Raised phenytoin levels have been reported with co-trimoxazole (n = 1, Gillman and Sandyk, Arch Intern Med 1985;**102**:559).

DEXAMETHASONE + PHENYTOIN

Phenytoin levels may be halved by dexamethasone (eg. n = 1, Lackner, Pharmacother 1991;**11**:344–7; n = 1, Griffiths and Taylor, Can J Hosp Pharm 1999;**52**:96–8) and very high doses of phenytoin may be necessary (eg. 900mg/d) to maintain

levels (case and review by Recueno et al, Ann Pharmacother 1995;**29**:935). Regular and frequent monitoring of phenytoin levels is thus essential.

Dextropropoxyphene + phenytoin

See propoxyphene + phenytoin.

DIAZOXIDE + PHENYTOIN

Reduced phenytoin levels occur via increased metabolism (Turck et al, Presse Med 1986;**15**:31) so monitor carefully.

DICOUMAROL + PHENYTOIN

Phenytoin levels may rise rapidly by over 100% (Hansen et al, Acta Med Scand 1971;**189**:15–9) via enzyme inhibition. Avoid the combination if at all possible or monitor very carefully.

Digoxin + phenytoin

Phenytoin reduces digoxin half-life by 30% (n = 6, RCT, open, c/o, Rameis et al, Eur J Clin Pharmacol 1985;**29**:49–53) so monitor both carefully.

DISOPYRAMIDE + PHENYTOIN

Phenytoin reduces the plasma levels of disopyramide, possibly to below therapeutic levels (Kessler et al, Clin Pharm 1982;**1**:263–4).

Disulfiram + phenytoin

Phenytoin toxicity and delirium may occur via enzyme inhibition (eg. n = 1, Brown et al, Ann Emerg Med 1983;**12**:310–3).

Dopamine + phenytoin

Hypotension may occur in patients on dopamine if phenytoin is added (n = 5, Bivins et al, Arch Surg 1978;**113**:245–9), although lack of interaction has been reported in a well studied case (n = 1, Torres et al, Ann Pharmacother 1995;**29**:1300–1).

Doxifluridine + phenytoin

Elevated phenytoin levels have been reported (n = 1, Konishi et al, Ann Pharmacother 2002; **36**: 831–4).

DOXYCYCLINE + PHENYTOIN

Doxycycline metabolism is accelerated by phenytoin to give a reduced effect, with a halved half-life (Penttila et al, Br Med J 1974;ii:470). Other tetracyclines appear not to interact, so make dosage adjustments or use an alternative.

Enteral feeds + phenytoin

See nasogastric feeds + phenytoin.

Ethosuximide + phenytoin

See ethosuximide (4.5.2).

FLUCONAZOLE + PHENYTOIN

Oral fluconazole inhibits phenytoin metabolism producing rapid and severe toxicity (Mitchell and Holland, Br Med J 1989;**298**:1315; reviewed by Cadle et al, Ann Pharmacother 1994;**28**:191–5).

Continuous phenytoin plasma monitoring is recommended with doses of fluconazole at 200 mg/d or above (n = 20, RCT, p/c, Blum et al, Clin Pharmacol Ther 1991;**49**:420–5).

Fluorouracil + phenytoin

Cases exist of elevated phenytoin levels 11 weeks after starting fluorouracil and leucovorin, possibly via CYP2C9 inhibition (n = 1, Gilbar and Brodribb, Ann Pharmacother 2001;**35**:1367–70; n = 1, Rosemergy and Findlay, N Z Med J 2002; **115**:U124).

FLUVOXAMINE + PHENYTOIN

Fluvoxamine may triple phenytoin levels with associated toxicity, probably by 2C9/19 inhibition (n = 1, Mamiya et al, Ther Drug Monit 2001;**23**:75–7).

FLUOXETINE + PHENYTOIN

Phenytoin levels raised by 66% have been reported two weeks after fluoxetine was added, with levels falling back to nearly normal within a week of stopping fluoxetine (n = 1, Woods et al, N Z Med J 1994;**107**:19). Conversely, loss of phenytoin efficacy as a result of fluoxetine discontinuation has been reported (n = 1, Shad and Preskorn, J Clin Psychopharmacol 1999; **19**:471).

Folic acid + phenytoin

Serum folate decreases when phenytoin is started and folic acid supplementation is usually used to counteract this folate deficiency. However, folic acid supplementation in folate-deficient patients changes the kinetics of phenytoin and plasma phenytoin levels are then reduced (n = 4, open, Berg et al, Ther Drug Monit 1983;**5**:389–99). Folate supplementation should thus be started with phenytoin. If started later, phenytoin levels should be monitored and changes in seizure activity looked for (extensive review by Lewis et al, Ann Pharmacother 1995;**29**:726–35).

Furosemide + phenytoin

The diuretic effect may be reduced by up to 50% by phenytoin (eg. Bissoli et al, Recenti Prog Med 1996;**87**:227–8) so larger doses may be needed.

Gabapentin + phenytoin

See gabapentin (4.5.3).

Gingko biloba + phenytoin *

There is a case of a fatal seizure with the combination, probably due to reduced phenytoin levels via CYP2C19 induction (n = 1, Kupiec and Raj, J Anal Toxicol 2005;**29**:755–8).

Glucagon + phenytoin

Patients on phenytoin may get false negatives with glucagon stimulation tests.

Glucocorticoids + phenytoin

A reduced steroid effect via enzyme induction is possible.

Griseofulvin + phenytoin

It is postulated that reduced griseofulvin levels may occur, via enzyme induction (Am J Hosp Pharm 1986;**16**:52).

H2-blockers + phenytoin

Phenytoin toxicity has occurred with cimetidine (n = 1, Phillips and Hansky, Med J Aus 1984; **141**:602), with a 30% increase in phenytoin levels in other reports (Pharm Int 1985;**6**:223–4; n = 9, open, Salem et al, Epilepsia 1983;**24**:284–8) and so toxicity may occur, even with OTC cimetidine (n = 9, Rafi et al, Ann Pharmacother 1999;**33**:769–74). The effect is rapid and can occur within two days. An alternative is ranitidine, where lack of interaction has been shown (eg. Watts et al, Br J Clin Pharmacol 1983;**15**:499–500). There have been reports of elevated phenytoin levels with ranitidine (eg. Tse et al, Ann Pharmacother 1993;**27**:1448–51), including one case where oral ranitidine produced toxic phenytoin levels, which remained high for a week even though the phenytoin was stopped, and only dropped when the ranitidine was also stopped (Tse and Iagmin, Ann Intern Med 1994;**120**:892–3). It is best to monitor phenytoin levels or use an alternative, eg. famotidine (n = 10, RCT, open, c/o, Sambol et al, Br J Clin Pharmacol 1989;**27**:83–7) or nizatidine (Bachmann et al, Br J Clin Pharmacol 1993;**36**:380–2).

Indinavir + phenytoin

Plasma indinavir levels may be reduced by phenytoin (BNF).

Influenza vaccine + phenytoin

This is reported to reduce total and free phenytoin levels (Smith et al, Clin Pharm 1988;**7**:828–32), although one study showed only a transient 60% increase in levels (Jann and Fidone, Clin Pharm 1986;**5**:817–20).

Irinotecan + phenytoin

Phenytoin appears to decrease plasma levels of irinotecan (Murry et al, J Pediatr Hematol Oncol 2002;**24**:130–3).

ISONIAZID + PHENYTOIN

Phenytoin toxicity may occur via enzyme induction (n = 1, Witmer and Ritschel, Drug Intell Clin Pharm 1984;**18**:483–6) so observe for toxicity and reduce phenytoin doses if necessary.

KETOCONAZOLE + PHENYTOIN
Phenytoin toxicity may occur via enzyme inhibition. Ketoconazole may also have a reduced effect.

Lamotrigine + phenytoin
See lamotrigine (4.5.4).

Levetiracetam + phenytoin
See levetiracetam (4.5.5).

Levodopa + phenytoin
Levodopa can be completely antagonised by phenytoin (Mendez et al, Arch Neurol 1975; 32:44–6), and so increased levodopa doses may be necessary.

Levothyroxine (thyroxine) + phenytoin
Levothyroxine metabolism is accelerated by phenytoin, increasing requirements (Blackshear et al, Ann Int Med 1983;99:341–2).

Lidocaine + phenytoin
Phenytoin's CNS effects may be enhanced if used concurrently (Karlsson et al, Eur J Clin Pharmacol 1974;7:455–9). Sinoatrial arrest has been reported (Wood, Br Med J 1971;i:645) which was reversed by isoproterenol. The mechanism is probably enhanced cardiac depression.

Lithium + phenytoin
See lithium (4.4).

Lopinavir + phenytoin
Phenytoin increases lopinavir clearance, and lopinavir and ritonavir reduce phenytoin levels through 2C9 induction (n = 24, Lim et al, J Acquir Immune Defic Syndr 2004;36:1034–40).

Losartan + phenytoin
Losartan has no effect on phenytoin, but losartan levels may rise via 2C9 inhibition (n = 16, RCT, c/o, Fischer et al, Clin Pharmacol Ther 2002; 72:238–46).

Memantine + phenytoin
See memantine (4.6.9).

Methadone + phenytoin
See methadone (4.6.10).

Methotrexate + phenytoin
An increased antifolate effect with phenytoin may occur.

Methylphenidate + phenytoin
See methylphenidate (4.6.11).

METRONIDAZOLE + PHENYTOIN
Mild phenytoin toxicity via enzyme inhibition is possible (Blyden et al, J Clin Pharmacol Ther 1988; 28:240–5).

MEXILITINE + PHENYTOIN
Mexilitine levels are reduced by up to 50% via enzyme induction so adjust dosage as necessary

(n = 6, open, Begg et al, Br J Clin Pharmacol 1982;14:219–23).

MICONAZOLE + PHENYTOIN
Phenytoin toxicity via enzyme inhibition has been reported (n = 2, Rolan et al, Br Med J 1983; 287:1760).

Mirtazapine + phenytoin
See mirtazapine (4.3.3.3).

Modafinil + phenytoin
See modafinil (4.6.12).

Nasogastric feeds + phenytoin
Reduced phenytoin levels have been reported with nasogastric feeds (eg. Osmolite®, Ensure® [Abbott]) and other enteral feeds (Pharm J 1989;243:181; Hosp Pharm 1989;24:562). One study showed that the absolute bioavailability of phenytoin was unaffected by enteral feeds but that the absorption patterns were significantly different, with phenytoin sodium more rapidly absorbed (n = 10, RCT, Doak et al, Pharmacother 1998;18:637–45). Phenytoin dosage should be spaced to one hour before feeding or two hours after feeding (tube may need to be clamped). Monitor plasma levels frequently (see comment by Au Yeung and Ensom, Ann Pharmacother 2000;34:896–905, 32 refs).

Neuromuscular blocking agents + phenytoin
Phenytoin reduces the effects of most NMBAs, eg. pancuronium (n = 1, Hickey et al, Anesthesia 1988;43:757–9; n = 1, Liberman et al, Int J Clin Pharmacol Ther Toxicol 1988;26:371–4) and vecuronium, by several mechanisms (n = 22, Wright et al, Anesthesiology 2004;100:626–33), although atracurium appears unaffected.

NICOUMALONE + PHENYTOIN
Nicoumalone metabolism is induced by phenytoin, reducing its effect, although enhancement has also been reported.

Nitrofurantoin + phenytoin
There is a report of a stable epileptic developing seizures when nitrofurantoin was added, requiring increased phenytoin dosage (n = 1, Heipertz and Pilz, J Neurol 1978;218:297–301).

NSAIDs + phenytoin
One study shows no interaction to occur with ibuprofen (n = 10, open, Bachmann, Br J Clin Pharmacol 1986;21:165–9), but toxicity has been reported (n = 1, Sandyk, S Afr Med J 1982;62:592). Phenytoin levels may be increased by aspirin via binding displacement (n = 10, open, 11/7, Leonard et al, Clin Pharmacol Ther 1981;29:56–60), free levels

seeming to remain constant. Transient toxicity may be the only effect and then only at high (900 mg, four-hourly) aspirin doses. Plasma phenytoin levels may be increased by azapropazone via enzyme inhibition (n=5, open, Geaney et al, Br J Clin Pharmacol 1983;**15**:727–34).

ORAL CONTRACEPTIVES + PHENYTOIN

Contraceptive failure via enzyme induction has been reported many times (eg. JAMA 1986;**256**:238–40). Any OC needs to contain at least 50 mcg ethinylestradiol, Depot Provera given every 10 rather than 12 weeks (Crawford, CNS Drugs 2002;**16**:263–72), or alternative contraceptive methods used. In the UK, one tablet each of Marvelon® and Mercilon® (Organon) or two tablets of Ovranette® (Wyeth) are often recommended as daily oral contraception.

Oxcarbazepine + phenytoin
See oxcarbazepine (4.5.6).

Paroxetine + phenytoin
See paroxetine (4.3.2.4).

Pethidine + phenytoin
Attenuation of pethidine's effect via enzyme induction is possible, with increased metabolite levels (n=4, open, Pond and Kretschzmar, Clin Pharmacol Ther 1981;**29**:273).

Phenindione + phenytoin
No interaction is thought to occur (n=54, open, Skovsted et al, Acta Med Scand 1976;**199**:513).

Pregabalin + phenytoin
See pregabalin (4.5.10).

PHENYLBUTAZONE + PHENYTOIN

Phenytoin toxicity may occur via enzyme inhibition and plasma protein displacement (n=6, open, Neuvonen et al, Eur J Clin Pharmacol 1979;**15**:263–8). Dosage adjustment may be necessary.

PROGABIDE + PHENYTOIN

Phenytoin levels may rise by up to 40% (n=6, open, Bianchetti, Epilepsia 1987;**28**:68–73).

Propoxyphene + phenytoin
Large doses of propoxyphene may raise phenytoin levels (Kutt et al, Ann N Y Acad Sci 1971;**179**:704) but normal doses have little or no effect (n=16, open, Hansen et al, Acta Neurol Scand 1980;**61**:357).

Proton pump inhibitors + phenytoin
A lack of effect of omeprazole on phenytoin kinetics has been reported, as has a mild rise in phenytoin levels (n=10, RCT, d/b, c/o, 9/7, Prichard et al, Br J Clin Pharmacol 1987;**24**:543–

5). The SPC for omeprazole states that there are no significant changes in plasma levels, but patients should be monitored and doses adjusted if necessary. Lack of interaction has been reported with pantoprazole (n=23, RCT, d/b, p/c, c/o, Middle et al, Int J Clin Pharmacol Ther 1996;**34**:S72–S75).

Pyridoxine + phenytoin
Large doses of pyridoxine (eg. 200 mg/d) can reduce phenytoin levels by up to 40–50% (Hansson and Sillanpaa, Lancet 1976;**i**:256). Monitoring levels would thus be wise.

Quetiapine + phenytoin
See quetiapine (4.2.5).

QUINIDINE + PHENYTOIN

A reduced quinidine effect may occur via enzyme induction (Anon, N Engl J Med 1983;**308**:724–5), so monitoring of quinidine levels or effect may be necessary.

RIFAMPIN + PHENYTOIN

Significant reductions in phenytoin levels may occur via enzyme induction (Abajo, Br Med J 1988;**297**:1048).

Ritonavir + phenytoin
See lopinavir + phenytoin.

Sertindole + phenytoin
See sertindole (4.2.7).

Sertraline + phenytoin
See sertraline (4.3.2.5).

Shankhapushpi + phenytoin
It has been recommended to avoid the Ayurvedic herbal mixture shankhapushpi, as decreased plasma phenytoin levels may occur (mentioned by Fugh-Berman, Lancet 2000;**355**:134–8).

Sodium oxybate + phenytoin *
See sodium oxybate (4.6.13).

Statins + phenytoin
There is a case of phenytoin reducing the therapeutic effect of simvastatin and atorvastatin, probably via CYP3A4 induction (n=1, Murphy and Dominiczak, Postgrad Med J 1999;**75**:359–60).

St John's wort + phenytoin
See St John's wort (4.3.3.9).

SUCRALFATE + PHENYTOIN

One study showed a small reduction in phenytoin bioavailability (n=9, open, Hall et al, Drug Intell Clin Pharm 1986;**20**:607–11) by decreased absorption. This can be avoided by giving phenytoin two hours or more after sucralfate.

Sulphonamides + phenytoin
Phenytoin toxicity is known to be possible via

P450 inhibition by co-trimoxazole (Gillman and Sandyk, *Ann Intern Med* 1985;**102**:559) and other sulphonamides, so monitor plasma levels and reduce phenytoin doses if necessary.

Theophylline + phenytoin

Phenytoin produces a 45% increase in clearance of theophylline, so higher doses may be needed (n = 8, open, Adebayo, *Clin Exp Pharmacol Physiol* 1988;**15**:883–7). Phenytoin absorption may also be reduced (*Int Pharm J* 1989;**3**:98–101). Separating the doses by 1–2 hours may reduce the effect.

Tiagabine + phenytoin

See tiagabine (*4.5.11*).

Ticlopidine + phenytoin

Ticlopidine 500 mg/d inhibits phenytoin clearance so dose adjustment and careful monitoring should be considered (n = 6, Donahue *et al*, *Clin Pharmacol Therapeut* 1999;**66**:563–8; n = 1, Privitera and Welty, *Arch Neurology* 1996;**53**:1191–2), especially since the onset of phenytoin toxicity may be delayed by several weeks (n = 1, Dahm and Brors, *Tidsskr Nor Laegeforen* 2002;**122**:278–80).

Tolbutamide + phenytoin

Mild phenytoin toxicity may occur via increased free levels (n = 18, Tassaneeyakul *et al*, *Br J Clin Pharmacol* 1992;**34**:494–8).

Topiramate + phenytoin

See topiramate (*4.5.12*).

Trazodone + phenytoin

There is a report of phenytoin toxicity developing when relatively high dose trazodone was added (n = 1, Dorn, *J Clin Psychiatry* 1986;**47**:89).

TRIMETHOPRIM + PHENYTOIN

Plasma phenytoin levels and the antifolate effect may be increased by trimethoprim.

TRICYCLICS + PHENYTOIN

Phenytoin levels may be raised by imipramine (Perucca and Richens, *Br J Clin Pharmacol* 1977;**4**:485–6), but not nortriptyline (Houghton and Richens,*Int J Clin Pharmacol* 1975;**12**:210–6) or amitriptyline (*Clin Pharmacol Ther* 1975;**18**:191–9), probably due to CYP2C19 inhibition (Shin *et al*, *Drug Metab Dispos* 2002;**30**:1102–7). Phenytoin levels may need to be monitored frequently. Tricyclics may lower the seizure threshold.

VALPROATE + PHENYTOIN

Valproate inhibits phenytoin metabolism and competes for its binding sites. If enzyme saturation has not occurred then this displacement of phenytoin leads to decreased bound, but increased free phenytoin (n = 12, Lai and Huang, *Biopharm Drug Dispos* 1993;**14**:365–70). More phenytoin is then metabolised so the net result is reduced total and bound concentrations. The free concentration will remain about the same and lower plasma levels will still contain about the same amount of active/free drug. Thus, beware of raising the dose of phenytoin to bring the total plasma concentration into the 'therapeutic range' as it would then be toxic (Keys, *Drug Intell Clin Pharm* 1982;**16**:737–9). If the enzyme is saturated, then displacement may lead to a stable total concentration but decreased bound and increased free phenytoin (n = 6, open, Johnson *et al*, *Br J Clin Pharmacol* 1989;**27**:843–9). This could lead to toxic effects within the therapeutic range. In practice, phenytoin levels tend to fall initially by up to 50%, then return to normal over about five weeks. Toxicity is possible if levels were higher at the start. Reports of a toxic interaction are not common, but monitoring is essential. Finally, changing valproate from a standard tablet to a slow-release tablet has been shown to result in a 30% rise in phenytoin levels and toxicity (n = 11, Suzuki *et al*, *Eur J Clin Pharmacol* 1995;**48**:61–3).

VIGABATRIN + PHENYTOIN

Vigabatrin produces a mean 20–30% reduction in phenytoin levels (n = 8, open, Rimmer and Richens, *Br J Clin Pharmacol* 1989;**27**:27S–33S) and may compromise seizure control (eg. n = 89, s/b, Browne *et al*, *Neurology* 1987;**37**:184–9).

Vincristine + phenytoin

Phenytoin significantly increases the clearance of vincristine, probably by CYP3A4 induction (n = 15, open, Villikka *et al*, *Clin Pharmacol Therapeut* 1999;**66**:589–93).

WARFARIN + PHENYTOIN

Warfarin metabolism is accelerated by phenytoin, reducing its effect, although enhanced levels of both and deaths have been reported (n = 1, Panegyres and Rischbieth, *Postgrad Med J* 1991;**67**:98; Meisheri, *J Ass Physicians India* 1996; **44**:661–2).

Zinc + phenytoin

One case exists of reduced phenytoin levels probably caused by zinc (*Am J Hosp Pharm* 1988; **18**:297–8).

Zonisamide + phenytoin *

See zonisamide (*4.5.15*).

Zotepine + phenytoin
See anticonvulsants + zotepine (4.2.9).

4.5.9 PIRACETAM

Warfarin + piracetam
Significantly prolonged prothrombin time has been reported with piracetam and warfarin (n = 1, Pan and Ng, *Eur J Clin Pharmacol* 1983;**24**:711).

4.5.10 PREGABALIN

Pregabalin is excreted by the kidneys, undergoes little metabolism, has no effect on P450 enzymes, and is not bound to plasma proteins so interactions are unlikely. Lack of interaction has also been shown with antidiabetics, diuretics and insulin.

Alcohol + pregabalin
Pregabalin may potentiate the sedative effects of alcohol (SPC).

Benzodiazepines + pregabalin
Pregabalin may potentiate the sedative effects of lorazepam (SPC).

Carbamazepine + pregabalin
Lack of interaction has been shown (UK SPC).

Gabapentin + pregabalin
Lack of interaction has been shown (UK SPC), although pregabalin displaces gabapentin from receptors.

Lamotrigine + pregabalin
Lack of interaction has been shown (UK SPC).

Oral contraceptives + pregabalin
Lack of interaction has been shown (UK SPC).

Oxycodone + pregabalin
Pregabalin may enhance the cognitive and motor effects of oxycodone (SPC).

Phenobarbital + pregabalin
Lack of interaction has been shown (UK SPC).

Phenytoin + pregabalin
Lack of interaction has been shown (UK SPC).

Tiagabine + pregabalin
Lack of interaction has been shown (UK SPC).

Topiramate + pregabalin
Lack of interaction has been shown (UK SPC).

Valproate + pregabalin
Lack of interaction has been shown (UK SPC).

4.5.11 TIAGABINE

Tiagabine appears to be metabolised by CYP3A4.

Alcohol + tiagabine
Lack of interaction has been shown (n = 20, RCT, d/b, p/c, c/o, Kastberg et al, *Drug Metabol Drug Interact* 1998;**14**:259–73), although some caution is still advised.

Benzodiazepines + tiagabine
No interaction with triazolam has been detected (n = 12, RCT, Richens et al, *Drug Metabol Drug Interact* 1998;**14**:159–77).

Carbamazepine + tiagabine
Tiagabine clearance is 60% greater with carbamazepine, with plasma levels reduced by a factor of 1.5–3, probably by CYP3A4 induction. There is no effect on carbamazepine.

Cimetidine + tiagabine
No interaction has been detected.

Digoxin + tiagabine
Lack of interaction has been shown (n = 13, open, Snel et al, *Eur J Clin Pharmacol* 1998;**54**:355–7).

Erythromycin + tiagabine
Lack of significant interaction has been shown (n = 13, open, c/o, Thomsen et al, *J Clin Pharmacol* 1998;**38**:1051–6).

Fosphenytoin + tiagabine
See phenytoin + tiagabine.

Oral contraceptives + tiagabine
No interaction has been detected.

Phenobarbital + tiagabine
Tiagabine clearance is 60% greater in people also taking phenobarbital, with plasma levels reduced by a factor of 1.5–3, probably by CYP3A4 induction. There is no effect on phenobarbital.

Phenytoin + tiagabine
Tiagabine clearance is 60% greater in people also taking phenytoin and plasma levels are reduced by a factor of 1.5–3, probably by CYP3A4 induction. There is no effect on phenytoin.

Pregabalin + tiagabine
See pregabalin (4.5.10).

Theophylline + tiagabine
No interaction has been detected.

Valproate + tiagabine
Tiagabine causes a 10–12% reduction in steady-state valproate levels while valproate increases free tiagabine levels by about 40% (n = 12, open, Gustavson et al, *Am J Ther* 1998;**5**:73–9).

Warfarin + tiagabine
No interaction has been detected.

Zotepine + tiagabine
See anticonvulsants + zotepine (4.2.9).

4.5.12 TOPIRAMATE

Topiramate is 13–17% bound to plasma proteins (and thus unlikely to interact with highly bound drugs) and not extensively metabolised. Excretion is mainly via the kidneys. *In vitro* data suggests that effects on hepatic enzyme metabolism are small and interactions with antipsychotics, tricyclics, antidepressants, caffeine and xanthines are unlikely via this mechanism. Concomitant use with drugs predisposing to nephrolithiasis (renal stone formation) is not recommended, eg. allopurinol, megadose ascorbic acid, furosemide, methyldopa, phenolphthalein abuse, steroids and Worcester Sauce overdose.

Reviews: Bailer *et al*, *Clin Pharmacokinet* 2004; **43**:763–80; Johannessen, *Epilepsia* 1997; **38**[Suppl 1]:S18–S23.

Acetazolamide + topiramate
There may be an increased risk of renal stone formation in susceptible patients.

Barbiturates + topiramate
Topiramate has been shown to have no effect on the plasma levels of phenobarbital or primidone (Floren *et al*, *Epilepsia* 1989;**30**:646). The effect of the barbiturates on topiramate has not been studied.

Carbamazepine + topiramate
Topiramate has been shown to have no effect on the plasma levels of CBZ or CBZ-E, although there is a suggestion that it may increase CBZ levels (n = 2 + 23, Mack *et al*, *Seizure* 2002;**11**:464–7). However, topiramate clearance is increased two-fold by CBZ and half-life reduced (n = 12 open, Britzi *et al*, *Epilepsia* 2005;**46**:378–84), and so topiramate doses may need to be lowered if CBZ is reduced or discontinued (n = 12, open, Sachdeo *et al*, *Epilepsia* 1996;**37**:774–80).

Digoxin + topiramate
Topiramate may decrease the plasma concentration of digoxin, with peak levels reduced by 16%, possibly by reduced bioavailability. Dose reduction or routine digoxin blood levels might be considered.

Lamotrigine + topiramate
See lamotrigine (*4.5.4*).

Lithium + topiramate
See lithium (*4.4*).

ORAL CONTRACEPTIVES + TOPIRAMATE
Serum estrogen levels are reduced by topiramate in patients taking combined oestrogen/ progesterone oral contraceptives. An oral contraceptive containing not less than 50mcg of estrogen or Depot Provera given every 10 rather than 12 weeks is recommended, or the use of alternative methods (n = 12, Rosenfeld *et al*, *Epilepsia* 1997;**38**:317–23; review by Crawford, *CNS Drugs* 2002;**16**:263–72). Any changes in bleeding patterns should be reported. There were no contraceptive failures reported in 52 patients in early clinical trials. In the UK, one tablet each of Marvelon® and Mercilon® (Organon) or two tablets of Ovranette® (Wyeth) are often recommended as daily oral contraception.

Phenytoin + topiramate
Decreases in phenytoin clearance may occur in a few patients with topiramate, probably via CYP2C19 inhibition (n = 12, Sachdeo *et al*, *Epilepsia* 2002;**43**:691–6). Conversely, topiramate plasma levels are reduced by about 40% by phenytoin, which could be important if phenytoin is withdrawn (Floren *et al*, *Epilepsia* 1989;**30**:646).

Pregabalin + topiramate
See pregabalin (*4.5.10*).

Triamterene + topiramate
There may be an increased risk of renal stone formation in susceptible patients.

Valproate + topiramate *
Topiramate has been shown to produce a small but significant increase in valproate clearance, reducing plasma levels, although enhanced valproate side-effects, eg. apathy, hypothermia and raised LFTs have also been reported (n = 3, Longin *et al*, *Epilepsia* 2002;**43**:451–4), as has reversible hepatic failure, which resolved on stopping valproate (n = 1, Bumb *et al*, *Epileptic Disord* 2003;**5**:157–9) and hyperammonemic encephalopathy (n = 1, Cheung *et al*, *J Child Neurol* 2005;**20**:157–60). Topiramate plasma levels are increased by about 15% by valproate, which could be important if valproate is withdrawn.

Zonisamide + topiramate *
See zonisamide (*4.5.15*).

Zotepine + topiramate
See anticonvulsants + zotepine (*4.2.9*).

4.5.13 VALPROATE (SODIUM VALPROATE, VALPROIC ACID, DIVALPROEX SODIUM, ETC) *

Valproate has a complex metabolism; 50% is metabolised by glucuronidation, 40% by mitochondrial beta-oxidation and 10% by P450 (CYP2C9 and 2C19) enzymes (Sheehan et al, Ann Pharmacother 2006;**40**:147–50).

Review: DeVane, Psychopharmacol Bull 2003; **37**(Suppl 2):25–42.

Antacids + valproate
A slight decrease in valproate absorption with antacids has been noted (n = 7, open, May et al, Clin Pharm 1982;**1**:244–7).

ANTIDEPRESSANTS + VALPROATE
Antidepressants lower the seizure threshold and may antagonise valproate's anticonvulsant effect. Tricyclic levels may be raised by 19% by valproate (n = 15, open, amitriptyline and nortriptyline, Wong et al, Clin Pharmacol Ther 1996;**60**:48–53) and status epilepticus has been reported, with valproate possibly elevating clomipramine to toxic levels (n = 1, DeToledo et al, Ther Drug Monit 1997;**19**:71–3; see also Fehr et al, J Clin Psychopharmacol 2000;**20**:493–4).

Aspirin + valproate
Valproate's effect and toxicity may be enhanced by repeated high-dose aspirin (n = 3, Goulden et al, Neurology 1987;**37**:1392–4), and levels may rise by 12–43% (n = 6, open, Orr et al, Clin Pharmacol Ther 1982;**31**:642–9).

Bupropion + valproate
See bupropion (4.6.6).

CARBAMAZEPINE + VALPROATE
See carbamazepine (4.5.1).

Charcoal, activated + valproate
Activated charcoal reduces the absorption of sodium valproate by 65% (n = 6, Neuvonen et al, Eur J Clin Pharmacol 1983;**24**:243–6) but has no effect on valproate elimination (n = 8, Al-Shareef et al, Br J Clin Pharmacol 1997;**43**:109–11).

Clozapine + valproate
See clozapine (4.2.3).

Erythromycin + valproate
Valproate levels may rise three-fold when erythromycin is started, resulting in CNS toxicity (n = 1, Redington et al, Ann Intern Med 1992;**116**:877–8).

Ethosuximide + valproate
See ethosuximide (4.5.2).

Fluoxetine + valproate
See fluoxetine (4.3.2.2).

Fluvoxamine + valproate
See fluvoxamine (4.3.2.3).

Gabapentin + valproate
See gabapentin (4.5.3).

Gingko biloba + valproate *
There is a case of a fatal seizure with the combination, probably due to reduced valproate levels via CYP2C19 induction (n = 1, Kupiec and Raj, J Anal Toxicol 2005;**29**:755–8).

H2-blockers + valproate
One study showed that cimetidine reduces the clearance and prolongs the half-life of valproate but ranitidine does not interact (n = 12, RCT, Webster et al, Eur J Clin Pharmacol 1984;**27**:341–3).

Isoniazid + valproate
Enhanced hepatotoxicity has been reported (n = 1, Dockweiler, Lancet 1987;**2**:152).

LAMOTRIGINE + VALPROATE
See lamotrigine (4.5.4).

Levetiracetam + valproate
See levetiracetam (4.5.5).

Lopinavir/ritonavir (Kaletra®) + valproate *
Valproate levels decreased by 48% (resulting in manic relapse) have been reported with Kaletra®, (Abbott) probably via glucuronidation-induction (n = 1, Sheehan et al, Ann Pharmacother 2006;**40**:147–50).

MEROPENEM + VALPROATE *
Meropenem rapidly decreases valproate levels to potentially sub-therapeutic levels, a serious interaction (n = 3, Nacarkucuk et al, Pediatr Neurol 2004;**31**:232–4; n = 1, Coves-Orts et al, Ann Pharmacother 2005;**39**:533–7; n = 2, Sala Pinol et al, Ann Pediatr (Barc) 2006;**64**:93–5; Clause et al, Intensive Care Med 2005;**31**:1293–4).

Methylphenidate + valproate
See methylphenidate (4.6.11).

Olanzapine + valproate *
See valproate + olanzapine (4.2.7).

Oral contraceptives + valproate *
A reduced contraceptive effect has not been reported with valproate (Mattson et al, JAMA 1986;**256**:238–40; n = 6, Crawford et al, Contraception 1986;**33**:23–9), but valproate plasma levels may be higher during drug-free weeks of combined hormonal oral contraceptives than during the 3/52 on it. There is a wide inter-individual variation and monitoring valproate may be prudent if adding or discontinuing OCs or steroids (n = 9, RCT, c/o, Galimberti et al, Epilepsia 2006;**47**:1569–72).

Oxcarbazepine + valproate
See oxcarbazepine (4.5.6).

Paroxetine + valproate
See paroxetine (4.3.2.4).

PHENOBARBITAL + VALPROATE
See phenobarbital (4.5.7).
PHENYTOIN + VALPROATE
See phenytoin (4.5.8).
Pregabalin + valproate
See pregabalin (4.5.10).
Sodium oxybate + valproate *
See sodium oxybate (4.6.13).
Thiopental + valproate
An animal study suggested that the effects of thiopental may be slightly enhanced (Aguilera et al, Br J Anaesth 1986;**58**:1380–3).
Tiagabine + valproate
See tiagabine (4.5.11).
Topiramate + valproate
See topiramate (4.5.12).
Tricyclics + valproate
See antidepressants + valproate.
Vigabatrin + valproate
See vigabatrin (4.5.14).
Warfarin + valproate
Rapidly raised INR (to 3.9) has been reported after a single dose of valproate (Guthrie et al, J Clin Psychopharmacol 1995;**15**:138–9). Care is thus needed.
Zidovudine + valproate
Valproate produces a dose-dependent inhibition of AZT glucuronidation, leading to raised zidovudine levels (Trapnell et al, Antimicrob Agents Chemother 1998;**42**:1592–6), possibly by up to three-fold (n = 1, Akula et al, Am J Med Sci 1997;**31**:244–6). This is a new UK SPC warning, with severe anaemia reported (n = 1, Antoniou et al, Clin Infect Dis 2004;**38**:38–40).
Zolpidem + valproate
See zolpidem (4.1.5).
Zonisamide + valproate *
See zonisamide (4.5.15).

4.5.14 VIGABATRIN

Vigabatrin is not metabolised, does not induce enzymes and is not protein bound. It is renally excreted.
Carbamazepine + vigabatrin
A 10% rise in carbamazepine levels has been reported with vigabatrin (n = 66, Jedrzejczak et al, Epilepsy Res 2000;**39**:115–20), as has an 18% reduction in steady-state carbamazepine plasma levels (n = 15, Sanchez-Alcaraz et al, J Clin Pharm Ther 2002;**27**:427–30).

Oral contraceptives + vigabatrin
Vigabatrin is unlikely to affect consistently the efficacy of oral contraceptives, although in one study two women showed reduced ethinyloestradiol levels (n = 113, Bartoli et al, Epilepsia 1997;**38**:702–7).
Phenobarbital + vigabatrin
One study reported non-clinically significant 7–11% reductions in barbiturate levels (n=89, s/b, 12/52, Browne et al, Neurology 1987;**37**:184–9).
PHENYTOIN + VIGABATRIN
See phenytoin (4.5.8).
Valproate + vigabatrin
Lack of interaction has been shown (eg. McKee et al, Epilepsia 1993;**34**:937–43), but a small rise in levels may occur (Lisart et al, Eur Hosp Pharm 1996;**2**:33–6; disputed by Mumford, Eur Hosp Pharm 1996;**2**:190–1).
Zotepine + vigabatrin
See anticonvulsants + zotepine (4.2.9).

4.5.15 ZONISAMIDE *

Zonisamide does not inhibit 1A2 nor 2D6, and only weakly inhibits 2A6, 2C9, 2C19 and 2E1. It is partly metabolised by 3A4 and partly by N-acetyl transferases and glucuronidation.
Carbamazepine + zonisamide *
Zonisamide does not significantly effect carbamazepine, but 3A4 induction by CBZ reduces zonisamide half-life from 65–36 hours (n = 18, Ragueneau-Majlessi et al, Epilepsy Res 2004;**62**:1–11).
Cimetidine + zonisamide *
Lack of interaction has been shown (SPC).
Ketoconazole + zonisamide *
Lack of interaction has been shown (SPC).
Lamotrigine + zonisamide *
Lack of clinically significant interaction has been shown (n = 20 [c = 18], open, Levy et al, Ther Drug Monit 2005;**27**:93–8).
Oral contraceptives + zonisamide *
No apparent interaction (SPC).
Phenytoin + zonisamide *
Lack of clinically relevant interaction has been shown (SPC).
Rifampicin + zonisamide *
An interaction is theoretically possible via 3A4 induction (SPC).
Topiramate + zonisamide *
The UK SPC recommends caution with the use

of zonisamide with carbonic anhydrase inhibitors such as topiramate.

Valproate + zonisamide *
Lack of significant interaction has been shown so no dosage adjustments would appear necessary (n = 22[c = 17], open, Ragueneau-Majlessi et al, Clin Pharmacokinet 2005;**44**:17–23).

4.6 OTHER DRUGS

4.6.1 ACAMPROSATE

Acamprosate is not protein bound, is excreted in the urine and is not significantly metabolised and so probably has a low liability for drug-drug interactions by these mechanisms.

Alcohol + acamprosate
See alcohol (4.7.1).

Benzodiazepines + acamprosate
Lack of interaction with diazepam has been shown.

Disulfiram + acamprosate
Lack of interaction has been shown (n = 118, RCT, p/c, 2 years, Besson et al, Alcohol Clin Exp Res 1998;**22**:573–9).

Food + acamprosate
Food reduces acamprosate's oral absorption.

Naltrexone + acamprosate
Naltrexone significantly increases plasma acamprosate levels, with some increase in ADRs with the combination (n = 23, RCT, d/b, p/c, c/o, 23/7, Johnson et al, J Clin Psychopharmacol 2003;**23**:281–93).

Tricyclics + acamprosate
There is a lack of interaction with imipramine.

4.6.2 ANTICHOLINERGIC OR ANTISCARINIC AGENTS

Anticholinesterases + anticholinergics
Some antagonism would be expected.
Antipsychotics + anticholinergics
See antipsychotics (4.2.1).
Benzodiazepines + anticholinergics
See benzodiazepines (4.1.1).
Beta-blockers + anticholinergics
Propantheline increases atenolol bioavailability by 36%, increasing its effect (open, Regardh et al, Biopharm Drug Dispos 1981;**2**:79–87) but not that of metoprolol (n = 15, open, Briant et al, Eur J Clin Pharmacol 1983;**25**:353).

Betel nut + anticholinergics
Heavy betel nut consumption has resulted in severe EPSE, possibly by antagonising the effect of procyclidine (n = 1, Deahl, Mov Disord 1989; **4**:330–2).

H2-blockers + anticholinergics
A single-dose study showed possible reduced cimetidine absorption (Kanto et al, Br J Clin Pharmacol 1981;**11**:629–31), but not with ranitidine (n = 12, open, Donn et al, Pharmacother 1984;**4**:89–92) or nizatidine (Knadler et al, Clin Pharmac Ther 1987;**42**:514–20).

Levodopa + anticholinergics
Anticholinergics may reduce the peak blood levels of levodopa and reduce total absorption (Algeri et al, Eur J Pharmacol 1976;**35**:293–9), possibly by slowed gut motility and increased gut metabolism.

MAOIs + anticholinergics
See MAOIs (4.3.4).
Memantine + anticholinergics
See memantine (4.6.9).
Nitrofurantoin + anticholinergics
Nitrofurantoin bioavailability may be increased by anticholinergics (n = 10, Mannisto, Int J Clin Pharmacol Biopharm 1978;**16**:223–8).

Olanzapine + biperiden
See olanzapine (4.2.4).
Paracetamol + anticholinergics
Propantheline delays the absorption of paracetamol (Nimmo et al, Br Med J 1973;**i**:587–9).
Procarbazine + anticholinergics
Increased sedation could occur.

SSRIs + anticholinergics
There are several cases of the combination probably causing delirium, eg. sertraline and benzatropine (n = 1, Byerly et al, Am J Psychiatry 1996;**153**:965–6), paroxetine and benzatropine (Armstrong and Schweitzer, Am J Psychiatry 1997;**154**:581–2, where paroxetine definitely raised benzatropine levels) and a variety of adverse effects (n = 5, Roth et al, J Clin Psychiatry 1994;**55**:491–5). CYP2D6 inhibition seems the likely mechanism.

Thiazide diuretics + anticholinergics
Thiazide bioavailability may be enhanced (open, Beermann et al, Eur J Clin Pharmacol 1978;**13**:385–7).

Tricyclics + anticholinergics
See tricyclics (4.3.1).
Ziprasidone + anticholinergics
See ziprasidone (4.2.8).

Zotepine + anticholinergics

See zotepine (4.2.9).

4.6.3 ANTICHOLINESTERASES

Review: anticholinesterase interactions (Bentue-Ferrer et al, CNS Drugs 2003;**17**:947–63).

4.6.3.1 DONEPEZIL

Donepezil is metabolised slowly by CYP2D6 and 3A4 to multiple metabolites, only one of which appears to be pharmacologically active.

Anticholinergics + donepezil

See anticholinesterases + anticholinergics (4.6.2).

Antipsychotics + donepezil *

Donepezil 5 mg/d had no effect on risperidone pharmacokinetics in schizophrenia and was well tolerated (n = 31, open, 7/7, Reyes et al, Br J Clin Pharmacol 2004;**58**(Suppl 1):50–7) although NMS with bromperidol (n = 1, Ueki et al, Nippon Ronen Igakkai Zasshi 2001;**38**:822–4) and severe EPSE with risperidone (n = 1, Magnuson et al, Am J Psychiatry 1998;**155**:1459) have been reported.

Cimetidine + donepezil

Lack of significant pharmacokinetic interaction has been reported (n = 19, open, Tiseo et al, Br J Clin Pharmacol 1998;**46**[Suppl 1]:25–9).

Digoxin + donepezil

Lack of significant pharmacokinetic interaction has been reported (n = 12, open, Tiseo et al, Br J Clin Pharmacol 1998;**46**[Suppl 1]:40–4).

Ketoconazole + donepezil

Donepezil levels may rise by around 25% over a week (n = 21, open, Tiseo et al, Br J Clin Pharmacol 1998;**46**[Suppl 1]:30–4).

Memantine + donepezil

See anticholinesterases + memantine (4.6.9).

NMBAs + donepezil

A synergistic effect could be predicted.

NSAIDs + donepezil

The manufacturers of donepezil recommend additional monitoring of patients at risk of developing ulcers, eg. if taking concomitant NSAIDs.

SSRIs + donepezil *

Lack of interaction has been shown between donepezil 5 mg/d and sertraline 100 mg/d (n = 19 [c = 16], RCT, open, c/o, Nagy et al, Br J Clin Pharmacol 2004;**58**(Suppl 1):25–33), although case reports exist with paroxetine (Carrier, J Am Geriatr Soc 1999;**47**:1037).

Suxamethonium + donepezil

Donepezil is a cholinesterase inhibitor and would be likely to enhance the effect of suxamethonium-type muscle relaxants (n = 1, Crowe and Collins, Anesthiology 2003;**98**:574–5), eg. during ECT (letter: Walker and Perks, Anesthesia 2002;**57**:1041).

Theophylline + donepezil

Lack of significant pharmacokinetic interaction has been reported (n = 12, open, Tiseo et al, Br J Clin Pharmacol 1998;**46**[Suppl 1]:35–9).

Warfarin + donepezil

Lack of significant pharmacokinetic interaction has been reported (n = 12, open, Tiseo et al, Br J Clin Pharmacol 1998;**46**[Suppl 1]:45–50).

4.6.3.2 GALANTAMINE

Galantamine is 90% bioavailable, has a large VD, low protein binding, and is metabolised by CYP2D6 and 3A4. Galantamine has a minimal effect on P450 enzymes (review by Farlow, Clin Pharmacokinet 2003;**42**:1383–92).

Anticholinergics + galantamine

See anticholinesterases + anticholinergics (4.6.2).

Antipsychotics + galantamine

Lack of interaction has been reported with risperidone (n = 16, RCT, open, c/o, Huang et al, J Clin Pharmacol 2002;**42**:1341–51).

Beta-blockers + galantamine

As galantamine may cause bradycardia, the SPC recommends care with drugs that significantly reduce heart rate, eg. beta-blockers.

Digoxin + galantamine

As galantamine may cause bradycardia, the SPC recommends care with drugs that significantly reduce heart rate, eg. digoxin. Galantamine has been shown to have no effect on the kinetics of digoxin.

Erythromycin + galantamine

A 12% increase in galantamine plasma levels has been reported, probably by CYP3A4 inhibition.

Ketoconazole + galantamine

A 30% increase in galantamine plasma levels has been reported, probably by CYP3A4 inhibition, and so a reduced maintenance dosage might be appropriate.

Memantine + galantamine

See memantine (4.6.9).

Paroxetine + galantamine

A 40% increase in galantamine plasma levels has been reported, probably by CYP2D6 inhibition, and so a reduced maintenance dosage might be appropriate.

Suxamethonium + galantamine

Galantamine is likely to enhance the effect of suxamethonium-type muscle relaxants.

Warfarin + galantamine

Galantamine has been shown to have no effect on the kinetics of warfarin.

4.6.3.3 RIVASTIGMINE

Rivastigmine has minimal protein binding, a short half-life, is metabolised by esterases (but with little effect on P450 enzymes) and lack of significant interaction has been shown with 22 different therapeutic classes (Grossberg et al, Int J Geriatr Psychiatry 2000;15:242–7).

Anticholinergics + rivastigmine

See anticholinesterases + anticholinergics (4.6.2).

Benzodiazepines + rivastigmine

No interaction in healthy volunteers has been seen.

Digoxin + rivastigmine

No interaction in healthy volunteers has been seen.

Fluoxetine + rivastigmine

No interaction in healthy volunteers has been seen.

Memantine + rivastigmine

See anticholinesterases + memantine (4.6.9).

Suxamethonium + rivastigmine

Rivastigmine may enhance the effect of suxamethonium-type muscle relaxants during anaesthesia.

Warfarin + rivastigmine

No interaction in healthy volunteers has been seen.

4.6.4 ATOMOXETINE

Atomoxetine is metabolised by CYP2D6 and half-life may be longer (five hours vs 21 hours) and peak levels five times higher in poor metabolisers but doesn't usually need dose reduction, although accumulation can occur (Sauer et al, Clin Pharmacokinet 2005;44:571–90). It has no clinically significant effect on CYP1A2, 3A4, 2D6 or 2C9.

Antacids + atomoxetine

Antacids and omeprazole have no effect on atomoxetine bioavailability (UK SPC).

Aspirin + atomoxetine

Lack of interaction has been shown (UK SPC).

Benzodiazepines + atomoxetine

Lack of interaction has been shown with diazepam (UK SPC).

MAOIs + atomoxetine

These should not be used together and a two-week gap is needed after stopping an MAOI before starting atomoxetine (UK SPC).

Methylphenidate + atomoxetine

Lack of additive cardiovascular effects has been shown (UK SPC).

Noradrenergic drugs + atomoxetine

The UK SPC recommends caution with the potential for potentiation with other nor-adrenergic drugs, eg. tricyclics, venlafaxine, mirtazapine, pseudoephedrine or phenylephrine.

Phenytoin + atomoxetine

Lack of interaction has been shown (UK SPC).

PPIs + atomoxetine

See antacids + atomoxetine above.

Salbutamol + atomoxetine

Caution is needed with high-dose salbutamol (any route) or other beta-blockers, as the cardiovascular effects of salbutamol can be potentiated (UK SPC).

SSRIs + atomoxetine

Fluoxetine and paroxetine may increase atomoxetine levels via 2D6 inhibition (UK SPC).

Warfarin + atomoxetine

Lack of interaction has been shown (UK SPC).

4.6.5 BUPRENORPHINE *

Buprenorphine has an extensive first-pass metabolism, but sub-lingual bioavailability is sufficient to allow administration by this route. Half-life can vary widely (3–44 hours). It is highly protein bound (96%), metabolised by CYP2D6 and 3A4. It is a major inhibitor of 2D6 and 3A4, and a weak inhibitor of 1A2, 2B6, 2C9, 2C19 and 2E1, although this is yet to be confirmed in human data (review by Elkader and Sproule, Clin Pharmacokinet 2005;44:661–80).

Atazanavir/ritonavir + buprenorphine *

There are cases of clinical pharmacokinetic interaction (n=3, Bruce and Altice, AIDS 2006; 20:783–4).

Benzodiazepines + buprenorphine

See benzodiazepines (4.1.1).

Cocaine + buprenorphine

No notable interaction has been observed (SPC).

Ketoconazole + buprenorphine
Start with half doses of buprenorphine due to CYP3A4 inhibition (SPC).
Methadone + buprenorphine
See methadone (4.6.10).
Tricyclics + buprenorphine
See trcyclics (4.3.1).

4.6.6 BUPROPION

Bupropion is primarily metabolised by CYP2B6, with a significant first-pass metabolism, although poor metabolisers may accumulate hydroxy-bupropion, leading to reduced efficacy (n = 12, Pollock et al, Ther Drug Monit 1996;**18**:581–5).
Review: interactions with anticonvulsants (Popli et al, Ann Clin Psychiatry 1995;**7**:99–101).
Alcohol + bupropion
There is an increased risk of seizures, so alcohol should be avoided or minimised. Extreme care is needed in overdose, chronic use and in alcohol withdrawal states.
Antipsychotics + bupropion
The CSM recommends caution due to the possible increased risk of seizures.
Carbamazepine + bupropion
Carbamazepine induces bupropion metabolism, markedly decreasing bupropion plasma levels (n = 17, RCT, Ketter et al, J Clin Psychopharmacol 1995;**15**:327–33).
Ciclosporin + bupropion
A life-threatening decrease in ciclosporin levels has been reported with bupropion (n = 1, Lewis et al, J Child Adolesc Psychopharmacol 2001;**11**:193–8).
Cimetidine + bupropion
Cimetidine may inhibit the metabolism of bupropion, and increase adverse effects, although no effect on bupropion SR was seen in one study (n = 24, RCT, open, Kustra et al, J Clin Pharmacol 1999;**39**:1184–8).
Clonidine + bupropion
Lack of interaction has been reported (n = 8, RCT, d/b, c/o, Cubeddu et al, Clin Pharmacol Ther 1984;**35**:576–84).
Clopidogrel + bupropion *
A single-dose study showed clopidogrel to significantly inhibit the metabolism of bupropion, increasing AUC by 60% (n = 12, Turpeinen et al, Clin Pharmacol Ther 2005;**77**:553–9).
Fluoxetine + bupropion
Bupropion produces no significant changes in fluoxetine levels (open, 8/52, Kennedy et al, J Clin Psychiatry 2002;**63**:181–6). Panic disorder has been reported with the combination (Young, J Clin Psychiatry 1996;**57**:177–8).
Fosphenytoin + bupropion
See phenytoin + bupropion.
Guanfacine + bupropion
There is a report of a grand mal seizure with the combination (n = 1, Tilton, J Am Acad Child Adolesc Psychiatry 1998;**37**:682–3).
MAOIs + bupropion
Animal studies have indicated that acute bupropion toxicity might occur, and the combination is contraindicated.
Lamotrigine + bupropion
See lamotrigine (4.5.4).
Levodopa + bupropion
An increased incidence of side-effects has been reported with the combination.
Moclobemide + bupropion
See MAOIs + bupropion.
Paroxetine + bupropion
Bupropion produces no significant changes in paroxetine levels (open, 8/52, Kennedy et al, J Clin Psychiatry 2002;**63**:181–6), but the CSM recommends caution.
Phenobarbital + bupropion
Phenobarbital may induce the metabolism of bupropion, which would reduce its efficacy.
Phenytoin + bupropion
Phenytoin may induce the metabolism of bupropion, which would reduce its efficacy.
Pseudoephedrine + bupropion
There is a report of acute myocardial ischaemia with the combination (n = 1, Pederson et al, Can J Cardiol 2001;**17**:599–601).
Rifampicin + bupropion *
Rifampicin may reduce bupropion's half-life by 50%, reducing plasma levels, probably by CYP2B6 induction (n = 18, Loboz et al, Clin Pharmacol Ther 2006;**80**:75–84).
Ritonavir + bupropion
Ritonavir may decrease the metabolism of bupropion, which would increase side-effects.
Selegiline + bupropion
See MAOIs + bupropion.
Sertraline + bupropion *
A marked adverse reaction has been reported with the combination, where mood appeared to deteriorate and venlafaxine was added, but was later recognised as serotonin syndrome (n = 1,

Munhoz, *Clin Neuropharmacol* 2004;**27**:219–22).

Smoking + bupropion

In a single-dose study, cigarettes had no detectable effect on bupropion kinetics (open, Hsyu *et al*, *J Clin Pharmacol* 1997;**37**:737–43).

Ticlopidine + bupropion *

A single-dose study showed that ticlopidine significantly inhibited the metabolism of bupropion, increasing AUC by 85% (n=12, Turpeinen *et al*, *Clin Pharmacol Ther* 2005;**77**:553–9).

Tricyclics + bupropion

Bupropion has been reported to increase imipramine and desipramine levels, through decreased clearance (n=1, Shad and Preskorn, *J Clin Psychopharmacol* 1997;**17**:118–9). Also reported with bupropion are seizures with trimipramine (n=1, Enns, *J Clin Psychiatry* 2001;**62**:476–7), prolonged seizures with clomipramine (n=1, Shin *et al*, *Clin Neuropharmacol* 2004;**27**:192–4) and nortriptyline toxicity (n=1, Weintraub, *Depress Anxiety* 2001;**13**:50–2).

Valproate + bupropion

Valproate does not seem to induce bupropion metabolism, but raised metabolite levels are possible (n=17, RCT, Ketter *et al*, *J Clin Psychopharmacol* 1995;**15**:327–33).

Venlafaxine + bupropion *

Bupropion has been shown to produce a significant increase in venlafaxine but decrease O-desmethylvenlafaxine levels (open, 8/52, Kennedy *et al*, *J Clin Psychiatry* 2002;**63**:181–6). See also sertraline + bupropion.

Zolpidem + bupropion

There are some reported cases of antidepressants and zolpidem causing short-lived hallucinations (eg. Elko *et al*, *Clin Toxicol* 1998;**36**:195–203).

4.6.7 CLOMETHIAZOLE

Clomethiazole inhibits CYP2E1.

Alcohol + clomethiazole

See alcohol (*4.7.1*).

Cimetidine + clomethiazole

Cimetidine inhibits the metabolism of clomethiazole, raising plasma levels.

Methadone + clomethiazole

See methadone (*4.6.10*).

4.6.8 DISULFIRAM

Disulfiram is a potent inhibitor of CYP1A2 and 2E1 (the enzyme that metabolises ethanol), but chronic use could affect other enzymes too (n=7, Frye and Branch, *Br J Clin Pharmacol* 2002;**53**:155–62).

Review: disulfiram interactions (*Acta Psychiatr Scand* 1992;**86**[Suppl 369]:59–66).

Acamprosate + disulfiram

See acamprosate (*4.6.1*).

ALCOHOL + DISULFIRAM

See disulfiram under 'Alcohol abuse and dependence' treatment options (*1.4*) and alcohol (*4.7.1*).

Antipsychotics + disulfiram

There is a report of psychotic symptoms reappearing when disulfiram was started and an increased first-pass metabolism of perphenazine has been noted (n=1, Hansen *et al*, *Lancet* 1982;**2**:1472).

Benzodiazepines + disulfiram

Disulfiram may inhibit the metabolism of diazepam, chlordiazepoxide and temazepam (n=1, Hardman *et al*, *Lancet* 1994;**344**:1231–2), leading to lengthened half-lives, but not with oxazepam (open, MacLeod, *Clin Pharmacol Ther* 1978;**24**: 583–9) or alprazolam (n=11, 2/52, Diquet *et al*, *Eur J Clin Pharmacol* 1990;**38**:157–60).

Caffeine + disulfiram

Disulfiram may reduce caffeine clearance by 50% (n=21, open, Beach *et al*, *Clin Pharmacol Ther* 1986;**39**:265–70).

Cannabis + disulfiram

See cannabis (*4.7.2*).

Carbamazepine + disulfiram

Lack of significant interaction has been shown (n=7, open, Krag *et al*, *Acta Neurol* 1981;**63**: 395–8).

Isoniazid + disulfiram

CNS toxicity has been reported in patients taking isoniazid who then took disulfiram (Rothstein, *JAMA* 1972;**219**:1216).

Lithium + disulfiram

These appear compatible, with no theoretical or clinical reasons why an interaction should occur.

MAOIs + disulfiram

Delirium has been reported with the combination (n=1, Blansjaar and Egberts, *Am J Psychiatry* 1995;**152**:296; n=1, Circulo, *J Clin Psychopharmacol* 1989;**9**:315–6).

Methadone + disulfiram

See methadone (*4.6.10*).

Metronidazole + disulfiram

Psychotic reactions have been reported (n = 2, Hotson and Langston, *Arch Neurol* 1976;**33**: 41–2).

NICOUMALONE + DISULFIRAM

An enhanced anticoagulant effect is possible.

Omeprazole + disulfiram

There is a report of confusion, disorientation and catatonia with the combination (n = 1, Hajela *et al*, *Can Med Assoc J* 1990;**143**:1207).

Paraldehyde + disulfiram

An enhanced disulfiram-reaction is possible (mentioned in Hadden and Metzner, *Am J Med* 1969;**47**:642).

Phenytoin + disulfiram

See phenytoin (*4.5.8*).

Theophylline + disulfiram

Theophylline levels may be increased via enzyme inhibition. Monitor and reduce the theophylline dose if necessary (n = 20, RCT, Loi *et al*, *Clin Pharmacol Ther* 1989;**45**:476–86).

Tricyclics + disulfiram

See tricyclics (*4.3.1*).

WARFARIN + DISULFIRAM

Prothrombin time can fall by about 10% (Rothstein, *JAMA* 1972;**221**:1051–2), with one study showing a marked effect with reduced warfarin doses sometimes necessary (n = 7, open, O'Reilly, *Clin Pharmacol Ther* 1981;**29**:332). The literature notes this to be a significant effect.

4.6.9 MEMANTINE

Memantine is only minimally metabolised, does not inhibit CYP1A2, 2A6, 2C9, 2D6, 2E1 or 3A, or the FMO system, or epoxide hydrolase or sulphation, and so metabolic interactions are unlikely. Raised urinary pH (eg. infections, diet change, excessive alkalising gastric buffers, etc.) may significantly reduce excretion. Plasma protein binding is 45%.

Alcohol + memantine

See alcohol (*4.7.1*).

Amantadine + memantine

Both are NMDA-antagonists and the combination should be avoided as CNS ADRs may be more frequent. The same may be true of ketamine and dextromethorphan.

Anticholinergics + memantine

The anticholinergic's effects may be enhanced by memantine.

Anticholinesterases + memantine *

Lack of interaction has been suggested, along with a possible synergistic effect (Wenk *et al*, *Life Sci* 2000;**66**:1079–83). A post-marketing survey of patients taking memantine with AChEs suggested that the combination was safe and well-tolerated (n = 158, open, mean 4/52, Hartmann and Mobius, *Int Clin Psychopharmacol* 2003;**18**:81–5). Lack of interaction has been shown between donepezil and memantine (n = 19, open, Periclou *et al*, *Ann Pharmacother* 2004;**38**:1389–94).

Antipsychotics + memantine

The antipsychotic effects may be reduced by memantine.

Antispasmodic agents + memantine

The effects may be modified by memantine and dose adjustment may be necessary.

Baclofen + memantine

The effects may be modified by memantine and dose adjustment may be necessary.

Barbiturates + memantine

The barbiturate's effects may be reduced by memantine.

Dantrolene + memantine

Dantrolene's effects may be modified by memantine and dose adjustment may be necessary.

Dextromethorphan + memantine

See amantadine.

Dopamine agonists + memantine

Dopamine antagonists such as bromocriptine may be enhanced by memantine.

H2-blockers + memantine

A theoretical interaction via competition for cationic transport system exists and there is the potential for increased plasma levels.

Hydrochlorthiazide + memantine

There is a theoretical possibility of reduced diuretic effect.

Ketamine + memantine

See amantadine.

Levodopa + memantine

The effects of levodopa may be enhanced by memantine.

Phenytoin + memantine

There is one case report of interaction.

Procainamide + memantine

A theoretical interaction via competition for cationic transport system exists and there is the potential for increased plasma levels.

Quinidine/quinine + memantine

A theoretical interaction via competition for cationic transport system exists and there is the potential for increased memantine plasma levels.

Smoking + memantine

A theoretical interaction via competition for cationic transport system exists and there is the potential for increased memantine plasma levels.

4.6.10 METHADONE

Methadone is readily metabolised mainly by CYP3A4 and partly by 2D6 and 1A2 (and possibly 2B6) and inhibits CYP2D6 and 3A4. Absorption is also variable according to P-glycoprotein status. The (R)-methadone is the active moiety, (S)-methadone being inactive.

Reviews: general (DeMaria, *J Maint Addictions* 2003;**2**:41–57), TDM (Moolchan et al, *J Addict Dis* 2001;**20**:55–73).

Alcohol + methadone

See alcohol (*4.7.1*).

Ascorbic acid + methadone

Vitamin C and other urine acidifiers (eg. ammonium chloride) can decrease plasma levels via increased renal excretion if the pH is less than 6. Methadone's half-life can be halved to around 19–20 hours.

Atazanavir + methadone *

Although atazanavir is a CYP3A4 inhibitor, one study showed no clinically relevant interaction with methadone and no dose adjustment needed (n=16, 2/52, Friedland et al, *AIDS* 2005; **19**:1635–41).

Barbiturates + methadone

Enhanced sedation and respiratory depression may occur. Reduced methadone levels have been reported with phenobarbital (eg. n=43, Bell et al, *Clin Pharmacol Ther* 1988;**43**:623–9; n=1, Liu and Wang, *Am J Psychiatry* 1984;**141**:1287–8).

Benzodiazepines + methadone

There is no proven pharmacokinetic interaction but additive sedation can occur (eg. n=5, RCT, Preston et al, *Drug Alc Dep* 1986;**18**:195–202).

Buprenorphine + methadone

An antagonistic effect would be predicted and buprenorphine might displace methadone from Mu-opioid receptors, precipitating withdrawal. Enhanced sedation and respiratory depression may occur.

Cannabis + methadone

An interaction would be possible through CYP3A4 induction.

Carbamazepine + methadone *

Reduced methadone levels can occur through CYP3A4 induction (Ketter et al, *J Clin Psychopharmacol* 1991;**11**:198–203; n=43, Bell et al, *Clin Pharmacol Ther* 1988;**43**:623–9), and methadone-induced respiratory depression has been reported after withdrawal of carbamazepine (n=1, Benitez-Rosario et al, *J Pain Symptom Manage* 2006;**32**:99–100).

Chloral + methadone

Additive sedation can occur.

Cimetidine + methadone

Raised methadone levels can occur.

Clomethiazole + methadone

Additive sedation can occur.

Cocaine + methadone

Cocaine may accelerate methadone elimination (Moolchan et al, *J Addict Dis* 2001;**20**:55–73).

Ciprofloxacin + methadone

A course of ciprofloxacin has caused sudden and profound methadone toxicity (n=1, Herrlin et al, *Lancet* 2000;**356**:2069–70).

Cyclizine + methadone

There are rare reports of hallucinations with the combination.

Dextromethorphan + methadone *

Delirium, hypersomnia and confusion has been reported with the combination in an elderly woman (n=1, Lotrich et al, *Am J Geriatr Pharmacother* 2005;**3**:17–20).

Didanosone + methadone

Serum levels of didanosone can be reduced by about 40% (n=27, open, Rainer et al, *J AIDS* 2000; **24**:241–8).

Diphenhydramine + methadone

There are rare reports of additional CNS effects with the combination.

Disulfiram + methadone

Lack of kinetic interaction has been shown (n=7, Tong et al, *J Clin Pharmacol* 1980;**20**:506–13).

Domperidone + methadone

Increased absorption has been reported.

Efavirenz + methadone

Efavirez can induce CYP3A4 and produce withdrawal symptoms from reduced methadone levels (n=1, Pinzani et al, *Ann Pharmacother* 2000;**34**:405–7; n=1, Marzolini et al, *AIDS* 2000; **14**:1291–2).

Erythromycin + methadone
Raised methadone levels could occur through CYP3A4 inhibition.

Fluconazole/ketoconazole + methadone
Methadone levels can rise by a mean of 27% through CYP3A4 inhibition, although one study did not detect any signs of toxicity (n = 25, RCT, d/b, p/c, 14/7, Cobb et al, Clin Pharmacol Ther 1998;**63**:655–62).

Fluoxetine + methadone
Lack of significant interaction has been shown (n = 16, open, 9/52, Batki et al, J Clin Psychopharmacol 1993;**13**:243–50).

Fluvoxamine + methadone
Fluvoxamine may inhibit methadone metabolism leading to raised levels (n = 1, DeMaria and Serota, J Addict Dis 1999;**18**:5–12; Perucca et al, Clin Pharmacokinet 1994;**27**:175–90) and severe hypoventilation has been reported (n = 1, Alderman and Frith, Aust N Z J Psychiatry 1999; **33**:99–101).

Fosphenytoin + methadone
See phenytoin.

Grapefruit juice + methadone
Raised methadone levels through CYP3A4 inhibition could theoretically occur.

Hypnotics + methadone
Enhanced sedation.

Indinavir + methadone
Slightly raised methadone levels have been reported.

MAOIs + methadone
See MAOIs (4.3.4).

Metapyrone + methadone
Metapyrone can cause a withdrawal-like syndrome with methadone (n = 15, open, Kennedy et al, Br J Addict 1990;**85**:1133–40).

Naltrexone + methadone
This opiate antagonist would block the effect of methadone.

Naloxone + methadone
This opiate antagonist would block the effect of methadone: this can occur within 5–10 minutes (Tornabene, Ann Intern Med 1974;**81**:349–51).

Nevirapine + methadone
Reduced methadone levels through CYP3A4 induction can occur, precipitating withdrawal (n = 4, Otero et al, AIDS 1999;**13**:1004–5; n = 7, Altice et al, AIDS 1999;**13**:957–62).

Phenytoin + methadone
Reduced methadone levels can occur through

CYP3A4 induction, with withdrawal symptoms occurring within four days (open, Tong et al, Ann Intern Med 1981;**94**:349–51; n = 43, Bell et al, Clin Pharmacol Ther 1988;**43**:623–9). Dosage adjustment may be needed.

Paroxetine + methadone
See paroxetine (4.3.2.4).

Reboxetine + methadone
See reboxetine (4.3.3.5).

Rifampin + methadone
Methadone levels reduce by 30–65% within 4–5 days in 70% patients given rifampin, through CYP3A4 induction (n = 30, Kreek et al, N Engl J Med 1976;**294**:1104–6).

Risperidone + methadone
There is a report of possible interaction, resulting in irritability and aches (n = 1, Wines and Weiss, J Clin Psychopharmacol 1999;**19**:65–7).

Ritonavir + methadone
Ritonavir may decrease methadone levels slightly (n = 1, Geletko and Erickson, Pharmacother 2000; **20**:93–4), although ritonavir/saquinavir has been used without dose adjustment in AIDS patients (n = 12, Gerber et al, J AIDS 2001;**27**:153–60).

Sodium bicarbonate + methadone
Sodium bicarbonate and other urinary alkalinisers can increase plasma levels via decreased renal excretion.

Tramadol + methadone
Tramadol may cause withdrawal in people already taking opioids (UK SPC).

Tricyclics + methadone
Additive sedation might occur. A small study showed desipramine blood levels can double with methadone (n = 5, Maany et al, Am J Psychiatry 1989;**146**:1611–3).

Zidovudine + methadone
Raised zidovudine levels have been reported (AUC increased by 41%) (n = 8, McCance-Katz et al, J Acquir Immune Defic Synd Hum Retrivirol 1998;**18**:435–43).

4.6.11 METHYLPHENIDATE

Review: interactions with psychostimulants (Markowitz et al, Int Clin Psychopharmacol 1999; **14**:1–18).

Atomoxetine + methylphenidate
See atomoxetine (4.6.4).

Carbamazepine + methylphenidate
Carbamazepine has been reported to cause

an extreme reduction of methylphenidate levels (n = 1, Behar et al, J Am Acad Child Adolesc Psychiatry 1998;**37**:1128–9).

Cocaine + methylphenidate *
No pharmacokinetic or physiological interaction seems to occur (n = 7, p/c, Winhusen et al, Pharmacol Biochem Behav 2006;**85**:29–38).

Ciclosporin + methylphenidate
A rise in ciclosporin levels has been reported with methylphenidate (n = 1, Lewis et al, J Child Adolesc Psychopharmacol 2001;**11**:193–8).

MAOIs + methylphenidate
See MAOIs (4.3.4).

Modafinil + methylphenidate
See modafinil (4.6.12).

Phenytoin + methylphenidate
Phenytoin toxicity has been reported (n = 3, Ghofrani, Dev Med Child Neurol 1988;**30**:267–8).

Tricyclics + methylphenidate
Mood and cognitive deterioration has been reported with imipramine and methylphenidate (n = 2, Grob and Coyle, J Dev Behav Pediatr 1986;**7**:265–7). Methylphenidate may inhibit the metabolism of tricyclics producing up to a four-fold increase in levels (eg. n = 2, Grob and Coyle, J Dev Behav Pediatrics 1986;**7**:265–7).

Valproate + methylphenidate
Rapid onset and severe dyskinesia and bruxism has been reported with the combination (n = 2, Gara and Roberts, J Child Adolesc Psychopharmacol 2000;**10**:39–43).

4.6.12 MODAFINIL

Modafinil is moderately bound to plasma proteins (62%), essentially to albumin. Renal excretion is the main route of elimination, but is also metabolised by CYP3A4. It produces a reversible inhibition of 2C19, small and concentration-dependent induction of 1A2, 2B6 and 3A4 and inhibition of 2D6 (Robertson and Hellriegel, Clin Pharmacokinet 2003;**42**:123–37). Modafinil is metabolised to two inactive metabolites.

Amfetamines + modafinil
Low dose amfetamines appear to have no significant effects on steady state modafinil (n = 32, RCT, open, Hellriegel et al, J Clin Pharmacol 2002;**42**:450–60).

Benzodiazepines + modafinil
Triazolam levels may be significantly reduced by modafinil, probably via 3A4 induction (n = 41,

RCT, 4/52, Robertson, Clin Pharmacol Ther 2002; **71**:46–56).

Carbamazepine + modafinil
Carbamazepine might reduce plasma modafinil levels (SPC).

Ciclosporin + modafinil
The UK SPC reports a case of a 50% reduction in ciclosporin levels with modafinil.

Cocaine + modafinil
Single dose IV cocaine has no apparent medical or cardiac interaction with modafinil, although the cocaine euphoria was significantly blunted (n = 7, open, Dackis et al, Drug Alcohol Depend 2003;**70**:29–37).

Dexamfetamine + modafinil
Dexamfetamine has no apparent effect on steady state modafinil levels (n = 32, RCT, open, Hellriegel et al, J Clin Pharmacol 2002;**42**:450–60).

Ethinylestradiol + modafinil
Ethinylestradiol levels may be reduced by modafinil, probably via 3A4 induction (n = 41, RCT, 4/52, Robertson, Clin Pharmacol Ther 2002;**71**:46–56).

MAOI + modafinil *
See MAOIs (4.3.4).

Methylphenidate + modafinil
Low-dose methylphenidate does not appear to interact with modafinil (n = 32, RCT, open, Hellriegel et al, J Clin Pharmacol 2002;**41**:895–904), although methylphenidate may slightly slow the absorption of modafinil (RCT, Wong et al, J Clin Pharmacol 1998;**38**:276–82).

Oral contraceptives + modafinil
Higher dose oral contraceptives containing 50 mcg ethinylestradiol should be used.

Phenobarbital + modafinil
Phenobarbital might reduce plasma modafinil levels (SPC).

Phenytoin + modafinil
Phenytoin's clearance might be reduced by modafinil (SPC).

Sodium oxybate + modafinil *
See sodium oxybate (4.6.13).

Tricyclics + modafinil
A single dose study showed a clinically important interaction with clomipramine 50 mg/d (n = 1, Grozinger et al, Clin Neuropharmacol 1998; **21**: 127–9).

Warfarin + modafinil
A single-dose study suggested no interaction (n = 28, Robertson et al, J Clin Pharmacol

2002;**42**:205–14) but the UK SPC recommends caution and additional monitoring as warfarin clearance may be reduced.

4.6.13 SODIUM OXYBATE *

Sodium oxybate is metabolised by GHB dehydrogenase, eventually to carbon dioxide and water, with no active metabolites. It does not appear significantly inhibit P450 enzymes 1A2, 2C9, 2C19, 2D6, 2E1, and 3A4 at therapeutic doses.

Alcohol + sodium oxybate *
Enhanced CNS depression can occur (SPC)

Benzodiazepines + sodium oxybate *
Respiratory depression might be increased and so the combination should be avoided (SPC).

Ethosuximide + sodium oxybate *
Ethosuximide inhibits GHB dehydrogenase, which metabolises oxybate, and so an interaction is theoretically possible but there are no human studies (SPC).

Modafinil + sodium oxybate *
Lack of interaction has been reported (SPC).

Phenytoin + sodium oxybate *
Phenytoin inhibits GHB dehydrogenase, which metabolises oxybate, and so an interaction is theoretically possible but there are no human studies (SPC).

Proton-pump inhibitors + sodium oxybate*
Lack of interaction has been reported with omeprazole (SPC).

Tricyclics + sodium oxybate *
Lack of interaction has been reported with protriptyline, but adverse effects may be increased with this combination (SPC).

Valproate + sodium oxybate *
Valproate inhibits GHB dehydrogenase, which metabolises oxybate, and so an interaction is theoretically possible but there are no human studies (SPC).

Zolpidem + sodium oxybate *
Lack of interaction has been reported (SPC).

4.7 NON-PRESCRIBED DRUGS AND 'VICES'

4.7.1 ALCOHOL

Alcohol/ethanol–psychotropic drug interactions can occur frequently and with varied outcome, depending upon:

- alcohol usage (eg. chronic and/or acute, leading to altered enzymes)
- consumption (amount, time span)
- type of interaction (eg. additive sedation, antagonism or cross-tolerance)
- what the individual then tries to do (eg. sleep, drive)
- comorbidity (eg. asthma).

These variables need to be considered when assessing the effect, or potential effect, of the interaction. Alcohol distribution is wide, with the direct central depressant effect impairing all central functions (eg. cognition and respiration) and contributing to many of the drug–drug interactions. Alcohol also promotes the action of GABA and may release other amines such as dopamine and endorphins.

Reviews: pharmacokinetic interactions (Fraser, *Clin Pharmacokinet* 1997;**33**:79–90, 151 refs), drug-alcohol interactions (Ferner, *Adv Drug React Bull* 1998;**189**:719–22, 40 refs).

Acamprosate + alcohol
Continued alcohol consumption may negate the therapeutic effect of acamprosate. There is no detectable pharmacokinetic interaction (review by Nalpas *et al*, *Encephale* 1990;**16**:175–9).

ANTIPSYCHOTICS + ALCOHOL

Enhanced CNS depression is well-documented, resulting in impaired concentration, coordination, judgement, drowsiness and lethargy, as well as hypotension and respiratory depression. Alcohol-related drowsiness is significant with **phenothiazines** and **flupentixol**. EPSE may also be enhanced (Freed, *Med J Aust* 1981;**2**:44–5), as can hepatotoxicity with, eg. **chlorpromazine** (Strubelt, *Biochem Pharmacol* 1980;**29**:1445–9). Single oral doses of **amisulpride** do not seem to enhance the effects of alcohol on the performance and memory of healthy subjects (n = 18, RCT, Mattila *et al*, *Eur J Clin Pharmacol* 1996;**51**:161). No significant difference in performance or gross motor skills has been shown with **aripiprazole**. Enhanced CNS sedation would be expected with **olanzapine**, and raised heart rate and increased postural hypotension have been reported. There is no published evidence that alcohol reduces antipsychotic efficacy (n = 31, open, Chetty *et al*, *Eur J Clin Pharmacol* 1994;**46**:523–6). Overall, this is a potentially important interaction, especially in the community. Accidental alcohol over-dosage, especially in people with asthma, respiratory depression or chest infections, could prove fatal if combined with antipsychotics.

BARBITURATES + ALCOHOL

Enhanced or prolonged CNS and respiratory depression can occur, seriously impairing concentration and performance. Acute alcohol ingestion may increase barbiturate levels but chronic alcohol use may decrease barbiturate levels (Mezey and Robles, *Gastroenterology* 1974;**66**:248–53). The lethal dose of barbiturates is up to 50% lower when alcohol is also present (Bogan and Smith, *J Forensic Sci* 1967;**7**:37–45), mainly due to additive respiratory depression.

BENZODIAZEPINES + ALCOHOL

Alcohol can enhance the sedation caused by benzodiazepines by 20–30%, a well-established, documented and predictable interaction. Synergistic sedation has been reported with **lorazepam** (d/b, c/o, Lister and File, *J Clin Psychopharmacol* 1983;**3**:66–71), **clorazepate** and **diazepam**. Larger quantities of alcohol may inhibit benzodiazepine metabolism, especially in those with impaired or borderline hepatic function (review by Guthrie and Lane, *Alcoholism* 1986;**10**:686–90). Acute ethanol consumption decreases diazepam clearance by up to 50%, (Laisi et al, *Eur J Clin Pharmacol* 1979;**16**:263–70). At low dose, alcohol and **temazepam** appear not to interact adversely (n = 24, p/c, c/o, Martin and Siddle, *Brain Cogn* 2003;**53**:58–65).

Beta-blockers + alcohol

Alcohol may slightly reduce propranolol absorption and increase clearance (n = 5, open, Grabowski et al, *Int J Clin Pharmacol Ther Toxicol* 1980;**18**:317–9; Sotaniemi et al, *Clin Pharmacol Ther* 1981;**29**:705–10).

Bupropion + alcohol

See bupropion (4.6.6).

Buspirone + alcohol

A minimal interaction and slightly increased sedation has been reported (n = 24, RCT, Erwin et al, *J Clin Psychopharmacol* 1986;**6**:199–209).

Cannabis + alcohol

See cannabis (4.7.2).

Carbamazepine + alcohol

There is virtually nothing published but additive sedation would be expected.

CHLORAL HYDRATE + ALCOHOL

Additive (or more) CNS depressant effects occur when alcohol is taken with chloral hydrate. Tachycardia, impaired concentration, disulfiram-like effects and profound vasodilation may also occur (Owen and Taberner, *Br J Pharmacol* 1978; **64**:400).

Clomethiazole + alcohol

Alcohol increases the bioavailability of oral clomethiazole, probably via inhibition of first-pass metabolism (Neuvonen et al, *Int J Clin Pharmacol Ther Toxicol* 1981;**19**:552–60).

Citalopram + alcohol

There is little published at present on this. The manufacturers state that citalopram does not enhance the sedation caused by alcohol.

Cocaine + alcohol

See cocaine (4.7.3).

DISULFIRAM + ALCOHOL

Disulfiram inhibits the aldehyde dehydrogenase enzyme, leading to accumulation of acetaldehyde from incomplete alcohol metabolism. The main symptoms of the 'Antabuse reaction' are flushing, sweating, palpitations, hyperventilation, increased pulse, hypotension, nausea and vomiting (often in that order). Arrhythmias and shock can follow. The reaction occurs within 5–15 minutes and can be fatal. Factors affecting the severity of the reaction include the dose of disulfiram, rate and dose of alcohol ingestion, sensitivity, individual aldehyde dehydrogenase activity, concurrent medication (see disulfiram, 4.6.4) and co-existing pulmonary or cardiac disease. Patients should be warned that reactions can occur with disguised sources of alcohol, eg. 'Listerine' mouthwash, sauces, pharmaceuticals (eg. cough mixtures) and topical preparations (eg. shampoo, Stoll and King, *JAMA* 1980;**244**:2045). Delirium has been reported with the combination (Park and Riggio, *Ann Pharmacother* 2001;**35**:32–5).

Escitalopram + alcohol

See citalopram + alcohol.

Fluoxetine + alcohol

Alcohol has no additional significant effect on drowsiness, sedation or task performance tests with fluoxetine 40 mg/d, compared with fluoxetine alone (eg. Shaw et al, *Hum Psychopharmacol* 1989;**4**:113–20).

Fluvoxamine + alcohol

Moderately enhanced sedation has been reported (*J Clin Pharmacol* 1989;**29**:91–5), but a later study showed no significant potentiation of the cognitive effects of 40 g IV alcohol by single and multiple doses of 50 mg fluvoxamine (n = 24, van Harten et al, *Clin Pharmacol Ther* 1992;**52**:427–35).

Levetiracetam + alcohol

See levetiracetam (4.5.5).

Lithium + alcohol

Impaired driving skills have been suggested (Linnoila et al, Eur J Clin Pharmacol 1974;**7**:337), although no clinically significant adverse interactions have actually been reported. Alcohol may produce a slight (12%) increase in peak lithium levels (n = 10, RCT, d/b, p/c, c/o, Anton et al, Clin Pharmacol Ther 1985;**38**:52–5).

MAOIs + ALCOHOL

As well as an interaction occurring with alcoholic and low alcoholic drinks (see MAOIs, 4.3.4), alcohol may increase central catecholamine synthesis and release, and MAOIs may inhibit alcohol dehydrogenase, potentiating alcohol (comprehensive review by Weller et al, Psychosomatics 1984;**25**:301–9).

Memantine + alcohol

Memantine has no effect on alcohol-induced performance impairment, but may increase some subjective symptoms (n = 18, 3 × 3/7, d/b, Bisaga and Evans, Psychopharmacol (Berl) 2003; **172**:16–24).

Methadone + alcohol

Predictably, increased sedation and respiratory depression may occur with the combination (Bellville et al, Clin Pharmacol Ther 1971;**12**:607-12), especially in overdose, as could hepatotoxicity. Chronic high use of alcohol may induce enzymes requiring higher methadone doses and binge drinking may increase methadone excretion via an enhanced diuretic effect.

MIANSERIN + ALCOHOL

Mianserin causes drowsiness, which is enhanced considerably by alcohol (n = 13, RCT, Seppala et al, Eur J Clin Pharmacol 1984;**27**:181–9).

Mirtazapine + alcohol

Lack of pharmacokinetic interaction has been shown, but additive sedation was noted (Mercer, mentioned in Timmer et al, Clin Pharmacokinet 2000;**38**:461–74).

Moclobemide + alcohol

Some degree of potentiation of the effects of alcohol has been noted, although less than with trazodone and clomipramine (Zimmer et al, Acta Psychiatr Scand 1990;**360**[Suppl]:84–6). There has also been a case of a fatality with a moclobemide overdose, plus half a bottle of whisky (n = 1, Bleumink et al, Neth J Med 2003; **61**:88–90).

Oxcarbazepine + alcohol

See oxcarbazepine (4.5.6).

Paraldehyde + alcohol

An enhanced sedative effect can be expected.

Paroxetine + alcohol

Lack of interaction has been shown (review by Boyer and Blumhardt, J Clin Psychiatry 1992;**53**[Suppl 2]:132–4).

PHENYTOIN + ALCOHOL

Alcohol has a variable effect on phenytoin so monitor plasma levels regularly. The half-life of phenytoin can be up to 50% shorter in an abstaining alcoholic than in a non-drinker (Kater et al, Gastroenterology 1969;**56**:412; See also n = 1, Bellibas and Tuglular, Therapie 1995;**50**:487–8).

Pregabalin + alcohol

See pregabalin (4.5.10).

Quetiapine + alcohol

Additive sedation would be expected.

Reboxetine + alcohol

No potentiation of alcohol's cognitive effects has been reported (UK SPC), and up to 4 mg/d showed no interaction with alcohol in one trial (n = 10, d/b, Kerr et al, Br J Clin Pharmacol 1996;**42**:239–41).

Sertraline + alcohol

The evidence for a lack of interaction has been reviewed by Warrington (Int Clin Psychopharmacol 1991;**6**[Suppl 2]:11–21).

Sodium oxybate + alcohol

See sodium oxybate (4.6.13).

Tiagabine + alcohol

See tiagabine (4.5.11).

TRAZODONE + ALCOHOL

Additive sedation has been reported (n = 26, d/b, c/o, Warrington et al, Neuropsychobiology 1986;**15**[Suppl 1]:31–7).

TRICYCLICS + ALCOHOL

Enhanced sedation with most tricyclics is known, but surprisingly little has actually been published and most studies refer to the effect on driving performance. Sedation caused by amitriptyline (Shaw et al, Hum Psychopharmacol 1989;**4**:113–20), maprotiline and doxepin is enhanced by alcohol, but less, or minimally so, with nortriptyline, clomipramine, desipramine and amoxapine. Both alcohol and tricyclics lower the seizure threshold and care is needed in patients susceptible to seizures. Concurrent alcohol may also increase the oral bioavailability of tricyclics by reducing first-pass metabolism (n=5, open, Dorian et al, Eur J Clin Pharmacol 1983;**25**:325–31).

Venlafaxine + alcohol

There appears to be no significant additive effect between alcohol and venlafaxine (n=16, RCT, d/b, p/c, c/o, Troy et al, J Clin Pharmacol 1997;**37**:1073–81).

Zaleplon + alcohol

While zaleplon enhances alcohol performance impairment, the effect appears short-lived and less than triazolam (n=18, c/o, Roehrs et al, Sleep Med 2001;**2**:323–32) and zolpidem, albeit less potent on a mg for mg basis (n=10, RCT, c/o, Drover et al, Clin Ther 2000;**22**:1443–61).

Zolpidem + alcohol

There is no published information available indicating an interaction.

Zopiclone + alcohol

There appears to be no significant interaction (n=9, RCT, Hindmarch, Int Clin Psychopharmacol 1990;**5**[Suppl 2]:105–13).

Zotepine + alcohol

See zotepine (4.2.6).

4.7.2 CANNABIS (TETRAHYDRO-CANNABINOL, SEE ALSO SMOKING)

Cannabis/marijuana is a frequently (and usually secretively) used drug, but, with the exception of perhaps tricyclics, has few known important adverse drug interactions.

Alcohol + cannabis

Decreased ethanol metabolism may occur, with enhanced CNS depression (n=10, RCT, p/c, d/b, c/o, Consroe et al, Psychopharmacol 1979;**66**:45–50). Cannabis may also reduce peak alcohol levels in modest doses (n=15, RCT, p/c, Lukas et al, Neuropsychopharmacology 1992;**7**:77–81). I've heard the combination of Champagne and cannabis described as 'supercalifragilisticexpialidocious', so it must be good — allegedly.

Antidepressants + cannabis

Mental status changes consistent with delirium and tachycardia and other clinically significant adverse events have been reported following use of marijuana and **tricyclics** (n=4, Wilens et al, J Am Acad Child Adolesc Psychiatry 1997;**36**:45–8; Lancet 1997;**349**:106). Increased heart rate has been reported, eg. marked sinus tachycardia, possibly via a combined beta-adrenergic effect (eg. n=2, Hillard and Vieweg, Am J Psychiatr

1983;**140**:626–7). Mania has been reported with **fluoxetine** and cannabis (n=1, Stoll et al, J Clin Psychiatry 1991;**52**:280–1).

Antipsychotics + cannabis

Chlorpromazine clearance has been shown to be increased by cannabis smoking, although the clinical significance is not known (n=31, Chetty et al, Eur J Clin Pharmacol 1994;**46**:523–6). Cessation of cannabis smoking can lead to **clozapine** intoxication through removal of CYP1A2 induction (n=1, Zullino et al, Int Clin Psychopharmacol 2002;**17**:141–3). Additive drowsiness has been reported (review by Benowitz and Jones, Clin Pharmacol Ther 1977;**22**:259–68).

Benzodiazepines + cannabis

Additive drowsiness with benzodiazepines and cannabis has been reported (review by Benowitz and Jones, Clin Pharmacol Ther 1977;**22**:259–68).

Cocaine + cannabis

See cocaine (4.7.3).

CNS depressants + cannabis

The combination has resulted in additive drowsiness (review by Benowitz and Jones, Clin Pharmacol Ther 1977;**22**:259–68), eg. anticholinergics and barbiturates.

Disulfiram + cannabis

There have been two reported reactions; a hypomanic episode in an alcoholic on disulfiram taking marijuana (n=1, Lacoursiere and Swatek, Am J Psychiatry 1983;**140**:242–4) and an acute confusional state (n=1, Mackie and Clark, Br J Psychiatry 1994;**164**:421).

Lithium + cannabis

There is a case of lithium levels raised into the toxic range by secretive use of cannabis (n=1, Ratey et al, J Clin Psychopharmacol 1981;**1**:32) and additive drowsiness has been reported (review by Benowitz and Jones, Clin Pharmacol Ther 1977;**22**:259–68).

Methadone + cannabis

See methadone (4.6.10).

4.7.3 COCAINE

Review: Ciraulo, J Clin Psychopharmacol 1992; **12**:49–55 (73 refs).

Alcohol + cocaine

Simultaneous cocaine and alcohol may produce changes in heart rate and blood pressure, increasing the risk of cardiovascular toxicity (Farre

et al, J Pharmacol Exp Ther 1993;**166**:1364–73).
Combined use has led to enhanced cocaine-
induced hepatotoxicity.

Antidepressants + cocaine
In combination with cocaine, desipramine may
reduce the effect, fluoxetine has no significant
effect (n = 5, Walsh et al, J Clin Psychopharmacol
1994;**14**:396–407), trazodone has minor physiological effects and MAOIs probably augment the
pressor effect.

Antipsychotics + cocaine
Flupentixol may reduce cocaine craving and
haloperidol may moderate the stimulant effects.
Clozapine increases cocaine levels but reduces
the cocaine 'high', and some cardiac events
(near-syncopal episode) have been reported,
so caution is necessary (n = 8, Farren et al, Drug
Alcohol Depend 2000;**59**:153–63).

Cannabis + cocaine
Enhanced cardiotoxicity (eg. increased heart
rate) may occur.

Carbamazepine + cocaine
Cocaine may enhance the cardiac effects of
carbamazepine.

Lithium + cocaine
Lithium probably has little effect on cocaine.

Methadone + cocaine
See methadone (4.6.10).

Methylphenidate + cocaine *
See methylphenidate (4.6.11).

Modafinil + cocaine
See modafinil (4.6.12).

4.7.4 SMOKING

Many people with mental health problems
smoke. There are over 3000 different known
chemicals in cigarette smoke, but which ones are
significant is not fully known. Only a few smoking
drug interactions are significant, and only brief
details of the more significant psychotropic
ones are included here (review by Schein, Ann
Pharmacother 1995;**29**:1139–48). The major
enzyme metabolising nicotine is probably
CYP2A6, with 2B6 and 2D6 playing lesser, but
still substantial, roles. Cigarette smoke contains
polycyclic aromatic hydrocarbons, which are
potent inducers of CYP1A2.
Reviews: general (Zevin and Benowitz, Clin
Pharmacokinet 1999;**36**:425–38, 128 refs; Desai
et al, CNS Drugs 2001;**15**:469–94, 100 refs).

Antipsychotics + smoking *
Schizophrenics who smoke tend to receive
higher doses of antipsychotics than non-smokers
(n = 78, open, Goff et al, Am J Psychiatry 1992;
149:1189–94), possibly via increased hepatic
metabolism and renal excretion (n = 90, RCT, d/b,
p/c, Salokangas et al, Schizophren Res 1997;**23**:55–
60). Plasma levels of **haloperidol** are around
23% lower in smoking than in non-smoking
schizophrenic patients (n = 66, open, Shimoda et
al, Ther Drug Monit 1999;**21**:293–6; confirmed by
another study, n = 63, Pan et al, Ther Drug Monit
1999;**21**:489). **Chlorpromazine** clearance may
be increased by cigarette smoking, but the clinical
significance is unclear (n = 31, Chetty et al, Eur J
Clin Pharmacol 1994;**46**:523–6). **Clozapine** levels
are lowered by smoking (n = 148, open, Haring
et al, Am J Psychiatry 1990;**147**:1471–5), the 1A2
induction leading to clozapine non-response, but
this usually takes two to four weeks to manifest
itself (Zullion et al, Int Clin Psychopharmacol
2002;**17**:141–3). Stopping smoking can be
dangerous for someone taking clozapine (n = 1,
Derenne and Baldessarini, Am J Ther 2005;
12:469–71; n = 2, Bondolfi et al, Ther Drug Monit
2005;**27**:539–43), one case being after admission
to a non-smoking ward. One study showed a
mean 72% **increase** in stable clozapine levels on
smoking cessation, with one case so extreme it
caused a significant ADR (n = 11, open, Meyer,
J Clin Psychopharmacol 2001;**21**:569–74). The
change in plasma clozapine levels can, in 80%
cases, be predicted by using the formula:

> Non-smoking level = 45.3 + (1.474 × smoking level)

Nomograms exist to help predict doses in
people on clozapine who smoke, but you'll
need a colour copy of the best paper (Rostami-
Hodjegan et al, J Clin Psychopharmacol 2004;**24**:1–
9) to make sense of it. **Olanzapine** clearance
may be higher and half-life 21% shorter in
smokers compared to non-smokers, probably
via CYP1A2 induction. Smoking cessation can
lead to olanzapine intoxication through removal
of CYP1A2 induction (n = 1, Zullino et al, Int
Clin Psychopharmacol 2002;**17**:141–3). Smoking
seems to have no effect on **zotepine** plasma
levels (n = 14, Kondo et al, Psychopharmacol

[Berl] 1996;**127**:311–4). Lack of interaction has been shown with **amisulpride** levels (n = 85, Bergemann *et al*, *Eur Neuropsychopharmacol* 2004;**14**:245-50), **ziprasidone** and **aripiprazole**. There is nothing reported with **risperidone**. Many schizophrenics may smoke to relieve subjective distress from the illness and treatment (review, McEvoy, *Curr Opin Psychiatry* 2000;**113**:115–9).

Benzodiazepines + smoking

Early studies suggested an increased clearance of benzodiazepines in smokers (review by Schein, *Ann Pharmacother* 1995;**29**:1139–48). One review noted increased clearance by smoking of alprazolam, lorazepam, oxazepam and diazepam but not chlordiazepoxide (mentioned in Desai *et al*, *CNS Drugs* 2001;**15**:469–94).

Bupropion + smoking

See bupropion (*4.6.6*).

Carbamazepine + smoking

There appears to be no interaction (mentioned in Desai *et al*, *CNS Drugs* 2001;**15**:469–94).

Duloxetine + smoking

See duloxetine (*4.3.3.1*).

Fluvoxamine + smoking

Fluvoxamine levels are significantly lower in smokers, probably due to CYP1A2 induction (n = 30, open, Yoshimura *et al*, *Neuropsychobiology* 2002;**45**:32–5).

Lithium + smoking

Smoking induces CYP1A2 and caffeine is metabolised by CYP1A2. Theoretically, ceasing smoking could raise xanthine levels, which could increase lithium excretion (as with theophylline), lowering levels.

Memantine + smoking

See memantine (*4.6.9*).

Phenobarbital + smoking

Smoking has been shown not to effect the drowsiness caused by phenobarbital (n = 12, d/b, Mirfazaelian *et al*, *Biopharm Drug Dispos* 2001; **22**:403–6).

Propranolol + smoking

Steady-state propranolol levels may be reduced in smokers, via 1A2 induction.

Tricyclics + smoking

Although serum levels of tricyclics fall in smokers, free levels rise, minimising the clinical significance (n = 24, open, Perry *et al*, *Ther Drug Monit* 1986; **8**:279–84).

Zolpidem + smoking

See zolpidem (*4.1.5*).

4.8 CYTOCHROME P450 DRUG METABOLISM

Knowledge of the role of the P450 enzyme system is rapidly developing. These tables may be of use in determining actual or potential interactions. There are, however, many discrepancies in the published literature and so these tables may inadvertently perpetuate some inaccuracies or incomplete knowledge. The author would be very happy to receive any advice on this.

Some points about P450/CYP interactions include:

1. Some drugs are metabolised by several enzymes, so if one enzyme is inhibited, another may compensate. There are over 40 known human P450 enzymes.

2. A drug may inhibit or induce one enzyme, but be metabolised by another.

3. Onset and offset of inhibition is dependent on the half-life and time to steady state of the inhibitory drug (may be 24 hours to several months) and the drug to be metabolised, but onset is frequently rapid.

4. Onset and offset of induction may take days or several weeks to become apparent, dependent on the inducing drugs half-life, enzyme turnover, age (induction reduces with age) and concurrent liver disease (reduced induction ability).

5. Other enzyme systems are also important. The **UGT** (uridine diphosphate glucuronosyltransferase) enzymes (de Wildt *et al*, *Clin Pharmacokinet* 1999;**36**:439–52) are induced by phenytoin, valproate, phenobarbital and carbamazepine, and lamotrigine is a weak UGT inducer. The Flavin Monoxygenase (**FMO**) system is also important. Humans have FMO1, FMO3, FM04 and FM05 enzymes in the liver; intestine and kidney. Imipramine, chloropromazine and orphenadrine are known to be metabolised by this enzyme system.

The general rules for avoiding metabolic interactions are:

1. Avoid reported and predictable interactions.

2. With potential interactions, use reduced doses where possible (ie. start low and go slow).

CYP1A2

Substrates, ie drugs metabolised by this enzyme

Agomelatine (90%)
Amiodarone
Caffeine
Carbamazepine (minor)
Chlordiazepoxide
Ciprofloxacin
Clarithromycin
Clozapine (most)
Dextropropoxyphene
Diazepam
Duloxetine
Erythromycin
Estradiol
Flecainide
Flutamine
Fluvoxamine (partly)
Haloperidol (partly)
Lidocaine
Mexiletine (minor)
Melatonin (partly)
Methadone (minor)
Mirtazapine (partly)
Naproxen
Norfloxacin
Olanzapine (partly)
Omeprazole
Ondansetron
Oxfloxacin
Paracetamol
Perphenazine
Pimozide (possibly)
Promazine

Propafenone
Propranolol
Ritonavir
Rofecoxib
Tacrine
Tamoxifen
Theophylin
Tizanidine (main)
Tricyclics (tertiary, eg.
  amitriptyline, clomipramine,
  desipramine, trimipramine
  imipramine)
Verapamil
Warfarin-R (major)
Zotepine
Ziprasidone (minor)

Significant enzyme inducers

Cabbage
Caffeine (weak, animal
  studies)
Charcoal-broiled food
Cigarette smoke (inc.
  cannabis)
Modafinil (small and
  dose-dependent)
Omeprazole
Phenobarbital (weak)
Phenytoin (weak)
Rifampin
Ritonavir

Significant enzyme inhibitors

Celery
Cimetidine
Clarithromycin
Diet (low protein/high
  carbohydrates)
Disulfiram (strong)
Erythromycin
Fluoroquinolones eg.
  ciprofloxacin and
  norfloxacin (strong)
Fluvoxamine (potent
  — other SSRIs only very
  weak inhibitors)
Grapefruit juice
Griseofulvin?
Isoniazid
Ketoconazole
Mirtazapine (very weak)
Moclobemide
Nefazodone (very weak/nil)
Norfloxacin
Omeprazole
Parsley
Parsnip
Rofecoxib (potent, dose-
  dependent)
Sertraline (weak)

CYP2B6

Substrates, ie drugs metabolised by this enzyme	Significant enzyme inducers	Significant enzyme inhibitors
Alfentanil	Modafinil (minor and	Clopidogrel
Bupropion	dose-dependent)	Glabridin (a liquorice
Carbamazepine	Rifampin	extract)
Carteolol		HRT (potent)
Clopidogrel		OCs (weak)
Cyclophosphamide		Ticopidine
Dexamethasone		Zolpidem (very weak)
Diazepam		
Ecstasy (MDMA)		
Efavirenz		
Estrone		
Ifosfamide		
Lidocaine		
S-methadone (major)		
R-methadone (minor)		
Midazolam		
Nevirapine		
Nicotine		
Orphenadrine		
Phenobarbital		
Procainamide		
Promethazine		
Propofol (main)		
Rifampicin		
Ropivacaine		
Sevoflurane		
Tamoxifen		
Thiotepa (minor)		
Valproic acid		

CYP2C9

Substrates, ie drugs metabolised by this enzyme	Significant enzyme inducers	Significant enzyme inhibitors
Agomelatine (10%)	Carbamazepine (weak)	Amiodarone
Alosetron	Phenobarbital (weak)	Cimetidine
Amiodarone	Phenytoin (weak)	Cyclizine
Amitriptyline	Rifampin	Fluconazole
Atorvastatin	St John's wort (weak?)	Fluorouracil
Bupropion (8/9)		Fluoxetine
Carbamazepine (minor)		Fluvastatin
Cimetidine		Fluvoxamine
Fluconazole		Gingko biloba (weak)
Fluoxetine		Ginseng (weak)
Flurbiprofen		Modafinil
Fluvastatin		Omeprazole
Irbesartan		Paroxetine (weak)
Losartan		Phenylbutazone
Miconazole		Promethazine
NSAIDs (eg. diclofenac, naproxen, piroxicam, tenoxicam 8/9)		Sertraline (moderate)
		Tamoxifen
Phenytoin		Topiramate
Phenobarbital		Tranylcypromine (part)
Rifampicin		Valproate
Sildenafil (partly)		Venlafaxine (weak)
Tolbutamide (8/9)		
Trimethoprim		
Valsartan		
Valproate		
S-warfarin (major)		

2C is a sub-family, containing many closely related enzymes, eg. 2C9, 2C10, 2C19, etc. About 20% Asians and 3–5% Caucasians are poor CYP2C19 metabolisers.

CYP2C19

Substrates, ie drugs metabolised by this enzyme	Significant enzyme inducers	Significant enzyme inhibitors
Barbiturates	Carbamazepine (weak)	Cimetidine
Carisoprodol	Gingko biloba?	Fluconazole
Cimetidine	Phenobarbital (weak)	Fluoxetine (moderate)
Citalopram (major 60%)	Phenytoin (weak)	Fluvoxamine
Diazepam (genotype important)		Isoniazid (potent)
Fluoxetine		Ketoconazole
Fluvoxamine		Moclobemide
Flunitrazepam		Modafinil
Lansoprazole		Omeprazole
Melatonin (partly)		Oxcarbazepine
Mephenytoin		Paroxetine (weak)
Moclobemide (major)		Sertraline (weak)
Nelfinavir		Ticlopidine
Omeprazole (major)		Topiramate
Perphenazine		Tranylcypromine (weak)
Phenytoin		Tricyclics
Promazine		Valproate
Proguanil		Venlafaxine (weak)
Propranolol (part)		
Rabeprazole		
Rifabutin		
Rifampicin		
Topiramate		
Tranylcypromine		
Tricyclics (tertiary, eg. amitriptyline, clomipramine, trimipramine, imipramine)		
R-warfarin (minor)		

CYP2D6

Substrates, ie drugs metabolised by this enzyme	Significant enzyme inducers	Significant enzyme inhibitors
Amfetamines	Carbamazepine (weak)	Amidarone
Amprenavir	Phenobarbital (weak)	Buprenorphine (very weak)
Antiarrhythmics type 1c	Phenytoin (weak)	Bupropion
(encainide, flecainide, etc)	Rifampin (weak)	Chloroquine
Aripiprazole	Ritonavir (weak)	Chlorphenamine
Beta-blockers (especially		Chlorpromazine
lipophilic, metoprolol,		Cimetidine
propranolol, timolol)		Citalopram (very weak/nil)
Buprenorphine		Cocaine
Carvedilol		Cyclizine
Chloroquine		Dextromethorphan
Chlorphenamine		Dextropropoxyphene
Cinnarizine		Diltiazem (weak)
Ciprofloxacin		Diphenhydramine
Citalopram (minor)		Fenfluramine?
Clozapine (minor and		Flecainide
unproven)		Fluoxetine (strong)
Codeine (to morphine)		Fluphenazine
Debrisoquine		Fluvoxamine (very weak)
Dexfenfluramine		Haloperidol (dose-
Dextromethorphan		dependent)
Diazepam		Indinavir
Donepezil		Levomepromazine
Duloxetine (partly)		Methadone (weak?)
Fenfluramine		Metoclopramide
Flecainide		Metoprolol
Fluoxetine (partly)		Mexiletine
Fluvoxamine (partly)		Mibefradil
Galantamine		Mirtazapine (very weak/nil)
Haloperidol		Moclobemide
Hydrocodone		Modafinil (small and
Indoramin		dose-dependent)
Loratadine		Nefazodone (very weak/nil)
Maprotiline (possibly)		Nicardipine
Methadone (part)		Norfluoxetine (strong)
Methamfetamine		Paroxetine (strong,
Mexiletine (main)		dose-related)
Mianserin		Perphenazine
Mirtazapine (minor)		Pindolol
Morphine derivatives		Primaquine
Nefazodone		Promethazine
Nicotine (partly)		Propafenone
Olanzapine (partly)		Propanolol
		Quinine

CYP2D6

Substrates, ie drugs metabolised by this enzyme	Significant enzyme inducers	Significant enzyme inhibitors
Ondansetron		Quetiapine
Oxycodone		Ritonavir
Paroxetine		Sertraline (weak, dose-
Phenothiazines		related, moderate at
(eg. perphenazine,		150 mg/d)
chlorpromazine,		Terbinafine (potent)
fluphenazine)		Thioridazine
Propafenone		Timolol
Quinidine		Tricyclics (all, strong)
Risperidone (major)		Venlafaxine (very weak/nil)
Sertindole (partly)		Yohimbine
Tamoxifen		
Tolterodine		
Tramadol		
Trazodone		
Tricyclics — secondary and		
tertiary tricyclics (eg.		
nortriptyline, imipramine,		
maprotiline, trimipramine,		
amitriptyline, clomipramine		
and desipramine [weak])		
Venlafaxine (major)		
Zuclopenthixol		

CYP2D6 metabolism occurs both in the liver and in the brain. An individual's CYP2D6 status can be determined by giving the probes debrisoquine or dextromethorphan and measuring the ratios of drug and metabolite. Around 5–8% Caucasians, 8.5% African-Americans and 2–10% Asians are slow metabolisers. Up to 29% North Africans and Middle East people (de Leon et al, Psychosomatics 2006;**47**:75-85) are ultra-rapid metabolisers (3 or more 2D6 allelles). All CYP2D6 inhibition is probably concentration-dependent and so inclusion in this list only predicts that an interaction could occur, not that it will occur.

References used include: Meyer et al, Acta Psychiatr Scand 1996;**93**:71–9; Nemeroff et al, Am J Psychiatry 1996;**153**:311–20; Callahan et al, Harvard Rev Psychiatry; 1996;**4**:153–8; Centorinno et al, Am J Psychiatry; 1996 **153**:820–2; Cohen and De Vane, Ann Pharmacother 1996;**30**:1471–80.

CYP3A3/4

Substrates, ie drugs metabolised by this enzyme

Alfentanil
Alosetron
Amiodarone
Amprenavir
Antihistamines, eg. astemizole
Aripiprazole
Benzodiazepines (eg. alprazolam, clonazepam, diazepam, flunitrazepam, midazolam, temazepam, but not lorazepam)
Bromocriptine
Budesonide
Buprenorphine
Buspirone
Busulfan
Calcium-channel blockers (eg. amlodipine, diltiazem, felodipine, isradipine, nicardipine, nifedipine, verapamil)
Cannabinoids
Carbamazepine
Chloramphenicol
Chloroquine
Ciclosporin
Cimetidine
Ciprofloxacin
Cisapride (restriced in UK)
Citalopram (minor, 30%)
Clindamycin
Clopidrogel
Clotrimazole
Clozapine (partly)
Cocaine
Codeine
Colchicine
Cortisol
Cyclophosphamide
Dapsone
Dexamethasone
Dextromethorphan
Digoxin
Disopyramide
Docetaxol
Donepezil
Doxorubicin
Doxycycline
Dutasteride

Efavirez
Ergotamine
Estradiol
Ethosuximide
Ethinylestradiol
Etoposide
Fentanyl
Fexofenadine
Fluconazole
Fluoxetine
Flutamine
Fluvoxamine
Galantamine
Glibenclamide
Glyburide?
Granisetron
Haloperidol
Indinavir
Irinotecan
Isoniazid
Isotretinoin
Itraconazole
Ivabradine
Ivermectin
Ketoconazole
Lansoprazole (weak)
Levonorgestrel
Lidocaine
Lisuride
Lopinavir
Loratadine
Losartan
Macrolides (eg. erythromycin, clarithromycin)
Meloxicam
Methadone (main)
Methylprednisolone
Mianserin
Mibefradil
Miconazole
Mifepristone
Mirtazapine (partly)
Modafinil
Nefazodone
Nelfinavir

CYP3A3/4

Substrates, ie drugs metabolised by this enzyme

Omeprazole
Ondansetron
Orphenadrine
Paclitaxel
Paracetamol
Perphenazine
Phenobarbital
Phenytoin
Pimozide (mostly)
Prednisone
Progesterone
Proguanil
Propafenone
Promazine
Quetiapine (mostly)
Quinidine
Quinine
Rabeprazole
Reboxetine
Rifampin
Rimonabant
Risperidone (partly)
Ritonavir
Saquinavir
Sertindole (partly)
Sertraline
Sildenafil (partly)
Sirolimus
Sodium fusidate

Statins (eg. atorvastatin, lovastatin, pravastin, simvastatin)
Steroids (eg. dexamethasone)
St John's wort
Tacrolimus
Tamoxifen
Testosterone
Theophylline
Tiagabine
Tolterodine
Tricyclics — tertiary (eg. imipramine, amitriptyline, clomipramine)
Topiramate (possibly)
Valproate
Vardenafil
Venlafaxine
Vinblastine
Vincristine
R-warfarin (minor)
Zaleplon (secondary route)
Ziprasidone (most)
Zolpidem (mainly)
Zotepine
Zopiclone (mostly)

CYP3A3/4 (very similar structures, and are often grouped together). CYP3A4 is an important P450 enzyme, metabolising at least 50% of all marketed medications, and may account for up to 50–60% of the total liver P450. There is little generic polymorphism so little inter-individual variation exits. CYP3A4 occurs in the liver, gut and, possibly, the brain. Ultra-rapid metabolisers have not yet been identified. Debrisoquine is a probe.

CYP3A3/4

Significant enzyme inducers (decrease levels of substrates)	Significant enzyme inhibitors (increase levels of substrates)	
Barbiturates (all)	Acetazolamide	Metronidazole
Carbamazepine	Amiodarone	Mibefradil
Cortisol	Atazaivir (moderate)	Miconazole (strong)
Dexamethasone	Buprenorphine (weak/ moderate)	Mirtazpine (very weak/nil)
Efavirez	Cannabinoids	Nefazodone (strong)
Ethosuximide	Cimetidine (moderate)	Nelfinavir
Flucloxacillin	Citalopram (weak)	Norfluoxetine (moderate)
Modafinil (small and dose-dependent)	Clotrimazole	Omeprazole (weak)
Nevirapine (?)	Danazol	Orange juice (weak)
Omeprazole	Diltiazem (weaker)	Paroxetine (weak)
Oxcarbazepine	Fluconazole (strong)	Quinine
Phenobarbital	Fluoxetine (weak)	Ritonavir (moderate)
Phenytoin	Fluvoxamine (moderate)	Sertindole (weak)
Prednisone	Grapefruit juice (weak)	Sertraline (minor/moderate)
Primidone	Indinavir (moderate)	St John's wort
Rifampin (rapid)	Itraconazole (strong)	Statins (atorvastatin, fluvastatin)
St John's wort (weak?)	Isoniazid (potent)	Stiripentol (variable)
Topiramate (dose-dependent, especially at high doses)	Ivabradine (very weak)	Terbinafine
Troglitazone	Ketoconazole (strong)	Trazodone
	Lopinavir	Tricyclics (moderate)
	Macrolides (some, eg. clarith-romycin, erythromycin, strong)	Troleandomycin (strong)
	Methadone (weak?)	Venlafaxine (very weak)
		Verpamil (weak)
		Zafirlukast

5 DRUG-INDUCED PSYCHIATRIC DISORDERS

The drugs listed in each section have been reported to cause that condition in some context (eg. standard dose, high dose, prolonged courses, etc). The main references at the end of this section and others (where known or where they exist) next to the drug should be consulted to ascertain the circumstances of reports. The references are offered without qualification and no indication of frequency or status of reports can be given as this information is not really available, except where a side-effect is well recognised. For completeness, drugs not available in Europe but which are available in Canada and/ or USA are also listed.

Review: psychiatric adverse effects of anti-convulsant drugs (Wong et al, CNS Drugs 1997; **8**:492–509), general (Bishop and Lee, Pharm J 1998;**261**:935–9).

5.1 AGITATION, ANXIETY AND NERVOUSNESS

● **Psychotropics, etc** *

Aripiprazole (n = 2, J Clin Psychiatry 2004;**65**:132–3)

Atomoxetine (n = 1, Pediatrics 2004;**114**:895–6)

Benzodiazepine withdrawal (eg. Am J Psychiatry 1984;**141**:848–52)

Bromocriptine

Bupropion (9.7% reported)

Carbamazepine (J Am Acad Child Adolesc Psychiatry 1988;**27**:500–3)

Clomethiazole

Citalopram (cases in Eur J Clin Pharmacol 1986;**31**:18–22)

Dexamfetamine

Fluoxetine (9% incidence? eg. J Clin Psychiatry 1985;**46**(3 Pt 2):32–7)

Memantine (n = 3, J Neurol Neurosurg Psychiatry 2006: Oct 9)

Modafinil (UK SPC)

Moclobemide (5–10% incidence, eg. J Neural Transm 1989;**28** [Suppl]:S77–S89)

Olanzapine (Can J Psychiatry 1998;**43**:1054)

Paroxetine (11%? incidence, Acta Psychiatr Scand 1989;**80**[Suppl 350]:117–37)

Phenobarbital and other barbiturates

Risperidone (n = 1, Am J Psychiatry 1995;**152**:1096–7)

Rivastigmine (< 5%)

Temazepam

Tricyclics (eg. amitriptyline, lofepramine at < 2%, review in Drugs 1989;**37**:123–40)

● **Anticonvulsants**

Carbamazepine

Clonazepam

Ethosuximide

Gabapentin

Gabapentin withdrawal (n = 1, J Clin Psychiatry 1998;**59**:131)

Lamotrigine

Valproate (n = 1, J Neuropsychiatry Clin Neurosci 2001;**13**:528–30)

Vigabatrin

Zonisamide (SPC)

● **Antiparkinsonian drugs**

Atropine eye drops (n = 1, J Ped Ophthalmol Strabis 1985;**22**:38–9)

Levodopa (common)

● **Gastrointestinal**

Famotidine (mentioned in Digestion 1985;**32** [Suppl 1]:24–31)

Omeprazole

● **Cardiovascular**

Doxazosin (2.4% incidence)

Hydralazine

Methyldopa (rare)

Nicardipine (rare)

● **NSAIDs and analgesics**

Ibuprofen (overdose, Am J Emerg Med 1998; **16**:549–50)

Indometacin (n = 1, South Med J 1983;**76**:679–80)

Mefenamic acid

Naproxen

Naproxen + chloroquine (Ann Pharmacother 1993;**27**:1058–9)

Nefopam

Pentazocine (eg. Br Med J 1974;**2**:224)

- Miscellaneous

Amantadine
Aminophylline
Baclofen (n = 2, Lancet 1977;**2**:44)
Bismuth intoxication (Postgrad Med J 1988;**64**:308–10)
Botulinum toxin A injection (South Med J 1999; **92**:738)
Caffeine OD
Co-trimoxazole (n = 1, J Clin Psychopharmacol 1991;**11**:144–5)
Dexamethasone and other glucocorticoids (eg. Arch Gen Psychiatry 1981;**38**:471–7)
Fentanyl transdermal
Flumazenil
Flunisolide
Gancyclovir (N Engl J Med 1990;**322**:933–4)
Ginseng (Arch Gen Psychiatry 1998;**55**:1033–44)
Granisetron (unconfirmed, eg. Eur J Cancer 1990;**26**[Supp 1]:S19–23)
Isoniazid (Lancet 1989;**ii**:735–6)
Levamisole (rare, N Engl J Med 1990;**322**: 352–8)
Levothyroxine
Mefloquine (Pharm J 1989;**243**:561)
Methoxamine
Methyltestosterone
Misoprostol
Morphine
Naltrexone
Neostigmine (cases in Dtsch Med Wochenschr 1966;**91**:699)
Octreotide
Phenylephrine (rare)
Phenylpropanolamine OD (Lancet 1979;**ii**:1367)
Piperazine (see Trans R Soc Trop Med Hyg 1976;**70**:358)
Prednisone (esp. in children, cases in Clin Paediatr 1990;**29**: 382–8)
Pseudoephedrine (n = 1, Eur J Clin Pharmacol 1978;**14**:253–9)
Pyridostigmine (rare)
Rimonabant (SPC)
Salbutamol
Sibutramine
Streptokinase (see Drugs 1973;**5**:357)
Theophylline
Yohimbine (see Arch Gen Psychiatry 1998; **55**:1033–44)

5.2 AGGRESSION, INCLUDING HOSTILITY AND VIOLENCE *

Review: Shaw and Fletcher, Adv Drug React Toxicolog Rev 2000;**19**: 35–45, 64 refs.

Alcohol withdrawal
Amantadine (cases in Br Med J 1972;**3**:50)
Amphetamine withdrawal
Anabolic steroid withdrawal
Barbiturate withdrawal
Benzodiazepines (during prolonged benzodiazepine use: Can J Psychiatry 2000;**45**:89–90; aggressogenic effect from diazepam, n = 60 male, Addict Behav 2002;**27**: 167–77; review CNS Drugs 1998;**9**:41–57; flunitrazepam: J Am Acad Psychiatry Law 1999;**27**:83–99)
Carbamazepine
Dapsone (Br Med J 1991;**4**:300)
Donepezil (eg. Am J Psychiatry 1998;**155**:1632–3)
Gabapentin (n = 1, J Neuropsychiatry Clin Neurosci 2001;**13**:424)
Lamotrigine (survey, n = 19, Epilepsia 1998;**39**:280–2)
Levetiracetam (SPC)
Modafinil (n = 2, J Clin Psychopharmacol 2005; **25**:628–9)
Naloxone IV (n = 2, Ann Pharmacother 1992;**26**:196–8)
Omeprazole
Olanzapine (Can J Psychiatry 1998;**43**:1054)
Oxandrolone (and other anabolic steroids)
Paroxetine withdrawal (Lancet 1995;**346**:57)
Tricyclics (rare)
Venlafaxine (n = 1, J Am Acad Child Adolesc Psychiatry 2003;**42**:383–4)
Vigabatrin (eg. Drugs 1991;**41**:889–926)

5.3 BEHAVIOURAL CHANGES

Anabolic steroids (Am J Psychiatry 1992; **149**:271–2)
Barbiturates
Benzodiazepines
Clonazepam (Dev Med Child Neurol 1991;**33**:362–5)
Bismuth (Acta Neurologica Belgica 1979;**79**:73)
Carbamazepine (J Paediatrics 1982;**101**:785–7)
Donepezil (eg. n = 7, Am J Psychiatry 1998; **155**:1632–3)
Levetiracetam (7% of n = 553, Neurology 2003; **61**:1218–21)

Levodopa
Levodopa + carbidopa
Lithium + antipsychotics
Methyldopa + haloperidol
Prednisone withdrawal (*JAMA* 1989;**261**: 1731)
Theophylline (disputed — not in children, *JAMA* 1992;**267**:2621–4)

5.4 DELIRIUM (ACUTE ORGANIC PSYCHOSIS) AND CONFUSION

Drug-induced delirium is usually an acute reaction and always with fluctuating levels of awareness of self and environment. It is most frequent in frail or dementing elderly, drug abusers and with pre-existing organic brain disease and strongly associated with anticholinergic activity:

- high risk drug groups are TCAs and typical antipsychotics
- medium risk drugs include benzodiazepines, sedatives, dopamine-activating drugs, anticonvulsants, histamine H2 receptor blockers, digoxin, beta-blockers and analgesics. Most of these do not have direct anticholinergic effects but in vitro have shown to bind to muscarinic receptors.

Reviews: drug-induced delirium, including management (Karlsson, *Dement Geriatr Cogn Disord* 1999;**10**:412–5; Brown, *Semin Clin Neuropsychiatry* 2000;**5**:113–24), in the elderly (Moore and O'Keeffe, *Drugs Aging* 1999;**15**: 15–28; Inouye, *Dement Geriatr Cogn Disord* 1999; **10**: 393–400).

- **Psychotropics etc** *
Alcohol + disulfiram (n = 1, *Ann Pharmacother* 2001;**35**:32–35)
Amfetamines
Anticholinergic drugs (particular association, *J Am Geriatr Soc* 1988;**36**:525; n = 278, *Arch Internal Med* 2001;**161**:1099–105)
Barbiturates
Benzodiazepines (common cause)
Bromides
Bupropion (cases, eg. *J Clin Psychiatry* 1990;**51**: 307–8)
Butyrophenones
Cannabis
Chloral and derivatives
Clomethiazole
Clozapine withdrawal (n = 3, *J Clin Psychiatry* 1997;**58**:252–5)

Clozapine (may occur in 10%, especially if older people, also taking other anticholinergics; n = 139, *Pharmacopsychiatry* 2003;**36**: 156–60)
Cocaine (*Am J Forensic Med Pathol* 1999;**20**: 120–7)
Disulfiram (*Am J Psychiatry* 1974;**131**: 1281)
Disulfiram + alcohol (n = 1, *Ann Pharmacother* 2001;**35**: 32–5)
Donepezil (n = 1, *J Clin Psychiatry* 2002;**63**: 250–1)
Fluoxetine (n = 1, *Am J Psychiatry* 1995; **152**: 295–6)
Lithium (eg. *Am J Psychiatry* 1983;**140**: 1612)
MAOIs eg. phenelzine (*J Clin Psychiatry* 1987;**48**: 340–1)
Mianserin (*Br Med J* 1988;**296**: 137)
Mirtazapine (n = 3, *Int Clin Psychopharmacol* 2000;**15**:239–43)
Olanzapine (n = 1, *J Pain Symptom Manage* 2004;**28**: 102–3, n = 1 [elderly], *J Clin Psychiatry* 2004;**65**;582–3; n = 1, *Ann Pharmacother* 2006;**40**:135–8)
Olanzapine + opioid (n = 2, *J Pain Symptom Manage* 2005;**29**: 330–2)
Paroxetine withdrawal (n = 1, *J Neuropsych Clin Neurosci* 2004;**16**: 119–20)
Paroxetine and benzatropine (*Am J Psychiatry* 1997;**154**:581–2)
Phenothiazines (esp. sedative ones)
Risperidone (n = 1, *Can J Psychiatry* 1998;**43**: 194; n = 1, *J Child Adolesc Psychopharmacol* 2005;**15**:520–5)
Rivastigmine (< 5%)
Sodium oxybate (SPC)
Solvent intoxication
Trazodone (n = 3, *Int Clin Psychopharmacol* 1998;**13**:225–8)
Tricyclics (*J Clin Psychiatry* 1983;**44**: 173–6)
Venlafaxine (n = 1, *Can J Psychiatry* 2003;**48**: 129)
Zolpidem (several cases eg. *J Clin Psychiatry* 2000;**61**:449–50; n = 1, *Ann Pharmacother* 2001;**35**: 1562–64; n = 1, elderly, *Psychosomatics* 2004;**45**:88–9)

- **Drug withdrawal/cessation etc** *
Alcohol (*Am J Psychiatry* 1997;**154**:846–51)
Baclofen (*Br Med J* 2001;**323**:870, letter)
Barbiturates
Benzodiazepines
Clomethiazole
Dextropropoxyphene
Nicotine (*J Pain Symptom Manage* 1998;**15**:S18;

n = 5, *Neurology* 2001;**57**:551–3)
Zopiclone withdrawal (n = 1, *Age Ageing*
2005;**34**:526–7)

- **Anticonvulsants**
Barbiturates (dose-related)
Carbamazepine (especially early in therapy)
Ethosuximide
Phenytoin (dose-related)
Primidone
Topiramate (n = 1, *Bipolar Disord* 2001;**3**:211–2)
Valproate (high dose)
Valproate + lamotrigine (n = 1, *Am J Psychiatry*
2004;**161**:1128–9)
Zonisamide (*J Clin Psychopharmacol* 2004;
4:110–1; SPC)

- **Antiparkinsonian drugs**
Amantadine (case in *Am J Psychiatry*
1980;**137**:240–2)
Anticholinergics (especially longer-acting ones,
eg. benzhexol)
Bromocriptine
Levodopa (*Lancet* 1973; ii:929)
Lysuride
Methixene
Pergolide withdrawal (*Clin Neuropharmacology*
1988;**11**:545–8)
Selegiline

- **Cardiovascular drugs**
Amiodarone (n = 1, *Am J Psychiatry*
1999;**156**:1119)
Amiloride
Beta-blockers (eg. *Postgrad Med J*
1990;**66**:1050–2; atenolol n = 1, *Br Med J*
1988;**297**:1048)
Clonidine (*Curr Med Res Opin* 1977; **4**:630)
Digoxin (*Am Heart J* 1983;106:419; *J Clin
Pharmacol* 1979;**19**:747)
Disopyramide
Diuretics (via severe K + loss)
Hydralazine
Lidocaine
Methyldopa
Mexilitine
Procainamide
Spironolactone

- **NSAIDs and analgesics**
Aspirin toxicity (*Lancet* 1971;**2**:242)

Fenoprofen
Ibuprofen (*Arthritis Rheum* 1982;**25**: 1013)
Indomethacin, inc. OD (*Drugs* 1980;**19**:220–42)
Nalbuphine
Naproxen (cases)
Narcotics
Papaveretum
Salicylate OD (rare cases)
Sulindac (*JAMA* 1980; **243**:1630)
Tramadol (n = 11, *Curr Problems* 1995;**21**:2)

- **Anticholinergics**
Antiparkinsonian drugs (separate section)
Atropine and homatropine eye drops
Scopolamine (transdermal) (*JAMA*
1988;**260**:478)

- **Anti-infection**
These may indirectly cause delirium if inducing
diarrhoea and dehydration.
Aciclovir (eg. *Nervenarzt* 1998;**69**:1015–8)
Cephalosporins (*Br Med J* 1989;**299**: 393)
Chloramphenicol (*Clin Pharmacol Ther* 1970;
11:194)
Chloroquine
Ciprofloxacin (eg. n = 1, *Ann Pharmacother*
1997;**31**: 252, letter)
Clarithromycin (*Psychosomatics* 1998;**39**:540–2)
Cicloserin
Isoniazid (*Br Med J* 1969;i:461)
Mefloquine (*Pharm J* 989;**243**:561)
Penicillin
Rifampicin
Streptomycin
Sulphadiazine
Sulphonamides

- **Miscellaneous**
Adrenocorticotrophin
Aminophylline
Anesthetic agents (56% incidence, *Br J Psychiatry*
2001;**178**: 360–6)
Baclofen
Caffeine (*Am J Psychiatry* 1978;**135**:855–6)
Cimetidine (eg. *Ann Intern Med* 1992;**115**:658–9)
Corticosteroids (11% incidence? review
by Ismail and Wessely, *Br J Hosp Pharm*
1995;**53**:495–9)
Diphenhydramine + linezolid (n = 1, *Ann
Pharmacother* 2004;**38**: 62–5)
Doxapram

Ergotamine-caffeine (n = 1, *Pharmacother* 2002;**22**;126–9)

Famotidine (n = 1, *Pharmacother* 1998;**18**: 404–7)

Gancyclovir (*N Engl J Med* 1990;**322**:933–4)

Hydroxychloroquine

Hypoglycaemics (oral)

Iodoform gauze (n = 1, *Lancet* 1997;**350**:1294)

Interferon Alfa (*Arch Intern Med* 1987;**147**:1557–80)

Mentholatum (n = 1, *Am J Psychiatry* 2000;**157**:483–4)

Methylprednisolone

Misoprostol (*Drug Intell Clin Pharm* 1991;**25**:133–44)

Nabilone

Nalbuphine

Phenylpropanolamine O/D (*Br Heart J* 1982; **47**:51–4)

Piperazine

Ranitidine (*Ann Intern Med* 1992;**115**:658–9; *Br Med J* 1987; **294**: 1616)

Theophylline (*Br Med J* 1982;**284**:939)

Triamcinolone

5.5 DEPRESSION

Occurs mainly in patients with a history of depression. An analysis of all FDA antidepressant trials was unable to find any link with increased suicide with any antidepressants compared to placebo (n = 49 277, Khan *et al*, *Am J Psychiatry* 2003;**160**:790–92).

Reviews: general (Patten and Love, *Psychother Psychosom* 1997;**66**:63–73), in elderly (Dhondt et al, *Int J Geriatr Psychiatry* 1996;**11**:141–8).

- **Psychotropics etc**

Benzodiazepines (especially resistant depression):

Alprazolam (*Am J Psychiatry* 1987;**144**:664–5)

Bromazepam (*Acta Psych Scand* 1989;**74**:451–8)

Clorazepate

Lorazepam (*Am J Psychiatry* 1989;**146**:1230)

Benzodiazepine withdrawal (*Psychol Med* 1984;**14**:937–40)

Buspirone (3% incidence? *J Clin Psychiatry* 1982;**43**[sect 2]:100–2)

Disulfiram (case in *Arch Neurol* 1976;**33**:141)

Flumazenil (< 1% incidence)

Fluphenazine depot (n = 1, *Br Med J* 1969;**3**:564–7)

MDMA ('Ecstasy') (case in *Lancet* 1991;338: 1520, letter; *Lancet* 1996;**347**:833; former chronic users report higher levels of depression than matched controls — n = 29, *J Psychopharmacol* 2001;**15**:181–6)

Modafinil (UK SPC)

Nortriptyline (n = 2, *Br Med J* 1964;**2**:1593)

Smoking cessation, especially if previous MDD (n = 1, *Acta Psych Scand* 1998;**98**:507–8; n = 304, *Am J Psychiatry* 2000;**157**:368–74; n = 100 with history of MDD, 2/12, *Lancet* 2001;**357**:1929–32; see also *Lancet* 2001; **357**:1900–1)

SSRIs (no association with risk of suicide: *Curr Problems* 2000;**26**:11–2)

Fluoxetine (intense suicidal ideation) (*Am J Psychiatry* 1990;**147**:570–2 etc), disproven (*Br Med J* 1991;**303**:685–92), as fluoxetine shows a slight reduction in suicidal behavior (n = 185, *Am J Psychiatry* 1999;**156**:195–201)

Tetrabenazine

Zuclopenthixol

- **Anticonvulsants**

Carbamazepine

Clobazam (n = 1, *Br Med J* 1983;**286**:1246–7)

Clonazepam

Ethosuximide

Lamotrigine (rare, *Epilepsia* 1991;**32**[Suppl 2]:S17–21; n = 1, *J Clin Psychiatry* 2006; **67**:1159–60)

Levetiracetam (n = 1, *J Clin Psychiatry* 2006; **67**:1159–60)

Phenobarbital (*Pediatrics* 1990;**85**:1086–91)

Phenytoin (n = 2, *Arch Phys Med Rehab* 1990; **71**:422–3)

Pregabalin (rare — SPC)

Topiramate (n = 1, *Am J Psychiatry* 2001;**158**:1736)

Vigabatrin (< 10%, *Neurology* 1991;**41**:363–4; *Lancet* 1990;**335**:970)

- **Antiparkinsonian drugs**

Amantadine (mentioned in *JAMA* 1972; **222**:792–5)

Alpha-adrenoceptor blockers (case-control study concluding no association, *Pharmacoepidemiol Drug Saf* 2002;**11**:55–61)

Anticholinergics

Levodopa (well known, review in *N Engl J Med* 1976;**295**:814–8)

- **Cardiovascular drugs**

One review has shown that users of medium and high lipid-soluble beta-blockers may have an increased risk of suicide, but there is no greater risk with calcium-channel blockers and ACE inhibitors (n = 58 529, *Br J Clin Pharmacol* 2001; **52**: 313–8).

Amiodarone (n = 1, *Br J Psychiatry* 1999;**174**: 366–7; n = 1, *J Pharm Technol* 1999; **15**:50–3)

Beta-blockers (*Drug Intell Clin Pharm* 1984;**18**:741–2). Lipophilic drugs may be more likely: atenolol, nadolol (low lipid solubility), labetalol, oxprenolol, timolol, acebutol (low/ moderate), pindolol (moderate), metoprolol (moderate/high), propranolol (high). Theory disputed in *JAMA* 1992;**267**: 1783–7; 1826–7)

Acebutol (mentioned in *Am J Med* 1987; **83**: 223–6)

Atenolol (*J Hum Hypertens* 1987;**1**:87–93)

Metoprolol (5% incidence? review in *Drugs* 1977;**14**: 321–48)

Nadolol (*Lancet* 1982;**i**: 1286)

Propranolol (*Am J Psychiatry* 1982;**139**: 1187–8)

Timolol

Calcium-channel blockers (no increased risk of suicide with use of calcium-channel blockers compared to other antihypertensives, n = 153 458, Gasse *et al*, *Br Med J* 2000;**320**: 1251)

Felodipine (*Br Heart J* 1987;**58**: 122–8)

Nicardipine (cases mentioned in *Br J Clin Pharmacol* 1985;**20**[Suppl]: 178–86)

Nifedipine (*Br J Psychiatry* 1991;**159**: 447–8)

Clonidine (1% incidence, case study in *Postgrad Med J* 1993;**150**: 1750)

Diltiazem (*Br Med J* 1989;**299**: 796)

Enalapril (n = 1, *South Med J* 1989;**82**: 402–3)

Hydralazine

Inositol (n = 3, *Am J Psychiatry* 1996;**153**:839)

Lisinopril (rare)

Methyldopa (review in *Am J Psychiatry* 1983; **140**: 534–8)

Procainamide

Quinapril (n = 1, *Am J Psychiatry* 1999;**156**: 1115)

Quinidine (several cases, eg. *J Am Geriatr Soc* 1985;**33**: 504–6)

Streptokinase (cases, eg. *Drugs* 1973;**5**: 357–445)

- **Gastrointestinal**

Cimetidine (several cases, eg. *Can J Psychiatry* 1981;**26**: 260–1)

Famotidine (rare reports)

Metoclopramide (cases, eg. *Am J Gastroenterol* 1989;**84**: 1589–90)

Omeprazole (unproven reports)

Ranitidine (n = 3, *Am J Psychiatry* 1986; **143**:915–6)

Sulphasalazine

- **NSAIDs and analgesics**

Diflunisal (< 1% incidence)

Etodolac (rare)

Flurbiprofen (> 1% incidence?)

Ibuprofen (uncommon, *Arthritis Rheum* 1982;**25**: 1013)

Indomethacin (4% incidence? *Br Med J* 1972; **4**:398)

Nabilone

Nalbuphine

Naproxen (rare)

Pentazocine (*South Med J* 1975;**68**: 808)

Sulindac

Tramadol (n = 1, *Am J Psychiatry* 1996;**153**: 843–4)

- **Anti-infection** *

Anti-TB drugs (*Lancet* 1989;**ii**:735–6)

Cephradine (n = 1, *Med J Aus* 1973;**2**:742)

Chloramphenicol (rare mild cases)

Ciprofloxacin (very rare)

Clotrimazole — oral (review in *Drugs* 1975; **9**: 424)

Co-trimoxazole (rare, but severe cases, eg. *Drug Intell Clin Pharm* 1988;**22**: 267)

Dapsone (*Br Med J* 1989;**298**: 1524)

Griseofulvin (as part of psychosis, case in *JAMA* 1974;**229**: 1420)

Interferon alpha (appears relatively common with hepatitis C; n = 39, 33% incidence, *Mol Psychiatry* 2002;**7**:942–7; n = 1, *Am J Psychiatry* 1999;**156**: 1120; n = 1, *J Clin Psychiatry* 2002;**63**:66–7; review Am *J Psychiatry* 2000;**157**:867–76; can be treated with paroxetine [*N Engl J Med* 2001;**344**:961–6], sertraline [*Med J Aus* 2000;**173**: 359–61] or methylphenidate n = 1, *J Psychopharmacol* 2006;**20**:687–9)

Mefloquine (*Am J Psychiatry* 1992;**149**: 712; CSM warning, *Curr Prob Pharmacovig* 1999;**25**: 15)

Metronidazole (n = 1, *Am J Psychiatry* 1977;**134**: 329–30)

Piperazine (cases, eg. *J Indian Med Assoc* 1976;**66**: 33)

Primaquine (n = 1, *Ann Int Med* 1980;**92**: 435)

Sulphonamides/sulfonamides

- **Respiratory**

Aminophylline (*Br Med J* 1980;**281**: 1322)

Ephedrine (as part of a psychosis, *Br Med J* 1968;**2**: 60)

Flunisolide (inhaled, 1–3% incidence)

Theophylline (*Br Med J* 1980;**281**: 1322)

- **Cytotoxics etc**

Mesna

Mithramycin

Octreotide (rare)

Plicamycin

Tamoxifen (n = 1, *Ann Int Med* 1984;**101**: 652)

Triamcinolone (up to 8%, see *Br Med J* 1969;i: 682)

- **Steroids**

Review: Ismail and Wessely, *Br J Hosp Med* 1995; **53**: 495–99.

Dexamethasone (up to 40% incidence, *Arch Gen Psychiatry* 1981;**38**: 471–7)

Methyltestosterone (rare)

Prednisolone (*J Assoc Physicians India* 1973;**21**: 909)

Prednisone (review in *Clin Paediatr* 1990;**29**: 382–8)

Stanozolol

- **Miscellaneous** *

Allopurinol

Anesthetic agents (in elderly, n = 140, *Br J Psychiatry* 2001;**178**: 360–6)

Astemizole (debatable, *Drugs* 1984;**28**: 38–61)

Baclofen (rare cases eg. *Arch Intern Med* 1985; **145**: 1717–8)

Botulinum toxin A injection (*South Med J* 1999; **92**: 738)

Caffeine withdrawal (review in *N Engl J Med* 1992;**327**: 1160–1)

Cholesterol-lowering drugs? (higher incidence of low cholesterol in parasuicide [n = 100, *Br J Psychiatry* 2000;**177**: 77–83] and suicide [n = 783, Bocchetta et al, *Acta Psych Scand* 2001;**104**: 37–41]; but high risk of violent suicide with high cholesterol, n = 37,635, *Am J Psychiatry* 2000;**157**: 648–50). Low cholesterol seems to be connected with higher suicide rates.

Cinnarizine (*Br Med J* 1988;**297**: 722)

Clomiphene

Codeine — long-term use (community survey, *J Clin Psychopharmacol* 1999;**19**: 373–6)

Danazol (rare cases, *Am J Obstet* 1977;**27**: 130)

Dianette (SPC)

Diphenoxylate

Etretinate (*Br Med J* 1989;**298**: 964)

Fentanyl (transdermal)

Hydroxyzine (some reports)

Interferon-alfa (13% incidence, n = 93, *J Clin Psychiatry* 2005;**66**: 1050–7)

Isotretinoin (very rare, *J Am Dermatol* 1988;**18**: 543–52; n = 132, unable to show any depressant effect, and in fact reduced depressive symptoms; *Arch Dermatol* 2005;**141**: 557–60; and in 2006, the UK MHRA concluded that there is no firm evidence of an association between isotretinoin and depression and suicide, although there are reported cases)

Naltrexone (probably doesn't cause it, n = 80, *J Psychiatry Neurosci* 2006;**31**: 38–45)

Omega-3 fatty acids (low plasma levels may be risk factor for suicide or depression: *Am J Psychiatry* 2006;**163**: 1100–2)

Ondansetron (n = 1, *Am J Psychiatry* 1995;**152**: 1101)

Oral contraceptives combined (16–56% incidence, review in *J Adolescent Health Care* 1981;**2**: 53–64)

Organophosphates (n = 761, *Ann Epidemiol* 2002;**12**: 389–94)

Pegylated Interferon-alpha and ribavirin (n = 162, moderate to severe depressive symptoms seem to be common, especially with higher doses of ribavirin; *J Clin Psychiatry* 2005;**66**: 41–8)

Phenylpropanolamine (*Am J Psychiatry* 1990; **147**: 367–68)

Pravastatin (n = 4, *Lancet* 1993;**341**: 910)

Progestogens (*Drug Treatment Psychiatry* 1982; **12**: 234–5)

Rimonabant (SPC)

Roaccutane

Sodium oxybate (SPC)

Simvastatin (*Curr Problems* 1992;**33**; n = 4, *Lancet*

1993;**341**: 14. Low cholesterol is a high risk factor for attempted suicide *Am J Psychiatry* 1995;**152**:419–23)

Tamoxifen (no increased risk, n = 11 064, *J Natl Cancer Inst* 2001;**93**: 1615–23)

Trimeprazine/alimemazine

Xylometazoline (case in child in *JAMA* 1970;**211**: 123–4)

5.6 HALLUCINATIONS (INCLUDING VISUAL DISTURBANCES, SEE ALSO PSYCHOSIS)

- **Psychotropics etc** *

Review of factors associated with visual hallucinations with antidepressants (*Hum Psychopharmacol* 2004;**19**:577–84).

Alcohol

Amfetamines (*Biol Psychiatry* 1980;**15**:749)

Benzodiazepines, eg. temazepam (n = 1, *J Am Geriatr Soc* 2006;**54**:1627–8)

Fluoxetine (case in *Am J Psychiatry* 1993;**150**:1750)

Fluoxetine + zolpidem (n = 1, *J Forensic Sci* 2004;**49**: 392–3)

Imipramine

LSD (*J Nerv Mental Dis* 1991;**179**: 173–4)

Maprotiline (n = 1, *Acta Psychiatr Scand* 2000;**101**:476–7)

Memantine (n = 3, *J Neurol Neurosurg Psychiatry* 2006;Oct; exacerbation, n = 3, *Neurology* 2005;**65**:481–2)

Methadone (*J Am Acad Child Adolesc Psychiatry* 1999;**38**: 355–6)

Midazolam IV (*Drug Intell Clin Pharm* 1989;**23**:671–2)

Moclobemide (pseudohallucinations, n = 1, *Pharmacopsychiatry* 2005;**38**: 179–81)

Olanzapine (n = 1, hypnopompic hallucinations, *Can J Psychiatry* 2004;**49**:496–7)

Paroxetine OD (*Psych Clin Neurosci* 2003; **57**:548–9)

Phenelzine (n = 1, *Am J Psychiatry* 1994;**151**:450)

Sertraline (n = 1, *J Clin Psychiatry* 2004;**65**:446–7)

Sodium oxybate (SPC)

Tricyclics

Zolpidem (n = 5, *J Toxicol Clin Toxicol* 1998;**36**:195–203; distorted perception, n = 1, *Ann Pharmacother* 2003;**37**:683–6)

Zolpidem + fluvoxamine (n = 1, *Int Psychogeriatr* 2006;**18**:749–51)

Zopiclone (*Pharm J* 1990;**245**:210)

- **Anticonvulsants**

Carbamazepine

Gabapentin

Lamotrigine (n = 1, *Am J Psychiatry* 2006; **163**:749–50)

Phenytoin (n = 1, *Drug Intell Clin Pharm* 1988;**22**:1003–4; n = 1, Gatzonis et al, *Epilepsy Behav* 1990;**71**:422–3)

Primidone (n = 241, 43% incidence; *Epilepsy Behav* 2005;**6**:413–6).

Valproate

Zonisamide (n = 3, *Pharmacotherapy* 2003;**23**:93–6; SPC)

- **Antiparkinsonian drugs**

Amantadine (n = 1, *Med J Aus* 1973;**1**: 444)

Anticholinergics

Bromocriptine (< 1% incidence — *Ann Int Med* 1984;**101**: 149)

Levodopa (< 26% incidence in elderly, eg. *Postgrad Med J* 1989;**65**: 358–61)

Levodopa-carbidopa + paroxetine (n = 1, *Ned Tijdschr Geneeskd* 2002;**146**:1056–7).

Pergolide (in up to 13%, eg. *Neurology* 1982;**32**: 1181–4)

Pergolide withdrawal (*Clin Neuropharmacology* 1988;**11**:545–8)

Riluzole added to memantine/bupropion (n = 1, *J Clin Psychopharmacol* 2006;**26**:218–20)

- **Cardiovascular drugs**

Beta-blockers (*Postgrad Med J* 1987;**63**:57–8)

Clonidine (n = 3, *Ann Int Med* 1980;**93**:456)

Digoxin (*Ann Int Med* 1979;**91**:865).

Diltiazem (*Psychiatr Prax* 1998;**25**:91–2)

Disopyramide

Procainamide

Streptokinase (reported in *Drugs* 1973;**5**: 357–445)

Timolol (*JAMA* 1980;**244**:768)

- **NSAIDs and analgesics**

Buprenorphine (rare < 1%, eg. *Br Med J* 1988; **296**:214)

Buprenorphine–epidural (*Br Med J* 1989; **298**:928)

Celecoxib (auditory n = 1, *Am J Psychiatry* 2000; **157**:1022–3)

Fenbufen (*Br Med J* 1985;**290**:822)

Indomethacin (rare, eg. *Br Med J* 1966;**1**:80 OD in *Drugs* 1980;**19**:220–42)

Nefopam (*Curr Probl* 24; **1**:89)

Oxycodone + sertraline (n = 1, *J Clin Pharmacol* 2001;**41**:224)

Pentazocine

Salicylates

Tramadol (n = 6, *Curr Probl* 1995;**21**:2)

- **Anti-infections**

Amoxicillin (*Practitioner* 1984;**228**:884)

Ciprofloxacin (*Arch Intern Med* 1989;**110**:170–1)

Gentamicin (*JAMA* 1977;**238**:53)

Itraconazole, oral (n = 1, *Clin Infect Dis* 1995; **21**:456

- **Miscellaneous**

Cimetidine (*Arch Intern Med* 1983;**98**:677)

Corticosteroids

Decongestants (*Br Med J* 1984;**288**:1688)

Dextromethorphan (n = 1, *Psychosomatics* 1996; **37**:71–4)

Erythropoietin (n = 5, *N Engl J Med* 1991; **325**:285; *J Neurol* 1999;**246**:614–6)

Famotidine (n = 1, *Pharmacother* 1998;**18**:404–7)

Ginseng (n = 1, *Acta Psych Scand* 2002;**105**:76–8)

Hydroxyurea

Khat chewing (n = 4, *Br J Hosp Med* 1995; **54**:322–6)

Ketamine (*Anaesthesia* 1990;**45**:422)

Mefloquine (*N Engl J Med* 1990;**322**:1752–3)

Phenylephrine (*JAMA* 1982;**247**:1859)

Phenylpropanolamine (*JAMA* 1981;**245**:601–2)

Promethazine (*Acta Paediatrica Scand* 1989; **78**: 131–2)

Pseudoephedrine

Radiocontrast media (n = 2, review, *Br J Clin Pharmacol* 1999;**47**:226–7)

Ranitidine (*Eur J Clin Pharmacol* 1985;**29**:375–6)

Salbutamol (nebulised) (*Br Med J* 1986; **292**:1430)

Steroid-induced mania (case, review, risk factors; *Can J Clin Pharmacol* 2001;**8**:109–12)

Sulphasalazine

Tolterodine (n = 1, *Br J Urol* 1999;**84**:1109)

5.7 MANIA, HYPOMANIA OR EUPHORIA

Antidepressant-induced mania may be a marker for increased vulnerability to antidepressant-induced cycle acceleration. The most common symptoms of drug-induced mania are increased activity, rapid speech, elevated mood and insomnia. The main risk factors are prior history, family history or concurrent mood disorder. Steroids, levodopa, triazolobenzodiazepines and hallucinogens are most commonly associated. A sudden switch to mania or hypomania may be indicative of the diagnosis of 'bipolar III'.

Reviews: antidepressant-induced mania (Altshuler et al, *Am J Psychiatry* 1995;**152**:1130–8), drug-induced mania (Peet and Peters, *Drug Saf* 1995; **12**:146–53).

- **Hallucinogens**

LSD (*Am J Psychiatry* 1981;**138**:1508–9)

- **CNS stimulants**

Amphetamine withdrawal (*J Clin Psychiatry* 1980;**41**:33–4)

Caffeine (*Gen Hosp Psychiatry* 2003;**25**:138–9)

Dexamfetamine (*Am J Psychiatry* 1976;**133**:1177–80)

Ephedrine (*J Clin Psychopharmacol* 1983;**3**:97–100; and in a Herbal Diet Supplement, case in *Am J Psychiatry* 1995;**152**:647)

Methylphenidate (*J Clin Psychiatry* 1986;**47**:566–7)

Pemoline (possible case in *Biol Psychiatry* 1981; **16**:987–9)

Phenylephrine (*Am J Psychiatry* 1981;**138**:837–8)

Phenylpropanolamine (*Am J Psychiatry* 1981;**138**:392)

Pseudoephedrine (*Psychiatr J Uni Ott* 1987; **12**:47–8)

- **Antidepressants** *

Antidepressant-induced mania is well known (especially in bipolar III), as is the spontaneous swing to hypomania from depression in bipolars. SSRIs and bupropion are generally considered less likely to induce. Depressed bipolar II patients may be less vulnerable than bipolar I to switch to mania/hypomania when treated with an antidepressants adjunctive to a mood stabiliser (n = 184, 10/52, Altshuler et al, *Am J Psychiatry* 2006;**163**:313–5). Risk factors include increased antidepressant trials and substance misuse (n = 53, Goldberg and Whiteside, *J Clin Psychiatry* 2002;**62**:792–5). There is significant risk switch to mania/hypomania during acute and maintenance antidepressants in bipolar depression; venlafaxine being worst, sertraline medium and bupropion lowest risk (n = 159, RCT, 10/52, Leverich et al, *Am J Psychiatry* 2006;**163**:232–9). Switching can be reduced by using adjunctive lithium (n = 44, review by Henry et al, *J Clin Psychiatry* 2001;**62**: 249–55). SSRI-induced hypomania may be dose-related (n = 2, Ramasubbu, *Acta Psychiatr Scand* 2001;**104**: 236–9) and may be similar with SSRIs and bupropion (retrospective, Joffe et al, *Acta Psychiatr Scand* 2002;**105**:427–30).

Reviews: general (Peet, *Br J Psychiatry* 1995; **164**:549–50; Benazzi, *J Affect Disord* 1997;**46**:73–7), avoiding drug-induced switching in bipolar depression (Henry et al, *Drug Saf* 2003;**26**:337–51; Andrade, *J Clin Psychiatry* 2004;**65**:987–93). See also chapter 1.10.3.

Amitriptyline (*Br Med J* 1991;**303**:331–2, 720, 1200; *Neurology* 1989;**39**: 305)

Amitriptyline withdrawal (*J Clin Psychiatry* 1980;**41**: 33–4)

Amoxapine (*Compr Psychiatry* 1982;**23**:590–2)

Bupropion (n = 1, within a week, *Bipolar Disord* 2001;**3**: 159–60)

Clomipramine (*Arch Gen Psychiatry* 1979; **36**:560–5)

Citalopram (n = 1, *Aust NZ J Psychiatry* 2003; **37**:776–7)

Citalopram + silbutramine (n = 1, *J Clin Psychiatry* 2002;**63**: 165)

Desipramine (*Am J Psychiatry* 1985;**142**: 386)

Desipramine withdrawal (*Am J Psychiatry* 1983; **140**: 624–5)

Duloxetine (rare in unipolar depression; *J Affect Disord* 2005;**87**: 115–9)

Escitalopram (n = 1, *Eur Psychiatry* 2004;**19**: 455–6; n = 1, *Mil Med* 2003;**168**: 2)

Fluoxetine (cases in *Ann Pharmacother* 1991; **25**: 1395–6; *Am J Psychiatry* 1991;**148**: 1403–4; n = 3, *J Child Adolesc Psychopharmacol* 1998; **8**:73–80)

Flupentixol (n = 6, *Eur Psychiatry* 2002;**17**: 349–52)

Fluvoxamine (*Am J Psychiatry* 1991;**148**: 1263–4; case series in *Ann Pharmacother* 1993; **27**:1455–7; n = 1, *World J Biol Psychiatry* 2001;**2**:201–4; n = 1, *J Psychiatry Neurosci* 2003;**28**: 134–5)

Imipramine (eg. *J Clin Psychopharmacol* 1985; **5**:342–3)

Imipramine withdrawal (*Am J Psychiatry* 1986; **143**:260)

Isocarboxazid (n = 3, *J Clin Psychiatry* 1986; **47**: 40–1)

Isocarboxazid withdrawal (n = 2, *J Clin Psychopharmacol* 1985;**5**: 340–2)

Maprotiline (cases in *Curr Ther Res* 1976; **19**:463–8)

Mianserin

Mirtazapine (n = 1, *J Neuropsychiatry Clin Neurosci* 1999;**11**: 115–6; n = 1, *Br J Psychiatry* 1999;**175**: 390; n = 1 + review, *Int Clin Psychopharmacol* 2002;**17**:319–22)

Mirtazapine withdrawal (n = 1, *Br J Psychiatry* 1999;**175**: 390)

Mirtazapine + sertraline (n = 1, *J Clin Psychiatry* 1998;**59**: 320)

Mirtazapine + fluoxetine (n = 1, *Depress Anxiety* 2002;**15**:46–7)

Paroxetine (case of psychotic mania, *Am J Psychiatry* 1995;**152**: 1399–440; incidence of mania with paroxetine is 8.86%; n = 79, *Hum Psychopharmacol* 2003;**18**:565–8).

Phenelzine (eg. *Biol Psychiatry* 1985;**20**: 1009–14)

Reboxetine (n = 3, *Am J Psychiatry* 2001;**62**:655–6)

Sertraline (cases in *Am J Psychiatry* 1994;**343**:606–7; n = 1, *Acta Psychiatr Scand* 2003;**108**: 70–4)

St. John's wort (n = 12, review in *Int J Clin Pharmacol Ther* 2004;**2**: 473–80)

Trazodone (eg. *Br J Psychiatry* 1991;**158**:275–8)

Trazodone withdrawal (*Br J Psychiatry* 1987; **151**:274)

Tryptophan + MAOI (*Am J Psychiatry* 1985; **142**: 1487–8)

Venlafaxine (*J Clin Psychopharmacol* 1999;**19**: 184–5; n = 1, *Can J Psychiatry* 2004;**49**: 496; n = 1, *Can J Psychiatry* 2004;**49**:786–7)

Venlafaxine withdrawal (n = 1, *Int J Neuropsychopharmacol* 2003;**6**:89–90)

Ziprasidone (n = 1, *J Clin Psychiatry* 2004;**65**: 132)

Ziprasidone + SSRI (n = 1, *J Clin Psychiatry* 2003; **64**: 1393–4)

• **Other psychotropics etc** *

Review that notes mania has been reported to be induced by full atypicals (olanzapine, risperidone, quetiapine and ziprasidone) but not (or only very rarely) with clozapine or typicals (including amisulpride) (Rachid et al, *J Clin Psychiatry* 2004;**11**: 1537–45; 57 refs).

Alprazolam (*J Clin Psychiatry* 1987;**48**: 117–8)

Atomoxetine (n = 1, *J Clin Psychopharmacol* 2004; **24**:567–8; n = 1, *Pediatrics* 2004;**114**:895–6)

Benzodiazepine withdrawal (*Acta Psychiatr Scand* 1989;**79**:406–7)

Buprenorphine (n = 1, *Aust N Z J Psychiatry* 2004;**38**:560–1)

Bupropion discontinuation (n = 1, *J Clin Psychiatry* 2004;**65**:277)

Bupropion (rare, *Am J Psychiatry* 1991;**148**:541)

Buspirone (*Br J Psychiatry* 1991;**158**:136–7)

Disulfiram (*J Clin Psychopharmacol* 1986;**6**:178–80; *J Am Acad Child Adolesc Psychiatry* 1988; **27**:500–3)

Fenfluramine (eg. *Med J Aus* 1976;**2**:537; *Am J Psychiatry* 1997;**154**:711)

Lithium + TCA (*Br J Psychiatry* 1988;**153**:828–30)

Lithium toxicity (*Drug Intell Clin Pharm* 1987; **21**:979)

Lorazepam withdrawal (*J Affect Disord* 1989; **17**:93–5)

Midazolam (euphoria possible)

Modafinil (n = 1, *Am J Psychiatry* 2005;**162**:813–4)

Olanzapine (review, concludes half of reports are poorly documented but, in the others, mood-elevating effects were prominent, n = 26, *J Clin Psychiatry* 2000;**61**:649–55; Lilly post-hoc analysis of two RCTs failed to show evidence of olanzapine-induced mania; n = 254, Baker et al, *J Affect Dis* 2003;**73**:147–53).

Olanzapine/fluoxetine combo (no greater risk than OLZ or placebo over 8/52, n = 370 + 377 + 86, *J Clin Psychiatry* 2005; **66**:611–6)

Quetiapine (n = 1, *Eur Neuropsychopharmacol* 2003;**13**:135–6; n = 1, *Can J Psychiatry* 2003;**48**:349–50; n = 1, *Eur Psychiatry* 2002; **17**:292–3)

Risperidone (review, concludes half of reports are poorly documented but, in the others, mood-elevating effects were prominent, n = 26, *J Clin Psychiatry* 2000;**61**:649–55; eg. *Ann Pharmacother* 1999;**33**:380–1).

Risperidone withdrawal (n = 1, *J Clin Psychiatry* 1998;**59**:620–1)

Ziprasidone (=14 worldwide, reviewed in *Clin Neuropharmacol* 2005;**28**:83–6)

- **Anticonvulsants** *

Carbamazepine (*J Clin Psychiatry* 1984;**45**:272–4)

Carbamazepine withdrawal (n = 1, *Br J Psychiatry* 1995;**167**:698)

Clonazepam (*Drug Intell Clin Pharm* 1991;**25**: 938–9)

Ethosuximide

Gabapentin (n = 1, *Br J Psychiatry* 1995;**166**:679–80; review in *Br J Psychiatry* 1995;**167**:549–54; n = 1, *Br J Psychiatry* 1999;**175**:291)

Lamotrigine (n = 1, *Am J Psychiatry* 2003; **160**:183–4; n=3, *Am J Psychiatry* 2006 **163**:159–60; n = 1, *Aust N Z J Psychiatry* 2006; **40**:718)

Phenobarbital (*Pediatrics* 1984;**74**:1133)

Pregabalin (SPC)

Topiramate (n = 1, *J Neurol Neurosurg Psychiatry* 2002;**73**:208–9; *J Clin Psychopharmacol* 2005; **25**:196–7)

Valproate

Vigabatrin (n = 1, *Lancet* 1994;**343**:606–7)

Zonisamide (*J Clin Psychopharmacol* 2004; **24**:110–1; n = 1, *J Clin Psychopharmacol* 2006; **26**:439–40)

- **Antiparkinsonian drugs** *

Amantadine (n = 1, *J Clin Psychiatry* 1989; **50**:143–4)

Bromocriptine (*Br Med J* 1984;**289**:1101–3; postpartum mania, n = 1, *J Gynecol Obstet Biol Reprod* [Paris] 2006;**35**:79–81)

Levodopa (eg. *N Engl J Med* 1971;**285**:1326)

Levodopa + carbidopa (*J Clin Psychopharmacol* 1985;**5**:338–9)

Procyclidine (eg. *Br J Psychiatry* 1982;**141**:81–4)

- **Cardiovascular drugs**

Captopril (*Am J Psychiatry* 1985;**142**:759–60; case in *Am J Psychiatry* 1993;**150**:1429–30)

Clonidine (*Am J Psychiatry* 1982;**139**:1083)

Clonidine withdrawal (*J Clin Psychopharmacol* 1981;**1**:93–5)

Digoxin (*Med J Rec* 1929;**130**:381–2)

Diltiazem (*Clin Cardiology* 1984;**7**:611–2)

Hydralazine

Methyldopa withdrawal (*Am J Psychiatry* 1989; **146**:1075–6)

Procainamide (*Am J Psychiatry* 1988;**145**:129–30)

Propranolol (*South Med J* 1984;**77**:1603)

Propranolol withdrawal (*Am J Psychiatry* 1986; **143**:1633)

- **NSAIDs and analgesics**

Buprenorphine (up to 1%, *Br J Clin Pract* 1980; **34**:144–6)

Codeine + paracetamol (n = 1, *Aust N Z J Psychiatry* 1998;**32**:586–8)

Indomethacin (*J Clin Psychopharmacol* 1987;**7**:203–4)

Nefopam IM (euphoria reported — *Br J Anaesth* 1979;**51**:691–5)

Pentazocine (*South Med J* 1975;**68**:808)

Gastrointestinal

Cimetidine (*J Clin Psychiatry* 1983;**44**:267–8)

Metoclopramide (case in *J Clin Psychiatry* 1984; **45**:180)

Ranitidine IV (case in *South Med J* 1987; **80**:1467)

- **Steroids**

Steroid-induced mania (case, review, risk factors; *Can J Clin Pharmacol* 2001;**8**:109–12)

ACTH (*Psychosomatic Med* 1953;**15**:280–91)

Beclomethasone aerosol (*Am J Psychiatry* 1989; **146**:1076–7)

Beclomethasone nasal spray (*Br J Psychiatry* 1989;**155**:871–2)

Corticosteroids (*Clin Pharm* 1987;**6**:186; n = 1, *Anesthesiology* 1996;**85**:1194–6)

Cortisone (*Psychosomat Med* 1953;**15**:589–97)

Dexamethasone (up to 31% incidence, *Arch Gen Psychiatry* 1981;**38**:471–7)

Hydrocortisone (*J Nerv Ment Dis* 1979; **167**:229–36; *Postgrad Med J* 1992;**68**:41–3)

Prednisone (*J Affect Disord* 1983;**5**:319–24)

Testosterone-patches (n = 1, *Am J Psychiatry* 1999;**156**:969)

Triamcinolone (rare cases)

- **Anti-infection**

Anti-TB drugs (*Lancet* 1989;**ii**:735–6)

Chloroquine (*Br J Psychiatry* 1991;**159**:164–5 + 735)

Clarithromycin (n = 1, *Am J Psychiatry* 1998; **155**:1626)

Dapsone (*Br Med J* 1989;**298**:1524)

Efavirenz overdose (n = 1, *Clin Infect Dis* 2001; **33**:270–1)

Isoniazid (*Br Med J* 1957;**ii**:743–6)

Mepacrine (*Mayo Clin Proc* 1989;**64**:129)

Ribavirin + pegylated interferon (n = 1, *Am J Psychiatry* 2004;**161**:429)

Zidovudine (*JAMA* 1988;**259**:3406)

- **Miscellaneous**

Alimemazine/trimeprazine (rare cases)

Aminophylline Baclofen (eg. *Biol Psychiatry* 1982; **17**:757–9)

Baclofen withdrawal (*Am J Psychiatry* 1980; **137**:1466–7)

Bromide (*Am J Psychiatry* 1976;**133**:228–9)

Calcium IV (*J Nerv Ment Dis* 1980;**168**:562–3)

Ciclosporin (*Biol Psychiatry* 1984;**19**:1161–2)

Cyclizine

Cyproheptadine (rare, eg. *Am J Psychiatry* 1980; **137**:378–9)

Decongestants

Dextromethorphan (n = 1, *Psychosomatics* 1996; **37**:71–4)

Dextromethorphan abuse (cases in *Br Med J* 1986;**293**:597; *Br Med J* 1993;**306**:896)

Dihydroepiandrosterone (*Biol Psychiatry* 1999;**45**:241–2)

Frovatriptan (n = 1, *J Neuropsychiatry Clin Neurosci* 2005;**17**:430–1)

Ginseng (n = 1, *Acta Psychiatr Scand* 2002; **105**:76–8)

Herbal remedies (n = 1, *Am J Psychiatry* 1998; **155**:1627)

Interferon-alpha (n = 1, *Postgrad Med J* 1997; **73**:834–5; 16% incidence, n = 93, *J Clin Psychiatry* 2005;**66**:1050–7)

Nicotine withdrawal (*Am J Psychiatry* 1990; **147**:1254–5; *Am J Psychiatry* 1992;**149**:708)

Omega-3 fatty acids (n = 1, *Arch Gen Psychiatry* 2000;**57**:715–6)

Procarbazine (*Br Med J* 1982;**284**:82)

Salbutamol

Sildenafil (relapse, n = 1, *Int J Neuro-psychopharmacol* 2004;**7**:525)

Silbutramine + citalopram (n = 1, *J Clin Psychiatry* 2002;**63**:165).

Thyroid (*Am J Psychiatry* 1970;**126**:1667–9)

Tramadol (n = 1, *Am J Psychiatry* 1997;**154**:1624)

Triptorelin (n = 1, *Br J Psychiatry* 1999;**175**:290–1)

Triiodothyronine (*J Clin Psychiatry* 1986;**47**:521–32)

Yohimbine? (see *Arch Gen Psychiatry* 1998; **55**:1033–44)

5.8 MOVEMENT DISORDERS, EXTRA-PYRAMIDAL DISORDERS

Four distinct types of drug-induced extra-pyramidal or movement disorders are common, especially by antipsychotics. These are dystonias, akathisias, pseudoparkinsonism and dyskinesias. All can occur acutely or be delayed (tardive). Acute reactions are usually at the start of treatment or after a dose increase and are usually reversible. The tardive forms are not invariably reversible on discontinuation of the drug or on dose reduction and can be aggravated by anticholinergics.

Reviews: calcium-channel blockers as cause of EPS (*Ann Pharmacother* 1995;**29**:73–5), general (Jimenez-Jimenez et al, *Drug Saf* 1997;**16**:, 180–204, 643 refs; n=1559, Muscettola et al, *J Clin Psychopharmacol* 1999;**19**:203–8), SSRI-induced movement disorders (Gerber and Lynd, *Ann Pharmacother* 1998;**32**:692–8), management of acute antipsychotic-induced EPS (Remington and Bezchlibnyk-Butler, *CNS Drugs* 1996;**5**[Suppl 1]:21–35), tardive EPS (Marsalek, *Pharmacopsychiatry* 2000;**33**[Suppl 1]:14–33).

5.8.1 PSEUDOPARKINSONISM

This is characterised by akinesia, tremor and rigidity, and generally occurs within a month of the start of treatment.

* **Psychotropics etc** *
Review of antipsychotic drug-induced movement disorders (Blanchet, *Can J Neurol Sci* 2003; **30**[Suppl 1]:S101–7)
Amoxapine (*Am J Psychiatry* 1983;**140**:1233–5)
Aripiprazole (n=2,*J Clin Psychiatry* 2005;**66**:135–6; n=1,*J Psychopharmacol* 2005;**19**:592–3; n=1, *Am J Psychiatry* 2006;**163**:160–1; n=1,*Aust N Z J Psychiatry* 2006;**40**:194–5; n=1,*Int Clin Psychopharmacol* 2006;**21**:127–9)
Antipsychotics (see 2.1.5).
Bromocriptine
Bupropion (n=1,*J Clin Psychiatry* 1992;**53**:157–9)
Clozapine (n=1,*Ann Pharmacother* 2000;**34**:615–18)
Cocaine abuse (*Arch Internal Med* 1997; **157**:241)
Dexamphetamine
Donepezil (n=1,*Ann Pharmacother* 1998; **32**:610–11)
Fluoxetine (*Am J Psychiatry* 1989;**146**:1352–3; case in *Neurology* 1993;**43**:211–13; n=21, *Parkinsonism Relat Disord* 2002;**8**:325–7; mean latency for tremor was 54 days, it was mild and remitted in 50% over a mean of 35 days on discontinuation)
Fluoxetine withdrawal (*Am J Psychiatry* 1991; **148**:1263)
Fluvoxamine (*Am J Psychiatry* 1989;**146**:1352–3)

Lithium-long-term (eg. *Br J Psychiatry* 1980;**136**: 191) and short-term (*J Neurol Sci* 2000;**176**: 78–9)
MAOIs
Olanzapine overdose (n=1, *Am J Psychiatry* 1998;**155**:1630–1)
Paroxetine (cases reported in *Current Problems* 1993;**19**:1; incidence as with other SSRIs, *Lancet* 1993;**341**:624)
Prochlorperazine
Risperidone (case with 2mg/d,*Lancet* 1995; **346**:226; probable case, *Am J Psychiatry* 1996; **153**:843)
Rivastigmine
Sertraline (n=1, *Am J Psychiatry* 1994;**151**:288)
Sertraline and oxycodone (n=1,*J Clin Pharmacol* 2001;**41**:224)
SSRIs (review, *Prescrire Internat* 2001;**10**:118–19; concluding annual incidence around 1 or 2 cases per 1000 patients)
Trazodone (*Clin Neuropharmacol* 1988;**11**:180–2; n=1, *Nephron* 2002;**90**:222–3)
Tricyclics
Ziprasidone IM (n=1, *Am J Psychiatry* 2005; **23**:92–3)

* **Anticonvulsants** *
Carbamazepine (tremor may occur in 22% of pts, *NEJM* 1992;**327**:765–71)
Lamotrigine (n=1, *Mov Disord* 2006;**21**:2269–70)
Levetiracetam (n=1, *Clin Neuropharmacol* 2005;**28**:188–90)
Valproate (n=10, *Pharmacopsychiatry* 2006;**39**:9–12; n=1, elderly, demented patient, *J Clin Psychiatry* 2002;**63**:75)

* **NSAIDs and analgesics**
Fenoprofen
Flurbiprofen (*Br Med J* 1990;**300**:549)
Ibuprofen (case in *Postgrad Med J* 1987;**63**:593–4)
Indomethacin
Mefenamic acid (n=1, *J Roy Soc Med* 1983; **76**:35)
Nabilone
Pethidine and other opioids
Sulindac (single case in *Ann Neurol* 1985; **17**:104–5)

* **Cardiovascular drugs**
Amiodarone (*Ann Neurol* 1989;**25**:630–2)

Diazoxide (n = 6, *Br Med J* 1973;**3**:474–5)
Diltiazem (*Am J Med* 1989;**87**:95–6)
Methyldopa (cases in *Can Med Assoc J* 1966;
  95:928)
Metirosine
Mexilitine
Nifedipine (*Br Med J* 1978;**i**:1619)
Tocainide

• **Gastrointestinal**
Cimetidine (possible case in *Postgrad Med J*
  1982;**58**:527–8)
Domperidone (rare, case in *Helv Paediatr Acta*
  1984;**39**:285–8)
Metoclopramide (2–30% incidence, cases
  in, eg. *Ann Int Med* 1989;**149**:2486–92)
Prochlorperazine (common, eg. *Lancet* 1984;
  2:1082–3)

• **Anti-infection**
Acyclovir
Cephaloridine
Chloroquine

• **Respiratory drugs**
Antihistamines
Brompheniramine (*NEJM* 1975;**293**:
  486)
Cinnarizine (*Lancet* 1987;**i**:1324)
Diphenhydramine (*NEJM* 1977;**296**:111)
Orciprenaline
Promethazine (*Clin Pharm* 1984;**3**:83)
Salbutamol
Terbutaline

• **Hormones**
Medroxyprogesterone

• **Cytotoxics**
Ciclosporin
Interferons

• **Miscellaneous**
Cyclizine
Levodopa
Ondansetron (cases in *Ann Pharmacother*
  1994;**28**:280 and *Ann Pharmacother*
  1996;**30**:196)
Prednisolone (increases incidence
  with neuroleptics, review in *JAMA*
  1973;**224**:889)

Tetrabenazine

5.8.2 AKATHISIA

Characterised by motor restlessness, with an
inability to stay still. Onset is around 6–60 days
and has been implicated with all antipsychotics,
but especially with the high potency ones.
Review: symptoms, classification, drug effects,
treatment, etc (Gattera *et al*, *Aus J Hosp Pharm*
1994;**24**:480–9).

• **Psychotropics etc** *
Alimemazine /trimeprazine
Alprazolam
Amoxapine (*Curr Ther Res* 1972;**14**:381–9)
Antipsychotics (*Psychopharmacol* 1989;**97**:1–11.
  Trifluoperazine and haloperidol more likely
  than less potent drugs, eg. chlorpromazine or
  thioridazine)
Aripiprazole
Buspirone (n = 1, *Ann Intern Med* 1983;**99**:94–5).
Citalopram (n = 1, *J Clin Psychiatry* 1988;
  49[Suppl]:18–22)
Clozapine (6% incidence claimed:
  Psychopharmacology 1995;**118**:52–6; but may
  be rarer, see *Biol Psychiatry* 1991;**29**:1215–19)
Fluoxetine (*J Clin Psychiatry* 1991;**52**:491–3; *J
  Clin Psychiatry* 1989;**50**:339–42; n = 1, dose
  dependent, *J Psychopharmacol* 2003;**17**:451–2)
Fluvoxamine (n = 1, resulting in suicide attempt, *J
  Clin Psychiatry* 1999;**60**:869)
Haloperidol (review in *Psychopharmacol* 1985;
  21:69–72)
Imipramine (n = 1, *J Clin Psychopharmacol* 1987;
  7:254–7)
Lithium (*J Neurol Sci* 2000;**176**:78–9)
Lorazepam (n = 1, *Oncology* 1990;**47**:415–17)
Mianserin (n = 3, *Br J Psychiatry* 1989;**155**:415–17)
Mirtazapine (*Med J Aust* 2002;**176**:242)
Olanzapine (6% incidence)
Paroxetine (*Can J Psychiatry* 2000;**45**:398)
Pipothiazine (study in *Curr Ther Res*
  1981;**29**:903–14)
Prochlorperazine (44% incidence with IV,
  n = 140, *Ann Emerg Med* 1999;**34**:469–75)
Promazine
Quetiapine (n = 1, *Mov Disord* 2003;**18**:712–13;
  n = 1, *Aust N Z J Psychiatry* 2006;**40**:607–8)
Risperidone (*Neurology* 1995;**45**:14–19)
Risperidone withdrawal (*Am J Psychiatry*

1997;**154**:437–8; n = 2, *Actas Esp Psiquiatr*
2002;**30**:195–7)

Risperidone + levomepromazine (n = 1, *Eur Psychiatry* 2002;**17**:294–5)

Sertraline (n = 1, *Am J Psychiatry* 1993;**150**:986–7; *J Clin Psychiatry* 1993;**54**:321; mistaken for panic attack, n = 1, *Psychiatr Serv* 2002; **53**:1477–8)

Tricyclics (*Br Med J* 1986;**282**:1529)

Venlafaxine withdrawal (n = 1, *Am Fam Physician* 1997;**56**:455–62)

Ziprasidone dose reduction (n = 5, *Am J Psychiatry* 2006;**163**:546)

Zuclopenthixol (study in *Pharmatherapeutica* 1989;**5**:380–86)

- Others *

Diltiazem (n = 1, *Ann Intern Med* 1983;**99**:794)

Interferon-alpha (*Gen Hosp Psychiatry* 1999; **21**:134–5)

Levodopa (review in *Neurology* 1990;**40**:340–5)

Melatonin withdrawal (*Mov Disord* 1999; **14**:381–2)

Metoclopramide (n = 1, *Milit Med* 1987; **152**:585–6)

Midodrine + promethazine (n = 1, *JAMA* 2006;**295**:2000–1)

Ondansetron (n = 1, *Cancer* 1992;**69**:1275)

Prochlorperazine (n = 1, *JAMA* 1985;**253**:635)

Verapamil (*Lancet* 1991;**338**:893)

5.8.3 DYSTONIAS

Includes oculogyric crisis, trismus and torticollis. May occur within 72 hours of start of therapy. Occurs more frequently with high-potency antipsychotics, where the incidence may be as high as 10% (*Applied Therapeutics*, Koda-Kimble, 2004).

Review: van Harten *et al*, *Br Med J* 1999;**319**:623–6, 34 refs.

- Psychotropics, etc *

Amoxapine (*Psychosomatics* 1984;**25**:66–9)

Aripiprazole (n = 1, *J Neuropsychiatry Clin Neurosci* 2006;**18**:426–7; n = 1, *Am J Psychiatry* 2006;**163**:1112–3; n = 1, *Ann Pharmacother* 2006;**40**:775–7)

Benzatropine (case in child in *Ann Emerg Med* 1986;**15**:594–6)

Bupropion (n = 1, *J Clin Psychiatry* 1997;**58**:218; n = 1, *Ann Pharmacother* 2002;**36**:251–4)

Buspirone (possible case in *Neurology* 1990;**40**:1904; discussion in *Neurology* 1991;**41**:1850)

Carbamazepine (n = 1, *Postgrad Med J* 1994;**70**:54; n = 1, *N Z Med J* 1994;**107**:360–1)

Clozapine (rare, n = 1, *Am J Psychiatry* 1995; **152**:647–8)

Clozapine withdrawal, abrupt (cases, *J Clin Psychiatry* 1998;**59**:472–7)

Citalopram (Dystonic rabbit syndrome; n = 2, *Clin Neuropharmacol* 2005;**28**:289–91)

Cocaine (risk factor for neuroleptic-induced acute dystonia, *J Clin Psychiatry* 1998;**59**:128–30)

Cocaine withdrawal (*Neurology* 1989;**39**:996)

Disulfiram (n = 1, *Mov Disord* 1991;**6**:166–70)

Escitalopram (n = 1, *Int Arch Allergy Immunol* 2006;**140**:27–9)

Fluoxetine (*Am J Psychiatry* 1994;**151**:149; n = 1, *Mov Disorder* 2001;**16**:767–9; n = 1, *Rev Neurol* 2004;**38**:99)

Flupentixol decanoate (n = 1, *Br Med J* 1981; **282**:1756)

Gabapentin (n = 1, *Ann Pharmacother* 2005; **39**:380–2)

Lithium (n = 1, *Neurol India* 2002;**50**:473–5)

Loxapine

Midazolam (*Br Med J* 1990;**300**:614)

Mirtazapine (n = 1, *J Clin Psychiatry* 2002;**63**:452–3; n = 1, *Tijdschr Psychiatr* 2006;**48**:153–7)

Olanzapine (n = 1, *Am J Psychiatry* 1999; **156**:1662; tardive n = 1, *Neurol Sci* 2001; **22**:331–2)

Paroxetine (cases reviewed in *Curr Prob* 1993; **19**:1; n = 1, *J Psychopharmacol* 2002;**16**:395–7)

Phenelzine (n = 1, *J Clin Psychopharmacol* 1990; **10**:144–5)

Pimozide (n = 1, delayed by 12 hours in child, *J Toxicol Clin Toxicol* 2004;**42**:977–81)

Prochlorperazine

Quetiapine (n = 1, *Ann Pharmacother* 2004;**38**:719–20; n = 1, *Aust N Z J Psychiatry* 2006;**40**:607–8)

Risperidone (n = 1, *Am J Psychiatry* 1996;**153**:577; *Can J Psychiatry* 1999;**44**:507–8; n = 1, *Lancet* 1999;**353**:981, letter)

Sertraline (n = 1, *J Clin Psychopharmacol* 1999;**19**:98–100; mistaken for panic attack, n = 1, *Psychiatr Serv* 2002;**53**:1477–8)

Tiagabine (n = 3, *Epilepsia* 2001;**42**:944–6)

Tricyclics

Venlafaxine

Zuclopenthixol (study in *Acta Psychiatr Scand* 1991;**84**:14–16)

Ziprasidone (n = 1, *Am J Psychiatry* 2005; **162**: 625–6; Ziprasidone (n = 2, *J Clin Psychiatry* 2006;**67**:326–7; n = 1, *Am J Psychiatry* 2005; **162**:2191)

- **Others**

Alimemazine/trimeprazine

Amiodarone (isolated case in *Lancet* 1979;**1**:81–2)

Azapropazone (n = 1, *J Neurol Neurosurg Psychiatry* 1988;**51**:731–2)

Diphenhydramine oral (*Clin Pharm* 1989;**8**:471)

Diphenhydramine IV (*Ann Intern Med* 1989; **111**:92–3)

Domperidone

Ergotamine (*Mov Disord* 1991;**6**:263–4)

Indomethacin (n = 1, *J Neurol Neurosurg Psychiatry* 1988;**51**:731–2)

Metoclopramide (3% incidence, see *NEJM* 1983;**309**:433; cases in, eg. *Ann Intern Med* 1989;**149**:2486–92)

Nifedipine (*Ann Intern Med* 1985;**104**:125)

Penicillamine (review *Arch Neurol* 1987;**44**:490–3)

Prochlorperazine (many cases)

Promethazine (n = 1, *Clin Pharm* 1984;**3**:83–5)

Propofol (n = 45, *Anesth Analg* 2002;**94**:1237–40)

Propranolol

Sumatriptan (possible case in *Ann Pharmacother* 1994;**28**:1199)

Verapamil (n = 1, *J Clin Pharmacy Ther* 1998; **23**:79–80)

5.8.4 DYSKINESIAS *

If of late onset, tardive dyskinesia (TD) can be a potentially irreversible movement disorder with possible relationship to drug, dose and duration (see 6.5). The risk of developing definitive TD is half with the use of atypicals than with conventional antipsychotics, even among patients at high risk of the condition. 110 were receiving atypicals (risperidone, olanzapine or quetiapine) and 130 conventional (haloperidol or thioridazine) antipsychotics (n = 240, Dolder

and Jeste, *Biol Psychiatry* 2003:**53**:142–5).

Amoxapine (mentioned in *J Clin Psychopharmacol* 1987;**7**:243–6)

Amisulpride (n = 1, *Schizophr Res* 2006;**88**:232–4)

Aripiprazole (n = 1, after 18/12 for refractory depression, *CNS Spect* 2006;**11**:435–9)

Benzatropine (study showed worsening TD — *Neuropsychobiology* 1980;**6**:109)

Bupropion (*J Clin Psychiatry* 1997;**58**:218)

Buspirone? (*Pharm J* 1989;**243**:480)

Clomipramine (*Am J Psychiatry* 1993;**150**:165–6)

Clozapine (n = 1, *J Clin Psychiatry* 2002;**63**:167–8; n = 3, *Eur Psychiatry* 2003;**18**:260–1; n = 1, after 10 years, *Am J Psychiatry* 2003;**160**:588; n = 1, *PNBP* 2005;**29**:633–65)

Clozapine withdrawal, abrupt (cases, *J Clin Psychiatry* 1998;**59**:472–7)

Cocaine (n = 1, *Neurology* 2001;**56**:964–5)

Donepezil (*Ann Pharmacother* 2000;**34**:1347, letter)

Doxepin (10% incidence in study in *J Clin Psychopharmacol* 1987;**7**:243–6)

Diphenhydramine (n = 1, *Can J Psychiatry* 1985; **30**:370–1)

Fluoxetine (*Am J Psychiatry* 1991;**148**:1403; *Am J Psychiatry* 1995;**152**:122–5)

Fluvoxamine (n = 1, *J Clin Psychopharmacol* 1993; **13**:365–6)

Fluoxetine + low dose neuroleptics (*Am J Psychiatry* 1991;**148**:683)

Flupentixol decanoate (*Psychopharmacol* 1983; **81**:359–62)

Gabapentin (n = 1, *J Clin Psychopharmacol* 2001; **21**:623–4)

Haloperidol (many cases)

Lithium (*Am J Psychiatry* 1979;**136**:1229–30; *Br J Psychiatry* 1990;**156**:128–9)

Loxapine

Metoclopramide (BNF, many cases, eg. *Neurology* 1984;**34**:238–39)

Methylphenidate (n = 1, *Prim Care Companion J Clin Psychiatry* 2002;**4**:158–9)

Olanzapine (n = 2, *Ann Intern Med* 1999;**131**:72; n = 1, *J Clin Psychiatry* 1999;**60**:870; *J Neuropsychiatry Clin Neurosci* 2006;**18**:132)

Phenytoin (n = 1, *NEJM* 1978;**298**:457)

Pimozide (35% incidence reported, probably rarer — see *Neurology* 1982;**32**:335–6)

Quetiapine (n = 1, *Am J Psychiatry* 1999; **156**:796–7; n = 1, *Am J Psychiatry* 2001; **158**:1737)

Risperidone (n = 1, *Pharmacopsychiatry* 1998;**31**:68–9; n = 1, *Ann Pharmacother* 2000;**34**:1487–8; clear case, *Am J Psychiatry* 1999;**156**:1290; n = 1, *J Clin Psychiatry* 1999; **60**:485–7; although a lower incidence in the elderly with low-dose has been reported, n = 330, open, 12/52, RCT, *Am J Psychiatry* 2000;**157**:1150–5)

Risperidone/citalopram abrupt withdrawal (n = 1, *Ann Pharmacother* 2000;**34**:269)

Sulpiride (*Clin Neuropharmacol*1990;**13**:248–52)

Venlafaxine

Ziprasidone (n = 1, *Am J Psychiatry* 2002;**159**: 1436; n = 1, *Am J Psychiatry* 2004; **161**:175–6; *Can J Psychiatry* 2005;**50**:567–8)

5.8.5 OTHER MOVEMENT DISORDERS

5.8.5.1 CATATONIA *

Review: in young people (*J Am Acad Child Adolesc Psychiatry* 1999;**38**:1040–6)

Allopurinol (n = 1, *Br Med J* 1991;**302**:970)

Azithromycin (n = 1, *J Clin Psychiatry* 2006; **67**:492)

Baclofen (cases, *Clin Neuropharmacol* 1992; **15**:56–62)

Benzodiazepine withdrawal (n = 5, *J Clin Psychopharmacol* 1996;**16**:315–19)

Bupropion (n = 1, *J Clin Psychiatry* 1992;**53**:210)

Clozapine (*Can J Psychiatry* 2001;**46**:458)

Clozapine-withdrawal (n = 1, *Clin Neuro-pharmacol* 2004;**27**:216–8)

Cicloserin

Cocaine (n = 1, *Am J Psychiatry* 1998;**155**:1629)

Disulfiram (n = 1, *Arch Neurol* 1989;**46**:798–804; possible case in *Am J Psychiatry* 1992;**149**:1279–80)

Fluphenazine (n = 1, *Br J Psychiatry* 1973; **122**: 240)

Hydroxyzine (n = 1, *No To Shinkei* 2005;**57**:45–9)

Levetiracetam (n = 1, *Epilepsy Behav* 2006; **8**:303–7)

Loxapine (n = 1, *J Clin Psychiatry* 1983;**44**:10–12)

Morphine epidural (n = 1, *Lancet* 1980;**2**:984)

Phenelzine + haloperidol (n = 1, *Can J Psychiatry* 1988;**33**:633–4)

Piperazine (mentioned in *Trans Roy Soc Trop Med Hyg* 1976;**70**:358)

Prochlorperazine (n = 1, *Postgrad Med* 1976; **60**:171–3)

Zotepine (n = 1, *Pharmacotherapy* 2005;**25**: 1156–9)

5.8.5.2 CHOREAS *

- **Psychotropics etc**

Amoxapine

Amfetamines/amfetamines (chronic abuse, eg. *J Clin Psychopharmacol* 1988;**8**:146)

Chlorpromazine (n = 1, *Postgrad Med J* 1970;**540**: 633–4)

Cocaine (cases in *Am J Emerg Med* 1991;**9**: 618–20)

Donepezil? (n = 1, *Ann Pharmacother* 2000;**34**: 1347)

Fluoxetine (n = 1, *J Clin Psychiatry* 1999;**60**:68–9)

Haloperidol (many cases)

Lamotrigine (n = 1, *J Child Neurol* 2003;**18**:479–80; *J Child Neurol* 2006;**21**:357–8)

Lamotrigine + phenytoin (n = 3, *Seizure* 2001;**10**: 596–9)

Methadone

Methylphenidate

Mianserin (case in *Br J Psychiatry* 1989;**154**:13–14)

Oral contraceptives (n = 2, *Rev Med Chil* 1999; **127**:468–71)

Paroxetine (n = 1, after a single dose, *Br J Psychiatry* 1997;**170**:193–4)

Phenytoin (review in *Pediatr* 1983;**72**:31–4)

Risperidone (n = 1, *J Clin Psychiatry* 1999;**60**:85–7)

Sulpiride (n = 1, *J Psychopharmacol* 1993;**7**:290–2; n = 6, *Clin Neuropharmacol* 1990;**13**:248–52)

Trihexyphenidyl (benzhexol)

Valproate (n = 3, *Arch Neurol* 1994;**51**:702–4; n = 1, *Seizure* 2002;**11**:205–6)

- **Others**

Anabolic steroids

Cimetidine (pos. case in *Ann Intern Med* 1982;**96**:531)

Cyclizine (n = 1, *J Neurol Sci* 1977;**31**:237–44)

Dienoestrol/dienestrol

Metoclopramide (n = 1, *Lancet* 1982;**2**:1153)

Oral Contraceptives (cases in *Drugs* 1983;**26**:124)

Ranitidine (n = 1, *Lancet* 1988;**2**:158)

5.8.5.3 TICS (inc. Tourette's syndrome) *

Amfetamines (*JAMA* 1982;**247**:1729–31)

Amisulpride (n = 1, *Clin Neuropharmacol* 2006; **29**:163–4)

Androgenic steroids (eg. stanozolol, methandros-tenolol, testosterone) (*NEJM* 1990;**322**:1674)

Atomoxetine (n = 1, *J Child Adolesc Psychopharmacol* 2005;**15**:331–3)

Carbamazepine (*Clin Neuropharmacol* 1989;**12**:298–302)

Clozapine (n = 1, *Am J Psychiatry* 1995;**152**:649)

Cocaine (*NEJM* 1986;**315**:398; n = 1, *Am J Psychiatry* 1996;**153**:965)

Dexamphetamine (see amphetamine)

Escitalopram (n = 1, *Int Clin Psychopharmacol* 2005;**20**:177–8)

Fluoxetine (cases in *Drug Intell Clin Pharm* 1993; **27**:725–6; *Am J Psychiatry* 1994; **151**:946–7)

Haloperidol (*Am J Psychiatry* 1986;**143**:176–7)

Lamotrigine (n = 3, *Neurology* 1999;**52**:1191–4; n = 5, *Epilepsia* 2000;**41**:862–7; n = 1, vocal and motor tics, *Am J Psychiatry* 2006; **163**:159))

Methylphenidate (*JAMA* 1982;**247**:1729–31)

Ofloxacin (n = 1, *Ann Pharmacother* 1996;**30**: 138–41)

Risperidone withdrawal (n = 1, *J Am Acad Child Adolesc Psych* 1997;**36**:162–3)

Sertraline (n = 1, *Int Clin Psychopharmacol* 2005; **20**:177–8)

Thioridazine + methylphenidate (n = 1, *J Clin Psychiatry* 1986;**47**:44–5)

5.9 NEUROLEPTIC MALIGNANT SYNDROME

NMS is mostly related to the use of therapeutic or high doses of neuroleptics, particularly phenothiazines and high potency drugs. It frequently occurs within 4–11 days of initiation, or alteration of dosages, of neuroleptic therapy (*Am J Psychiatry* 1989;**146**:717–25). NMS may be due to a sudden and profound reduction in dopaminergic function, caused by dopamine blocking drugs. See 6.6.

Reviews: NMS with risperidone, clozapine and other novel antipsychotics (Hasan and Buckley, *Am J Psychiatry* 1998;**155**:1113–16), atypicals as causes (*Expert Opin Drug Saf* 2003;**2**:21–35)

- Antidepressants *

Amoxapine (pos. cases in *Br J Psychiatry* 1991; **159**:889; *Drug Intell Clin Pharm* 1989;**23**: 50–1)

Amoxapine + lithium (n = 1, *Ann Clin Psychiatry* 2000;**12**:107–9)

Clomipramine (n = 1, *Br Med J* 2004;**329**:1333–5)

Desipramine (n = 1, *Neurology* 1990;**40**:1797–8)

Phenelzine (many cases, eg. *Can Med Assoc J* 1991;**145**:817–19)

Trimipramine (n = 1, *J Clin Psychiatry* 1989;**50**: 144–5)

Venlafaxine (n = 1, *J Formos Med Assoc* 2006;**105**: 90–3)

Venlafaxine + trifluoperazine (n = 1, *Lancet* 2000;**354**:289–90)

- Antipsychotics *

Aripiprazole (n = 1, *Int Clin Psychopharmacol* 2004;**19**:351–3; n = 1, *J Clin Psychopharmacol* 2006;**26**:534; n = 1, *J Clin Psychopharmacol* 2006;**26**:94–5; n = 1 without fever, *J Okla State Med Assoc* 2006;**99**:435–8)

Aripiprazole + fluoxetine (possible case, *Am J Psychiatry* 2005;**162**:397–8)

Bromperidol + donepezil (n = 1, *Nippon Ronen Igakkai Zasshi* 2001;**38**:822–4)

Chlorpromazine (eg. n = 2, *Biol Psychiatry* 1983; **18**:1441–6)

Clozapine + risperidone (n = 1, *PNBP* 2002;**26**: 407–9)

Clozapine (rare, but cases exist, eg. n = 2 and review, *Ann Pharmacother* 1999;**33**:623–30; long-term n = 1, *Chang Gung Med J* 2001;**24**: 522–5; n = 1, *Ann Intern Med* 2002;**137**:374; after 30 years uneventful treatment; n = 1, *Anasthesiol Intensivmed Notfallmed Schmerzther* 2006;**41**:125–7; n = 1, *J Am Acad Child Adolesc Psychiatry* 2005;**44**:1101–2)

Clozapine + paroxetine (n = 1, *Aging Clin Exp Res* 2006;**18**:266–70)

Flupentixol (possible case in *Br J Psychiatry* 1988; **152**:558–9)

Fluphenazine (reviewed in *Compr Psychiatry* 1985;**26**:63–70)

Haloperidol (many cases, eg. *J Trauma* 1989;**29**: 1595–7; in pregnancy, n = 1, *Obstet Gynecol* 2001;**98**:906–8; following clozapine discontinuation, n = 1, *Aust NZ J Psychiatry* 2005;**39**:947–8).)

Haloperidol + olanzapine (n = 1, *Am J Psychiatry* 2001;**158**:650–1)

Lithium + amoxapine (n = 1, *Ann Clin Psychiatry* 2000;**12**:107–9)

Lithium + risperidone (possible case in *Am J Psychiatry* 1995;**152**:1096)

Lithium + ziprasidone (n = 1, *Ann Pharmacother* 2006;**40**:139–42)

Loxapine (*Br J Psychiatry* 1991;**159**:572–3)

Methylphenidate (n = 1, *Prim Care Companion J Clin Psychiatry* 2006;**8**:47)

Olanzapine (n=1, *Am J Psychiatry* 1999;**156**: 1836; atypical syndrome, n = 1, *Pharmaco-therapy* 2002;**22**:641–4; n = 1, with severe hypernatraemia, *Hum Psychopharmacol* 2001; **16**:279–81; 2.5 mg/d, n = 1, *Am J Psychiatry* 2003;**160**:796; n = 1, atypical with CK not raised, *Acta Psychiatr Scand* 2005;**112**:238–40; *Actas Esp Psiquiatr* 2006;**34**:144–5)

Olanzapine + fluphenazine (n = 1, *J Clin Psycho-pharmacol* 2003;**23**:672–4)

Olanzapine + levomepromazine (n = 1, *Acta Psychiatr Scand* 2000;**102**:231–3)

Olanzapine + lithium (n = 1, *Pharmacother* 2003; **23**:255–9)

Paroxetine + alprazolam (n = 1, Naranjo = 6, *Prog Neuropsychopharmacol Biol Psychiatry* 2006;**30**:1176–8)

Promazine

Quetiapine (n = 1, Stanley and Hunter, *Br J Psychiatry* 2000;**176**:497; n = 1, *J Neuropsych Clin Neurosci* 2002;**14**:87; n = 1, *Am J Psychiatry* 2002;**159**:149–50)

Quetiapine + fluvoxamine (n = 1, *Am J Psychiatry* 2005;**162**:812)

Risperidone (many cases, eg. n = 1, *J Child Adolesc Psychopharmacol* 2005;**15**:844–5)

Risperidone + haloperidol (during switch, *Ann Pharmacother* 2001;**35**:698–701)

Risperidone + lithium (*J Clin Psychopharmacol* 2003;**23**:315–17; n = 1, *J Clin Psychiatry* 2004; **65**:724)

Thioridazine (several cases, eg. *Biol Psychiatry* 1987;**22**:1293–7)

Ziprasidone (*J Clin Psychopharmacol* 2002;**22**:624–6; n = 1, adolescent, *Clin Ther* 2004;**26**:1105–8)

Zotepine (n = 1, *Pharmacotherapy* 2005;**25**: 1156–9)

Zotepine + valproate + BDZ (n = 2, *Psychiatr Clin Neurosci* 2003;**57**:369–71)

Zuclopenthixol (n = 1, *Br J Psychiatry* 1989;**154**: 562–3)

● **Others** *

Alimemazine (n = 1, *Eur J Pediatr* 2002;**161**:259–61)

Amantadine

Amantadine, abrupt withdrawal (n = 1, *Am J Psychiatry* 1994;**151**:451–2)

Anticholinergic withdrawal (n = 1, *Int Clin Psycho-pharmacol* 1996;**11**:207–9)

Bromocriptine to pergolide (rapid switch, n = 1, *Parkinsonism Relat Disord* 2002;**9**:116–16)

Carbamazepine (may also complicate symptoms, *Br J Psychiatry* 1990;**157**:437–8; n = 1, *Br J Psychiatry* 1994;**164**:270)

Carbamazepine withdrawal (*Am J Psychiatry* 1990;**147**:1687)

Donepezil (n = 1, *Int J Neuropsychopharmacol* 2004;**7**:101–3)

Ganciclovir (n = 1, *Pharmacother* 2000;**20**:479–83)

Iron (low levels? *Am J Psychiatry* 1991;**148**:148–9)

Levodopa

Levodopa withdrawal (n = 3, *JAMA* 1985;**254**: 2792–5)

Lithium (possible cases in *J Clin Psychopharmacol* 1987;**7**:339–41)

Methylphenidate (n = 1, *Pediatr Neurol* 1998;**19**: 299–301)

Metoclopramide (several cases, eg. *Arch Intern Med* 1987;**147**:1495–7; *Ann Pharmacother* 1999;**33**:644–5)

Oral contraceptives (possible case in *Drug Intell Clin Pharm* 1989;**23**:811)

Promethazine (n = 1, *Aust N Z J Psychiatry* 2005; **39**:113–14)

5.10 OBSESSIVE-COMPULSIVE SYMPTOMS *

Review of atypical-antipsychotic induced OCD (*Prog Neuropsychopharmacol Biol Psychiatry* 2003: **27**;333–46)

Clozapine (n = 1, *Am J Psychiatry* 1998;**155**: 1629–30; especially early in schizophrenia, n = 121, *J Clin Psychiatry* 1999;**60**;364–5; n = 1, *Psychiatr Clin Neurosci* 2005;**59**:219–22; although one study showed it might be of some use for OCD symptoms in people with schizophrenia; n = 15, Reznik *et al*, *Pharmacopsychiatry* 2004;**37**:52–6)

Gabapentin withdrawal (n = 1, *J Clin Psychiatry* 1998;**59**:131)

Methamphetamine (*J Clin Psychiatry* 1999;**60**: 337–8; n = 1, *J Am Acad Child Adolesc Psychiatry* 1998;**37**:135)

Methylphenidate (n = 1, *CNS Spectr* 2003;**8**:612–3)

Olanzapine (n = 2, *Am J Psychiatry* 1999;**156**: 799–800; severity associated with duration of treatment: n = 113, *J Clin Psychiatry* 2002; **63**:104–7)

Quetiapine (n = 1, *Prog Neuropsychopharmacol Biol Psychiatry* 2006;**30**:724–7; n = 5, *J Clin Psychopharmacol* 2006;**26**:396–400)

Risperidone (dose dependent case, *Aust N*

Z J Psychiatry 1998;**32**:299–301; n = 1, Br
 J Psychiatry 1999;**174**:559; see also J Clin
 Psychiatry 1999;**60**:261–3 for an obsessive
 discussion; n = 2, children, J Child Adolesc
 Psychopharmacol 2003;**13**[Suppl 1]:S89–92)
Risperidone and olanzapine — no differences
 in incidence but severity associated with
 longer duration of olanzapine (n = 113, J Clin
 Psychiatry 2002;**63**:104–7)
Stimulants (n = 1, Biol Psychiatry 1985;**20**:1332–7)
Topiramate (n = 1, Psychiatry Clin Neurosci 2006;
 60:394)

5.11 PANIC DISORDER

- **Psychotropics etc** *

Alprazolam (J Am Board Fam Pract 2002;**15**:69–72)
Amfetamines (n = 3, Biol Psychiatry 1992;**32**:91–5)
Buspirone (case + correspondence in Lancet
 1989;**2**:46–7, 615, 682–3)
Citalopram (n = 1, South Med J 2002;**95**:1088–9)
Clobazam (withdrawal, Br Med J 1981;**282**: 1931)
Clozapine (n = 1, Am J Psychiatry 2000;**157**:2056)
Cocaine (review in J Addict Dis 1992;**11**:47–58)
Flumazenil (mentioned in Psychiatr Res 1991;
 6:115)
Fluoxetine (unless initial doses kept very low, eg.
 J Clin Psychopharmacol 1987;**7**:329–32)
Fluoxetine + bupropion (J Clin Psychiatry 1996;
 57:177–8)
Marijuana (n = 1, Acta Psychiatr Scand 1998;**98**:
 254–5)
Naltrexone (Am J Psychiatry 1998;**155**:447)
Olanzapine (eg. hyperventilation, n = 1, J Psych
 Neurosci 2002;**27**:360–3)
Topiramate (n = 1, J Clin Psychopharmacol
 2001;**21**:461–2; n = 1, J Clin Psychiatry 2006;
 67:326–7)
Trazodone

- **Others**

Aspartame (unproven case with high doses in
 Lancet 1986;**12**:631)
Carvedilol (n = 1, Ann Pharmacother 2002;**36**:
 1736–40)
Co-trimoxazole (n = 1, J Clin Psychopharmacol
 1991;**11**:144–5)
Lactate oral (eg. in calcium lactate tablets, case in
 Ann Pharmacother 1995;**29**:539–40)
Oxymetazoline (case in abuse, J Clin Psychiatry
 1987;**48**:293)

Phenylephrine (n = 1, Br J Psychiatry 1980;**136**:
 297–9)
Sibutramine (n = 1, Am J Psychiatry 2002;**159**:
 1793–4)
Smoking cessation (n = 2, J Clin Psychiatry 2002;
 63:594–5)
Sodium lactate (study in Arch Gen Psychiatry
 1989;**46**:135–40)
Steroids (mentioned in J Psychiatry Neurosci
 1997;**22**:346–7)
Sumatriptan (7%, panic being interpretation of
 side-effects such as chest pain, palpitations,
 etc, Am J Psychiatry 1996;**153**:1505)
Yohimbine (see Arch Gen Psychiatry
 1998;**55**:1033–44)

5.12 PARANOID OR SCHIZOPHRENIC-LIKE PSYCHOSES

(See also hallucinations 5.6.) Characterised by
paranoid delusions and hallucinations in a person
with little clouding of consciousness. The literature
on drug-induced psychosis is extensive but mainly
case reports and short uncontrolled studies. A
classification has been proposed:

- **Intoxication mimicking functional:** (eg.
  drug-induced), eg. stimulants and cannabis.
  Persists for several days until the drug
  has cleared.

- **Psychoactive drugs altering the clinical
  presentation of an existing psychosis:** eg.
  cannabis or amfetamines, etc. creating a
  more aggressive and disturbed schizophrenic
  patient (Davison and Roth, Br J Psychiatry
  1996;**168**:651).

- **Chronic hallucinations induced by
  substance abuse:** insight usually present,
  no clouding of consciousness, continue
  despite long-term abstinence, eg. alcoholic
  hallucinosis, LSD or cannabis flashbacks.

- **Drug-induced relapse of functional
  psychosis:** eg. schizophrenia.

- **Withdrawal states:** eg. delirium tremens,
  benzodiazepine or barbiturate withdrawal.

- **Others:** acute intoxication/confusion with
  clouding of consciousness, post-intoxication
  depression, eg. post-amphetamine crash,
  panic/anxiety attacks, eg. from hallucinogens
  such as LSD.

- **True drug-induced psychosis:** any psychotic
  symptoms which occur with drug intoxication

and then persist after elimination of the causing drug, eg. one to two drug-free weeks. There is surprisingly little, if any proof that such causal link can be made firmly between drug use and later psychosis, eg. there is no direct proof that cannabis causes schizophrenia rather than schizophrenics trying to self-medicate before symptoms become clear to others.

- **Hallucinogens etc (major cause)**
Cannabis (acute onset, usually resolves in 2–7 days, *Acta Psychiatr Scand* 1991;**83**:34–6). At higher doses, canabis is a risk factor for the development or relapse of schizophrenia, eg. there is a two-fold increase in relative risk for later schizophrenia. Cannabis itself, however, is neither a sufficient nor necessary cause for psychosis but should be discouraged in vulnerable youths (Arseneault et al, *Br J Psychiatry* 2004;**184**:110–17; see also *Br J Psychiatry* 2001;**178**:116–22)
Dimethoxy-methylamphetamine (DOM)
Lysergic acid diethylamide (LSD)
Khat chewing (n = 4, *Br J Hosp Med* 1995;**54**: 322–6)
Mescaline
MDMA/Ecstasy (*Br Med J* 1991;**302**:1150, *Br J Psychiatry* 1991;**159**:713–15; *Arch Gen Psychiatry* 1993;**50**:75)
Petrol (*Am J Psychiatry* 1964;**126**:757)
Phencyclidine (angel dust)
Psilocybin (magic mushrooms) (*Br J Psychiatry* 1978;**132**:602)
Volatiles (*Br Med J* 1962;**ii**:1448)

- **CNS stimulants (major cause)** *
Amfetamines/amfetamines (eg. treatment/ review in *Topic Emerg Med* 1985;**7**:18–32)
Cocaine (*Am J Psychiatry*, 1991;**148**:495–8)
Ephedrine (review in *Br J Psychiatry* 1987;**150**: 252–5)
Methamphetamine (n = 1, *Am J Psychiatry* 1999;**4**:662; *Australas Psychiatry* 2006;**14**:86–9)
Phenylephrine (eg. *JAMA* 1982;**247**:1859–60)
Phenylpropanolamine (*Am J Psychiatry* 1990;**147**:367–8; n = 1, *Am J Psychiatry* 2000;**157**:1021–2)
Pseudoephedrine (many cases, eg. *South Med J* 1990;**83**:64–5)
Solvent abuse (*Br J Psychiatry* 1989;**152**:132)

- **Other CNS drugs***
Alcohol
Alcohol, caffeine and 'vigueur fit' (n = 1, *Med Sci Law* 2001;**41**:331–6)
Aripiprazole (n = 1, *J Clin Psychiatry* 2005;**66**: 1339; n = 4, *Int Clin Psychopharmacol* 2004; **19**:45–8; as both add-on and during tapered crossover)
Antihistamines
Barbiturates
Benzodiazepines:
    Alprazolam
    Lorazepam (*Br J Psychiatry* 1985:**147**:211)
    Midazolam (possible case in *Drug Intell Clin Pharm* 1989;**23**:671–2)
    Triazolam (eg. *Pharmacopsychiatry* 1989;**22**: 115–19)
Benzodiazepine withdrawal (*Int J Geriatr Psychiatry* 1995, **10**, 901–2)
Buspirone (*Am J Psychiatry* 1991;**148**:1606; *J Psychopharmacol* 1993;**7**:295–300)
Chloral
Chlorpromazine (n = 1, *Can Med Assoc J* 1970: **102**:642; n = 1, *Brain Inj* 1993;**7**:77–83)
Clozapine withdrawal (eg. rebound psychosis, study in *Psychopharmacol* 1988;**24**:260–3; n = 3, *J Clin Psychiatry* 1997;**58**:252–5)
Codeine OD (n = 1, *Neurobehavioral Toxicol Teratol* 1985;**7**:93–4)
Disulfiram (n = 1, *Br Med J* 1992;**305**:763; n = 1, *Ned Tijdschr Geneeskd* 2002;**146**:965)
Haloperidol (*Drug Intell Clin Pharm* 1981; **15**:209)
Lorazepam (pre-operative, n = 1, *Anaesthesia* 2003;**58**:1036)
Methadone withdrawal (eg. *J Clin Psychiatry* 1995;**56**:73–6)
Memantine (n = 1, *J Clin Psychiatry* 2005;**66**:658–9; n = 3, *Neurology* 2005;**65**:481–2)
Modafinil (may exacerbate: n = 1, *Arch Gen Psychiatry* 2002;**59**:292–3; n = 1, *Am J Psychiatry* 2005;**162**:1983)
Morphine (rare, *Br J Psychiatry* 1990;**157**: 758–9)
Promethazine (rare but possible, eg. *NEJM* 1960; **263**:747)
Risperidone (n = 1, *J Child Adolesc Psychopharmacol* 2005;**15**:520–5)
Sodium oxybate (SPC)
Zopiclone (some cases reported — *WHO Drug Information* 1990;**4**:179)

- Antidepressants

Bupropion (many cases, eg. n = 1, Am J Psychiatry 1999;**156**:2017–18; n = 1, Pharmacopsychiatry 2002;**35**:247–8)

Fluoxetine (J Nerv Mental Dis 1990;**178**:55–8)

Fluvoxamine (n = 1, Can J Psychiatry 2000;**45**:762; n = 1, Hum Psychopharmacol 2003;**18**:477–8)

Imipramine (eg. Am J Psychiatry 1974;**131**:21)

Mirtazapine + levodopa (n = 1, Pharmacopsychiatry 1997;**30**: 263–5)

Paroxetine (case of psychotic mania, Am J Psychiatry 1995;**152**:1399–440)

Phenelzine, eg. Br J Psychiatry 1991;**159**:716–17)

Trazodone (n = 1, J Neuropsych Clin Neurosci 2005;**17**:253–4)

St. John's wort (n = 1, Hum Psychopharmacol 2004;**19**:27–76)

Zolpidem (Lancet 1992;**339**:813)

Venlafaxine + propafenone (Int J Psychiatr Med 2001;**31**:427–32)

- Anticonvulsants *

Psychosis induced by anticonvulsants may be the result of 'forced normalisation'. Risk factors include TLE (treatment resistance), past history of psychosis or affective disorder, and becoming suddenly seizure-free (best to do this gradually). Drug regimens should be changed gradually and compliance should be maintained to prevent epileptic psychoses (n = 44, Matsuura, J Neurol, Neurosurg Psychiatry 1999;**67**:231–3).

Carbamazepine toxicity (Lancet 1989;i:167)

Clonazepam (n = 1, J Nerv Ment Dis 1982;**170**: 117)

Ethosuximide

Gabapentin (exacerbation of psychosis in schizophrenic, n = 1, Can J Psychiatry 2002; **47**:975–6)

Levetiracetam (n = 1, Epileptic Disord 2003;**5**: 117–19; n = 1, long-term, Can J Psychiatry 2004;**49**:868; Can J Psychiatry 2005;**50**:948; comment on Can J Psychiatry 2004;**49**:868)

Phenytoin (n = 1 for trigeminal neuralgia, Epilepsy Behav 2003;**4**:771–2; Clin Pediatr (Phila) 1993;**32**:107–10))

Pregabalin (n = 1, Seizure 2006;**15**:208–10)

Tiagabine (RCT shows no significant risk; n = 554, Epilepsia 2002;**43**:394–8)

Topiramate (discussion in J Clin Psychiatry 2004;**65**:1145–6; n = 2, Expert Opin Drug Saf 2006;**5**:741–2; n = 1, > 400 mg/d, Am J Psychiatry 2005;**162**:1542; n = 2, Clin Neuropharmacol 2006;**29**:168–9)

Valproate (isolated cases, eg. Clin Electroencephalography 1982;**13**:50–3)

Vigabatrin (2% incidence, eg. J Neurol Neurosurg Psychiatry 1989;**52**: 467–71; cases in Lancet 1994;**343**:606–7; Ann Pharmacother 1995; **29**:1115–17)

Vigabatrin withdrawal (letter in Lancet 1990; **335**:1279)

- Antiparkinsonian drugs (excess DA) *

Amantadine (Drugs 1981;**21**:341–53)

Anticholinergic withdrawal (Am J Psychiatry 1980;**137**:1613)

Bromocriptine (< 1% chance, review in Biol Psychiatry 1985;**20**:326–8)

Levodopa (esp. hallucinations — Arch Neurol 1970;**23**:193–200)

Lisuride (a few cases, eg. Lancet 1986;**2**:510)

Pergolide (esp. hallucinations, in up to 13%, eg. Neurology 1982;**32**:1181–4)

Ropinirole (n = 1, Am J Psychiatry 2006;**163**:546–7)

Selegiline (a few cases, eg. Neurology 1981;**31**: 19–23)

Trihexyphenidyl (benzhexol)

- NSAIDs and analgesics

Aspirin (JAMA 1965;**193**:555–8)

Ibuprofen (J Clin Psychiatry 1982;**43**:499–500)

Indomethacin (rare, eg. South Med J 1983;**76**:679–80; Br Med J 1977;**2**:994)

Pentazocine (esp. hallucinations, eg. Br Med J 1974;**2**:224)

Sulindac (JAMA 1980;**243**:1420)

- Cardiovascular drugs

Amyl nitrate (Martindale, 1993)

Beta-blockers (see under depression for differentials), eg: Atenolol (rare, n = 1, Am J Psychiatry 1983;**140**:1382) and propranolol (well known, eg. Biol Psychiatry 1989;**25**: 351–4)

Clonidine (n = 1, Prog Neuropsychopharmacol 1980;**4**:21)

Clonidine withdrawal (Am J Psychiatry 1982;**139**: 110–11)

Digoxin toxicity (rare, J Nerv Mental Dis 1978; **166**:817)

Diltiazem (n = 1, Arch Internal Med 1991;**151**:373–4)

Disopyramide (isolated cases, eg. *Lancet* 1978;**1**: 858 + 1152)

Doxazosin (n = 1, *Br Med J* 1997;**314**:1869; n = 1, *Br Med J* 1997;**314**:1869)

Enalapril (n = 1, *Drug Intell Clin Pharm* 1991;**25**: 558–9)

Hydralazine

Lidocaine IV (n = 6, *Ann Intern Med* 1982;**97**: 149–50)

Methyldopa

Mexilitine (n = 1, *Am Heart J* 1984;**107**:1091–8)

Nifedipine (possible case in *J Am Geriatr Soc* 1984;**32**:408)

Procainamide

Tocainide (*Br Med J* 1984;**288**:606–7)

- **Anti-infection** *

Amphotericin B IV (n = 1, *Ariz Med* 1972; **29**:322)

Antituberculous drugs (*Lancet* 1989;**ii**:105 + 735–6)

Cefuroxime (*Lancet* 1984;**i**:965)

Cephalexin (n = 1, *Med J Aust* 1973;**i**:497)

Cephalothin (*Drug Intell Clin Pharm* 1974;**8**:71)

Chloroquine (cases in *Lancet* 1985;**2**:37)

Ciprofloxacin (n = 1, *Ann Pharmacother* 1992;**26**: 930–1; n = 1, *Postgrad Med J* 1998;**74**:189–90)

Clarithromycin (*Eur J Clin Microbiol Infect Dis* 1999; **18**:70–1; n = 1, *Psychiatr Bull* 2004;**28**: 98–9)

Colistin (esp. with large doses)

Dapsone (*Br Med J* 1989;**299**:324)

Erythromycin (*Arch Internal Med* 1986;**146**:897)

Ganciclovir (n = 1, *Pharmacother* 2000;**20**:479–83)

Isoniazid (rare — *Am J Psychiatry* 1991;**148**: 1402; *Ann Pharmacother* 1998;**32**:889–91)

Ketoconazole (*Am J Psychiatry* 1990;**147**:677)

Levofloxacin (rare but can be serious, SPC)

Mefloquine (n = 179, more common in females and first-time users; *Eur J Clin Pharmacol* 2002;**58**:441–5; n = 1, after single therapeutic dose, responded to quetiapine, *Malar J* 2006;**5**:74)

Metronidazole (case in *Am J Psychiatry* 1997;**154**: 1170–1)

Nalidixic acid (many cases, eg. *Br Med J* 1965;**2**: 590)

Primaquine (n = 1, *Ann Intern Med* 1980;**92**:435)

Procaine

Penicillin G (several cases, eg. *Br J Psychiatry* 1990;**156**:554)

Sulphonamides

Tobramycin (a few cases, eg. P*ediatr Pulmonol* 1988;**4**:201–4)

- **Steroids** (*Postgrad Med J* 1984;**60**:467–70)

Adrenocorticotrophin

Clomiphene (n = 2, *Am J Psychiatry* 1997; **154**:1169–70)

Corticosteroids (11% incidence? Review by Ismail and Wessely, *Br J Hosp Pharm* 1995;**53**: 495–9)

Cortisone

Methylprednisolone

Methyltestosterone (*Lancet* 1987;**i**:863)

Prednisone (usually >40mg/d, eg. *J Clin Psychiatry* 1982;**43**:75–6 inc. brief overview; case and discussion in *Br J Psychiatry* 1993; **162**:549–53)

Triamcinolone (possible but no specific reports)

- **Miscellaneous**

Antidiarrheals (OTC) (*Br J Psychiatry* 1990; **157**:758–9)

Atropine (oral, IV, eye drops. Many cases, eg. *DICP Ann Pharmacother* 1990;**24**:708–9)

Baclofen

Carbaryl (n = 1, *Am J Psychiatry* 1995;**152**:46–7)

Carbimazole

Chlorphenamine OD (case in child in *Med J Aust* 1973;**1**:382–6)

Cimetidine (*Am J Psychiatry* 1980;**137**:1112)

Desmopressin (n = 1, *Lancet* 1981;**2**:808)

Dextromethorphan (n = 1, *Am J Psychiatry* 2000;**157**:304)

Dicyclomine

Diphenhydramine (n = 1, *JAMA* 1968;**203**:301)

Disulfiram

Estrogen withdrawal (review, n = 26, *J Acta Psychiatr Scand* 2001;**104**:323)

Hyoscine-transdermal (*Postgrad Med* 1988;**84**: 73–6)

Insulin abuse (*Br Med J* 1971;**4**:792–3)

Interferon alpha (n = 1, *Addiction* 2000;**95**:1101– 4; n = 1, persistent, *J Clin Psychopharmacol* 2006;**26**:446–7)

Isotretoin (possible case, *J Clin Psychiatry* 1999; **60**:407–8; n = 5, *Int Clin Psychopharmacol* 2005;**20**:39–41)

Ketamine (discussion, *Am J Psychiatry* 1997; **154**:805–11)

Lactate oral (eg. in calcium lactate tablets, case in *Ann Pharmacother* 1995;**29**:539–40)

Lariam (severe is extremely low, eg. 1 in 6000, *Pharm J* 1996;**256**:184)

Melatonin (n = 1, *Ann Pharmacother* 1997;**31**:1408)

Nabilone

Nicotine, abrupt withdrawal of (*Am J Psychiatry* 1994;**150**:452)

Oxymetazoline (several cases, eg. *Scott Med J* 1982;**27**:175–6)

Phenylephrine (*JAMA* 1982;**247**:1859)

Phenylpropanolamine (n = 1, *Am J Psychiatry* 2000;**157**:1021–2)

Promethazine (n = 1, *Psychosomatics* 2004;**45**: 89–90)

Pyridostigmine (case in German in *Deutsch Med Wschr* 1966;**9**:699)

Quinine (*Br J Psychiatry* 1988;**153**:575)

Quinidine (*Br Med J* 1987;**294**:1001–2; *Med J Aust* 1990;**153**:47–9)

Salbutamol (*Biol Psychiatry* 1989;**26**:631–3)

Scopolamine (transient to transdermal, n = 3, *Can J Hosp Pharm* 1994;**47**:67–9)

Silbutramine (*Am J Psychiatry* 2000;**157**:2057–8)

Yohimbine (unproven, see *Arch Gen Psychiatry* 1998;**55**:1033–44)

5.13 SEIZURES

These are rare at normal doses and occur mostly where seizure threshold is reduced, in at-risk patients or in overdose. The list of drugs that could induce seizures is enormous and so a literature search would be needed to clarify the current situation for any one drug.

Reviews: drug-induced seizures: controversies in their identification and management (Alldredge, *Pharmacotherapy* 1997;**17**:857–60, editorial, 26 refs), general review (*Drug Saf* 2002;**25**:91–110, 166 refs), assessment, management and prevention, (Murphy and Delanty, *CNS Drugs* 2000;**14**:135–46), antipsychotics as causes of seizures (*Drugs Today* [Barc] 2003;**39**:551–7).

- **Psychotropics etc** *

Alcohol (*NEJM* 1989;**320**:596–7)

Amitriptyline (*Am J Psychiatry* 1980;**137**:1461–2)

Amoxapine (*J Clin Psychiatry* 1981;**42**:238–42)

Antipsychotics (esp phenothiazines)

Aripiprazole (n = 1, *Can J Psychiatry* 2005;**50**:186; n = 1, *J Clin Psychiatry* 2006;**67**:995–6)

Atomoxetine overdose (n = 1, *Am J Psychiatry* 2004;**161**:757)

Bupropion (see *3.4*, eg. n = 1, *Clin Neuropharmacol* 2001;**24**:304–6)

Bupropion overdose (n = 1, *Lancet* 2001;**357**: 1624, letter)

Bupropion + trimipramine (n = 1, *J Clin Psychiatry* 2001;**62**:477–8)

Citalopram (n = 1, non-CSE, *Eur J Neurol* 2002;**9**: 319–20)

Citalopram overdose (n = 1, *J Emerg Med* 2004; **26**:177–81)

Clomipramine + bupropion (n = 1, *Clin Neuropharmacol* 2004;**27**:192–4)

Clozapine (*Neurology* 1991;**41**:369–71; *CSM Current Problems* 1991, no 31; *Am J Psychiatry* 1993;**150**:1128. Higher incidence with rapid upward titration, recent ECT, head trauma with loss of consciousness and concurrent use of seizure threshold-lowering drugs. They may be due to hyponatremia: *Lancet* 1992;**340**:672)

Donepezil (*Curr Prob Pharmacovig* 1999;**25**:7; *J Neurol, Neurosurg Psychiatry* 1999;**66**:410)

Duloxetine (*Neurology* 2006;**66**:773–4)

Fluoxetine (*Clin Pharm* 1989;**8**:296–8; *Am J Psychiatry* 1992;**149**:273; prolonged seizure reported in *Postgrad Med J* 1994;**70**:383–4)

Fluvoxamine (n = 1, *Ann Pharmacother* 2000; **34**:1276–8; n = 1, *Gen Hosp Psychiatry* 2005;**27**:148–50)

Imipramine

Levomepromazine + fluvoxamine (*Int Clin Psychopharmacol* 1993;**8**:61–2)

Lithium (*Biol Psychiatry* 1987;**22**:1184–90)

MAOIs

Maprotiline (*J Clin Psychiatry* 1982;**43**:117–18)

Memantine (*Am J Health Syst Pharm* 2005;**62**: 420–1)

Mianserin

Olanzapine (fatal case, *Ann Pharmacother* 1999; **33**:787–9; non-fatal case *Ann Pharmacother* 1999;**33**:554–6; myoclonic status, n = 1, *Clin Neuropharmacol* 2005;**28**:145–7)

Quetiapine (n = 1, *Ann Pharmacother* 2003;**37**: 1224–7)

Quetiapine + olanzapine (n = 1, *Ann Pharmacother* 2002;**36**:437–9)

Sertraline (n = 1, *Am J Psychiatry* 1996;**153**:732)

Sodium oxybate (SPC)

Tacrine (n = 6, *Lancet* 1996;**347**:1339–40)

Venlafaxine OD (*Ann Pharmacother* 1997;**31**: 178–80)

Venlafaxine + trimipramine (n = 1, *Ann Pharmacother* 2000;**34**:1402–5)
Zolpidem (review, *Lancet* 1998;**352**:83–90; n = 1, *Eur Psychiatry* 2003;**18**:140–1)

- **Drug withdrawal** *

Alcohol (*NEJM* 1989;**320**:596–7)
Anticonvulsants (ie. non-compliance)
Barbiturates
Benzodiazepines:
Alprazolam (*J Nerv Mental Dis* 1990;**178**: 208–9)
Carbamazepine (*J Clin Psychiatry* 1988;**49**[Suppl]: 410)
Zolpidem withdrawal (*JAMA* 1994;**272**:1721–2; n = 1, *Prog Neuropsychopharmacol Biol Psychiatry* 2007;**31**:539–40)
CNS stimulants
Cocaine (*Neurology* 1990;**40**:404–7)
Ephedrine (*Lancet* 1977;**1**:587–8)

- **Anticonvulsants** *

Reviews: general (Perucca et al, *Epilepsia* 1998; **39**:5–17; 155 refs, editorial by Loiseau, *Epilepsia* 1998;**39**:2–4, 43 refs), partial seizures (*Neurology* 2002;**59**:79–83)
Carbamazepine (n = 1, *Clin Electroencephalogr* 2002;**33**:174–7; auditory, n = 1, *Pharmacopsychiatry* 2006;**39**:192–3)
Carbamazepine OD (n = 2, *J Toxicol Clin Toxicol* 2002;**40**:81–90)
Carbamazepine withdrawal (*Ther Drug Monit* 2000;**22**:753–6)
Ethosuximide
Levetiracetam (myoclonic status epilepticus, n = 1, *Epileptic Disord* 2006;**8**:21–8)
Oxcarbazepine (myoclonic seizures, n = 2, *Epilepsy Behav* 2006;**8**:289–93)
Phenobarbital
Phenytoin (*Epilepsia* 1989;**30**:230–4)
Pregabalin (n = 1, *Seizure* 2006;**15**:208–10)
Tiagabine (n = 2, *Epilepsia* 1999;**40**:1159–62; n = 3 non-CSE, and review, *Seizure* 2002;**11**: 57–9 and 243–9)
Tiagabine OD (status; *Epilepsia* 2002;**43**: 773–4)
Valproate
Zonisamide (SPC)

- **NSAIDs and analgesics** *

Dextroproxyphene (*Arch Intern Med* 1973;**132**: 191–4)

Fentanyl (*Anesth Anal [Cleve]* 1982;**61**:1020–1)
Indomethacin (rare, eg. *Br Med J* 1966;**1**:80)
Mefenamic Acid (*Drug Intell Clin Pharm* 1983;**17**: 204–5)
Oxycodone (n = 1, *Clin Ther* 2005;**27**:1815–8)
Penicillamine
Pentazocine (eg. *Ann Emerg Med* 1983;**12**:28–31)
Pethidine (*Ann Neurol* 1983;**13**:180–5)
Propoxyphene (*Arch Intern Med* 1973;**132**:191–4)
Salicylates OD (*Lancet* 1998;**352**:383–90)
Sulindac
Tramadol (reviews in *JAMA* 1997;**278**:1661 and *Pharmacother* 1998;**18**:607–11; the latter concluding that seizures seem rarely attributable to tramadol)

- **Cardiovascular drugs**

Beta-blockers, eg:
　　Oxprenolol (*Lancet* 1972;**i**:587–8)
　　Propranolol (*Lancet* 1972;**i**:587–8)
Digoxin toxicity (rare eg. *Br Med J* 1982; **284**:162–3)
Disopyramide
Enoximone Inf (*Br Med J* 1990;**300**:613)
Lidocaine (*Eur J Clin Pharmacol* 1989;**36**:583–6) — s/c (*Clin Pharm* 1989;**8**:767–8)
Metolazone (*Br Med J* 1976;**i**:1381)
Mexilitine
Thiazide diuretics (review, *Lancet* 1998;**352**:383–90)
Tocainide

- **Anti-infection** *

Ampicillin? (*Lancet* 1982;**ii**:617)
Benzylpenicillin (*Lancet* 1977;**i**:587)
Carbenicillin (*JAMA* 1971;**218**:1942)
Cefazolin (*Am J Hosp Pharm* 1980;**37**:271)
Cefepime (non-convulsive status epilepticus, n = 1, Maganti et al, *Epilepsy Behav* 2006;**8**:312–4)
Ceftazidime (editorial in *Lancet* 1990;**340**:400–1)
Cephalexin (n = 1, *Med J Aust* 1973;**1**:497)
Cephalosporins (high dose in renal failure)
Chloroquine (*Br Med J* 1989;**299**:1524)
Ciprofloxacin (*Pharm J* 1989;**242**:340)
Gatifloxacin (n = 1, *Ann Pharmacother* 2004;**38**: 235–7)
Gentamicin (*J Neurol Orthop Med Surg* 1985;**6**: 123)
Imipenem (*Ann Int Med* 1989;**149**:1881–3)
Isoniazid (review in *J Clin Pharm Ther Toxicol* 1987;**25**:259–61)

Mefloquine (*Pharm J* 1989;**243**:561; CSM warning, *Curr Prob Pharmacovig* 1999;**25**:15)

Metronidazole (*Drug Intell Clin Pharm* 1982;**16**:409)

Nalidixic Acid (*Br Med J* 1977;**2**:1518)

Niridazole

Ofloxacin (n = 1, *Ann Pharmacother* 1997;**31**: 1475–7; *J Pharm Technol* 1997;**13**:174)

Penicillins (reviewed in *Ann Pharmacother* 1992; **26**:26–9, 30–1)

Piperazine

Piperacillin (*Clin Pediatr* 1997;**36**:475–6)

Pyrimethamine

Zudovudine (case in *Lancet* 1995;**346**:452)

- **Respiratory drugs**

Aminophylline (*Lancet* 1977;i:587)

Doxapram

Phenylpropanolamine (*J Med Soc New Jersey* 1979;**76**:591–2)

Terbutaline (*Am J Dis Child* 1982;**136**:1091–2)

Theophylline (*Ann Int Med* 1975;**82**:784)

Theophylline toxicity (*J Toxicol Clin Toxicol* 1999; **37**:99–101)

- **Hormones**

Glucocorticoids

Insulin

Oral contraceptives (exacerbate pre-existing)

Oxytocin

Prostaglandins

- **Cytotoxics**

Alprostadil

Busulphan (*Ann Intern Med* 1989;**111**:543–4; *Ann Pharmacother* 1992;**26**:30–1)

Chlorambucil (*Postgrad Med J* 1979;**55**:806–7)

Ciclosporin (*J Neurol Neurosurg Psychiatry* 1989; **55**:1068–71; *Psychosomatics* 1991;**32**:94–102)

Cisplatin (*Br Med J* 1991;**302**:416)

Methotrexate

Vinblastine

Vincristine

- **Anaesthetics**

Alfentanil (*Anesth Analg* 1989;**68**:692–3)

Enflurane (*Anaesthesia* 1992;**47**:79–80)

Ether

Etomidate (pre-ECT, n = 1, *Br J Psychiatry* 2000; **177**:373)

Halothane

Ketamine

Local anaesthetics

Bupivacaine (*Anesthesiology* 1979;**50**:454–6)

Lidocaine (mentioned in *Drugs Aging* 1995;**7**: 38–48)

Etidocaine (*Anesthesiology* 1979;**50**:51–3)

Procaine

Methohexital

Propofol (*Anaesthesia* 1990;**45**:255–6, can be delayed by up to six days — *CSM Curr Prob* 1992;**35**:2; systematic review concluding that rapid changes in cerebral concentration may be causal; n = 81, *Neurology* 2002;**58**:1327–32)

Propofol withdrawal (*Anaesthesia* 1990;**45**:741–2)

- **Miscellaneous** *

Allopurinol withdrawal (*Ann Neurology* 1990; **27**:691)

Aluminium toxicity (unproven, *Ann Intern Med* 1989;**111**:543–4)

Amantadine (unproven, *Ann Intern Med* 1989; **110**:323–4; *Drugs Aging* 1995;**7**:38–48)

Baclofen IT (*Lancet* 1992;**339**:373–4)

Baclofen withdrawal (*Neurology* 1992;**42**:447–9)

Brompheniramine

Bupivacaine epidural (case in 4 years: *Anaesthesia* 1995;**50**:563–77)

Caffeine (*Acta Psychiatr Scand* 1959;**15**:331–4)

Camphor (*Clin Pediatr* [Phila] 1977;**16**:901–2)

Clomiphene (n = 1, *Br Med J* 1994;**309**:512)

Colchicine OD

Cyclopentolate eye drops (*J Paed Child Health* 1990;**26**:106–7)

Diphenhydramine (*J Pediat* 1977;**90**:1017–18)

Diptheria-tetanus-pertussis vaccine (*JAMA* 1990; **263**:1641–5)

Flumazenil (n = 49, *Epilepsia* 2000;**41**:186–92)

Fluorescin IV (*Annals Opthal* 1989;**21**:89–90; *Acta Neurol Scand* 1999;**100**:278–80)

Ginkgo biloba (review of anecdotal reports: *Ann Intern Med* 2001;**134**:344)

Hepatitis B vaccine (*J Paed Child Health* 1990; **26**:65)

Ifosfamide (non-convulsive status epilepticus, n = 2, Kilickap et al, *Ann Pharmacother* 2006; **40**:332–5)

Interferon (n = 1, *Pediatrics* 1994;**93**:511–12)

Ketamine

Ketotifen (n = 19, *Epilepsia* 1998;**39**[Suppl 5]:64)

Levodopa (mentioned in *Drugs Aging* 1995;**7**: 38–48)

Levothyroxine (n = 1, *Ann Pharmacother* 1993; **27**:1139)

Lindane, topical (*Br J Dermatol* 1995; **133**:1013)

Measles/mumps/rubella vaccine (review in *Pediatrics* 1991; **88**:881–5)

Naftidrofuryl

Naloxone (rare)

Ondansetron (*Clin Pharm* 1993; **12**:613–15)

Pertussis vaccine

Phenylpropanolamine (n = 1, *J Pediatr* 1983; **102**: 143–5)

Pyridoxine (n = 1 and review, *J Paed Child Health* 2001; **37**:592–6)

Pyrimethamine radiographic contrast media (eg. metrizamide)

Sodium bicarbonate (*JAMA* 1989; **262**:1328–39)

Steroids, eg:

    Dexamethasone

    Hydrocortisone

    Prednisolone

    Prednisone (with hypocalcaemia) (mentioned in *Lancet* 1977; **1**:587–8)

Sulphasalazine

Sulphonylureas

Yohimbine (unproven, see *Arch Gen Psych* 1998; **55**:1033–44)

5.14 SEROTONIN SYNDROME

Serotonin syndrome has been reported with a variety of antidepressants, buspirone, carbamazepine, pethidine, dextromethorphan and levodopa, usually in combination but can be single drugs or in overdose.

Reviews: Mir and Taylor, *Psychiatr Bull* 1999; **23**: 742–7; Chan *et al, Med J Aust* 1998; **169**:523–5; Lane and Baldwin, *J Clin Psychopharmacol* 1997; **17**:208–21.

- Individual drugs

Amitriptyline (n = 1, *Postgrad Med J* 2000; **76**: 254–6)

Clomipramine (*J Clin Psychopharmacol* 1999; **19**:285–7; possible case after withdrawal of clozapine: *Ann Pharmacother* 2001; **35**:180–2)

Citalopram (n = 1, *Kaohsiung J Med Sci* 2005; **21**:326–8; at low dose *J Clin Psychopharmacol* 2000; **20**:713–4)

Dexfenfluramine (n = 1, *JAMA* 1996; **276**:1220–1)

Dothiepin overdose (*J Child Adolesc Psychopharmacol* 1998; **8**:201–4)

Ecstasy (*JAMA* 1993; **269**:869–70; review *Clin Neuropharmacol* 1996; **19**:157–64)

Fluoxetine (n = 1, *Psychiatr Pol* 1995; **29**:529–38)

Fluvoxamine (*Ann Emerg Med* 1999; **33**:457–9; after single dose n = 1, *Ann Emerg Med* 1999; **34**:806–7; mild syndrome may occur in 43% people on fluvoxamine alone, n = 37, *Int J Neurosci* 2001; **109**:165–72)

Mirtazapine (n = 1, *Ann Pharmacother* 2002; **36**: 641–3; n = 1, *Clin Neuropharmacol* 2003; **26**: 54–7)

Nefazodone (n = 8, *Br J Gen Pract* 1999; **49**: 871–4)

Paroxetine (*Am J Emerg Med* 1995; **13**:606–7)

Sertraline low dose (*J Clin Psychopharmacol* 2000; **20**:713–14)

Sertraline overdose (n = 1, *Arch Pediatr Adolesc Med* 1997; **151**:1064–7)

Trazodone (*Int J Geriatr Psychiatry* 1997; **12**:129–30)

Venlafaxine (n = 1, *J Emerg Med* 1997; **15**:491–3; n = 1, *Postgrad Med J* 2000; **76**:254–6; n = 1, *Psychiatry Clin Neurosci* 2006; **60**:121–2; 37.5 mg/d monotherapy, n = 1, *Ann Pharmacother* 2003; **37**:209–11)

Venlafaxine overdose (LD monotherapy 37.5 mg/d; n = 1, *Ann Pharmacother* 2003; **37**:209–11)

- Combinations, including SSRIs *

SSRIs + MAOIs (overview, *Lancet* 1994; **343**:607)

Citalopram + buspirone (n = 1, *Int Clin Psychopharmacol* 1997; **12**:61–3)

Citalopram/trazodone + linezolid (n = 1, *Ann Pharmacother* 2005; **39**:956–61)

Citalopram + linezolid (n = 1, *J Am Med Dir Assoc* 2004; **5**:111–13)

Citalopram + linezolid + mirtazapine (n = 1, *J Intensive Care Med* 2005; **20**:351–3)

Citalopram + moclobemide (*Med Clin [Barc]* 1999; **113**:677–8)

Citalopram overdose + moclobemide (*Lancet* 1993; **342**:1419)

Citalopram + moclobemide overdose (fatal, *J Anal Toxicol* 2001; **25**:147–51)

Citalopram + quetiapine (n = 1, *N Z Med J* 2006; **119**:2058)

Citalopram + tramadol (n = 1, *Am J Psychiatry* 2004; **161**:1129)

Fluoxetine/moclobemide/clomipramine

overdose (fatal case in *Anaesth Intensive Care* 1995;**23**:499–502)

Fluoxetine + buspirone (*Ann Pharmacother* 2000;**34**:871–4)

Fluoxetine + carbamazepine (n = 1, *Lancet* 1993; **42**:442–3)

Fluoxetine + dextromethorphan (n = 1, *Gen Hosp Psychiatry* 2006;**28**:78–80)

Fluoxetine + hydromorphone (n = 1, *Prescrire Int* 2004;**13**:57)

Fluoxetine + olanzapine (n = 1, *World J Biol Psychiatry* 2004;**5**:114–15)

Fluoxetine + lithium (n = 1, *Ugeskrift for Laeger* 1995;**157**:1204–5)

Fluoxetine + mirtazapine (*Int J Geriatr Psychiatry* 1998;**13**:495–6; n = 1, *Ann Pharmacother* 2001;**35**:1217–20)

Fluoxetine + moclobemide (eg. Benazzi, *Pharmacopsychiatry* 1996;**29**:162; n = 1, *Can J Anaesth* 2000;**47**:246–50)

Fluoxetine + nefazodone (n = 1, *J Clin Psychiatry* 2000;**61**:146)

Fluoxetine + paroxetine (n = 1, *Am Fam Physician* 1995;**52**:1475–82)

Fluoxetine + Parstelin (n = 1, *Anaesthesia* 1991; **46**:507–8)

Fluoxetine + sertraline (n = 1, *Clin Pharmacol Ther* 1993;**1**:84–8)

Fluoxetine + tramadol (n = 1, *J Royal Soc Med* 1999;**92**:474–5)

Fluoxetine + trazodone (*Biol Psychiatry* 1996; **39**:384–5)

Fluoxetine + venlafaxine (*Ann Pharmacother* 1998;**32**:432–6)

Fluvoxamine + oxycodone (n = 1, *Ann Pharmacother* 2006;**40**:155–7)

Paroxetine + lithium (n = 1, *Pharmaopsychiatry* 1997;**30**:106–7)

Paroxetine + moclobemide (fatal case, *J Anal Toxicol* 1997;**21**:518–20; *J Accid Emerg Med* 1999;**16**:293–5)

Paroxetine + nefazodone (n = 1, *Ann Emerg Med* 1997;**29**:113–19)

Paroxetine + OTC cold remedy (*Am J Emerg Med* 1994;**12**:642–4)

Paroxetine + risperidone (*J Clin Psychopharmacol* 2000;**20**:103–5)

Paroxetine + tramadol (n = 11, *Int Clin Psychopharmacol* 1997;**12**:181–2)

Paroxetine + trazodone (*Psychosomatics* 1995; **36**:159–60)

Sertraline + amitriptyline (*Ann Pharmacother* 1996;**30**:1499–500)

Sertraline + clomipramine (n = 1, *J Med Assoc Thai* 2005;**88**:993–6)

Sertraline + dolasetron (n = 1, *J Psychopharmacol* 2002;**16**:191)

Sertraline + erythromycin (*Pharmacotherapy* 1999;**19**:894–6)

Sertraline + linezolid (n = 1, *Clin Infect Dis* 2002;**34**:1651–2; n = 1, *Pharmacotherapy* 2006;**26**:269–76)

Sertraline + metoclopramide (n = 1, *Ann Pharmacother* 2002;**36**:67–71)

Sertraline + phenelzine (n = 1, *Ann Pharmacother* 1994;**28**:732–5)

Sertraline + tramadol (n = 1, *Ann Pharmacother* 1997;**31**:175–7; n = 1, *Aust Pres* 2002;**25**:19; n = 1, *Clin Neuropharmacol* 2004;**27**:150–1)

Sertraline + tranylcypromine (n = 1, *Clin Pharm* 1993;**12**:222–5)

Sertraline + buspirone + loxapine (n = 1, *Therapie* 1999;**54**:269–71)

SSRIs + risperidone (n = 2 [one fatal], *Ann Pharmacother* 2003;**37**:388–91)

- **Combinations, including MAOIs (see also above)**

MAOIs + TCAs (overview, Henry, *Lancet* 1994; **343**:607)

Phenelzine + clomipramine (n = 1, *Clin Pharmacol Therap* 1993;**53**:84–8)

Phenelzine + dextromethorphan (n = 1, *Clin Pharmacol Therap* 1993;**53**:84–8)

Tranylcypromine + venlafaxine (cases in *Vet Hum Toxicol* 1996;**38**:358–61 and *Hum Exp Toxicol* 1997;**16**:14–17)

- **Other combinations (see also above)**

Bupropion + sertraline + venlafaxine (n = 1, *Clin Neuropharmacol* 2004; **27**:219–22).

Mirtazapine + tramadol + olanzapine (n = 1, *Am J Psychiatry* 2002;**159**:672–3)

Moclobemide + clomipramine overdose (*Intensive Care Med* 1997;**23**:122–4; *J Toxicol Clin Toxicol* 1998;**36**:31–2)

Moclobemide + clomipramine (n = 1, *Br Med J* 1993;**306**:248)

Moclobemide + pethidine (possible case, *Med J Aust* 1995;**162**:554)

Nortriptyline + selegiline (n = 1, *J Neurol* 2000; **247**:811)

St John's wort + buspirone (n = 1, *J Psychopharmacol* 2002;**16**:401)

Tramadol + venlafaxine + mirtazapine (n = 1, *Ann Pharmacother* 2004;**38**:411–13)

Trazodone + amitriptyline (n = 1, *Int Clin Psychopharmacol* 1996;**11**:289–90)

Trazodone + nefazodone (n = 1, *Am J Psychiatry* 2000;**157**:1022)

Venlafaxine + amitriptyline (n = 1, *Postgrad Med J* 2000;**76**:254–6)

Venlafaxine + co-amoxiclav (n = 1, *J R Soc Med* 2003;**96**:233–4)

Venlafaxine + sour date nut (n = 1, *Am J Psychiatry* 2004;**161**:1129–30)

Venlafaxine + dexamphetamine (n = 1, *Med J Aust* 2002;**176**:240–1)

Venlafaxine + linezolid (n = 1, *J Antimicrob Chemother* 2004;**54**:289–90; n = 1, *Ann Pharmacother* 2005;**39**:956–61)

Venlafaxine + maprotiline + reboxetine (n = 1, *Eur Psychiatry* 2004;**19**:456–7)

Venlafaxine + metoclopramide (n = 1, *Ann Pharmacother* 2002;**36**:67–71)

Venlafaxine + mirtazapine (n = 1, *World J Biol Psychiatry* 2002;**3**:167)

Venlafaxine + trazodone (n = 1, *Am J Psychiatry* 2001;**158**:2088–9)

Venlafaxine + selegiline (n = 1, *J Clin Psychopharmacol* 1997;**17**:66–7)

Venlafaxine + St. John's wort? (*Presse Med* 2000; **29**:1285–6)

5.15 SLEEP PROBLEMS

5.15.1 SLEEP DISTURBANCES

Review of non-psychotropic causes: Novak and Shapiro, *Drug Saf* 1997;**16**:133–49.

- **Psychotropics etc** *
Benperidol
Biperiden withdrawal (n = 2, *Int Clin Psychopharmacol* 2000;**15**:357–9)
Bupropion (11%)
Chlorpromazine
Donepezil (n = 2, *J Am Geriatr Soc* 1998;**46**:119–20)
Fluoxetine
Fluspirilene
Lamotrigine (dose dependent, n = 7, *Epilepsia* 1999;**40**:322–5)

Levetiracetam (hypersomnia, n = 1, *Epilepsia* 2005;**46**:588–9)

Lorazepam
MAOIs (*Am J Psychiatry* 1989;**146**:1078)
Methysergide
Modafinil (UK SPC)
Nicotine (n = 252, *J Clin Psychiatry* 2001;**62**:319–24)
Olanzapine (somnambulism, n = 2, *Am J Psychiatry* 2001;**158**:1158)
Paroxetine (somnambulism, n = 1, *J Clin Psychiatry* 2003;**64**:483)
Phentermine (*Practitioner* 1970;**24**:423–5)
Phenytoin
Risperidone (sleep-related eating disorder, n = 1, *J Clin Psychiatry* 2004;**65**:273–4)
Rivastigmine (< 5%)
Sodium oxybate (SPC)
SSRIs (somnambulism, n = 1, *J Pharm Tech* 1999; **15**:204–7; paroxetine and fluvoxamine disrupt sleep architecture, RCT, n = 14, *J Clin Psychiatry* 2001;**62**:642–52)
Sulpiride
Stimulants (methylphenidate)
Trazodone
Tricyclics
Zolpidem (hypnagogic, on temporary withdrawal, n = 1, *J Toxicol Clin Toxicol* 2003; **41**:869–72)

- **Antiparkinsonian drugs**
Amantadine (4% incidence, see *J Clin Psychiatry* 1981;**42**:9)
Bromocriptine
Pramipexole (n = 6, *Mov Disord* 2000;**15**:658–63)
Ropinirole and/or pramipexole (n = 2, *Pharmacother* 2000;**20**:724–6)

- **Cardiovascular drugs**
Amiodarone (frequent, eg. *Am J Cardiol* 1983; **52**:975–9)
Beta-blockers (very common, especially with propranolol)
Atenolol (see *Adv Psychiatr Treat* 1999;**5**:30–8)
Carvedilol (n = 1, *Ann Pharmacother* 2002;**36**:1736–40)
Clonidine
Digoxin (see *Adv Psychiatr Treat* 1999;**5**:30–8)
Diltiazem (see *Adv Psychiatr Treat* 1999;**5**:30–8)
Isradipine (up to 3%, *Am J Med* 1989;**86**[Suppl 4A]:98–102)
Methyldopa

Nifedipine (see *Adv Psychiatr Treat* 1999;**5**:30–8)

- **NSAIDs and analgesics**
Diclofenac
Diflunisal
Fenoprofen
Indomethacin
Naproxen (*Eur J Rheumatol Inflamm* 1981;**4**: 87–92)
Nefopam
Sulindac

- **Respiratory drugs**
Aminophylline
Brompheniramine
Clomiphene
Pseudoephedrine
Theophylline

- **Anti-infection**
Cinoxacin
Ciprofloxacin (n = 1, *Lancet* 1986;**1**:819–22)

- **Miscellaneous** *
Bismuth toxicity (*Postgrad Med J* 1988;**64**: 308–10)
Dexamethasone
Ginseng (see *Arch Gen Psychiatry* 1998; **55**:1033–44)
Lovastatin (*Lancet* 1994;**343**:973)

Nicotine (n = 252, *J Clin Psychiatry* 2001;**62**:319–24)
Propantheline
Ranitidine (see *Adv Psychiatr Treat* 1999;**5**:30–8)
Sibutramine
Simvastatin
Sulphasalazine
Tolazamide
Triamcinolone

5.15.2 VIVID DREAMS AND NIGHTMARES

Review: Thompson and Pierce, *Ann Pharmacother* 1999;**33**:93–8.
Baclofen
Beta-blockers:
  Atenolol (*Clin Pharm Ther* 1979;**25**:8)
  Propranolol (*Adv Drug React Bull* 1983;**99**:364)
Clonidine (*Adv Drug React Bull* 1983;**99**:364)
Digoxin toxicity (*Ann Intern Med* 1980;**93**:639)
Famotidine (n = 1, *Pharmacother* 1998;**18**:404–7)
Indomethacin (rare, eg. *Br Med J* 1965;**2**:1281)
Methyldopa (*Adv Drug React Bull* 1983;**99**:364)
Nalbumetone (*Pharm J* 1990;**244**:764)
Pergolide (eg. *Clin Neuropharmacol* 1986;**9**:160–4)
Nicotine patches (*Pharm J* 1992;**249**:384)
Stanozolol
Verapamil (*NEJM* 1988;**318**:929–30)
Withdrawal from barbiturates, benzodiazepines, narcotics, etc

MANAGEMENT OF
SIDE-EFFECTS

6

Without wishing to state the blindingly obvious, we know that all drugs have side-effects. These may range from being mild and transient to being intolerable or life-threatening. If switching or discontinuing the causative agent is not clinically possible (eg. patient preference, clinical response), managing undesirable adverse effects may allow continued treatment, improve compliance and lead to better outcomes.

STANDARD STRATEGIES TO TRY FIRST INCLUDE:

- Drug — alter formulation (ie. SR/MR, liquid, injection).

- Dose — adjust total daily dose (increasing rarely works, but a systematic and gradual decrease should be tried to determine the minimum effective dose).

- Dose — manipulate frequency and timings (eg. split, or load to one particular time).

- Dose — consider drug holiday (eg. omitting doses on particular days, although this is likely only to be helpful for some specific ADRs).

- Dose — consider slower dose escalation (including stopping and restarting more gently), particularly with buspirone, many tricyclics and SSRIs.

- Monitor plasma levels to optimise dose if possible, eg. tricyclic ADRs are clearly correlated with plasma levels (review for our Polish readers by Grzesiak et al, Psychiatr Pol 2003;**37**:825–37).

- Switch to a drug from a different chemical group.

- Discontinue completely.

- Discontinue any concurrent drugs that might be interacting.

- Wait for side-effect to wear off.

- Initiate adjunctive therapies (additional drugs, physical management strategies).

All of these routine strategies may be of some importance and relevance for each side-effect. This chapter comments on some of the above, along with additional strategies. Data in this area of therapy is notably sparse, and the author would be grateful for any additional ideas.

Disclaimers:
- Some drug doses are quoted as total daily doses but many will need to be given as divided doses.
- Drugs and strategies are not in any particular order within each section, and are in alphabetical order where possible.

Reviews:
Antidepressant side-effects (Pollack and Rosenbaum, J Clin Psychiatry 1987;**48**:3–8)
Haddad, Dursun and Deakin (2005) Adverse Syndromes and Psychiatric Drugs. Oxford University Press, Oxford (ISBN 0-19-852748-9)

Anticholinergic, blurred vision

Antidepressants	**Switch** to antidepressant with less anticholinergic side-effects (see *2.1.2*). Beware of glaucoma developing (see *3.6*). **Bethanechol** 30–90 mg/d may be effective but often poorly tolerated. **Pilocarpine** 1% drops QDS may restore pupilary responsiveness and has been used if desipramine-induced (Salah and Cameron, *Am J Psychiatry* 1996;**153**:579).

Anticholinergic, constipation

Antidepressants (usually tricyclics)	Ensure adequate fluid intake. Usually requires bran or a bulking or lubricating laxative, eg. lactulose, docusate. **Bethanechol** 30–90 mg/d may be effective but often poorly tolerated.
Clozapine	As for tricyclics, but it is important to take this seriously as it may lead on to potentially fatal paralytic ileus, with or without previous abdominal symptoms (eg. review of fatal cases by Levin *et al*, *Psychosomatics* 2002;**43**:71–3; n = 1, Townsend and Curtis, *BMC Psychiatry* 2006;**19**:43).

Anticholinergic, dry mouth (xerostomia)

- **Stimulate salivary flow** — sugarless gum and other sugarless confectionary (eg. wine gums) stimulate salivary flow (avoid those with sugar as this can promote dental caries and weight gain).
- Artificial **saliva sprays** (most contain methylcellulose or glycerin, eg. Glandosane® [Fresenius Kabi]).
- Ensure adequate **hydration**.
- **Distigmine** bromide, but this has its own notable adverse effects, eg. digestive, urinary and dermatological (n = 25, open, Wolpert *et al*, *Fortschr Neurol Psychiatr Grenzgeb* 1980;**48**:224–33).
- **Pilocarpine** 10–30 mg/d, as 2–3 times a day, may resolve the problem within a day if caused by clozapine, olanzapine, benzatropine, tricyclics or mirtazapine, with no significant side-effects (naturalistic overview, Masters, *Am J Psychiatry* 2005;**162**:1023).

Review: dietary and dental advice to avoid dental consequences (Boyd *et al*, *Nutr Rev* 1997;**55**:362–8).

SSRIs	**Switching** to fluvoxamine may be effective if paroxetine-induced (n = 1, Arima *et al*, *Ann Pharmacother* 2005;**39**:567–71). Stop olanzapine, which may enhance the effect (n = 1, Hori *et al*, *Prog Neuro-psychopharmacol Biol Psychiatry* 2006;**30**:758–60).
Tricyclics	**Coffee** — chewing 15 g Cappuccino coffee for five minutes (n = 10, open, Chodorowski, *Przegl Lek* 2002;**59**:392–3). **Pilocarpine** (peripheral cholinergic) may not be effective but **bethanechol** has been used at 5–10 mg at night, or up to 60 mg/d sublingually to promote salivation (titrate dose slowly upwards, may be poorly tolerated). **Yohimbine** 4 mg/d may be effective for 3–4 hours (Bagheri *et al*, *Br J Clin Pharmacol* 1994;**37**:93–6).

Anticholinergic, urinary retention

Tricyclics	Once other physical causes have been excluded, the best course of action is probably to discontinue and/or switch. Can be a medical emergency (Tueth, *Am J Emerg Med* 1994;**12**:212–6) so take seriously. **Bethanechol** 30–90 mg/d may be effective, but may be poorly tolerated (Hermesh *et al*, *Drug Intell Clin Pharm* 1987;**21**:877–9).

Urinary hesitancy (see also anticholinergic effects)

Reboxetine	**Doxazosin** 1 mg/d (n = 1, Szabadi, *Br J Psychiatry* 1998;**173**:441–2). **Tamsulosin** 0.4 mg/d may be rapidly successful (within 20 minutes) and well tolerated (n = 6 males, open, Demyttenaere *et al*, *Int Clin Psychopharmacol* 2001;**16**:353–5; n = 8 males, Kasper and Wolf, *Eur Neuropsychopharmacol* 2002;**12**:119–22; n = 1, Kasper, *Psychopharmacol* 2002;**159**:445–6).

Urinary incontinence

Venlafaxine   Sertraline, switch to (n = 1, Polimeni et al, Clin Neuropharmacol 2005;**28**:247–8). Duloxetine might be an alternative if stress-related.

6.2 Cardiac effects

Hypertension

Antipsychotics   Beta-blockers and other general strategies are often adequate, eg. **propranolol** has been used if the hypertension is aripiprazole-induced (n = 1, Borras et al, Am J Psychiatry 2005;**162**:2392). **Pindolol** 5 mg BD has been used when clozapine-induced (where nifedipine was ineffective; n = 1, Shiwach, Clin Neuropharmacol 1998;**21**:139–40; see also review of 82 cases with clozapine; Henderson et al, J Clin Psychiatry 2004;**65**:686–9).

Clozapine   Hypertension is usually transient over the first month, so reduce the dose or rate of upward titration.
    If persistent or severe, antihypertensives may be necessary (n = 82, retrospective chart, Henderson et al, J Clin Psychiatry 2004;**65**:686–9).
    Review: management (Shiwach, Clin Neuropharmacol 1998;**21**:139–40).

MAOIs   For hypertensive crisis, refer to a specialist unit immediately for specialist care, eg. using British Hypertension Society guidelines for malignant hypertension (see also Elliot, J Clin Hypertens [Greenwich] 2004;**6**:587–92).

Hypotension

Hypotension occurs in about 10% people on MAOIs (n = 61, Remnick et al, Prog Neuropsychopharmacol Biol Psychiatry 1989;**13**:497–504) and usually involves specialist medical care.

MAOIs   **Metoclopramide** (Patterson, J Clin Psychopharmacol 1987;**7**:112–3).
    Plasma expansion, eg. salt tablets or fludrocortisone (review by Cockhill and Remick, Can J Psychiatry 1987;**32**:803–8).

Postural (orthostatic) hypotension

Initial strategies:

- Self-care (eg. if lying down, dangle legs for a minute before rising slowly and attempting to stand).
- Use support stockings.
- Slower dose titration.
- Plasma volume expansion, eg. fluid and increased sodium chloride intake.
- Desmopressin, indomethacin and erythropoietin can be used in extreme cases.
- Midodrine, an alpha-adrenergic agonist, is licensed and available in some countries (review by McClellan et al, Drugs Aging 1998;**12**:76–86), eg. for tricyclics (n = 1, Maskall and Lam, J Psychiatry Neurosci 1993;**18**:276–7).

Review: general (Freeman, Semin Neurol 2003;**23**:435–42).

Additional strategies:

Tricyclics   **Fludrocortisone** has been used but obviously has long-term side–effects (Chobanian et al, N Engl J Med 1979;**301**:68–73).
    Yohimbine 12 mg/d (n = 12, d/b, c/o, p/c, Lacomblez et al, Clin Pharmacol Ther 1989;**45**:241–51).

MAOIs   **Brewed coffee** (mentioned in Pollack and Rosenbaum, J Clin Psychiatry 1987;**48**:3–8).
    Fludrocortisone (Simonson, Am J Psychiatry 1964;**120**:1118–9).
    Levothyroxine or liothyronine has been suggested (see review, Whybrow and Prange, Arch Gen Psychiatry 1981;**38**:106–13).
    Methylphenidate 10–15 mg (case series, Feighner et al, J Clin Psychiatry 1985;**46**:206–9; mentioned in Pollack and Rosenbaum, J Clin Psychiatry 1987;**48**:3–8), but beware of ADRs.

	Salt tablets 600–1800 mg BD (n = 1, Munjack, *J Clin Psychiatry* 1984;**45**:89–90; mentioned in Pollack and Rosenbaum, *J Clin Psychiatry* 1987;**48**:3–8).
	Review: general (Cockhill and Remick, *Can J Psychiatry* 1987;**32**:803–8).
Antipsychotics	The effect is probably alpha-adrenergic-related so slower dose titration and lower dose are logical. Tolerance usually develops.
	Bovril and moclobemide has been used for severe clozapine-induced postural hypotension (n = 1, Taylor et al, *Br J Psychiatry* 1995;**167**:409–10).
	Fludrocortisone if clozapine-induced (n = 1, Testani, *J Clin Psychiatry* 1994;**55**:497–8).

QTc prolongation

See *Chapter 3.2* for risk factors and short review.

All drugs	**Switching** drugs is usually essential. If not possible, use the lowest doses in simple drug regimens. Avoiding metabolic interactions minimises the impact.
	Magnesium ion (Mg^{++}) orally at a mean dose of magnesium oxide 15 mg/kg/d shortens QTc, and can be given long term with appropriate monitoring.
	Magnesium sulphate by IV injection has been used and recommended by the American Heart Association (n = 24, Bachman, *J Clin Psychiatry* 2003;**64**:733–4).
	Beta-blockers can be used but are often ineffective (mentioned by Bachman, *J Clin Psychiatry* 2003;**64**:733–4).

Reviews: antipsychotics and QTc prolongation (Vieweg, *Prim Care Companion J Clin Psychiatry* 2003; **5**:205–15; Taylor, *Acta Psychiatr Scand* 2003;**107**:85–95; Zareba and Lin, *Psychiatr Q* 2003;**74**:291–306).

Tachycardia

Clozapine	Tachycardia is common (up to 67%) early in treatment, but usually resolves over 4–6 weeks (n = 100, Marinkovic et al, *Prog Neuropsychopharmacol Biol Psychiatry* 1994;**18**:537–44). It may be the first, or only presenting symptom of (often fatal) cardiomyopathy (eg. n = 1, Tanner and Culling, *Postgrad Med J* 2003;**79**:412–3; n = 26, Hagg et al, *J Clin Psychopharmacol* 2001;**21**:382–8), and so this must be fully excluded first. If the tachycardia is persistent and/or associated with chest pain, this may also indicate myocarditis (review of n = 26 where it was fatal in 46% of cases, Hagg et al, *J Clin Psychopharmacol* 2001;**21**:382–8), which can occur even six years after therapy (n = 1, Tanner and Culling, *Postgrad Med J* 2003;**79**:312–3) where discontinuation would be essential.
	Slower dose escalation may help.
	Discontinuation usually results in rapid resolution (eg. n = 1, Stampfer and Swanepoel, *Australas Psychiatry* 2005;**13**:80–2).
	Beta-blockers may help if tachycardia is anticholinergic/noradrenergic-related, although the literature on this is minimal.

6.3 Central adverse effects

Delirium

Discontinue any causative agent (see *5.4*).

Review: management of delirium from all causes (Carter et al, *Drug Saf* 1996;**15**:291–301).

Antidepressants	**Donepezil** if tricyclic overdose-induced (rapidly effective in n = 1, Noyan et al, *Prog Neuropsychopharmacol Biol Psychiatry* 2003;**27**:885–7).
Antipsychotics	Reduce any concurrent anticholinergics.
	Reduce dose, eg. clozapine-induced delirium appears to be dose-related (n = 139, Centorrino et al, *Pharmacopsychiatry* 2003;**36**:156–60).
	Propofol has been used successfully for post-ictal delirium with clozapine-ECT therapy (n = 1, Sienaert et al, *J ECT* 2004;**20**:254–7).

Switch drugs:

Switch to an antipsychotic with low anticholinergic effects (*Table 2.1.4*) or discontinue if no clear indication.

Quetiapine has been used if delirium is risperidone-induced (n=1, Kato *et al*, *Psychosomatics* 2005;**46**:374–5).

Haloperidol has been used if delirium is clozapine-induced (Spisla and Bunter, *Psychiatr Prax* 1997;**24**:308).

Depression

Tetrabenazine

Discontinue, or use antidepressants.

Reboxetine (n=1, Schreiber *et al*, *J Neurol Neurosurg Psychiatry* 1999;**67**:550).

Drowsiness (see also sedation)

Levetiracetam

Can be minimised by starting at a lower dose.

Mirtazapine

Start at higher dose: 30 mg/d, as this may produce less drowsiness than 15 mg/d (mirtazapine is a highly potent H1 receptor blocker, and at 30 mg/d the noradrenergic enhancement may counteract some of the histamine blockade).

SSRIs

Modafinil, used adjunctively to SSRIs at the start of treatment, may enhance the onset of action in people with MDD and fatigue (n=29, open, 6/52, Ninan *et al*, *J Clin Psychiatry* 2004;**65**:414–20, MS).

Valproate

Investigate immediately and discontinue if necessary. May be indicative of impending hepatic failure or encephalopathy.

Dysphoria

Antipsychotics

Procyclidine may be effective (n=51, King *et al*, *Br J Psychiatry* 1995;**167**:480–2).

Review: Voruganti and Awad, *Can J Psychiatry* 2004;**49**:285–9.

Fatigue

Antipsychotics

Adjust dose or spread the doses out throughout the day.

Modafinil has limited efficacy. A small study failed to show any differences vs placebo on fatigue, attention, working memory and executive functioning (n=24[c=20], 8/52, d/b, p/c, Sevy *et al*, *J Clin Psychiatry* 2005;**66**:839–43), although a smaller study showed it may be effective in some people (n=11, open, 4/52, Rosenthal and Bryant, *Clin Neuropharmacol* 2004;**27**:38–43).

Topiramate

Modafinil (Berigan, *Prim Care Companion J Clin Psychiatry* 2002;**4**:249–50).

Hypomania

Antidepressants

Discontinuation is the absolute priority, with short-term management of the manic episode.

Mania with antidepressants is restricted to people with bipolar disorder (review by Chun and Dunner, *Bipolar Disord* 2004;**6**:32–42). Beware of inducing rapid-cycling with antidepressants, which may be more prevalent in people given multiple antidepressant trials.

May be dose-related with SSRIs (n=1, Ramasubbu, *Acta Psychiatr Scand* 2001;**104**:236–8) but may only be transient with trazodone (n=3, Jabeen and Fisher, *Br J Psychiatry* 1991;**158**:275–8).

Once resolved, switch antidepressant; venlafaxine appears to have the highest risk of inducing mania, sertraline intermediate and bupropion the lowest risk (n=159, RCT, 10/52, Leverich *et al*, *Am J Psychiatry* 2006;**163**:232–9).

Adjunctive mood stabilisers, eg. lithium, may be protective.

Review: Goldberg and Truman, *Bipolar Disord* 2003;**5**:407–20.

Insomnia

Antidepressants (MAOIs, SSRIs, bupropion, venlafaxine)

Standard hypnotic therapy (time-limited) may be adequate, eg. zolpidem 5–10 mg/d if SSRI-induced (n=190, RCT, d/b, 5/52, Asnis *et al*, *J Clin Psychiatry* 1999;**60**:668–76).

Adjust time of doses, eg. take last dose of the day in the evening rather than late at night. For MAOIs, the last dose should be before 3.00 PM.

Quetiapine 50 mg/d was effective for phenelzine-induced insomnia non-responsive to BDZs, Zs and antihistamines (n = 1, Sokolski and Brown, *Ann Pharmacother* 2006;**40**:567–70).

Trazodone 50–75 mg was effective in nearly all patients on MAOIs (n = 21, open, Jacobsen, *J Clin Psychiatry* 1990;**51**:298–302; n = 13, open, Nierenberg and Keck, *J Clin Psychopharmacol* 1989;**9**:42–5). It was also highly effective at 100 mg at night for insomnia induced by SSRIs (n = 12, d/b, p/c, c/o, 2 × 7/7, Kaynak et al, *Sleep Med* 2004;**5**:15–20), bupropion (67% improved, n = 17, RCT, p/c, d/b, c/o, Nierenberg et al, *Am J Psychiatry* 1994;**151**:1069–72) and venlafaxine (especially in people with increased inner tenson; n = 50 [c = 42], open, 4/52, Bertschy et al, *Pharmacol Res* 2005;**51**:79–84).

Lamotrigine	Insomnia is probably dose-related so reduce dose, switch (n = 109, Sadler, *Epilepsia* 1999;**40**:322–5) or use hypnotics.

Nausea

Antidepressants
Slower dose increase helps initially. See *Table 2.1.2* for advice on antidepressants with a lower incidence of nausea. Short-term antinauseants may have a role. **Cisapride** (5–10 mg BD) has been used (n = 6, Russell, *J Clin Psychopharmacol* 1996;**16**:35–7), so presumably similar antiemetics may be effective.

Slow-release tablets/capsules reduce the peak plasma level effect, as does splitting dose throughout the day.

Gorei-san (TJ-17), a Japanese herbal medicine if SSRI-induced (n = 3, open, Yamada et al, *Psychiatr Clin Neurosci* 1999;**53**:681).

Mirtazapine may help if the nausea is SSRI-induced (Pedersen and Klysner, *Int Clin Psychopharmacol* 1997;**12**:59–60) and 15 mg at night may be effective within four days (n = 1, Caldis and Gair, *Can J Psychiatry* 2004;**49**:707; n = 3, Pedersen et al, *Int Clin Psychopharmacol* 1997;**12**:59–60).

Antipsychotics
Antiemetics, eg. ondansetron may be effective but **avoid** metoclopramide or prochlorperazine for the first 1–2 months, or if there is a history of EPSE.
Prochlorperazine has been effective for quetiapine-withdrawal nausea, where ondansetron had failed (n = 1, Kim and Staab, *Am J Psychiatry* 2005;**162**:1020).

Nocturnal enuresis (see also urinary incontinence)

Clozapine
Avoid or reduce fluids at night or after 6.00 PM, have planned night awakenings, enuresis alarms, and voiding before going to bed.
Adjust dose and bias towards morning if possible.
Desmopressin can be used intranasally at 10 mcg in each nostril at bedtime (n = 1, Aronowitz et al, *Am J Psychiatry* 1995;**152**:472; Steingard, *J Clin Psychiatry* 1994;**55**:315–6), although hyponatraemia can occur (n = 1, Sarma et al, *Aust N Z J Psychiatry* 2005;**39**:949).
Oxybutinin (mentioned in Lurie and Hosmer, *J Clin Psychiatry* 1997;**58**:404).
Tolterodine (there is one case where it did **not** work, whereas desmopressin did: n = 1, English et al, *Ann Pharmacother* 2001;**35**:867–9).
Trihexyphenidyl 5 mg/d at bedtime (n = 2, Poyurovsky et al, *Int Clin Psychopharmacol* 1996;**11**:61–3).

Obsessive-compulsive symptoms

Antipsychotics
Standard treatments may be adequate eg. **fluoxetine** if quetiapine-induced (n = 1, Ozer et al, *Prog Neuropsychopharmacol Biol Psychiatry* 2006;**30**:724–7).

Panic

SSRIs	Discontinue if panic symptoms are citalopram-induced (n = 1, Brauer et al, *South Med J* 2002;**95**:1088–9).

Sedation (see also drowsiness)

Antipsychotics	Tolerance partly develops.
	Adjust dose, eg. lower dose, bias full dose to night or early evening or spread out throughout the day.
	Avoid other concurrent CNS depressants.
	Methylphenidate 20–40 mg/d has been used if clozapine-induced (with great care; Miller, *Am J Psychiatry* 1996;**153**:1231–2).
	Modafinil 200 mg/d has been used if sedation is induced by clozapine (n = 3, Makela et al, *J Clin Psychiatry* 2003;**64**:485–6; comment by DeQuardo, *J Clin Psychiatry* 2004;**65**:278–9), risperidone or olanzapine, with no exacerbation of psychosis.
SSRIs	**Modafinil** has been used as an adjunct (n = 16, 3/52, open, Schwartz et al, *J Clin Psychiatry* 2004;**65**:1223–7).
Topiramate	**Modafinil** (Berigan, *Prim Care Companion J Clin Psychiatry* 2002;**4**:249–50).
Valproate	**Modafinil** (Berigan, *Can J Psychiatry* 2004;**49**:72–3).

Seizures

Clozapine	Clozapine-induced seizures are usually dose-related, so reduce the dose or rate of increase, or stop and restart if seizures occur. The incidence rises markedly above 600 mg/d.
	Stop any other drugs likely to reduce the seizure threshold.
	Carry out an **EEG** to test for ictal activity, as abnormal EEGs are not uncommon with clozapine or olanzapine (n = 323, Centorrino et al, *Am J Psychiatry* 2002;**159**:109–15).
	Valproate is standard management (case of successful concurrent valproate at low-dose clozapine 125 mg/d; n = 1, Foster and Olajide, *J Psychopharmacol* 2005;**19**:93–6) but the literature is remarkably sparce on this.
	Gabapentin up to 2100 mg/d is an alternative (n = 1, Usiskin et al, *Am J Psychiatry* 2000;**157**:482–3; Landry, *Am J Psychiatry* 2001;**158**:1930–1).
	Topiramate (Navarro et al, *Am J Psychiatry* 2001;**158**:968–9).
	Review: Devinsky and Pacia, *J Clin Psychiatry* 1994;**55**(Suppl B):153–6.

6.4 Endocrine effects

Diabetes insipidus

- Diabetes insipidus (not related to diabetes mellitus) is caused by poor kidney function or inadequate antidiuretic hormone production. It is most commonly reported with lithium and clozapine.
- Discontinuing the causative drug if possible is the obvious strategy.
- If urine volumes exceed 4 L/day, use thiazides and/or amiloride.
- NSAIDs (eg. indometacin) may help in severe cases.

Review: Bendz and Aurell, *Drug Saf* 1999;**21**:449–56.

Diabetes mellitus

Diabetes mellitus has two types:

Type 1: person is unable to produce any insulin (previously known as insulin-dependent diabetes).

Type 2: person is unable to produce enough insulin or when that insulin fails to work (insulin resistance, previously known as non-insulin dependent diabetes/NIDDM, mature-onset diabetes).

- May be caused by decreased insulin sensitivity and weight gain.

- Monitor carefully if there is a family history or risk factors exist.

General management includes:

- Adjust lifestyle changes, eg. manage obesity, smoking, exercise and diet.
- Oral hypoglycaemics, eg. metformin (n = 40, RCT, d/b, 14/52, Baptista et al, Can J Psychiatry 2006;1:192–6) or insulin should be considered.

Reviews: diabetes and atypicals (Clarke and Burge, Diabetes Technol Ther 2003;5:669–83), general (Lindermayer et al, J Clin Psychiatry 2001;62[Suppl 23]:30–8).

Clozapine	Discontinue clozapine (may not always resolve, n = 2, Tovey et al, J Psychopharmacol 2005;19:207–10).
	Orlistat has been used (Pavlovic, Eur Psychiatry 2005;20:520).
	Reviews: Haupt and Newcomer, J Clin Psychiatry 2001;62(Suppl 27):15–26; Henderson, CNS Drugs 2002;16:77–89.
Olanzapine	Discontinue drug (may not always resolve, see Koller and Doraiswamy, Pharmacotherapy 2002;22:841–52).
	Reduced dosage may help (n = 237, Koller and Doraiswamy, Pharmacotherapy 2002;22:841–52).
	Switch to an alternative antipsychotic, eg. quetiapine (n = 6 and review, Ashim et al, J Psychopharmacol 2004;18:128–32), risperidone (n = 1, Wu et al, Psychiatry Clin Neurosci 2006;60:115–6), aripiprazole (De Hert et al, Diabetes Care 2006;29:2329–30) or ziprasidone (Spivak et al, Am J Psychiatry 2002;159:1606).

Hepatotoxicity

Valproate	Early discontinuation and supportive therapy is usually vital (Konig et al, Epilepsia 1999;40:1036–40), although dose reduction may be possible if monitored with extreme care (n = 1, Lackmann, Pharmacology 2004;70:57–8).
	L-carnitine can help, especially if given IV and within the first five days (n = 92, Bohan et al, Neurology 2001;56:1405–9; n = 1, Romero-Falcon et al, Eur J Intern Med 2003;14:338–40), and it can also be given prophylactically (Raskind and El-Chaar, Ann Pharmacother 2000;34:630–8; review of evidence by Leheureux et al, Crit Care 2005;9:431–40).
	Garlic organosulfur and **gingko biloba** use has been postulated (Sabayan et al, Med Hypotheses 2007;68:512–4).

Hyperammonaemia

Valproate	This usually rapidly reversible (eg. n = 2, Panda and Radhakrishnon, J Assoc Physicians India 2004;52:746–8) but can lead to coma.
	Stop other drugs that may exacerbate, eg. phenobarbital, topiramate (Segura-Bruna et al, Acta Neurol Scand 2006;114:1–7) and pivmecillinam (n = 1, Lokrantz et al, Acta Neurol Scand 2004;109:297–301).
	L-carnitine can correct carnitine deficiency (n = 69, Bohles et al, Acta Paediatr 1996;85:446–9; Segura-Bruna et al, Acta Neurol Scand 2006;114:1–7) and be well tolerated (n = 19, LoVecchio et al, Am J Emerg Med 2005;23:321–2).
	Review: Stewart, J Am Geriatr Soc 2005;53:1080.

Hypercholesterol

Antipsychotics	Standard treatments for raised cholesterol.
	Switch drugs.
	Discontinue any beta-blockers, which may enhance clozapine's effect on cholesterol (n = 50, Batmiller et al, Schizophr Res 2003;59:49–57).

Hyperglycaemia

Clozapine	Orlistat has been used (Pavlovic, Eur Psychiatry 2005;20:520).
	Reviews: Haupt and Newcomer, J Clin Psychiatry 2001;62(Suppl 27):15–26; Henderson, CNS Drugs 2002;16:77–89.

Hyperlipidaemia

Antipsychotics

Manage risk factors, such as weight gain, dietary changes and glucose intolerance (Koro and Meyer, *Essent Psychopharmacol* 2005;**6**:148–57). Discontinue any beta-blockers which enhance the effects on lipids (n = 50, Batmiller *et al*, *Schizophr Res* 2003;**59**:49–57).

Lipid-lowering therapy, eg. rosuvastatin (n=100, 3/12, De Hert *et al*, *J Clin Psychiatry* 2006;**67**:1889–96).

Switch drugs:

Amisulpride or ziprasidone (Rettenbacher *et al*, *Int Clin Psychopharmacol* 2006; **21**:369–72) and **risperidone** (n = 15, Su *et al*, *Psychopharmacology (Berl)* 2005; **183**:383–6) may be alternatives if olanzapine or clozapine-induced.

Aripiprazole has resolved clozapine-induced hyperlipidaemia (n = 1, Ball *et al*, *Ann Pharmacother* 2005;**39**:1570–2) and may be the best option (n = 13,133, Olfson *et al*, *Am J Psychiatry* 2006;**163**:1821–5).

Fluvoxamine 50 mg/d has been used for clozapine-induced effects, partly by altering the clozapine:norclozapine ratio and possibly partly by facilitating a reduced clozapine dose via CYP1A2 inhibition (n = 68, RCT, 12/52, Lu *et al*, *J Clin Psychiatry* 2004;**65**:766–71; see also *Chapter 4.2.3*).

Hyperprolactinaemia

Antipsychotics

Reducing the dose of the causative agent may be effective.

Check clinical relevance or importance (remembering the potential long-term effects of raised prolactin), especially if it is resulting in amenorrhoea in women or testosterone deficiency in men.

HRT/combined oral contraceptive in women and exogenous testosterone in men (see Molitch, *Mayo Clin Proc* 2005;**80**:1050–7) may help, and avoid the need to switch drugs (Miller, *CNS Spectr* 2004;**9**[8 Suppl 7]:28–32).

Can test for a lesion by stopping the drug temporarily (or switching to a prolactin-sparing antipsychotic) to see if prolactin returns to normal, and/or performing a CT scan (Molitch, *Mayo Clin Proc* 2005;**80**:1050–7).

Switch drugs:

Switching to a prolactin sparing drug (*Table 2.1.4*) is first-line strategy:

Aripiprazole may be an alternative as it can reduce prolactin in its own right, but is not always successful (Paulzen and Grunder, *Int J Neuropsychopharmacol* 2006;**10**:149–51).

Quetiapine has a low incidence of hyperprolactinaemia (20%; n = 70, Stevens *et al*, *J Child Adolesc Psychopharmacol* 2005;**15**:893–900) and switching to quetiapine from typicals may be successful in about 65% (n = 69, Nakajima *et al*, *Pharmacopsychiatry* 2005;**38**:17–9).

Adjunctive therapies:

Aripiprazole augmentation may be successful (15 mg/d for risperidone depot, Wahl and Ostroff, *Am J Psychiatry* 2005;**162**:1542–3) but may exacerbate hallucinations in some patients (n = 7, Lee *et al*, *Prog Neuropsychopharmacol Biol Psychiatry* 2006;**30**:714–7).

Dopamine agonists should generally be avoided as they may precipitate psychosis, but with careful monitoring and dose adjustment may be successful in selected cases where other strategies have failed, eg:

- **Amantadine** has been successful on all measures of hyperprolactinaemia in 90% patients (n = 10, open, 7/52, Correa *et al*, *J Clin Psychopharmacol* 1987;**7**:91–5).

- **Bromocriptine** may reverse the hyperprolactinaemia and galactorrhoea from olanzapine (n = 1, Miller and Sebastian, *J Clin Psychiatry* 2005;**66**:269–

70) and amisulpride (n = 1, Bliesener *et al*, *Pharmacopsychiatry* 2004;**37**:189–91).

- **Cabergoline** is longer-acting, better tolerated and may be superior to bromocriptine in efficacy (Biller *et al*, *J Reprod Med* 1999;**44** [12Suppl]: 1075–84). Cabergoline 0.125–0.25 mg/d has been used if risperidone-induced (58% had a statistically significant reduction, with no adverse affects and no deterioration in psychosis; n = 19, 8/52, Cavallaro *et al*, *J Clin Psychiatry* 2004;**65**:187–90; n = 4, mean dose 0.3 mg/d, Cohen and Biederman, *J Child Adolesc Psychopharmacol* 2001;**11**:435–40).
  - **Pergolide** – mentioned in some reviews (see below).

Reviews: management of antipsychotic-induced hyperprolactinaemia (Haddad and Wieck, *Drugs* 2004;**64**:2291–314; Miller, *CNS Spectr* 2004;**9**[8 Suppl 7]:28–32; see also Gillam *et al*, *Pediatr Endocrinol Rev* 2004;**2**[Suppl 1]:108–14), general (Verhelst and Abs, *Treat Endocrin* 2003;**2**:23–32; Bankowski and Zacur, *Clin Obstet Gynecol* 2003;**46**:349–62).

Hyperthyroidism

Lithium

This is relatively unusual.

Carbimazole (n = 9 and review, Barclay *et al*, *Clin Endocrinol* [Oxf] 1994; **40**:759–64).

Radioactive iodine (n = 3, Dwarakanathan, *Endocr Pract* 1998;**4**:201–3).

Hyponatraemia

- Risk factors for hyponatraemia include older age, female gender, low body weight, concurrent drugs (eg. diuretics, NSAIDs, carbamazepine, cancer chemotherapy), reduced renal function, co-morbidity (eg. hypothyroidism, diabetes, COPD), and hotter weather (review Jacob and Spinler, *Ann Pharmacother* 2006; **40**:1618–22), so monitor serum sodium over several weeks in higher risk patients. Rapid correction is extremely hazardous.
- Smoking may exacerbate hyponatraemia.
- If necessary, restart at low dose, increase slowly and monitor carefully. On drug withdrawal, sodium usually returns to normal within two weeks.
- If sodium > 125 mmol/l, monitor daily until above 135 mmol/L. If < 125 mmol/L, refer for urgent specialist medical care.
- Loop diuretics at variable doses have been used (Jacob and Spinler, *Ann Pharmacother* 2006;**40**:1618–22).
- Restrict fluid intake.
- Rechallenge may be possible without recurrence, so it may be a transient effect (review, Kirby and Ames, *Int J Geriatr Psychiatry* 2001;**16**:484–93).

Antidepressants

May be due to inappropriate antidiuretic hormone secretion.

Mirtazapine appears to have the lowest risk based on current evidence and the level of reported problems, although all antidepressants have reported associations. Reboxetine and lofepramine are also possibilities.

If it recurs on rechallenge and antidepressants are essential, consider water restriction and/or careful use of demeclocycline.

Review: Spigset and Hedenmalm, *Drug Saf* 1995;**12**:209–25.

Antipsychotics

Can be caused by water intoxication, SIADH or severe hyperlipidaemia and/or hyperglycaemia.

If caused by water intoxication (serum and urine osmolality both low):

- Fluid restriction (refer to DGH if sodium < 125 mmol/L).
- Switch drugs, eg. clozapine (may reverse hyponatraemia/hypoosmolemia; n = 8, 18–24/52, open, Canuso and Goldman, *J Neuropsychiatry Clin Neurosci* 1999;**11**:86–90), olanzapine, risperidone or quetiapine.
- There is no evidence that altering doses is effective.

- Use of demeclocycline is controversial and some texts recommend avoiding it with antidepressants.

If caused by SIADH (high urine but low serum osmolality):

- Fluid restriction (refer to DGH if sodium < 125 mmol/L).
- Switch antipsychotic as soon as possible .
- Consider demeclocycline (probably directly blocks the renal tubule effect of antidiuretic homone; usual dose range is 0.9–1.2 g daily, reduced to 600–900 mg/d for maintenance, see standard texts).
- Discontinue any concurrent desmopressin (n = 1, Sarma et al, Aust N Z J Psychiatry 2005;**39**:1726–31).
- Lithium has been used (mentioned in Madhusoodanan et al, Adverse Drug React Toxicol Rev 2002;**21**:17–29).

Review: Spigset and Hedenmalm, Drug Saf 1995;**12**:209–25.

Hypothyroidism

Lithium
Lithium inhibits thyroid release but compensatory mechanisms normally operate in most patients.
Euthyroid or hypothyroid goitres tend to resolve with lithium withdrawal.
Supplementary thyroxine therapy is indicated for overt hypothyroidism.
Treatment with thyroxine for subclinical hypothyroidism is controversial.
Manage weight, especially during the first year, which can be highly predictive of hypothyroidism (Henry, J Psychiatry Neurosci 2002;**27**:104–7).
Refer to endocrinologist if TSH levels are repeatedly abnormal.
Reviews: general (Fagiolini et al, Epidemiol Psichiatr Soc 2006;**15**:123–7), mechanisms (Bocchetta and Loviselli, Clin Pract Epidemol Ment Health 2006;**12**:23; Johnson and Eagles, Br J Psychiatry 1999;**175**:336–9).

Polyuria (often a symptom of diabetes insipidus)

Lithium
Dose reduction is logical (although there is little data to support this).
Refer to renal physicians for assessment (although they are likely to recommend discontinuation).
Substitute with an alternative mood stabiliser (eg. valproate has been used; n = 7, Stoll et al, J Clin Psychiatry 1996;**57**:356–9).
Stop any serotonergic antidepressants that may enhance polyuria (n = 75, Movig et al, Br J Psychiatry 2003;**182**:319–23).
Diuretics such as amiloride have been used (n = 1, Finch et al, Pharmacotherapy 2003;**23**:546–50), but great care is needed with interactions, see Chapter 4.4 (mentioned in van Gerven and Boer, Ned Tijdschr Geneeskd 2006;**150**:1705–9).
NSAIDs such as ketoprofen 100 mg IV has been effective in acute lithium toxicity presenting as severe nephrogenic diabetes mellitus (n = 1, Tran-Van et al, Presse Med 2005;**34**:1137–40), as has indomethacin 150 mg (rapidly effective, within 36 hours; n = 1, Lam and Kjellstrand, Ren Fail 1997;**19**:183–8; 50 mg TDS, n = 1, Martinez et al, South Med J 1993;**86**:971–3; n = 1, Allen et al, Arch Intern Med 1989;**149**:1123–6), probably by blocking lithium's prostaglandin-inducing activity. Adequate hydration is essential.
Reviews: general (van Gerven and Boer, Ned Tijdschr Geneeskd 2006;**150**:1705–9), risk factors (n = 75, Movig et al, Br J Psychiatry 2003;**182**:319–23), clinical management (Martin, Hosp Com Psychiatry 1993;**44**:427–8).

Renal impairment (see also diabetes insipidus)

Lithium
About 20% of people on lithium develop decreased renal function, but this is probably only progressive in a few, with a change in therapy only recommended if the serum creatinine concentration rises

above 200 micromol/l (van Gerven and Boer, *Ned Tijdschr Geneeskd* 2006;**150**:1715–8). It may be due to lithium's effect on vasopressin at a hypothalamic level and a decrease in GFR. The main strategies are:

* reduce dose to the lowest possible, making it once daily (if not already)
* switch to an alternative drug if possible
* discontinue any other drugs that might be contributing
* refer to renal specialists for advice.

Reviews: effect of lithium on renal function (n = 20, Turan *et al*, *Prog Neuropsychopharmacol Biol Psychiatry* 2002;**26**:561–5), avoiding lithium toxicity based on renal clearance (Thomsen and Schou, *Pharmacopsychiatry* 1999;**32**:83–6).

Weight gain

Numerous mechanisms for drug-induced weight gain have been proposed, including:

* Sedation — leading to decreased activity.
* Thirst — anticholinergic dry mouth may lead to an increased intake of fluids and calories.
* Reduced metabolism — fat and carbohydrate oxidation.
* Increased food intake via neurotransmitter-mediated increase in appetite, eg. via blockade of receptors such as 5-HT2A, 5-HT2C (n = 123, Reynolds *et al*, *Lancet* 2002;**359**:2086–7), H1 or H2 (n = 92, males, retrospective, Wirshing *et al*, *J Clin Psychiatry* 1999;**60**:358–63) and perhaps D2, and polypeptides such as CCK (review by Stahl, *J Clin Psychiatry* 1998;**59**:500–1).
* Changes in levels of leptin (Baptista and Beaulieu, *Can J Psychiatry* 2002;**47**:742–9). Leptin is a multifunctional polypeptide produced by fat cells to reduce appetite (by signalling the size of the adipose tissue to the brain) and to increase energy expenditure (Friedman and Halass, *Nature* 1998;**395**:763–70). Weight gain induced by clozapine or olanzapine (n = 44, Kraus *et al*, *Am J Psychiatry* 1999;**156**:312–4) and other antipsychotics (n = 59 + 59, o/p, Herran *et al*, *Br J Psychiatry* 2001;**179**:59–62) seems related to an increase in leptin levels. Other polypeptides may also be implicated, eg. reductin and cytokines, mainly tumour necrosis factor alpha (TNF-alpha).
* Induction of abdominal fat deposition, combined with a dysfunction of the normal leptin control of weight (n = 46, 10/52, Zhang *et al*, *Br J Psychiatry* 2004;**184**:58–62).
* Fluid retention — via peripheral oedema, a minor effect.
* Endocrine effects — increased prolactin levels (which may promote adiposity and is related to weight gain in men; open, p/c, Baptista *et al*, *Pharmacopsychiatry* 1997;**30**:250–5), variation in cortisol or altered insulin secretion.

Reviews: general (Faulkner and Cohn, *Can J Psychiatry* 2006;**51**:502–11; Ness-Abramof and Apovian, *Drugs Today (Barc)* 2005;**41**:547–55; Ruetsch *et al*, *Encephale* 2005;**31**:507–16; Schwarz *et al*, *Obes Rev* 2004;**5**:115–21), aetiological factors (Virk *et al*, *Obes Rev* 2004;**5**:167–70).

Antidepressants	**Switch** antidepressants. SSRIs have the lowest short-term weight gain potential, although there is a tendency for weight gain after 6–12 months treatment.
	Tricyclics should be **avoided** as they cause carbohydrate craving (Paykel, *Br J Psychiatry* 1973;**123**:501–7) *and* a decreased metabolic rate (Fernstein *et al*, *Biol Psychiatry* 1985;**20**:688–92), a double whammy.
	Naltrexone can produce a reduction in continuous hunger and a small weight loss at eight weeks for tricyclic-induced weight gain (open, Zimmermann *et al*, *Biol Psychiatry* 1997;**41**:47–9).
Antipsychotics	Education; **WWW** (**w**arn, **w**eigh, **w**atch):
	Warn: counsel patients with a higher risk of weight gain, eg. female, prone to overeating under stress, narcissistic personality traits, family or personal history of obesity and a greater than 6.5 kg difference between adult maximum and minimum weights (Kalucy, *Drugs* 1980;**19**:268–78).

Weigh: take a baseline weight, warn of the unpredictable nature of the potential effect, that the effect plateaus after several months, and the need to optimise calorie intake.

Watch: most weight is gained in the first few months, so ensure the patient seeks advice from a dietician early, since it is easier to prevent weight gain than lose it once it has happened. Moderate physical exercise may be helpful and excessive intake of high calorie fluids should be avoided. As David Taylor once said, weight management includes all possible variations on 'eat less, move more' (see Sharpe *et al, J Clin Psychiatry* 2005;**66**:951–2 for explanation of the 'move more').

Behavioural interventions may be effective, including dietary interventions via regular dietician visits, and self-directed diet with weight loss as a treatment goal (n = 53, O'Keefe *et al, J Clin Psychiatry* 2003;**64**:907–12; n = 35 [c = 29], 15/12, Kalarchian *et al, J Clin Psychiatry* 2005;**66**:1058–63; n = 70, RCT, 4/12, Littrell *et al, J Nurs Scholar* 2003;**35**:237–41). Individual nutritional education for 3–6/12 after starting olanzapine may be successful, (although the studies have small sample sizes, excluded obese and diabetic people and had no dietary analysis; n = 51, RCT, open, 3–6/12, Evans *et al, Aust N Z J Psychiatry* 2005;**39**:479–86; critical review by Isaacs, *EBMH* 2006;**9**:11; programme focused on nutrition, exercise and motivation; n = 31 [c = 21], 12/12, Menza *et al, J Clin Psychiatry* 2004;**65**:471–7).

Reduce dose, although only a major reduction is likely to help.

A slower introduction has been postulated to lead to a lower final weight gain. Intermittent antipsychotic use is not recommended but has been suggested (Buchanan and Carpenter, *CNS Drugs* 1996;**5**:240–5).

Switch drugs:

See *2.1.3* for a table of the relative risks.

If olanzapine-induced, **aripiprazole** (n = 1, Luebbe *et al, Pharmacopsychiatry* 2006;**39**:76) and **risperidone** (n = 15, Su *et al, Psychopharmacology(Berl)* 2005; **183**:383–6; n = 121, Meyer *et al, Clin Ther* 2005;**27**:1930–41) have been used.

Adjunctive therapies:

Few, if any, adjunctive therapies have been shown to have any sustained and/or robust effect. The following, in alphabetical order, are the best of the bunch:

- **Amantadine** 100–300 mg/d may be well-tolerated and attenuated weight gain or modestly promoted weight loss in some patients who had already gained weight with olanzapine 5–20 mg/d (n = 125, RCT, d/b, p/c, 16/52, Deberdt *et al, Eur Neuropsychopharmacol* 2005;**15**:13–21). It may stabilise weight with olanzapine (n = 21, RCT, p/c, d/b, Graham *et al, Am J Psychiatry* 2005;**162**:1744–6), although was ineffective in an earlier trial (n = 25, Bahk *et al, Psychiatr Clin Neurosci* 2004;**58**:163–7).

- **Bupropion** 150–300 mg/d as an adjunct to olanzapine (mean duration 26/12) has produced modest weight loss, with 50% losing > 3% (n = 8 [c = 7], open, 24/52, Gadde *et al, J Clin Psychopharmacol* 2006; **6**:409–13).

- **Modafinil** significantly reduced weight over one year, maintained for three years, in a patient on clozapine, possibly by reducing clozapine-induced fatigue, reversed on discontinuation (n = 1, Henderson *et al, Ann Clin Psychiatry* 2005;**17**:95–7).

- **Orlistat** may be useful but requires compliance with a low-fat diet (Pavlovic, *Eur Psychiatry* 2005;**20**:520).

- **Quetiapine** has been used as an adjunct to clozapine; after six months on clozapine (200–800mg/d), patients had 25% of their dose converted to quetiapine (using ratio 1mg clozapine:2mg quetiapine) for 10 months. The average weight loss was 0.22–10.5kg after one month, and maintained, with 100% user satisfaction reported (n=65, open, 10/12, Reinstein *et al*, *Clin Drug Invest* 1999;**18**:99–104). Review by Werneke *et al*, *Int Clin Psychopharmacol* 2002;**17**:145–60.

- **Reboxetine** co-prescribing when starting olanzapine may reduce olanzapine-induced weight gain (n=26[c=20], RCT, p/c, d/b, 6/52, Poyurovsky *et al*, *Am J Psychiatry* 2003;**160**:297–302).

- **Sibutramine** 15mg/d significantly reduced olanzapine-induced weight gain (8lb vs 2lb) but increased bp and disturbed sleep in some patients (n=37, RCT, d/b, p/c, 12/52, Henderson *et al*, *Am J Psychiatry* 2005;**162**:954–62). It was ineffective for clozapine-induced weight gain (n=21, RCT, d/b, p/c, 12/52, Henderson *et al*, *Acta Psychiatr Scand* 2007; **115**:101–5), but is contraindicated in 'psychiatric illness' and should not be used with another serotonergic drug.

- **Switching** to orodispersible olanzapine (bizarre, but you can't ignore a reported mean weight loss 6.6kg; n=17, open, 16/52, de Haan *et al*, *Psychopharmacol* 2004;**175**:389–90).

- **Topiramate** 200mg/d may be effective (100mg/d is ineffective; n=66, RCT, d/b, p/c, 12/52, Ko *et al*, *Clin Neuropharmacol* 2005;**28**:169–75) but has helped with olanzapine-induced weight gain (n=1, Levy *et al*, *J Clin Psychiatry* 2002;**63**:1045; n=3, Lin *et al*, *Psychiatr Clin Neurosci* 2005;**59**:613–5) and has significantly reduced adiposity in women treated with olanzapine (n=43, RCT, d/b, p/c, 10/52, Nickel *et al*, *J Clin Psychopharmacol* 2005;**25**:211–7; n=26[c=13], open, 12/12, Vieta *et al*, *J Clin Psychopharmacol* 2004;**24**:374–8).

Less useful strategies:

Other drugs have been tried but those listed below are either of no use or theoretical prospects only:

- **Appetite suppressants** may exacerbate psychosis or fail to work.

- **Estrogen** (which promotes weight loss by several mechanisms) shows a possible preventative role in animal studies (see Baptista, *Acta Psychiatr Scand* 1999;**100**:3–16).

- **Fluoxetine** is ineffective if olanzapine-induced (n=30, RCT, d/b, 8/52, Poyurovsky *et al*, *Am J Psychiatry* 2002;**159**:1058–60; n=31, RCT, d/b, Bustillo *et al*, *Neuropsychopharm* 2003;**28**:527–9).

- **Fluvoxamine** (50mg/d) may allegedly attenuate weight gain and metabolic disturbances from clozapine, perhaps by allowing lower doses to be used, although the interaction can be dramatic and dangerous (n=68, RCT, 12/52, Lu *et al*, *J Clin Psychiatry* 2004;**65**:766–71).

- **H2-antagonists** such as famotidine (n=14, d/b, p/c, 6/52, Poyurovsky *et al*, *Eur Neuropsychopharmacol* 2004;**14**:332–6) and nizatidine are ineffective for olanzapine-induced weight gain (n=175, d/b, p/c, 16/52, Cavazzoni *et al*, *Eur Neuropsychopharmacol* 2003;**13**:81–5) but may have some effect (n=59, RCT, d/b, 8/52, Atamaca *et al*, *Hum Psychopharmacol* 2003;**18**:45 7–61). Ranitidine reduced the weight gain from olanzapine in 60% cases (RCT, open, Lopez-Mato *et al*, *Vertex* 2003;**14**:85–96). They may stop weight gain with quetiapine although will not reduce any weight already gained (n=47, RCT, Atmaca *et al*, *Hum Psychopharmacol* 2004;**19**:37–40).

- **Melatonin** augmentation helps in rats, but human data is currently unavailable (Raskind *et al*, *Neuropsychopharmacol* 2007;**32**:284–8).
- **Metformin** does not aid loss of olanzapine-induced weight gain (n = 40, RCT, d/b, p/c, 14/52, Baptista *et al*, *Can J Psychiatry* 2006;**51**:192–6), although glucose levels may decrease (n = 19, open, 12/52, Morrison *et al*, *Am J Psychiatry* 2002;**159**:655–7; n = 5, p/c, 12/52, Baptista *et al*, *J Clin Psychiatry* 2001;**62**:653–5). It has been shown to prevent weight gain when started *with* atypicals (n=39, RCT, d/b, p/c, Klein *et al*, *Am J Psychiatry* 2006;**163**:2072–9).
- **Phenylpropanolamine** is ineffective for clozapine-induced weight gain (n = 16, RCT, d/b, 12/52, Borovicka *et al*, *J Clin Psychiatry* 2002; **63**:345–8).
- **Tamoxifen** (no human studies yet but prevents sulpiride-induced weight gain in female rats; Baptista *et al*, *Pharmacol Biochem Behav* 1997;**57**:215–22).

Reviews: general (Faulkner and Cohn, *Can J Psychiatry* 2006;**51**:502–11; Gentile, *Drug Saf* 2006;**29**:303–19, Faulkner *et al*, *Acta Psychiatr Scand* 2003;**108**:324–32; Ananth *et al*, *Ann Clin Psychiatry* 2004;**16**:75–85), genetics (Muller and Kennedy, *Pharmacogenomics* 2006;**7**:863–87).

Lithium	Weight gain occurs predominantly during the first 1–2 years of treatment, occurs more often in people already overweight and may be more common in women than men.

Manage thirst, as increased thirst has been noted in 89% and strongly correlates with weight gain. Increased hunger/food intake has not been directly shown (*J Psychopharmacol* 1990;**4**:303) and so the predominant mechanism may be increased intake of high-calorie drinks.

Thyroid status should also be assessed as a possible contributory cause.

Counselling, eg. use of plain/low-calorie beverages, along with normal sodium intake, dietary advice and monitoring, particularly during the first year, may be adequate (general review by Baptista *et al*, *Pharmacopsychiatry* 1995;**28**:35–44).

Lamotrigine may be an alternative as it is associated with weight loss, there being no significant differences in non-obese patients (n = 155 + 399, s = 2, d/b, p/c, one year, Bowden *et al*, *Am J Psychiatry* 2006;**163**:1199–201).

Mirtazapine	This is difficult to manage, and it may be that switching is the only option. Ranitidine at night is probably of no use.
SSRIs	Weight gain tends to occur later in the first year of therapy.

Topiramate up to 250 mg/d has produced a mean 4 kg loss of weight (n = 15, open, 10/52, Van Ameringen *et al*, *J Clin Psychiatry* 2002;**63**: 981–4).

Valproate	Valproate-induced weight gain may have a variety of mechanisms, but seems more common in people with normal or below normal weight prior to starting (n = 70, Corman *et al*, *Can J Neurol Sci* 1997;**24**:240–4) and so warning people in advance may be advantageous.

Get a new set of genes (n = 5 twin pairs, Klein *et al*, *Obes Res* 2005;**13**:1330–4). OK, it's not realistic but may help to explain to some people that weight gain with valproate isn't all their 'fault'.

Lamotrigine may be an alternative (n = 222, open, Morrell *et al*, *Epilepsy Res* 2003;**54**:189–99) but carbamazepine may not be suitable (n = 211, Easter *et al*, *Seizure* 1997;**6**:121–5).

6.5 Movement disorders

Blepharospasm (see also tardive dystonia)

Blepharospasm is a sustained, forced, involuntary closing of the eyelids, often a presenting symptom of tardive dystonia.

Antipsychotics	Switching antipsychotics is usually the main effective strategy, eg. to **clozapine**, (n = 4, Levin and Reddy, *J Clin Psychiatry* 2000;**61**:140–3) or **quetiapine** (n = 1, Reeves and Liberto, *Mov Disord* 2003;**18**:1072–3).
	ECT has been used (n = 1, Sienaert and Peuskens, *J ECT* 2005;**21**:132–4).

Dysphagia

Difficulty in swallowing or painful swallowing has been reported with many antipsychotics.

Reviews: drug-induced (Bulling, *Aust N Z J Med* 1999;**29**:748) and neuroleptic dysphagia (Sokoloff and Pavlakovic, *Dysphagia* 1997;**12**:177–9).

Antipsychotics	Dysphagia generally responds rapidly to discontinuation (eg. n = 1, Stewart, *Dysphagia* 2003;**18**:274–5).
	In life-threatening dysphagia, **benzodiazepines** (clonazepam) or oral **anticholinergics** may be effective (trihexyphenidyl, n = 2, Hayashi *et al*, *Clin Neuropharmacol* 1997;**20**:77–81; benzatropine, n = 1, Nair *et al*, *Gen Hosp Psychiatry* 2001;**23**:231–2), although if used regularly, anticholinergics may be a causative or exacerbating factor.

Laryngospasm (see also dystonia)

Benzodiazepines	**Flumazenil** may be effective in 25 minutes if laryngospasm is midazolam-induced (n = 1, Davis *et al*, *Ann Emerg Med* 1998;**32**:263–5).

EPSE, akathisia

Neuroleptic-induced akathisia (NIA) is a subjective unpleasant feeling of inner restlessness and the urge to move, with rocking while standing or sitting, lifting feet as if marching on the spot, and crossing and uncrossing legs while sitting. NIA has been associated with suicidal behaviour (review of 83 reports, Hansen, *Hum Psychopharmacol* 2001;**16**:495–505) and is probably an imbalance of cortical and nigrostriatal dopaminergic innervation. Akathisia has been reported with other drugs.

Reviews: * general (Miller and Fleischhacker, *Drug Saf* 2000;**22**:73–81;71 refs), effect on clinical outcome (n = 34, Luthra *et al*, *Gen Hosp Psychiatry* 2000;**22**:276–80), use of serotonin-based drugs (Poyurovsky and Weizman, *Br J Psychiatry* 2001;**179**:4–8; including an algorithm), NIA and violence (Leong and Silva, *J Forensic Sci* 2003;**48**:187–9).

Antidepressants	**Reduce** the dose, as it is dose-related at least for fluoxetine (n = 1, Hansen, *J Psychopharmacol* 2003;**17**:451–2).
	Switch antidepressants, eg. **paroxetine** for fluoxetine-induced (n = 1, Bauer *et al*, *J Clin Psychiatry* 1996;**57**:593–4) or **mianserin** 15 mg/d (n = 1, Poyurovsky *et al*, *Int Clin Psychopharmacol* 1995;**10**:111–4).
	Propranolol has also been used if fluoxetine-induced (Fleischhacker, *Biol Psychiatry* 1991;**30**:531–2).
	Review: Lane, *J Psychopharmacol* 1998;**12**:192–214.
Antipsychotics	Reduce dose or switch antipsychotics is the main strategy.
	Adjunctive therapies:
	The following drugs may be useful in the short or long-term if the dose and drug cannot be changed:
	• **Anticholinergics** may have some efficacy if the akathisia forms part of an EPSE but are generally considered less useful. Biperiden 5 mg iv may be rapidly effective (within 10 minutes) for severe akathisia (n = 23, open, Hirose and Ashby, *Int J Psychiatry Med* 2000;**30**:185–94). Cochrane concludes there is no reliable evidence to support or refute the use of anticholinergics in acute NIA (Lima *et al*, *CDSR* 2006;**4**:CD003727).

- **Benzodiazepines**, eg. clonazepam 0.5–3 mg/d (mean 1.7 mg/d) have been used and 81% patients in one study improved, with the effect prominent in two days (n = 21, open, *Acta Psychiatr Scand* 1989;**80**:106–7). Diazepam 10–17 mg IV (at 5 mg/30sec) has also provided rapid relief of acute NIA (n = 18, open, Hirose and Ashby, *J Clin Psychiatry* 2002;**63**:524–7).
- **Beta-blockers**, eg. propranolol 30–80 mg/d can produce a dramatic and persistent improvement (especially if not part of an EPSE), but may take up to three months to act in chronic cases (d/b, p/c, Kramer et al, *Biol Psychiatry* 1988;**24**: 823–7). Other lipophilic beta-blockers eg. metoprolol (RCT, Adler et al, *Biol Psychiatry* 1990;**27**:673–5) and betaxolol (n = 19, RCT, p/c, c/o, *Am J Psychiatry* 1992;**149**:647–50) may be effective for olanzapine-induced akathisia (n = 1, Kurzthaler et al, *Am J Psychiatry* 1997;**154**:1316). Nadolol, sotalol and atenolol are probably ineffective.
- **Cyproheptadine** 16 mg/d may be effective, supported by a robust trial (n = 30, RCT, d/b, 7/7, Fischel et al, *J Clin Psychopharmacol* 2001;**21**:612–5).
- **Diphenhydramine** IV may rapidly (over 30 minutes) reduce the symptoms of acute NIA from IV prochlorperazine (n = 87, open, Vinson, *J Emerg Med* 2004;**26**:265–70; comment by Baden et al, *J Emerg Med* 2005;**28**:347–8).
- **Gabapentin**, where a dose-related response has been reported (n = 1, Pfeffer et al, *Int Clin Psychopharmacol* 2005;**20**:179–81).
- **Mianserin** 5 mg/d may produce a significant improvement in NIA and dysphoria (n = 15, RCT, 5/7, Poyurovsky et al, *Br J Psychiatry* 1999;**174**:238–42; n = 1, Stryjer et al, *Eur Psychiatry* 2004;**19**:237–8).
- **Mirtazapine** may be useful for NIA, probably via 5HT2A/2C antagonism (n = 26, RCT, d/b, 5/7, Poyurovsky et al, *J Clin Psychopharmacol* 2003;**23**:305–8; Wilson, *J Clin Psychopharmacol* 2005;**25**:394–5).
- **Thiamine** (vitamin B1) high-dose (1.2 g/d) may be useful for acute NIA (n = 20, RCT, p/c, d/b, 5/7, Lerner et al, *J Clin Psychiatry* 2004;**65**:1550–4).
- **Trazodone** 100 mg/d may produce a marked improvement (n = 9, 5/7, Stryjer et al, *Clin Neuropharmacol* 2003;**26**:137–41).
- **Zolmitriptan** (a selective 5HT1D inhibitor) 7.5 mg/d produced a significant and rapid improvement in NIA, even in chronic and resistant cases, warranting further trials (n = 8, open, 3/7, Gross-Isseroff et al, *Int Clin Psychopharmacol* 2005;**20**:23–5).

Less use:

Other drugs tried, usually without success, include:

- **Amantadine** (n = 4, Zubenko et al, *J Clin Psychopharmacol* 1984;**4**:218–20).
- **Apomorphine** low dose may reduce objective (movement) effects but not subjective distress (Karstaedt and Pincus, *Neurology* 1993;**43**:611–3).
- **Buspirone** has only a minor effect, with only 20% showing any effect (n = 10, Poyurovsky and Weizman, *Int Clin Psychopharmacol* 1997;**12**:263–8).
- **Granisetron** is ineffective (n = 10, 4/7, Poyurovsky and Weizman, *Int Clin Psychopharmacol* 1999;**14**:357–60).
- **Iron supplements**, via a disputed similarity with Ekbom's syndrome (Nemes et al, *Biol Psychiatry* 1991;**29**:411–3), have been proposed, although no relationship between plasma iron and chronic akathisia has been found (Barnes et al, *Br J Psychiatry* 1992;**161**:791–6).
- **Moclobemide** (n = 1, Ebert and Demling, *Pharmacopsychiatry* 1991; **24**: 29–31).
- **Tryptophan** (n = 6, open, *Biol Psychiatry* 1990;**27**:671–2).

EPSE, dyskinesias (acute or tardive)

Tardive dyskinesia (TD) is an involuntary hyperkinesia, which increases with anxiety, goes away during sleep and in some cases may be irreversible. Symptoms include choreas, tics, dystonias and orolingual dyskinesias, but not tremor. It is generally seen as repetitive, involuntary and purposeless movements of, eg. the tongue, neck and jaw. It may be a late symptom of schizophrenia and antipsychotics might in fact just bring such symptoms forward (rather than cause them), eg. brain structures are similar (n=93, McCreadie et al, Arch Gen Psychiatry 2002;**59**:332–6) and TD fluctuates with time (n=37, McCreadie et al, Br J Psychiatry 2002;**181**:135–7).

Risk factors include the length of exposure to antipsychotics in the elderly, alcohol consumption, advancing age, being male, previous head injury, presence of organic brain disease, structural brain damage, earlier drug-induced Parkinsonism, akathisia or dystonias, being non-right-handed, being diabetic, concurrent affective or negative symptoms and having a parent with schizophrenia who themselves has or had a dyskinesia.

Reviews: general (Tarsy, Curr Treat Options Neurol 2000;**2**:205–14; Sachdev, Aust N Z J Psychiatry 2000;**34**:355–69; Simpson, J Clin Psychiatry 2000;**61**[Suppl 4]:39–44), 'miscellaneous' treatments (McGrath and Soares, CDSR 2000;**2**:CD000208).

Antidepressants	**Mirtazapine** has been used for bupropion-induced TD (n=1, Kohen and Sarcevic, Movement Disord 2006;**21**:584–5).
Antipsychotics	**Withdrawal** or **dose reduction** are the usual strategies, although the risk of relapse may be high.

Drug 'holidays' seem detrimental.

Transient dose increases may help occasionally, but only in the short-term.

Withdraw or reduce any anticholinergic drugs if possible, as these can provoke or exacerbate TD, although are not a risk factor as such (Soares and McGrath, CDSR 2000;**2**:CD000204).

Switching antipsychotics:

Switching to an atypical is usually considered the main strategy, either through having a lower incidence or just being better antipsychotics. Options include:

* **Aripiprazole** (n=1, Grant and Baldessarini, Ann Pharmacother 2005;**39**:1953; Witschy and Winter, Can J Psychiatry 2005;**50**:188).

* **Clozapine** may improve TD, especially with dystonic features, eg. >50% reduction in symptoms has been seen (n=30, Lieberman et al, Br J Psychiatry 1991;**158**:503–10; see also n=7, open, Bassitt et al, Eur Arch Psychiatr Clin Neurosci 1998;**248**:209–11). It may also be effective for TD over the longer term (n=7, open, five years, Louza and Bassitt, J Clin Psychopharmacol 2005;**25**:180–2).

* **Olanzapine**, where there are several case reports of a marked reduction in pre-existing symptoms of TD (n=4, Littrell, Arch Gen Psychiatry 1998; **55**:279–80; n=2, Soutullo et al, J Clin Psychopharmacol 1999;**19**:100–1; n=2, Agarwal and Kumar, J Clin Psychiatry 2001;**62**:298–9).

* **Quetiapine**, where in a switch study, quetiapine maintained psychosis symptom control but reduced TD compared to haloperidol (n=45, RCT, 12/12, s/b, Emsley et al, J Clin Psychiatry 2004;**65**:696–701; see also n=3, Alptekin and Kivircik, Int Clin Psychopharmacol 2002;**17**:263–4). Adjunctive quetiapine has been used for risperidone-induced TD (n=1, Nelson et al, Clin Neuropharmacol 2003;**26**:297–8).

* **Risperidone**, where the response may occur in a few weeks and then be maintained (n=40, 48/52, Bai et al, Int Clin Psychopharmacol 2005;**20**:79–85; n=9, open, 52/52, Chen et al, Am J Psychiatry 2001;**158**:1931–2; n=49, RCT, d/b, p/c, 16/52, Bai et al, J Clin Psychiatry 2003;**64**:1342–8; MS; review by Tandon, EBMH 2004;**7**:83).

Adjunctive therapies:

Adjunctive therapies are usually considered to be of low efficacy, although tetrabenazine is licensed:

- **Tetrabenazine** is licensed in the UK, with a starting dose of 12.5 mg, titrated to 25–75 mg/d (maximum 200 mg/d). In refractory TD, tetrabenazine (mean 58 mg/d) has significantly improved AIMS scores over 20 weeks (n = 20, Ondo et al, Am J Psychiatry 1999;**156**:1279–81; see informal follow-up of 400 patients: n = 526, Jankovic and Beach, Neurology 1997;**48**:358–62).
- **Amantadine** was superior to placebo in one study (d/b, c/o, p/c, 18/52, Angus et al, J Clin Psychopharmacol 1997;**17**:88–91).
- **Buspirone** at up to 180 mg/d may be useful (n = 8, open, 12/52, Moss et al, J Clin Psychopharmacol 1993;**13**:204–9; n = 1, Neppe, Lancet 1989; **2**:1458).
- **Cyproheptadine** at 8–24 mg/d has significantly improved haloperidol-induced TD (n = 10, open, Lee et al, J Serotonin Res 1994;**1**:91–5).
- **Donepezil**, where a pilot study indicated that 5–10 mg/d might suppress symptoms of TD (n = 10, open, 8/52, Caroff et al, J Clin Psychiatry 2001;**62**:772–5).
- **Gabapentin** has improved long-term TD, with an average improvement of 47.5% (n = 25, open, one year, Hardoy et al, J Affect Disord 2003;**75**:125–30).
- **Levetiracetam** (mean 2300 mg/d, range 1–3 g) may significantly improve AIMS scores (n = 16 [c = 15], open, 3/12, Meco et al, Clin Neuropharmacol 2006;**29**:265–8).
- **Melatonin** 10 mg/d has been shown to decrease AIMS scores in TD (n = 22, d/b, p/c, c/o, 6/52, Shamir et al, Arch Gen Psychiatry 2001;**58**:1049–52).
- **Naltrexone** plus clonazepam have reduced TD scores compared with each drug individually (n = 23, RCT, d/b, p/c, Wonodi et al, J Clin Psychopharmacol 2004;**24**:441–5).
- **Ondansetron** (a 5-HT3 antagonist) 12 mg/d has been used successfully (n = 12, open, 12/52, Sirota et al, Am J Psychiatry 2000;**157**:287–9; although this could have been an interaction).
- **Pyridoxine** 200 mg/d has produced a rapid and sustained reduction in TD symptoms (eg. n = 1, Lerner and Liberman, J Clin Psychiatry 1998;**59**:623–4).
- **Thiamine** was effective in one small but careful study (n = 15, RCT, d/b, p/c, 4/52, Lerner et al, Am J Psychiatry 2001;**158**:1511–4).

Less useful:

Many adjunctive therapies have been tried but few have any real use. The following aren't in the useful group:

- **Baclofen**, see GABA agonists.
- **Benzodiazepines** have been used. Cochrane concludes that they have no proven advantage over placebo (McGrath and Soares, CDSR 2000;**2**:CD000205), although clonazepam may decrease some dystonic symptoms (n = 19, RCT, Thacker et al, Am J Psychiatry 1990;**147**:445–51).
- **Calcium-channel blocker** use is not supported by any robust studies (s = 0, Soares-Weiser and Rathbone, Cochrane Database Syst Rev 2004;**1**: CD000206), although older reviews were more positive (review by Cates et al, Ann Pharmacother 1993;**27**:191–6, 14 refs).
- **Cholinergic drugs** (eg. choline, lecithin, ACEIs) are probably ineffective (see systematic review; n = 261, s = 11, RCTs, Tammenmaa et al, Prog Neuropsychopharmacol Biol Psychiatry 2004;**28**:1099–107).

- **Citalopram** was ineffective in one study (n = 13, Korsgaard *et al*, *Clin Neuropharmacol* 1986;**9**:52–7).
- **GABA agonists/enhancers** such as baclofen and valproate. Cochrane concludes from the eight small, short-term studies that the evidence is inconclusive and unconvincing (Soares *et al*, *Cochrane Database Syst Rev* 2004;**4**:CD000203).
- **Insulin** (low-dose) has been suggested as superior to placebo (see McGrath and Soares, *Cochrane Database Syst Rev* 2000;**2**:CD000208).
- **Lithium** has no consistent positive effect (eg. Yassa *et al*, *Can J Psychiatry* 1984;**29**:36–7) and may even be detrimental.
- **Piracetam** has been used TD (n = 1, Fehr *et al*, *J Clin Psychopharmacol* 2001;**21**:248–9).
- **Valproate**, see GABA agonists.
- **Vitamin E** probably has no significant effect (up to 1600 iu/d; n = 40, RCT, 20/52, Dorevitch *et al*, *Biol Psychiatry* 1997;**41**:114; n = 158, RCT, up to two years, Adler *et al*, *Arch Gen Psychiatry* 1999;**56**:836–41; Soares and McGrath, *CDSR* 2000;**2**:CD000209) but may perhaps be effective in a small subgroup of patients (18-trial review, Boomershine *et al*, *Ann Pharmacother* 1999;**33**:1195–202).

EPSE, Parkinsonism

Pseudoparkinsonism or Parkinsonian side-effects include akinesia, rigidity, bradykinesia and coarse tremor at rest. They are usually associated with antipsychotics but can occur with many drugs (see *Chapter 5.8*).

Antidepressants, (especially tricyclics)	**Switch drugs** or treat as per antipsychotics is the best plan. **Benzodiazepines**, eg. diazepam (mentioned in Pollack and Rosenbaum, *J Clin Psychiatry* 1987;**48**:3–8). **Propranolol** 40–120 mg/d has been used (mentioned in Pollack and Rosenbaum, *J Clin Psychiatry* 1987;**48**:3–8). **Review:** Gill *et al*, *J Clin Psychopharmacol* 1997;**17**:377–89.
Antipsychotics	**Dose reduction** of any antipsychotic, or switch to an antipsychotic with lower EPS, eg. quetiapine, olanzapine, sertindole or aripiprazole. **Anticholinergics** (antimuscarinics) are first-line treatments. They include **benzatropine** (also has antihistaminic properties and a long half-life of up to 24 hours), **orphenadrine** (but overdose is associated with greater death rates than with other anticholinergics, and also of overuse [Slørdal and Gjerden, *Br J Psychiatry* 1999;**174**:275–6]), **procyclidine** (with a disputed abuse potential) and **trihexyphenidyl** (benzhexol; with a reported abuse and dependence potential; Frauger *et al*, *Therapie* 2003;**58**:541–7). They may improve survival (n = 88, 10-year prospective study, Waddington *et al*, *Br J Psychiatry* 1998;**173**:325–9) and compliance. Although they have had a bad press, they may actually only be detrimental to positive symptoms during acute phases (when excess dopaminergic activity is thought to occur) but not during stable phases (Tandon and Dequardo, *Am J Psychiatry* 1995;**152**:814–5). Anticholinergics may adversely effect memory, exacerbate TD, and abrupt withdrawal can produce rebound EPS, cholinergic rebound, myalgia, depression, anxiety, insomnia, headaches, g/i distress, vomiting, nightmares and malaise. They are best prescribed only for overt symptoms and discontinued gradually after three months, reinstated only if symptoms reappear. If, however, they aid long-term compliance then that may be a benefit that outweighs the risks.

Reviews: managing antipsychotic-induced parkinsonism (Mamo *et al*, *Drug Saf* 1999;**20**:269–75, 49 refs; Holloman and Marder, *Am J HealthSys Pharm* 1997;**54**:2461–77).

Adjunctive therapies:

- **Diphenhydramine** 25–300 mg (oral or parenteral) may rapidly be effective (within minutes) and maintenance doses of 25–50 mg TDS have been widely used (n = 5, RCT, Granana *et al*, *Medicina (B Aires)* 1999;**59**:38–42).
- **Donepezil** may have some use in treating EPSE in the elderly (n = 7, open, Bergman *et al*, *J Clin Psychiatry* 2005;**66**:107–10).
- **Estrogen** at high plasma levels has been reported to reduce hyperkinetic symptoms of EPSE in women with psychosis (n = 25, RCT, Thompson *et al*, *Acta Psychiatr Scand* 2000;**101**:130–4).
- **Iron supplementation** may help EPSE if associated with iron-deficient anaemia (n = 1, Yoshida *et al*, *Nihon Shinkei Seishin Yakurigaku Zasshi* 2004;**24**:29–31).
- **Kava special extract** WS1490 has been claimed to significantly improve EPSE (n = 42, open, Boerner and Klement, *Wien Med Wochenschr* 2004;**154**:508–10).
- **Zolpidem** 5 mg QDS has been used successfully to treat persistent and unresponsive EPSE (n = 1, Farver and Khan, *Ann Pharmacother* 2001;**35**:435–7).

Less use:

Some drugs that have been tried but failed include:

- **Amantadine** is not recommended for EPSE but may be effective (d/b, c/o, Silver *et al*, *J Clin Psychiatry* 1995;**56**:167–70) and better tolerated than anticholinergics in elderly patients (review by Mamo *et al*, *Drug Saf* 1999;**20**:269–75).
- **Calcium** orally.
- **Mianserin** is ineffective (Korsgaard and Friis, *Psychopharmacol (Berl)* 1986;**88**:109–11).
- **Quinine**.

EPSE, dystonia

Dystonia is a syndrome of sustained or slow involuntary muscular contractions, resulting in twisting of the neck, limbs, trunk or face. Acute dystonia from antipsychotics is more likely to occur in younger and more severely ill people, especially if antipsychotic-naïve. It can present as an oculogyric crisis (review by Abe, *World J Biol Psychiatry* 2006;**7**:70–4).

Reviews: * general (Adityanjee *et al*, *Biol Psychiatry* 1999;**45**:715–30; Balash and Giladi, *Eur J Neurol* 2004;**11**:361–70).

Antidepressants	**Switching drugs** is the main strategy.

Switching drugs is the main strategy.

Epinephrine 0.3 mg has been used for escitalopram-induced oculogyric dystonia (n = 1, Patel and Simon, *Int Arch Allergy Immunol* 2006;**140**:27–9).

Mianserin has been used at low dose for fluoxetine-induced dystonia (Poyurovsky *et al*, *Mov Disord* 1997;**12**:1102–5).

Antipsychotics

Acute dystonia:

- **Anticholinergics** are usually effective for acute dystonias (eg. laryngeal dystonia: Christodoulou and Kalaitzi, *J Psychopharmacol* 2005;**19**:307–11) and **procyclidine** is the standard UK treatment.
- **Diphenhydramine** (oral or parenteral) can be used and has been reported to produce rapid reversal of dystonic reactions, eg. oculogyric crisis (Leigh *et al*, *Ann Neurol* 1987;**22**:3–17).

Tardive dystonia:

Switching antipsychotic, usually to an atypical, is the first choice strategy:

- **Clozapine** may improve severe and persistent TD (n = 1, *J Nerv Ment Dis* 1993;**181**:137–8; n = 1, Sieche and Giedke, *J Clin Psychiatry* 2000;**61**:949).
- **Olanzapine** may have some role in improving TD (n = 4, s/b, Lucetti *et al*, *Clin Neuropharmacol* 2002;**25**:71–4; n = 1, 7/12, Jaffe and Simpson, *Am J Psychiatry* 1999;**156**:2016).
- **Quetiapine** has been used if TD is induced by risperidone, olanzapine (n = 2, Gourzis *et al*, *Clin Neuropharmacol* 2005;**28**:195–6; n = 1, Sasaki *et al*, *J Clin Psychiatry* 2004;**65**:583–4) or amisulpride (n = 1, Fountoulakis *et al*, *Schizophr Res* 2006;**88**:232–4).

Others:

In resistant cases, other strategies may be worth trying:

- **Benzodiazepines** — a multiple drug-resistant disabling TD responded partly to clozapine and virtually completely when clonazepam was added (n = 1, Shapleske *et al*, *Br J Psychiatry* 1996;**168**:516–8).
- **Botulinum toxin** may possibly relieve the pain and symptoms of TD (n = 34, open, Tarsy *et al*, *Clin Neuropharmacol* 1997;**20**:90–3).
- **Levodopa** combined with an anticholinergic has been used (n = 1, Looper and Chouinard, *Can J Psychiatry* 1998;**43**:646–7).
- **Levetiracetam** has helped generalised dystonia (n = 1, 20/52, Sullivan *et al*, *Parkinsonism Relat Disord* 2005;**11**:469–71).

Less useful:

- **Anticholinergics** are less effective in chronic dystonia (eg. n = 32, Wojcik *et al*, *Am J Psychiatry* 1991;**148**:1055–9).
- **Carbamazepine** is ineffective (*Psychopharmacol Bull* 1985;**21**;345–6).

Other drugs tried include baclofen, bromocriptine and tetrabenazine.

Myoclonus

- Myoclonus presents as shock-like, involuntary movements. It can also be caused by CNS infections, systematic metabolic disorders or neurodegenerative disorders.
- **Discontinuation, switching** or **dose reduction** usually resolves myoclonus.
- It can be a symptom of serotonin syndrome and akathisia, so exclude these first.
- **Discontinue** any other causative drugs, eg. levodopa, tricyclics, lamotrigine (n = 1, Rosenhagen *et al*, *J Clin Psychopharmacol* 2006;**26**:346–7) and bismuth salts (including OTC products).

Review: Jimenez-Jimenez, *CNS Drugs* 2004;**18**:93–104.

Other strategies:

Antidepressants	**Valproate**, if sertraline-induced (n = 1, Ghaziuddin *et al*, *J Child Adolesc Psychopharmacol* 2001;**11**:199–202).
Antipsychotics	**Carbamazepine**, if clozapine-induced, but beware of potential interaction (n = 5, Bak *et al*, *J Clin Psychiatry* 1995;**56**:418–22)
	Valproate, if clozapine-induced (n = 1, Meltzer and Ranjan, *Am J Psychiatry* 1994;**151**:1246–7).
	Haloperidol may be an alternative if olanzapine-induced (n = 1, Camacho *et al*, *Clin Neuropharmacol* 2005;**28**:145–7).

Restless legs (may also be akathisia)

Antidepressants	Although there are anecdotal reports, there is not a clear association between antidepressants and restless legs (n = 200, Brown *et al*, *Sleep Med* 2005;**6**:443–50).
	Re-exposure may be without recurrence with mirtazapine (n = 1, Pae *et al*, *Psychiatr Clin Neurosci* 2004;**58**:669–70).
	Exclude other drugs, eg. D2 receptor antagonists such as domperidone (n = 1,

Chang et al, Prog Neuropsychopharmacol Biol Psychiatry 2006;**30**:316–8).
Bupropion may be a therapy in its own right (n = 3, Kim et al, Clin
Neuropharmacol 2005;**28**:298–301).

Antipsychotics	**Benzodiazepines, eg. clonazepam** have been used (n = 1, Horiguchi et al, Int Clin Psychopharmacol 1999;**14**:33–6).

Tremor (see Others)

Bruxism (teeth grinding)

Bruxism is defined as grinding, clenching and forceful teeth or jaw movements, usually during sleep.
Almost everyone bruxes, and bruxism is where it is severe enough to cause damage or distress.
General review: (Lobbezoo et al, J Oral Rehabil 2006;**33**:293–300).

Antidepressants	**Dose reduction** usually leads to resolution (n = 4, Ellison and Stanziani, J Clin Psychiatry 1993;**54**:432–4).
	Buspirone has been used if bruxism is induced by venlafaxine (40mg/d, significantly effective over 4/52: Pavlovic, Int J Neuropsychopharmacol 2004;**7**:523–4; Jaffee and Bostwick, Psychosomatics 2000;**41**:535–6) or SSRIs (n = 4, Bostwick and Jaffee, J Clin Psychiatry 1999;**60**:857–60).
	Gabapentin, if venlafaxine-induced (n = 1, Brown and Hong, J Am Dent Assoc 1999;**130**:1467–9).
	ECT, if fluvoxamine-induced (n = 1, Miyaoka et al, J ECT 2003;**19**:170–2).
Antipsychotics	**Dose reduction** usually leads to resolution.
	Propranolol (case where concurrent akathisia also improved; n = 2, Amir et al, Clin Neuropharmacol 1997;**20**:86–9).

6.6 Neuroleptic malignant syndrome (NMS)

NMS is a rare and potentially fatal idiosyncratic dose-independent ADR resulting in a sudden loss
in control of body temperature. The main symptoms are hyperthermia or fever and severe muscle
rigidity, with two or more of: diaphoresis, dysphagia, tremor, incontinence, altered consciousness,
tachycardia, altered blood pressure, leucocytosis and raised creatinine phosphokinase concentration.
Body temperature rises rapidly and can be fatal in 1–3 days, although death rates are reducing
due to increased awareness, early intervention, and the use of atypicals (n = 68, Ananth et al, J Clin
Psychiatry 2004;**65**:464–70). It is probably caused by a sudden over-blockade of dopaminergic
function, resulting in a disruption to the thermoregulatory centre.

Risk factors include:

* **History** (previous NMS, known cerebral compromise, previous ECT).
* **Mental state** (agitation, overactive and/or in need of restraint or seclusion, catatonia, affective
  disorder [Berardi et al, Hum Psychopharmacol 2002;**17**:99–102], mental retardation).
* **Physical state** (dehydration, postpartum, Parkinson's disease, young and male, high serum
  creatinine phosphokinase [n = 32, Hermesh et al, J Clin Psychopharmacol 2002;**22**:252–6]).
* **Drugs** (see Chapter 5.9, eg. high potency antipsychotics, IM therapy, high doses over short periods,
  abrupt or recent changes, rapid neuroleptisation, and concurrent MAOIs and carbamazepine).

Neuroleptic re-challenge:

Rechallenge with antipsychotics may show a high rate of recurrence, although the majority may
be able to tolerate antipsychotics again if monitored carefully and a two-week recovery period is
allowed (n = 15, Rosebush et al, J Clin Psychiatry 1989;**50**:295–8). Rechallenge with clozapine has been
successful (Weller and Kornhuber, Br J Psychiatry 1992;**161**:855–6). Depots are contraindicated.
Reviews: risk factors (Gupta et al, Int J Psychiatry 2003;**45**:30–5; n = 20, Berardi et al, Hum
Psychopharmacol 2002;**17**:99–102; n = 15, controls n = 45, Viejo et al, Acta Psychiatr Scand
2003;**107**:45–9), general (Prescriber 2006;**17**:18–23; Khan and Farver, SDJ Med 2000;**53**:395–400;
Andreassen and Pedersen, Ugeskr Laeger 2000;**162**:1366–70; McDonough et al, Ir Med J
2000;**93**:152–4).

Antipsychotics

Immediate management is essential.

Withdraw any antipsychotics, lithium and antidepressants.

Correct any dehydration and hyperpyrexia, eg. using ice packs, re-hydration and sedation with benzodiazepines if necessary.

Measure WCC, U&E, LFT and CPK to assess diagnosis, cause and response. Manage acute symptoms, initially using a first-line agent below:

First line strategies:

- **Dantrolene** IV (a skeletal muscle relaxant used for malignant hyperthermia) is usually the treatment of choice. It reduces the duration and mortality of NMS (n = 9, Nisijima and Ishiguro, *Biol Psychiatry* 1993;**33**:45–8) and reduces body temperature in 2–24 hours. There are some views that it might prolong the course of symptoms compared to supportive therapy (Rosebush *et al*, *Br J Psychiatry* 1991;**148**:709–12).
- **Bromocriptine** 7.5–60 mg/d reduces the duration and mortality of NMS (Sakkas *et al*, *Psychopharmacol Bull* 1991;**27**:381–4). There are some views that it might prolong the course of symptoms compared to supportive therapy (Rosebush *et al*, *Br J Psychiatry* 1991;**148**:709–12).
- **Amantadine** 100 mg BD may be the third-line choice (mentioned by Waldorf, *AANA J* 2003;**71**:389–94).

Other strategies:

- **Anaesthetics** have been used for emergency treatment in a person recovering from NMS (Parke and Wheatley, *Anesthesia* 1992;**47**:908–9).
- **Anticoagulants** used to provide complete anticoagulation have been suggested as adjunctive therapy to reduce death as a result of pulmonary embolism (van Harten and van Agtmael, *Am J Psychiatry* 1995;**152**:1103).
- **Apomorphine** s/c 2 mg three-hourly for three days then 2 mg QD for two days can improve NMS significantly (n = 1, Lattanzi *et al*, *Am J Psychiatry* 2006;**163**:1450–1) and as rapidly as monotherapy (n = 1, Wang and Hsieh, *Mov Disord* 2001;**16**:765–7; n = 1, Gambassi *et al*, *Aging Clin Exp Res* 2006;**18**:266–70).
- **Benzodiazepines** (IV lorazepam or diazepam) can be been used if dantrolene and bromocriptine have failed. Predominantly catatonic symptoms may rapidly respond to diazepam, including via continuous IV administration (Miyaoka *et al*, *Am J Psychiatry* 1997;**153**:882), although its longer half-life may complicate recovery (Velamoor, *Br J Psychiatry* 1992;**160**:135–6).
- **ECT** has been used for low-dose quetiapine-induced NMS (n = 1, Bora *et al*, *Eur Psychiatry* 2003;**18**:323).
- **Levodopa** IV may be an effective alternative to dantrolene (Nisijima *et al*, *Biol Psychiatry* 1997;**41**:913–4), as may carbidopa/levodopa (Shoop and Cernek, *Ann Pharmacother* 1997;**31**:119).
- **Nifedipine** 25 mg s/l has been used (Talley and Taylor, *Psychosomatics* 1994;**35**:168–70).

Aftercare:

1. Review NMS symptoms to confirm diagnosis.
2. Review psychiatric diagnosis and the need for further antipsychotics.
3. Consider alternative management strategies.
4. Leave as long a gap as possible before restarting antipsychotics (eg. 14 days), considering also the risks of untreated psychosis.
5. Choose an antipsychotic from a different group to the causative agent, particularly of low potency or any previously used without problem. Start low and go slow. Contraindicate depots.

6. Perform alternate day CPK monitoring, interpreted in the context of the global clinical picture.
7. Perform daily temperature, pulse and muscle tone measures, weekly wbcs and ensure adequate hydration and nutrition.
8. Obtain an informal or formal second opinion, as informed consent for re-exposure may not be possible. Inform family and carers of the decisions and risks (and document this).
9. Educate patients, carers and care team of the symptoms of early NMS and of the appropriate action to take, ie. seek urgent medical advice.
Review: guidelines for the re-introduction of antipsychotics following NMS (Williams and MacPherson, *Irish J Psychiatr Med* 1997;**14**:147–8).

6.7 Serotonin syndrome

This potentially dangerous adverse reaction is attributed to a toxic hyperserotonergic state from hyperstimulation of the brain stem and spinal chord 5HT1A and 5HT2 receptors. Onset is usually within a few hours of drug or dose changes and usually resolves in about 24 hours. Deaths have been reported.

Sternbach's diagnostic criteria

1. At least three of the following: mental state changes (eg. confusion), agitation/restlessness, sweating, diarrhoea, fever, hyperreflexia, tachycardia, myoclonus, lack of co-ordination, shivering, and tremor. Other symptoms can include nausea, vomiting, tachycardia, myoclonus, hypertension, convulsions and multiple organ failure.
2. Other causes ruled out, eg. infection, metabolic disturbances, substance abuse or withdrawal.
3. No concurrent antipsychotic dose changes.

Reviews: general (Boyer and Shannon, *N Engl J Med* 2005;**352**:1112–20; Gillman, *Biol Psychiatry* 2006;**59**:1046–51; Mason *et al, Medicine* [Baltimore] 2000;**79**:201–9), Serotonin Syndrome Rating Scale to aid diagnosis (Hegerl *et al, Eur Arch Psych Clin Neurosci* 1998;**248**:96–103).

All drugs	**Discontinue** all serotonergic drugs (see *Chapter 5.14*), including over-the-counter sympathomimetics (usually adequate management in mild cases).
	Symptomatic support, eg. cooling blankets and fans.
	Benzodiazepines, eg. lorazepam (1–2 mg by slow IV injection every 30 minutes until excessive sedation occurs) can be used and may be superior to clonazepam, which has a lower affinity for peripheral benzodiazepine receptors (eg. Nierenberg and Semprebon, *Clin Pharmacol Ther* 1993;**53**:84–8).
	Chlorpromazine has been used for its sedative effect (n = 1, Graham, *Med J Aust* 1997;**166**:166–7).
	Cyproheptadine (a non-specific 5-HT blocker) at 4–8 mg orally (but perhaps as high as 10–20 mg), repeated every 2–4 hours up to 0.5 mg/kg/d maximum (beware of urinary retention) has been claimed to be the best antiserotonergic drug strategy, with case reports of rapid success (Lappin and Auchincloss, *N Engl J Med* 1994;**331**:1021–2; n = 3, McDaniel, *Ann Pharmaother* 2001;**35**:870–3; Baigel, *Eur J Anaesthiol* 2003;**20**:586–8).
	Mirtazapine blocks 5-HT2 and 5-HT3 receptors and may reduce serotonergic toxicity (Hoes, *Pharmacopsychiatry* 1996;**29**:81).
	Nitroglycerin (2 mg/kg/min) has been reported to be rapidly successful in severe SS (n = 1, Brown and Skop, *Ann Pharmacother* 1996;**30**:191).
	Propranolol (1–3 mg every five minutes, up to 0.1 mg/kg) may be useful, as it blocks 5-HT1A and 5-HT2 receptors (Guze and Baxter, *J Clin Psychopharmacol* 1986;**6**:119–20).

6.8 Sexual side-effects

General
The main stages of sexual activity that can be affected by psychotropics (as well as, of course, the conditions they may be treating) are libido, arousal/lubrication, erectile issues and orgasmic disorders. Many studies do not differentiate between these stages and refer to 'sexual dysfunction'. This initial section includes general advice and stage-specific strategies.

Review: female sexual dysfunction (Clayton, *J Clin Psychiatry* 2006;**67**:991–2).

General sexual dysfunction

Anticonvulsants	**Switching drugs**: lamotrigine improves sexual function, testosterone levels and gonadal efficiency compared to carbamazepine and phenytoin (n=85, Herzog *et al*, *Neurology* 2005;**65**:1016–20). It improves most measures of sexual function, especially in women, including people both starting on lamotrigine as a first anticonvulsant (n=79) and those switching (n=62) onto it (n=141, open, 8/12, Gil-Nagel *et al*, *Seizure* 2006;**15**:142–9). **Exogenous testosterone and aromatase inhibitors** (to reduce testosterone's metabolism) have been used experimentally for male sexual dysfunction. **Reviews:** general (Stimmel and Gutierrez, *CNS Spectr* 2006;**11**[8 Suppl 9]:31–7; Montouris *et al*, *Epilepsy Behav* 2005;**7** Suppl 2:S7–14; Penovich, *Epilepsia* 2000;**41** Suppl 2:S53–61).
Antidepressants	**General interventions** include behavioural strategies, psychotherapy, delaying drug intake until after sexual activity, reduction in dosage, drug holidays, adjuvants and switching. Sexual side-effects from SSRIs do not seem to abate with time (n=119, Landén *et al*, *J Clin Psychiatry* 2005;**66**:100–6). *Switch drugs:* Switching antidepressants is often the main strategy, including:

- **Bupropion** has placebo-level sexual ADRs (s=7, n=1463, RCT, d/b, Thase *et al*, *J Clin Psychiatry* 2005;**66**:974–81; n=11 [c=6], open, 8/52, Clayton *et al*, *J Clin Psychiatry* 2001;**62**:185–90), but is probably not effective as an adjunct in SSRI-induced sexual dysfunction (n=41, RCT, p/c, 6/52, DeBattista *et al*, *J Clin Psychiatry* 2005;**66**:844–8).
- **Escitalopram** has been claimed to have less sexual ADRs than similar antidepressants (Ashton *et al*, *J Sex Marital Ther* 2005;**31**:257–62).
- **Mirtazapine** has lower sexual ADRs than other antidepressants, apart from the potentilly counter-productive sedation (n=78, open, 6/12, Saiz-Ruiz *et al*, *Hum Psychopharmacol* 2005;**20**:435–40; n=102, open, 6/12, Osvath *et al*, *Neuropsychopharmacol Hung* 2005;**7**:177–86; n=19, open, 6/52, Gelenberg *et al*, *J Clin Psychiatry* 2000;**61**:356–60).
- **Moclobemide** may have lower sexual ADRs (n=5, open, Ramasubbu, *J Psychiatr Neurosci* 1999;**224**:45–50)
- **Reboxetine**, which lacks serotonin-related sexual ADRs (n=450, RCT, d/b, 8/52, Clayton *et al*, *Int Clin Psychopharmacol* 2003;**18**:151–6).

Adjunctive therapies:
- **Ephedrine** 50mg has been effective for SSRI-induced sexual dysfunction, but in this study placebo also improved all measures of sexual function (n=19 women, RCT, p/c, c/o, 8/52, Meston, *J Sex Marital Ther* 2004;**30**:57–68)
- **Gingko biloba** (some spectacular individual responses have been noted but no statistically significant differences; n=24 [c=11], RCT, t/b, p/c, 12/52, Wheatley, *Hum Psychopharmacol* 2004;**19**:545–8).

- **Ropinirole** up to 2–4mg/d was effective in 54% using ASES (n=13[3F, 10M], open, 4/52, Worthington et al, Int Clin Psychopharmacol 2002; 17:307–10).

No efficacy:

- **Granisetron** (n=12, RCT, d/b, p/c, 14/7, Jespersen et al, Int Clin Psychopharmacol 2004;19:161–4).

Reviews: managing antidepressant-induced sexual dysfunction (Gregorian et al, Ann Pharmacother 2002;36:1577–89; Taylor, Curr Psychiatry Rep 2006;8:431–6; Rudkin et al, Cochrane Database Syst Rev 2004;4:CD003382; Baldwin, Expert Opin Drug Saf 2004;3:457–70; Woodrum and Brown, Ann Pharmacother 1998;32:1209–15; Worthington and Peters, Drugs Today (Barc) 2003;39:887–96; Tayor et al, J Affect Disord 2005;88:241–54).

Antipsychotics Sexual dysfunction occurs at higher rates in schizophrenia (86–96%) than in the general population (n=98+81 controls, MacDonald et al, Br J Psychiatry 2003;182:50–6), and 40–60% feel that psychotropics cause their sexual problems. 42% men and 15% women admit that they had stopped their medication at some point due to this side-effect (n=51, Rosenberg et al, J Sex Marital Ther 2003;29:289–96). Sexual dysfunction may occur in 45% people on typicals, with hyperprolactinaemia being the predominant cause (n=101, Smith et al, Br J Psychiatry 2002;181:49–55).

General principles:

Normalise prolactin, eg. by switching to an atypical such as olanzapine (Ahl et al, Ann N Y Acad Sci 2004;1032:289–90) or quetiapine (cf risperidone and fluphenazine; n=27, RCT, d/b, Kelly and Conley, Psychoneuroendocrinology 2006;31:340–6).

Reviews: in men (Khawaja, J Ayub Med Coll Abbottabad 2005;17:73–5) and in women (Smith, J Clin Psychopharmacol 2003;23[3 Suppl 1]:S27–32).

Libido (see also introduction above)

Libido and desire is controlled by the mesolimbic dopamine reward pathway and facilitated by NA and 5-HT. Testosterone is essential for male, and estrogen and progesterone for female sexual behaviour. It is unclear to what extent psychotropics effect libido specifically.

Antidepressants **Switch drugs** to, eg. **moclobemide** (n=5, open, Ramasubbu, J Psychiatr Neurosci 1999;224:45–50), **bupropion** or **mirtazapine**.

Antipsychotics **Raised prolactin** may be the predominant effect, so check and, if raised, see the hyperprolactinaemia section for options.

Arousal (lubrication and erection)

Arousal mechanisms involve acetylcholine (facilitates erection/lubrication), adrenergic fibres (cause detumescence), cAMP (smooth muscle relaxation), dopamine (stimulates sexual arousal in females) and nitric oxide (activates the production of cGMP).

Review: options for oral pharmacotherapy in ED (Vitezic and Pelcic, Int J Clin Pharmacol Ther 2002; 40;393–403).

Antidepressants **Switching drugs** is the main strategy, eg. to:

- **Bupropion** (n=18 ethnic minority women, open, 10/52, Dobkin et al, J Clin Psychopharmacol 2006;26:21–6).
- **Moclobemide** (n=5, open, Ramasubbu, J Psychiatr Neurosci 1999;224: 45–50).
- **Mirtazapine**.

Adjunctive therapies:

- **Sildenafil** and similar drugs are effective for drug-induced erectile dysfunction (s=15, n=904, Taylor et al, J Affect Disord 2005;88:241–54), including men with ED at the time of diagnosis of MDD that then persists, despite the resolution of the depressive symptoms (RCT, 12/52, Tignol et al, *Int Clin Psychopharmacol* 2004;**19**:191–9).

- **Pentoxifylline** may improve ED caused by borderline arterial insufficiency (n = 36, Peskircioglu et al, *Br J Urol* 1996;**77**:563–5).
- **Yohimbine** given 1–2 hours pre-intercourse has been shown to improve antidepressant-induced ED (review by Labbate et al, *J Clin Psychiatry* 2003; **64**[Suppl 10]:11–9).

| Antipsychotics | **Switching drugs** is the main strategy, eg. to: |

Switching drugs is the main strategy, eg. to:

- **Quetiapine** (n = 28) may improve erectile function and lubrication compared to other antipsychotics (n = 86, 6/12, open, Montejo-Gonzalez et al, *J Clin Psychopharmacol* 2005;**25**:533–8; n = 8, open, Byerly et al, *J Sex Marital Ther* 2004;**30**:325–32).
- **Olanzapine**, if haloperidol-induced (n = 1, Tsai and Hong, *Gen Hosp Psychiatry* 2000;**20**:391–2; n = 570, Bitter et al, *Int Clin Psychopharmacol* 2005;**20**:19–21; part of SOHO study).

Adjunctive therapies:

- **Amantadine** 100 mg/d may help (n = 6, open, 6/52, Valevski et al, *Clin Neuropharmacol* 1998;**21**:355–7).
- **Sildenafil/tadalafil** can be effective if ED is induced by olanzapine (n = 10, 4/52, Atmaca et al, *Int J Impot Res* 2002;**14**:547–9) or risperidone (n = 32 [c = 31], RCT, d/b, p/c, c/o, Gopalakrishnan et al, *Am J Psychiatry* 2006;**163**:494–9; n = 12, open, Aviv et al, *J Clin Psychiatry* 2004;**65**:97–103).

| Carbamazepine | **Oxcarbazepine**, switch to (n = 4, Sachdeo and Sathyan, *Curr Med Res Opin* 2005;**21**:1065–8). |

Anorgasmia (see also introduction above)

Noradrenaline exerts an excitatory or facilitatory action on orgasm. Serotonin 5HT2A receptor agonism is inhibitory on orgasm.

Antidepressants — Anorgasmia from antidepressants is a common phenomenon. A minor effect can be advantageous in some men (by delaying ejaculation), but almost invariably considered disadvantageous in women.

Dose adjustment:

- reduce dose
- omit selected doses (eg. at weekends)
- use a single daily dose, eg. one taken at night will give trough levels the next evening, useful if that is when sexual activity occurs
- partial drug holiday (ie. missing specific days, although as David Baldwin once said, you'd need a sabbatical for fluoxetine, due to its long half-life).

Wait for spontaneous resolution (occurs in less than a third).

Withdraw drug — problem seems rapidly reversible on drug withdrawal.

Switch drugs:

Switching drugs may often be the main choice, but frequently a major problem if the patient has responded to the causative agent:

- **Bupropion** (probably fairly useful as it has a low serotoninergic effects). Switching to bupropion SR may be successful for escitalopram-induced anorgasmia (n = 830, s = 2, RCT, d/b, p/c, 8/52, Clayton et al, *J Clin Psychiatry* 2006;**67**:736–46).
- **Duloxetine** is alleged to have a lower anorgasmic effect (s = 4, RCT, d/b, p/c, n = 1466, Delgado et al, *J Clin Psychiatry* 2005;**66**:686–92).
- **Escitalopram** (better than paroxetine: Bielski et al, *Ann Clin Psychiatry* 2005;**17**:65–9).

- **Mirtazapine** (placebo-level effects on orgasmic capacity, probably because although it increases serotonin, it blocks the anorgasmic effect on 5HT2A receptors).
- **Trazodone** (if you can stay awake long enough) and 150–200 mg/d may help men with psychogenic ED (s = 6, n = 396 men, RCTs, > 1/52, Fink *et al*, *BJU Int* 2003;**92**:441–6) although another study found no effect, either positive or negative (n = 34, RCT, p/c,4/52, Enzlin *et al*, *Int J Impot Res* 2000;**12**:223–8).
- **Venlafaxine** 75 mg daily had no effect on premature ejaculation and therefore might be better than an SSRI at not causing it (n = 31, p/c, s/b, c/o, Kilic *et al*, *Int J Androl* 2005;**28**:47–52).

Adjunctive therapies:

Many adjunctive therapies have been tried and may work for some individuals. These are purely in alphabetical order as there is no robust way of assessing their relative efficacies:

- **Bethanechol** taken 1–2 hours prior to intercourse has been claimed to relieve tricyclic-induced anorgasmia, but may only occasionally be successful.
- **Bupropion** was effective in 46% of women and 75% of men, most improvement occurring in the first two weeks (open, n = 24, 7/52, Gitlin *et al*, *J Sex Marital Ther* 2002;**28**:131–8), but an RCT failed to show an effect in SSRI-induced anorgasmia (n = 30, RCT, p/c, Masand *et al*, *Am J Psychiatry* 2001;**158**:805–7).
- **Buspirone**: 58% patients taking an SSRI who reported sexual problems improved on buspirone 20–60 mg/d, whereas only 30% improved on placebo (n = 117, p/c, > 4/52, Landen *et al*, *J Clin Psychopharmacol* 1999;**19**:268–71).
- **Cyproheptadine** 2–4 mg 30–60 minutes before sex (provided one can then stay awake) may help if SSRI-induced, although relapse of depression has been reported (see *4.3.2.2*). Citalopram-induced anorgasmia has been treated with cyproheptadine 4 mg (but not 2 mg) the day before intercourse, this being referred to by the male patient as 'the catapult pills' (Lauerma, *Acta Psychiatr Scand* 1996;**93**:69–70), as has fluvoxamine (n = 1, Arnott and Nutt, *Br J Psychiatry* 1994;**164**:838–9) and MAOI-induced anorgasmia (Decastro, *Am J Psychiatry* 1985;**142**:783).
- **Dronabinol**, a synthetic cannabinol, one hour before sex has increased libido, arousal, lubrication, orgasm and overall quality, but beware of patients wandering around with a grin on their faces in case they get drug-tested (n = 1, Salerian, *J Clin Psychiatry* 2004;**665**:1146–7).
- **Loratadine** 15 mg/d may rapidly reverse SSRI-induced anorgasmia in men and women (n = 10, case series, Brubaker, *J Clin Psychiatry* 2002;**63**:534).
- **Methylphenidate** (Roeloffs *et al*, *J Clin Psychiatry* 1996;**57**:548) and dextroamfetamine (15–20 mg/d) have been used successfully for SSRI-induced anorgasmia (n = 5, Bartlik, *J Sex Marital Ther* 1995;**21**:264–71).
- **Mianserin** 7.5–15 mg/d as add-on to SSRI for SSRI 'sexual dysfunction' may be successful in 65% within 1–2 weeks, with no adverse effects (n = 16, open, 3/52, Aizenberg *et al*, *Clin Neuropharmacol* 1999;**22**:347–50; n = 11, open, Koutouvidis *et al*, *Int Clin Psychopharmacol* 1999;**14**:253–5; n = 17, open, 3/12, Dolberg *et al*, *Psychopharmacol* [Berl] 2002;**161**:404–7; n = 15 male, open, 4/52, Aizenberg *et al*, *Clin Neuropharmacol* 1997;**20**:210–4) although the only RCT showed no significant difference in women (n = 75, RCT, d/b, p/c, 4/52, Michelson *et al*, *J Psychiatr Res* 2002;**36**:147–52).

- **Mirtazapine** improved function in premenopausal females with SSRI-induced sexual side-effects (n=148, RCT, p/c, 6/52, Michelson et al, J Psychiatr Res 2002;**36**:147–52). Stimulation of the 5HT2A receptor inhibits orgasm, but mirtazapine blocks 5HT2A receptors, reversing the anorgasmic effect, and this may happen at relatively low doses, eg. 7.5–15mg/d.
- **PDE-5** inhibitors such as sildenafil 50–100mg, 30–60 minutes pre-sex may help SSRI-induced anorgasmia in men (n=90, RCT, p/c, 6/52, Nurnberg et al, JAMA 2003;**289**:56–64; n=98, d/b, p/c, Nurnburg et al, Am J Psychiatry 2001;**158**:1926–8) and in women (n=1, Shen et al, J Reprod Med 1999;**44**:535–42), but high doses may be needed (150–200mg/d) to overcome the problem (n=21, open Seidman et al, J Clin Psychiatry 2003;**64**:721–5).
- **Yohimbine** 5.4–10.8mg has been used if SSRI-induced and a retrospective chart review and survey showed it to be more effective than amantadine and cyproheptadine (n=596, Keller Ashton et al, J Sex Marital Ther 1997;**23**:165–75), although it was no better than placebo in the main RCT (n=148, RCT, p/c, 6/52, Michelson et al, J Psychiatr Res 2002;**36**:147–52). Yohimbine can cause insomnia, so rolling over and going to sleep afterwards may be trickier.

Less useful:
- **Amantadine** 200–300mg/d was ineffective in the main study (n=57, RCT, p/c, 8/52, Michelson et al, Am J Psychiatry 2000;**157**:239–43), but there are cases of use in SSRI-induced anorgasmia (n=596, Keller Ashton et al, J Sex Marital Ther 1997;**23**:165–75).
- **Ginkgo biloba** has failed to show any significant reversal of SSRI-induced sexual dysfunction (n=37, RCT, p/c, 2/12, Kang et al, Hum Psychopharmacol 2002;**17**:279–84).
- **Granisitron** (5-HT3 antagonist) has been used to treat fluoxetine-induced anorgasmia, but 1–2mg was ineffective in one study, although a significant placebo response was noted (n=20, p/c, c/o, Nelson et al, J Clin Psychiatry 2001;**62**:469–73).

Antipsychotics

Switch drugs:
- **Quetiapine** has a lower incidence of problems than risperidone and fluphenazine (n=27, RCT, d/b, Kelly and Conley, Psychoneuroendocrinology 2006;**31**:340–6).

Adjunctive therapies:
- **Amantadine** 100mg/d did not help in one study (n=6, open, 6/52, Valevski et al, Clin Neuropharmacol 1998;**21**:355–7).

Opiates

Buprenorphine probably has less sexual ADRs than methadone as it causes less plasma testosterone suppression (n=105, Bliesener et al, J Clin Endocrinol Metab 2005;**90**:203–6).

Methadone produces a dose-dependent inhibition of orgasm (n=92, Brown et al, J Addict Disord 2005;**24**:91–106), so dose reduction may help.

Anticonvulsants

Topiramate-induced anorgasmia responds to dose reduction or discontinuation (n=7, Sun et al, Headache 2006;**46**:1450–3).

Ejaculation problems

All drugs

Discontinue or reduce dose, eg. if tricyclic-induced (Aizenberg et al, J Clin Psychiatry 1991;**52**:461–3). Retrograde ejaculation from risperidone 8mg/d promptly responds to dose reduction (n=1, Loh et al, Int Clin Psychopharmacol 2004;**19**:111–2). Discontinuation generally works for clozapine (n=3, Talmon et al, Harefuah 1994;**126**:509–10).

Tamsulosin has been used for reboxetine-induced painful ejaculation (n = 2, Demyttenaere and Huygens, *Eur Neuropsychopharmacol* 2002;**12**:337–41), and intermittent use may help with other causes (n = 405, Goktas *et al*, *J Urol* 2006;**175**:650–2).

Priapism

Early treatment (within 4–6 hours before local hypoxemia) reduces morbidity, the need for invasive procedures and impotence, and may prevent or minimise long-term complications.

Immediate short-term treatment includes conservative measures, eg. pain control, vigorous hydration, and cold compress before urology consultation.

Active treatments include cavernosal penile aspiration, irrigation, instillation of vasoactive agents, intracavernosal injection of phenylephrine (n = 1, Davol and Rukstalis, *Urology* 2005;**66**:880) and, if necessary, shunting procedures.

Terbutaline orally may be effective for about 40% (cf. 15% with placebo), so may be worth a try (n = 68, RCT, p/c, Priyadarshi, *Int J Impot Res* 2004;**16**:424–6).

If antipsychotic related, switch to one with a lower propensity to cause priapism (highest with chlorpromazine, and risperidone; see review by Compton and Miller, *J Clin Psychiatry* 2001;**62**:362–6).

Review: typicals and atypicals (Compton and Miller, *J Clin Psychiatry* 2001;**62**:362–6), shunting procedures (review: Kalsi *et al*, *Hosp Med* 2002;**63**:224–5).

6.9 Others, side-effects

Abnormal dreams and nightmares

Antidepressants	**Alter time** of dose from night to morning if appropriate.
	Switching drugs or **discontinuation** may be the only option.
	Discontinue tramadol (n = 1, Devulder *et al*, *Acta Clin Belg* 1996;**51**:184–6) and possibly other similar drugs that may exacerbate the effect.

Alopecia

- Check trace minerals, eg. copper and zinc levels, as low plasma levels may pre-dispose to hair loss so oral supplementation may be effective (Ftemi and Calabrese, *Ann Pharmacother* 1995;**29**:1302; Tasaki *et al*, *J Dermatol* 1993;**20**:21–4).
- Other standard management includes hair care techniques and minoxidil.

Review: McKinney *et al*, *Ann Clin Psychiatry* 1996;**8**:183–5.

Carbamazepine	May occur in 6%.
	May resolve after withdrawal, but can take several months.
Lithium	Alopecia may resolve with continued treatment (Ghadirian *et al*, *J Clin Psychiatry* 1986;**47**:212–3) or withdrawal (but might take several months). Exclude hypothyroidism as a causative factor.
SSRIs	Occurs more in women and there may be an association with sertraline so switch if appropriate eg. to paroxetine or trazodone (may help if sertraline-induced; n = 1, Gautam, *Ann Pharmacother* 1999;**33**:631–7).
	Review: Hedenmalm *et al*, *Pharmacoepidemiol Drug Saf* 2006;**15**:719–25.
Valproate	**Dose reduction** may help as alopecia is considered to be dose-dependent (Mercke *et al*, *Ann Clin Psychiatry* 2000;**12**:35–42).
	Check copper and zinc levels as low levels may pre-dispose to hair loss with valproate (Ftemi and Calabrese, *Ann Pharmacother* 1995;**29**:1302; Tasaki *et al*, *J Dermatol* 1993;**20**:21–4).

Anorexia

Valproate	Could be a sign of impending hepatic failure. Investigate immediately and discontinue if necessary.

Ataxia

Lithium	Usually a sign of lithium toxicity and neurotoxicity, requiring immediate

action, eg. discontinuation or dose reduction. If acute, dialysis may be needed. Consider also the global clinical picture, as ataxia may occur with 'normal' therapeutic lithium plasma levels.

Discontinue any exacerbating drugs, eg. clozapine (Lee and Yang, *Zhonghua Yi Xue Za Zhi* [Taipei] 1999;**62**:184–7).

Buspirone (high-dose) has been used for ataxia due to lithium toxicity (n = 1, Megna and O'Dell, *Arch Phys Med Rehabil* 2001;**82**:1145–8).

Bleeding
SSRIs

Discontinuing or **switching** to a non-SSRI may be the best option.

Stop any NSAIDs (inc. aspirin) or prescribe a less gastrotoxic NSAID or co-prescribe gastroprotective drugs (Dalton *et al*, *CNS Drugs* 2006;**20**:143–51; Mort *et al*, *Pharmacotherapy* 2006;**26**:1307–13).

Vitamin C 500 mg/d has been used (n = 1, Tielens, *Am J Psychiatry* 1997;**153**:883; Rasker, *Ned Tijdschr Geneesk* 1993;**137**:618).

Blood dyscrasias (neutropenia, agranulocytosis)
Clozapine

Immediate cessation is mandatory as even a major dose reduction is unlikely to help in the short-term. The incidence peaks at 8–10 weeks on first exposure.

Exclude any interacting or contributing drugs, eg. carbamazepine (case reports, Imbarlina *et al*, *Eur Psychiatry* 2004;**19**:506–9; see *Chapter 4.2.3*), antibiotics, etc.

GCSF/filgrastim may be effective and logical (eg. n = 1, Schuld *et al*, *Acta Psychiatr Scand* 2000;**102**:153–5; Sperner-Unterweger *et al*, *Br J Psychiatry* 1998;**173**:82–4; n = 3, Lamberti *et al*, *J Clin Psychiatry* 1995;**56**:256–9), and may shorten the duration of hospitalisation (n = 11, Chengappa *et al*, *Psychopharmacol Bull* 1996;**32**:111–21). It can also be used long-term (11–48 months, n = 3, Hagg *et al*, *Int Clin Psychopharmacol* 2003;**18**:173–4).

Lithium (n = 2, Papetti *et al*, *Encephale* 2004;**30**:578–82) has been used to prevent a patient going red by reversing a low wbc, eg. during an 'amber' phase or raising baseline wbc where a low count exists, allowing clozapine to start. Although lithium protects against neutropenia (eg. Silverstone, *J Clin Psychopharmacol* 1998;**18**:86–8), it does not protect against neutropenia progressing to agranulocytosis (Paton and Esop, *Psychiatr Bull* 2005;**29**:186–8). Plasma levels of 0.4 mmol/l have been used.

After care and re-exposure:

In 53 patients rechallenged with clozapine after leucopenia or neutropenia, 38% had a further dyscrasia and, in most, it was more severe, longer-lasting and occurred more quickly (incidence peaks at 5.5 weeks), but 55% of these 53 were rechallenged successfully and remained in treatment (n = 53, Dunk *et al*, *Br J Psychiatry* 2006;**188**:255–63).

Review: management (Esposito *et al*, *Eur J Clin Pharmacol* 2005;**60**:759–64).

Gastric irritation or nausea
Valproate

Take with or after food.

Slow-release or enteric-coated tablets may help.

Avoid fizzy drinks with the liquid or soluble tablets.

Glaucoma
Topiramate

Discontinuation usually quickly leads to reversal (Anon, *Prescrire Int* 2003;**12**:61).

Methylprednisolone and mannitol may be rapidly effective if acute (n = 1, Rhee *et al*, *Am J Ophthalmol* 2006;**141**:1133–4).

Laser surgery or peripheral iridectomy may be longer-term options (n = 83, Fraunfelder *et al*, *Ophthalmology* 2004;**111**:109–11).

Hair loss

Venlafaxine   **Discontinue**, and it may resolve within a month (Pitchot and Ansseau, *Am J Psychiatry* 2001;**158**:1159–60).

Hypersalivation

Clozapine   See siallorrhoea.

Lithium   **Propantheline** may give some symptomatic relief (n = 1, Donaldson, *Am J Psychiatry* 1982;**139**:1350–1).

Incontinence (see also noctural enuresis)

Clozapine   This may be due to alpha-adrenergic antagonism and usually resolves spontaneously within 3/12 in nearly all cases (n = 16, Warner *et al*, *Int Clin Psychopharmacol* 1994;**9**:207–9).

                        Reducing fluid intake during the evening may help.

                        Alpha-adrenergic agonists; ephedrine was rapidly effective at 150mg at night in 16 patients with the problem, with response maintained over 12/12 (n = 57, Fuller *et al*, *J Clin Psychiatry* 1996;**57**:514–8).

                        DDAVP® (Ferring)/Desmopressin intranasally has been used symptomatically (Steingard, *J Clin Psychiatry* 1994;**55**:315–6; n = 1, English *et al*, *Ann Pharmacother* 2001;**35**:867–9).

                        Ephedrine 150mg/d was effective within 24 hours in 94% patients in one study, with 75% getting full remission (n = 16, Fuller *et al*, *J Clin Psychiatry* 1996;**57**:514–8).

                        Oxybutinin has been used (Lurie and Hosmer, *J Clin Psychiatry* 1997;**58**:404).

                        Tolterodine has been used, albeit unsuccessfully (n = 1, English *et al*, *Ann Pharmacother* 2001;**35**:867–9).

                        Review and case series: Warner *et al*, *Int Clin Psychopharmacol* 1994;**9**:207–9.

Jaundice (see also hepatotoxicity)

Valproate   Could be impending hepatic failure. Investigate immediately and discontinue if necessary.

Jitteriness or agitation, akathisia

Tricyclics   **Slower dose titration** usually helps, including stopping and restarting at a slower rate.

                        Iron supplements to resolve any low serum iron (Yeragani *et al*, *Neuropsychobiology* 1992;**25**:8–10).

                        Perphenazine was used once (n = 2, Pohl *et al*, *J Clin Psychiatry* 1986;**47**:427).

Mastalgia (see also hyperprolactinaemia)

Venlafaxine   **Check prolactin** and take appropriate action.

                        Bromocriptine 5mg/d has been used for mastalgia occurring in weeks 5–13 of therapy, with no recurrence on discontinuation (n = 1, Bhatia *et al*, *J Clin Psychopharmacol* 2000;**20**:590–1).

Megaloblastic anaemia

Anticonvulsants   Folic acid may be used if caused by, eg. phenytoin or phenobarbital.

Oedema

Lithium   This common effect may be dose-related so try a reduced dose.

                        Diuretics may be useful but see *Chapter 4.4* for interactions between lithium and thiazides or other diuretics.

Trazodone   **Reduction** in dose or **discontinuation** may be rapidly successful (n = 10, Barnett *et al*, *J Clin Psychopharmacol* 1985;**5**:161–4).

Osteopenia (see also hyperprolactinaemia)

Antipsychotics   **Correct** any raised prolactin abnormalities.

                        Treat with standard therapies, eg. alendronic acid 5mg/d has improved spine and hip T-scores by 7% and 9% respectively over a year (n = 1, Howes and Smith, *Am J Psychiatry* 2004;**161**:756).

Pain at site of injection

Depots

Warm baths and regular exercise can help.

Change site or systematically alternate injection sides.

Check injection technique, as Z-tracking technique may not always be meticulously followed (Belanger-Annable, *Canadian Nurse* 1985;**81**:1–3).

Photosensitivity

Antipsychotics

Exclude other causes, eg. SLE and porphyria.

Avoid direct sunlight or sun-lamps.

Use a high factor sun-block cream.

Reduce doses or switch drugs (there is no reliable comparative information but chlorpromazine is almost certainly the worst).

Reviews: antipsychotics (Warnock and Morris, *Am J Clin Dermatol* 2002; **3**:629–36), antipsychotics, antidepressants and anxiolytics (Harth and Rapoport, *Drug Saf* 1996;**14**:252–9).

Raised LFTs

Valproate

Raised LFTs are not uncommon but usually transient, so monitor LFTs (including prothrombin time) until it returns to normal.

Discontinue if abnormally prolonged prothrombin time.

Salicylates (inc. OTC) may exacerbate so should be discontinued.

Rash

Lamotrigine

Take seriously: although relatively rare, rash may be the first sign of a potentially fatal Stevens-Johnson syndrome (n = 1175, RCT, Ketter *et al*, *J Clin Psychiatry* 2006;**67**:400–6) and so must be taken very seriously. The risk is higher in people with a previous anticonvulsant rash and being under 13 years of age (n = 988, Hirsch *et al*, *Epilepsia* 2006;**47**:318–22).

Slow dose titration reduces the incidence, and should be even slower in people with risk factors.

Preventative dermatological advice should be given, eg. avoid other new medicines, foods, cosmetics, deodorants, detergents and fabric softeners, and avoid sunburn or exposure to poison ivy/oak (n = 100, Ketter *et al*, *J Clin Psychiatry* 2005;**66**:642–5). This may be effective in minimising the danger of this serious adverse reaction.

Valproate may not necessarily be an additional risk factor (n = 52, P-Codrea Tigaran *et al*, *Acta Neurol Scand* 2005;**111**:191–4) but does need extra care.

Careful (very) rechallenge may be possible in some patients, with a slower dose escalation (n = 52, P-Codrea Tigaran *et al*, *Acta Neurol Scand* 2005;**111**:191–4).

Phenytoin

Can be the presenting symptom of serious reactions (review by Scheinfeld, *Expert Opin Drug Saf* 2004;**3**:655–65).

If mild, can reintroduce cautiously but discontinue immediately if it recurs.

Siallorhoea (hypersalivation)

Clozapine

Hypersalivation may be a lack of the swallowing reflex or due to clozapine's pharmacology, eg. M4 activation or alpha-2 blockade. One study showed that hypersalivation is an inaccurate term for this side-effect. The dribbling is probably due to poor or inadequate swallowing, rather than excess saliva production (n = 17, Rabinowitz *et al*, *Biol Psychiatry* 1996;**40**:1132–4).

Physical strategies:
• Propping pillows up at night helps a little in some people.

- Reduce caffeine intake (n = 1, Odom-White and de Leon, *J Clin Psychiatry* 1996;57:175–6).

Adjunctive therapies:

With this common side-effect, adjunctive therapies are usually the only realistic option for this unpleasant, but not life-threatening ADR. The following are probably in descending order of efficacy:

- **Hyoscine** hydrobromide (Kwells®) 300 mcg sucked and swallowed up to TDS.
- **Pirenzapine**, an M1/M4 blocker at 25–100 mg/d is frequently used (n = 29, Schneider et al, *Pharmacopsychiatry* 2004;**37**:43–5) and has no interaction with clozapine, although it may not always be useful (n = 20, RCT, d/b, c/o, p/c, Bai et al, *J Clin Psychopharmacol* 2001;**21**:608–11).
- **Atropine** 1% eye drops, one drop given orally at bedtime may be rapidly effective (n = 3, Antonello and Tessier, *J Psychiatry Neurosci* 1999;**24**:250; Comley et al, *Aust N Z J Psychiatry* 2000;**34**:1033–4).
- **Tricyclics** (eg. amitriptyline; Praharaj and Arora, *Br J Clin Pharmacol* 2006;**63**:128–9) predominantly for their anticholinergic effect (Copp et al, *Br J Psychiatry* 1991;**159**:166).
- **Sulpiride** (150–300 mg/d) may have some efficacy (n = 18, open, 3/52, Kreinin et al, *Isr J Psych Relat Sci* 2005;**42**:61–3), as may amisulpride ('strong ameliorating effect'; n = 20, RCT, d/b, p/c, c/o, Kreinin et al, *Int Clin Psychopharmacol* 2006;**21**:99–103; Croissant et al, *Pharmacopsychiatry* 2005;**38**:38–9).
- **Quetiapine**, through allowing reduced clozapine dosage

Less use:

- **Anticholinergics** or antimuscarinics are generally ineffective, although trihexyphenidyl 5–15 mg/d at bedtime reduced secretions by 44% in one study (n = 14, open, Spivak et al, *Int Clin Psychopharmacol* 1997;**12**:213–5). Trihexyphenidyl and terazosin 2 mg/d (Reinstein et al, *Clin Drug Invest* 1999;**17**:97–102) may be better than either drug alone. **Biperiden** 6 mg/d has been effective in a case resistant to propranolol and clonidine (n = 1, Richardson et al, *Am J Psychiatry* 2001;**158**:1329–30).
- **Botulinum toxin** (injected into the parotid gland) has been used for sialorrhoea in neurological cases (n = 1, Kahl et al, *Psychopharmacol* [Berl] 2004;**173**:229–30; n = 1 and review, Kahl et al, *Nervenarzt* 2005;**76**:205–8).
- **Chewing gum** has been used to stimulate salivation and swallowing.
- **Clonidine** 50–100 mcg/d increases adrenergic tone and reduces patient-reported hypersalivation (wet area on pillow) without adverse effects (n = 12, open, 4/52, Parharaj et al, *J Psychopharmacol* 2005;**19**:426–8), although it might exacerbate depression and psychosis. Clonidine patches (0.1 mg/week) have been used.
- **Guanfacine** (Webber et al, *J Clin Psychopharmacol* 2004;**24**:675–6).
- **Ipratropium** (sublingually or intranasal spray) has limited efficacy (Freudenreich et al, *J Clin Psychopharmacol* 2004;**24**:98–100; n = 10, Calderon et al, *Int Clin Psychopharmacol* 2000;**15**:49–52).
- **Lofexidine** 0.2 mg BD has been used as an alpha-2 agonist in the short-term (testing the theory that hypersalivation is due to clozapine's alpha-2 antagonism; n = 1, 1/12, Corrigan et al, *Br J Psychiatry* 1995;**167**:412; rebuttal of theory by Szabadi, *Br J Psychiatry* 1996; **169**:380–1).
- **Propantheline** 7.5 mg/d has been used.

- **Scopolamine** patches (Gaftanyuk and Trestman, *Psychiatr Serv* 2004; **55**:318).
- **Septoplasty** was dramatically successful in one patient with a deviated septum causing him to breathe through his mouth (n = 1, Conry *et al*, *Am J Psychiatry* 1996;**153**:444).

Reviews: general (Praharaj *et al*, *Psychopharmacol [Berl]* 2006;**185**:265–73; Rogers and Shramko, *Pharmacotherapy* 2000;**20**:1092–95; Davydov and Botts, *Ann Pharmacother* 2000;**34**:662–5; Freudenreich, *Drugs Today [Barc]* 2005;**41**:411–8).

Sweating
Antidepressants
Discontinuation or dose-reduction improves this rapidly.

Adjunctive therapies:

This can be a significantly irritating ADR for patients, especially those on tricyclics. Drugs tried include:
- **Clonidine** 0.2 mg/d (dramatically effective within 24 hours, n = 1, Feder, *J Clin Psychiatry* 1995;**56**:35; Molnar, *Mod Med Aust* 1999;**42**:9), although stopping it sometimes helps (Leeman, *J Clin Psychiatry* 1990;**51**:258–9).
- **Cyproheptadine** 4 mg either BD or at night (n = 5, open, Ashton and Weinstein, *Am J Psychiatry* 2002;**159**:874–5).
- **Beta-blockers** (propranolol, atenolol, labetalol) probably make sweating worse and should be excluded before other therapies are tried (n = 1, Butt, *J Clin Psychiatry* 1989;**50**:146–7).
- **Benzatropine** 0.5–1 mg/d if venlafaxine-induced (Garber and Gregory, *J Clin Psychiatry* 1997;**58**:176–7; Pierre and Guze, *J Clin Psychopharmacol* 2000;**20**:269).
- **Mirtazapine** (dose-dependent, perhaps via 5-HT2/3 antagonism and influence on regulation of body temperature and diaphoresis; n = 1, Buecking *et al*, *Eur J Clin Pharmacol* 2005;**61**:543–4) has been successful for 'hot flushes' in women (n = 22 [c = 16], Perez *et al*, *J Support Oncol* 2004;**2**:50–6).

Terazosin 2 mg/d (n = 1, Leeman, *J Clin Psychiatry* 1990;**51**:258–9).

Review: case and brief review (Marcy and Britton, *Ann Pharmacother* 2005; **39**:748–52), general (Butt, *J Clin Psychiatry* 1989;**50**:146–7), pathophysiology of tricyclic-induced (Leeman, *J Clin Psychiatry* 1990;**51**:258–9)

Tremor (see also extra-pyramidal side-effects)
Lithium
Dose reduction is appropriate since tremor is dose/plasma level related. **Beta-blockers** are standard therapy, eg. **propranolol** 30–40 mg/d (n = 5, Lapierre, *Can Med Assoc J* 1976;**114**:619–20), **metoprolol** (comparison with propranolol, Zubenko *et al*, *Psychiatry Res* 1984;**11**:163–4), atenolol (n = 1, Dave, *Can J Psychiatry* 1989;**34**:132–3) and **nadolol** (for a hepatically-compromised patient; n = 1, Dave and Langbart, *Ann Clin Psychiatry* 1994; **6**:51–2).

Vitamin B6 900–1200 mg/d was completely effective in 80% patients (open, n = 5, Miodownik *et al*, *Int J Psychiatr Med* 2002;**32**:103–8).

Linoleic acid is ineffective (Schou, *Prostaglandins Med* 1980;**5**:343–4; Anton, *Prostaglandins Med* 1980;**5**:321–2).

Review: Gelenberg and Jefferson, *J Clin Psychiatry* 1995;**56**:283–7.

Vomiting
Valproate
Could be impending hepatic failure. Investigate immediately and discontinue if necessary.

7 MISCELLANEOUS INFORMATION

7.1 NEW PSYCHOTROPIC DRUGS EXPECTED

This is a list of drugs which are known to have a product licence application lodged in the UK, or where it is thought to be planned soon. The time between application and approval can be as short as six months or as long as two or more years, depending upon the data presented and perceived risks. Accurate marketing dates are thus not available.

The author would be grateful for any additional information or corrections to help with this section, which relies to a large extent on 'randomly acquired' information.

Drugs or preparations possible in 2007 *

Agomelatine (Valdoxan®, Servier) 2008? *
Agomelatine is a 5HT2C and 5HT2B antagonist and a melatonin M1 and M2 agonist for depression, anxiety and sleep disorders. Submitted for registration in EU. It was superior to placebo at 25 mg/d, with 50 mg/d effective (and as well-tolerated) in most patients who failed to respond to 25 mg/d after two weeks (n = 21, RCT, d/b, p/c, 6/52, Kennedy and Emsley, Eur Neuropsychopharmacol 2006;**16**:93–100). Agomelatine appears to have no sexual side-effects, no tolerability issues or discontinuation symptoms at a dose of 25 mg/d (n = 192, RCT, d/b, p/c, 2/52, Montgomery et al, Int Clin Psychopharmacol 2004;**19**:271–80).
Reviews: Rouillon, Int Clin Psychopharmacol 2006;**21**(Suppl 1):S31–5, den Boer et al, Int Clin Psychopharmacol 2006;**21**(Suppl 1):S21–4, Dubocovich, Curr Opin Investig Drugs 2006; **7**:670–80.

Armodafinil (Nuvigil®, Cephalon)
Armodafinil is the r-enantiomer of modafinil, presumably with similar effects but a longer half-life (12–15 hours). It is metabolised by 3A4.

Asenapine (Zydis, Organon/Pfizer)
A 5HT2 antagonist and D2 partial agonist in phase III trials for psychosis. Oral melt form of 'fragile wafer'. 15 mg dose proposed.

Bifeprunox (Lundbeck) *
A partial agonist and D2 receptor for schizophrenia (Cosi et al, Eur J Pharmacol 2006; **535**:135–44).

Desvenlafaxine (Pristiq®, Wyeth)
Metabolite of venlafaxine, for depression and anxiety. No reported adverse cardiac effects. Licenses being submitted.

Eszopiclone (Lunesta) *
An analogue of zopiclone, this drug has been licensed in the USA but with no limit to the time of treatment. Eszopiclone 2–3 mg appears to have no discontinuation, tolerance or rebound effects (n = 308, RCT, p/c, 7/52, Zemmit et al, Curr Med Res Opin 2004;**20**:1979–91).
Reviews: Najib, ClinTher 2006;**28**:491–516; Melton et al, Ann Pharmacother 2005;**39**:1659–66.

Fluoxetine (Prozac once-weekly, Lilly)
A 90 mg once-weekly oral form (slow-release to reduce peak levels) has been marketed in the USA. Since fluoxetine and norfluoxetine have long half-lives and 5 mg/d is the lowest effective dose, 90 mg a week should be therapeutically active. In an abrupt switch study from daily and established sertraline, citalopram or paroxetine, 79% completed successfully and 9.3% discontinued due to lack of efficacy. It was well-tolerated in all groups (n = 246, Miner et al, J Clin Psychiatry 2002;**63**:232–40). Slightly higher compliance has been shown over daily fluoxetine (86% vs 79%) (n = 117, 3/12, Claxton et al, J Clin Psychiatry 2000;**61**:92832, MS).

Gaboxadol (Merck/Lundbeck)
Gaboxadol (THIP) is a full or partial agonist at GABA-A receptors, for sleep disorders, and in phase III development. It acts on a delta-containing GABA(A) receptor subtype found exclusively outside of the synapse (Wafford, Curr Opin Pharmacol 2006;**6**:30–6).

Gepirone (Ariza®, Organon) *

Gepirone is a 5HT1A partial agonist with some alpha-2 activity, being developed as an antidepressant, with a launch planned 2008 in the USA. Gepirone needs an SR form to reduce g/i upset. The main ADR is lightheadedness (Leslie, Curr Opin Investig Drugs 2001;**2**:1120–07) and needs care in poor renal function (n = 37, Dogterom et al, Clin Drug Invest 2002;**22**:513–22; n = 209, RCT, p/c, 8/52, Feiger et al, J Clin Psychiatry 2003;**64**:243–9).

Guanfacine (Shire)

An alpha-2-adrenoceptor agonist for ADHD, submitted for approval in USA.

Iloperidone (Novartis)

Iloperidone is a D2 and 5HT2 antagonist, with some alpha-1 blocking activity, currrently undergoing phase III trials for schizophrenia.

Indiplon® (Neurocrine Biosciences, Pfizer)

GABA-A modulator at BDZ sites, for transient sleep disorders. Approval awaited in USA.

Melatonin (Genzyme) *

This may be licensed for insomnia, as it may produce a significant improvement in sleep (n = 24, Dolberg et al, Am J Psychiatry 1998;**155**:1119–21), following 510 mg at 9.00 PM ('interesting, but not miraculous' review, Anon, Prescrire Internat 1998;**7**:1807, 83 refs). However, a systematic review of the efficacy and safety of exogenous melatonin in managing secondary sleep disorders, and sleep disorders such as jet lag and shiftwork disorder, showed no evidence that melatonin had an effect on sleep onset latency in people with secondary sleep disorders (s = 32, RCT, Buscemi et al, Br Med J 2006;**332**:385–93).

Mifepristone (Corlux®, Concept)

A glucocorticoid type-II receptor (GRII) antagonist and progesterone receptor antagonist for depression and psychosis, approval awaited in USA.

Norclozapine (Acadia)

An active metabolite of clozapine, norclozapine is being investigated as an alternative to clozapine. It may have enhanced cognition, a unique effect on M1 receptors and it avoids the metabolic step from clozapine.

Paliperidone (J&J) 2007 *

Paliperidone is the 9-hydroxy derivative of risperidone and a full 5HT2/partial D2 antagonist with a high affinity for 5HT7 receptors, submitted for approval for psychosis in USA. It may be marketed in the OROS extended release system. The main advantages are smoother plasma levels, fewer side-effects and limited hepatic metabolism.

Phenserine (Axonyx) *

Phenserine is a potent and selective inhibitor of acetylcholinesterase which also inhibits the production of a toxic form of beta-amyloid protein in the brain. Phase III trials have not been conclusive though.

Quetiapine SR (Seroquel, Astra Zeneca) *

A sustained release tablet is projected for 2007-8, as is a bipolar depression licence.

Ramelteon (Rozerem®, Takeda) 2008? *

Melatonin M1 and M2 agonist for insomnia characterised by poor sleep onset. There is no physical dependence (Behavioural Neurosci 2006;**120**:535; review by Owen, Drugs Today [Barc] 2006;**42**:255–63). Phase III studies under way. Licensed in USA.

Tramiprosate (Alzhemed™, Neurochem) *

Undergoing phase III trials for Alzheimer's disease.

Xaliproden (Sanofi-Aventis) *

Xaliproden is a non-peptide compound that activates the synthesis of endogenous neurotropins, in phase III trials for Alzheimer's disease.

7.2 LABORATORY TEST INTERPRETATIONS

A guide to normal ranges, variations, causes and drug influences. Local ranges may differ slightly from these here.

Urea and electrolytes (U&Es)

Bicarbonate 2230 mmol/l

Calcium 2.252.6mmol/l

↑ malignancy (55%),
hyperparathyroidism (35%),
hyperthyroidism, vitamin D excess

↓ hypoparathyroidism, vitamin D deficiency

☐ OCs, lithium, thiazides

❏ barbiturates, cimetidine, corticosteroids,
phenytoin

Chloride 9105mmol/l

Glucose 3.35.6mmol/l

↑ >6.7 overnight =diabetes mellitus ?

☐ cimetidine, OCs, furosemide, lithium,
phenothiazines, thiazides, phenytoin,
some atypicals

■ ascorbic acid, levodopa, metronidazole

❏ dextropropoxyphene.

❏ ascorbic acid

Magnesium 0.71.2mmol/l

↑ renal failure

↓ severe diarrhoea

Phosphate 0.81.4mmol/l (adversely affects calcium metabolism)

↑ malnutrition (esp in alcoholics)

Potassium 3.55.3mmol/l

↑ dangerous. Treat as emergency.

↑ produces muscle weakness.

❏ salbutamol, insulin

Protein total 5070g/l

Albumin 35–55g/l

↑ = haemoconcentration

↓ = haemodilution, neuropathy, cirrhosis,
catabolism

Sodium 133–149mmol/l (rate of change is as important as the actual level)

↑ excess fluid loss/poor intake, renal failure.

↓ cardiac or renal failure, D&V, chest
disorders (infections or carcinoma),
hypoalbuminaemia, bulimia ?

☐ high dose sodium salt antibiotics, lithium

❏ diuretics (esp thiazides), steroids,
carbamazepine, oxcarbazepine, tricyclics,
SSRIs, chlorpropamide, clofibrate

Urea (2.5–8.0mmol/l)

↑ renal failure, catabolism, haemorrhage

☐ salicylates, tetracyclines

Renal function

Creatinine clearance

M97–140ml/min
F 85–125ml/min

(Best measure of GFR if collection of the 24-hour samples is accurate.)

Creatinine conc

M50–120mol/l
F 40–100mol/l

↑ catabolism, pregnancy. Should decrease
with age

■ ascorbic acid, methyldopa

☐ salicylates, captopril, cimetidine,
co-trimoxazole

Urea (BUN) 1–5mmol/l

↑ renal failure, high protein food, catabolism

Liver function tests (LFTS)

Ranges quoted by laboratories vary with the
method and conditions of the assay.

ALT (SGPT) 5–30iu/l

↑ hepatocellular damage, cholestasis,
occasionally cirrhosis

☐ alcohol, OCs, levodopa, phenothiazines,
phenytoin, valproate, antibiotics

❏ vigabatrin

❏ metronidazole

Albumin 35–55g/l

↓ oedema, neuropathy, cirrhosis

■ penicillins

❏ alcohol, phenytoin

Alkaline phosphatase (ALP), 20–100iu/l

↑ cholestasis, hepatocellular damage, bone
disease (eg. Pagets, carcinoma), pregnancy

☐ alcohol, carbamazepine, disulfiram,
phenothiazines, phenytoin

❏ nitrofurantoin, zinc

Aspartate transaminase (AST/SGOT) 5–40iu/l

↑ hepatocellular damage, cholestasis,
cirrhosis, infarction, muscle trauma,
respiratory failure

❏ vigabatrin

Bilirubin 2–20mmol/l

↑ liver cell damage, cholestasis,
haemolytic states

■ beta-blockers, valproate, isulfiram,
phenothiazines, alcohol, antibiotics

❏ ascorbic acid

Gamma-glutamyl transferase (GGT), 5–45iu/l

↑ cholestasis, hepatitis, cirrhosis,
cellular damage (eg. paracetamol
or disulfiram OD), enzyme

inducers (especially phenobarbital and phenytoin), excess alcohol, metastatic carcinoma

☐ alcohol, barbiturates, OCs, phenytoin, oxcarbazepine, simvastatin

Prothrombin ratio 1–1.2

Prothrombin time 10–135

↑ severe, usually chronic, liver damage

Blood

Blood pH 7.35–7.45

Outside range metabolic function is impaired

WBC/WCC 4.0–11.0 × 10⁹/l

↑↑ malignancy

↑ infection

↓ many drugs, some infections

RBC M 4.5–6 × 10¹²/l

F 4.3–5.5 × 10¹²/l

↑ fluid loss, polycythaemia

↓ fluid overload, anaemia, marrow aplasia

Hb M 13–18 g/dl

F 12–16 g/dl

↓ haemorrhage, iron deficiency, marrow depression

MCV (mean cell volume) 80–95 fl

↑ folate or B12 deficiency, liver disease, alcohol

↓ iron deficiency

ESR M 0–9 mm/h

F 0–20 mm/h

(viscosities now more usually used)

↑ infections, inflammatory diseases.

Lymphocytes 1–4 × 10⁹/l

↑ (lymphocytosis) mononucleosis, viral infections, TB, some leukaemias, auto-immune diseases, toxoplasmosis

↓ (lymphopenia) in marrow failure, plus treatment with corticosteroids and azathioprine

Platelets 100–450 × 10⁹/l

↓ marrow failure or toxicity, leukaemia, splenomegaly

Neutrophils 1.8–8 10⁹/l (45–75% of WBCs)

↑ infection, inflammation, carcinoma, leukaemia, gout

↓ viral infections, autoimmune disease, marrow failure drugs

☐ chlorpromazine, phenytoin, chloramphenicol, etc

Monocytes 0.1–1.1 × 10⁹/l

↑ (monocytosis) in TB, endocarditis, typhoid, leukaemia

Eosinophils 0.04–0.8 × 10⁹/l (1–4% of WBCs)

↑ (eosinophilia) in atopic asthma, hay fever, worm infestations, lymphomas, skin disease

Basophils 0.01–0.4 × 10⁹/l

↑ (basophil leucocytosis) leukaemia, ulcerative colitis

Miscellaneous

Amylase (serum) 60–300 μ/l

↑ acute pancreatitis, abdominal trauma, renal failure

☐ furosemide, morphine, valproate

Blood pressure (adult) ≤ 140/90

Systolic/diastolic, the latter more important. Possibly higher limit allowed in elderly.

Cortisol/Dexamethasone Suppression Test 200 nmol/l

↑ adrenal hyperplasia or tumour (or depression?)

CSF Protein 0.2–0.5 g/l

↑ infection, haemorrhage

CSF glucose 2.8–4 mmol/l

↑ haemorrhage

↓ infection

Folate serum 2.5–15 μg/l

↓ best guide to folate deficiency

Folate RBC 150–750 μg/l

↓ guide to long-term folate deficiency

☐ chloramphenicol, erythromycin, penicillins.

☐ barbiturates, OCs, phenytoin, alcohol

Iron serum M 10–30 μmol

F 7–25 μmol

↑ inflammation

↓ iron deficiency, rheumatoid arthritis

Iron binding capacity (serum) 45–72 μmol/l

↑ iron deficiency

↓ rheumatoid arthritis

Lipids:

~ cholesterol 4–7 mmol/l

↑ hyperlipidaemia, diabetes, nephrotic syndrome, biliary obstruction

☐ disulfiram, levodopa, OCs, phenytoin, oxcarbazepine

☐ metronidazole, tetracyclines

~ triglyceride 0.6–1.8 mmol/l (post 12-hour fasting)

↑ diabetes, nephrotic syndrome pancreatitis,

alcohol abuse

☐ alcohol, beta-blockers, clozapine, OCs, olanzapine, quetiapine

Osmolality 285–295 mOsm/kg

↑ fluid depletion

↓ fluid excess

pCO₂ 4.5–6 kPa or 34–45 mmHg

Measure of respiratory function.

Thyroxine-total 60–140 nmol/l

↑ hyperthyroidism (Grave's disease — confirm by TRH), varies with age.

↓ hypothyroidism

☐ beta-blockers, OCs

❑ carbamazepine, lithium, phenytoin, salicylates

T4/Thyroxine-Free 10–25 pmol/l

↑ hypothyroidism (Myxodema).

↓ hyperthyroidism

T3 1.1–2.3 nmol/l

↑ hypothyroidism

↓ hyperthyroidism

TSH 0.15–3.20 mIU/l

↑ hypothyroidism

↓ hyperthyroidism

Urate 150–500 umol/l

↑ purine metabolic defect, carcinoma, diminished excretion (eg. acidosis, renal failure, diuretics)

☐ alcohol, furosemide, salicylates, thiazides

Vitamin B12 160–900 ng/l

↓ diet deficiency, pernicious anaemia, ileitis or short bowel syndrome. May lead to macrocytic anaemia and peripheral neuropathy

KEY:

↑ increased level mainly caused by

↓ decreased level mainly caused by

▲ drugs which raise level include

▼ drugs which lower level include

■ drugs which appear to raise levels by test interference

❑ drugs which appear to lower levels by test interference

INDEX

All the main psychotropic drugs are indexed according to their BNF or other main indications in *Chapter 1*, but obviously may appear elsewhere. In order to keep the index down to a manageable size, you are then referred to the index listing for that drugs chemical or therapeutic group. Individual drugs should be looked up under their drug group.

Acamprosate
  for alcohol dependence 10
  interactions 349
  use in breast-feeding 213
  use in cardiac disease 221
  use in diabetes 229
  use in epilepsy 234
  use in glaucoma 238
  use in hepatic impairment 241
  use in old age 246
  use in pregnancy 253
  use in renal impairment 270
Acetazolamide
  for epilepsy 107
  see also anticonvulsants
Acute psychiatric emergency 1
Aggression
  drug-induced 374
  treatment of 6
Agitation
  drug-induced 373
  treatment of 17
Agoraphobia
  treatment of 8
Akathisia
  drug-induced 386
  management of side-effects 418
Alcohol dependence 9
Alcohol interactions 357
Alcohol misuse 9
Alcohol withdrawal syndrome 14
Alprazolam
  for anxiety 19
  for panic disorder 125
  see also benzodiazepines
Alzheimer's disease
  treatment of 57
Amisulpride
  for psychosis 141
  see also antipsychotics
Amitriptyline
  for depression 77
  see also tricyclics
Amoxapine
  for depression 77
  see also tricyclics
Amylobarbital
  for epilepsy 110
  see also barbiturates
Anorexia nervosa
  treatment of 95

Anorgasmia
  drug effects 430
Anticholinergics
  for extra-pyramidal side-effects 418
  interactions 349
  switching 179
  use in breast-feeding 213
  use in cardiac disease 221
  use in diabetes 229
  use in epilepsy 234
  use in glaucoma 238
  use in hepatic impairment 241
  use in old age 246
  use in pregnancy 253
  use in renal impairment 270
Anticholinesterases
  for Alzheimer's disease 58
  interactions 349
  use in breast-feeding 213
  use in cardiac disease 221
  use in diabetes 229
  use in epilepsy 234
  use in glaucoma 238
  use in hepatic impairment 241
  use in old age 246
  use in pregnancy 253
  use in renal impairment 270
Anticonvulsants
  for epilepsy 101
  interactions 325
  sexual side-effects 428
  therapeutic drug monitoring 102
  use in breast-feeding 213
  use in cardiac disease 221
  use in diabetes 229
  use in epilepsy 234
  use in glaucoma 238
  use in hepatic impairment 241
  use in old age 246
  use in pregnancy 253
  use in renal impairment 270
  weight changes 211
  withdrawal 100
Antidepressants
  for agoraphobia 8
  for anxiety disorder 18
  for benzodiazepine dependence
    and withdrawal 30
  for bulimia 97
  for depression 73
  for OCD 121

  for panic 126
  for PTSD 129–130
  for social phobia 166–167
  interactions 293
  pharmacokinetics 182
  relative side-effects 180
  sexual side-effects 428
  switching or stopping 180
  use in breast-feeding 213
  use in cardiac disease 221
  use in diabetes 229
  use in epilepsy 234
  use in glaucoma 238
  use in hepatic impairment 241
  use in old age 246
  use in pregnancy 253
  use in renal impairment 270
  weight changes with 209
Antihistamines
  for insomnia 116
  relative side-effects 179
Antimuscarinics
  see anticholinergics
Antipsychotics
  for acute psychiatric emergencies 3
  for anxiety 21
  for mania 41
  for Tourette's syndrome 169
  for psychosis 137
  equivalent doses 196
  injections, depot 148
  injections, depot kinetics 151–153
  interactions 281
  relative receptor blockades 186
  relative side-effects 184
  sexual side-effects 429
  switching or discontinuing 190
  use in breast-feeding 213
  use in cardiac disease 221
  use in diabetes 229
  use in ECT 175
  use in epilepsy 234
  use in glaucoma 238
  use in hepatic impairment 241
  use in old age 246
  use in pregnancy 253
  use in renal impairment 270
  weight changes with 208
Anxiety
  drug-induced 373
  treatment of 17

Anxiolytics
  for anxiety 18
  equivalent doses 179
  interactions 275
  relative side-effects 180
  sexual side-effects 428
  use in breast-feeding 213
  use in cardiac disease 221
  use in diabetes 229
  use in epilepsy 234
  use in glaucoma 238
  use in hepatic impairment 241
  use in old age 246
  use in pregnancy 253
  use in renal impairment 270
  weight changes with 208
Aripiprazole
  for psychosis 142
  use in breast-feeding 213
  use in cardiac disease 221
  use in diabetes 229
  use in epilepsy 234
  use in glaucoma 238
  use in hepatic impairment 241
  use in old age 246
  use in pregnancy 253
  use in renal impairment 270
  interactions 285
Atomoxetine
  for ADHD 24
  interactions 351
  use in breast-feeding 213
  use in cardiac disease 221
  use in diabetes 229
  use in epilepsy 234
  use in glaucoma 238
  use in hepatic impairment 241
  use in old age 246
  use in pregnancy 253
  use in renal impairment 270
Attention deficit disorder 23
Autism
  see autistic disorder
Autistic disorder
  treatment of 27
Barbiturates
  for epilepsy 107
  for insomnia 116
  interactions 336
  therapeutic drug monitoring 102
  use in breast-feeding 213
  use in cardiac disease 221
  use in diabetes 229
  use in epilepsy 218
  use in glaucoma 238
  use in hepatic impairment 241
  use in old age 246
  use in pregnancy 253
  use in renal impairment 270
  withdrawal of 100
Behavioural toxicity
  drug-induced 374
Benperidol

for psychosis 140
  for sexual deviancy 164
  see also butyrophenones
Benzodiazepine dependence 30
Benzodiazepine withdrawal 30
Benzodiazepines
  dependence 30
  for acute psychiatric
    emergency 4
  for alcohol withdrawal 15
  for anxiety 18
  for epilepsy 106
  for insomnia 114
  for panic disorder 126
  equivalent doses 179
  interactions 275
  relative side-effects 180
  switching/equivalent doses 179
  use in breast-feeding 213
  use in cardiac disease 221
  use in diabetes 229
  use in ECT 175
  use in glaucoma 238
  use in hepatic impairment 241
  use in old age 246
  use in pregnancy 253
  use in renal impairment 270
  weight changes with 211
  withdrawal 30
Benzhexol
  see trihexyphenidyl
Benzatropine
  for extra-pyramidal side-
    effects 418
  see also anticholinergics
Beta-blockers
  for anxiety 19
  relative side-effects 180
  use in breast-feeding 213
  use in cardiac disease 221
  use in diabetes 229
  use in epilepsy 234
  use in glaucoma 238
  use in hepatic impairment 241
  use in old age 246
  use in pregnancy 253
  use in renal impairment 270
Binge-eating disorder
  treatment of 99
Bipolar mood disorder
  prophylaxis, treatment of 33
  rapid-cycling, treatment of 51
Borderline personality disorder 53
Breast-feeding
  drugs in 213
Bromazepam
  for anxiety 20
  see also benzodiazepines
Bulimia nervosa
  treatment of 97
Buprenorphine
  use in breast-feeding 213
  use in cardiac disease 221

use in diabetes 229
  use in epilepsy 234
  use in glaucoma 238
  use in hepatic impairment 241
  use in old age 246
  use in pregnancy 253
  use in renal impairment 270
  interactions 351
Bupropion
  interactions 352
  use in breast-feeding 213
  use in cardiac disease 221
  use in diabetes 229
  use in ECT 176
  use in epilepsy 234
  use in hepatic impairment 241
  use in old age 246
  use in pregnancy 253
  use in renal impairment 270
Buspirone
  for anxiety 19
  interactions 278
  see also anxiolytics
Butyrophenones
  for acute psychiatric emergency 3
  for psychosis 140
  for Tourette's syndrome 169
  equivalent doses 196
  interactions 281
  relative side-effects 184
  sexual side-effects 428
  switching or discontinuing 198
  use in breast-feeding 213
  use in cardiac disease 221
  use in diabetes 229
  use in epilepsy 234
  use in glaucoma 238
  use in hepatic impairment 241
  use in old age 246
  use in pregnancy 253
  use in renal impairment 270
  weight changes with 208
Caffeine
  in ECT 176
Caffeinism 173
Cannabis
  interactions 361
Carbamazepine
  for alcohol withdrawal 16
  for bipolar disorder 34
  for epilepsy 103
  for mania 41
  interactions 326
  sexual side-effects 428
  therapeutic drug monitoring 102
  use in breast-feeding 213
  use in cardiac disease 221
  use in diabetes 229
  use in ECT 176
  use in hepatic impairment 241
  use in old age 246
  use in pregnancy 253
  use in renal impairment 270

weight changes with 211
withdrawal of 100
see also anticonvulsants
Cardiovascular disease
drugs in 222
Catatonia
drug-induced 389
treatment of 56
Changing psychotropics
see switching psychotropics
Chloral
for insomnia 116
interactions 279
see also hypnotics
Chlordiazepoxide
for anxiety 19
Chlormethiazole
see clomethiazole
Chlorpromazine
for acute psychiatric emergency 2
for psychosis 137
see also phenothiazines
Choreas
drug-induced 389
Citalopram
for agoraphobia 9
for depression 73
for panic disorder 126
interactions 297
see also SSRIs
Clobazam
for anxiety 19
for epilepsy 106
see also benzodiazepines
Clomethiazole
for alcohol withdrawal 15
for insomnia 116
interactions 353
relative side-effects 179
use in breast-feeding 213
use in cardiac disease 221
use in diabetes 229
use in epilepsy 234
use in glaucoma 238
use in hepatic impairment 241
use in old age 246
use in pregnancy 253
use in renal impairment 270
see also anticonvulsants
Clomipramine
for depression 77
for OCD 121
for panic disorder 125
see also tricyclics
Clonazepam
for epilepsy 106
for panic disorder 127
for status epilepticus 110
see also benzodiazepines
Clorazepate
for anxiety 19
see also benzodiazepines
Clozapine

for schizophrenia 142
interactions 285
use in ECT 176
see also antipsychotics
Cocaine
interactions 361
Confusion
drug-induced 375
Convulsions
drug-induced 396
treatment of 103
Cyproterone
for sexual deviancy 164
Cytochrome P450 enzymes 363
CYP1A2 364
CYP2B6 365
CYP2C9 366
CYP2C19 367
CYP2D6 368
CYP3A4 370
Delirium
drug-induced 375
Dementia
treatment of 57
Depression
drug-induced 377
treatment of 57
Depot injections
see antipsychotics
Dexamfetamine
for attention deficit disorder 24
use in breast-feeding 213
use in cardiac disease 221
use in diabetes 229
use in epilepsy 234
use in glaucoma 238
use in hepatic impairment 241
use in old age 246
use in pregnancy 236
use in renal impairment 270
Diabetes
drugs in 229
Diazepam
for acute psychiatric emergency 4
for anxiety 19
for benzodiazepine withdrawal 30
for epilepsy 107
for status epilepticus 110
see also benzodiazepines
Diphenylbutylpiperidines
for psychosis 141
interactions 281
relative side-effects 184
sexual side-effects 429
switching/equivalent doses 196
use in breast-feeding 213
use in cardiac disease 221
use in diabetes 229
use in epilepsy 234
use in glaucoma 238
use in hepatic impairment 241
use in old age 246
use in pregnancy 253

use in renal impairment 270
weight changes with 209
Disulfiram
for alcohol dependence 11
interactions 359
use in breast-feeding 213
use in cardiac disease 221
use in diabetes 229
use in epilepsy 234
use in glaucoma 238
use in hepatic impairment 241
use in old age 246
use in pregnancy 253
use in renal impairment 270
Dose equivalents 189
Donepezil
for Alzheimer's disease 59
interactions 350
see also anticholinesterases
Dosulepin
for depression 77
see also tricyclics
Dothiepin
see dosulepin
Doxepin
for depression 78
see also tricyclics
Drug-induced disorders 373
Drug interactions
acamprosate 349
alcohol 358
anticholinesterases 350
anticholinergics 349
anticonvulsants 326
antidepressants 293
antipsychotics 281
anxiolytics 275
aripiprazole 285
atomoxetine 351
benzodiazepines 275
buprenorphine 351
bupropion 352
buspirone 278
cannabis 361
carbamazepine 326
chloral 279
citalopram 297
clomethiazole 353
clozapine 285
cocaine 361
disulfiram 353
donepezil 350
escitalopram 297
ethosuximide 332
fluoxetine 299
fluvoxamine 301
gabapentin 332
galantamine 350
hypnotics 275
lamotrigine 332
levetiracetam 334
lithium 321
MAOIs 316

memantine 354
methadone 355
methylphenidate 356
mianserin 308
mirtazapine 308
moclobemide 309
modafinil 357
neuroleptics 281
olanzapine 288
oxcarbazepine 334
paroxetine 304
phenobarbital 336
phenytoin 338
piracetam 345
pregabalin 345
primidone 336
quetiapine 290
reboxetine 311
risperidone 290
rivastigmine 351
sertindole 291
sertraline 305
smoking 362
SSRIs 297
St John's wort 313
tiagabine 345
topiramate 346
trazodone 311
tricyclics 293
tryptophan 312
valproate 346
venlafaxine 312
vigabatrin 348
zaleplon 280
ziprasidone 292
zolpidem 280
zopiclone 281
zotepine 293
Duloxetine
    in depression 78
    drug interactions 307
    see also antidepressants
Dysthymia
    treatment of 93
Dystonia
    drug-induced 387
    management of side effects of 423
Eating disorders 95
ECT 174
Epilepsy
    drug-induced 396
    drug use in 234
    status epilepticus 110
    treatment of 100
Escitalopram
    for agoraphobia 8
    for depression 75
    for panic disorder 126
    interactions 297
    for social anxiety 168
    see also SSRIs
Equivalent doses 189–208
Ethosuximide

    for epilepsy 107
    interactions 332
    see also anticonvulsants
Euphoria
    see mania
Extra-pyramidal side-effects
    drug-induced 384
    management of side-effects of 418
Flunitrazepam
    for insomnia 114
    see also benzodiazepines
Fluoxetine
    for bulimia 97
    for depression 75
    for OCD 121
    interactions 299
    see also SSRIs
Flupentixol
    for psychosis 140
    see also thioxanthenes
Flupentixol decanoate
    for psychosis 149
    see also thioxanthenes
Fluphenazine
    for psychosis 137
    see also phenothiazines
Fluphenazine decanoate
    for psychosis 149
    see also phenothiazines
Flurazepam
    for insomnia 114
    see also benzodiazepines
Fluspirilene
    for psychosis 149
    see also diphenylbutylpiperidines
Fluvoxamine
    for depression 76
    for OCD 121
    interactions 301
    see also SSRIs
Fosphenytoin
    for status epilepticus 110
    see also anticonvulsants
Gabapentin
    for epilepsy 107
    interactions 332
    see also anticonvulsants
Galantamine
    for Alzheimer's disease 60
    interactions 350
    see also anticholinesterases
Gilles de la Tourette
    see Tourette's syndrome
Glaucoma
    drug use in 238
Hallucinations
    drug induced 380
Haloperidol
    for acute psychiatric emergency 3
    for psychosis 140
    for Tourette's syndrome 169
    see also butyrophenones
Haloperidol decanoate

    for psychosis 152
    see also butyrophenones
Hepatic impairment
    drugs in 241
Hydroxyzine
    for anxiety 20
    see also anxiolytics
Hyperactivity
    see Attention deficit disorder
Hypomania
    see mania
Hypnotics
    for insomnia 115
    interactions 275
    relative side-effects 179
    switching/equivalent doses 179
    use in breast-feeding 213
    use in cardiac disease 221
    use in diabetes 229
    use in epilepsy 234
    use in glaucoma 238
    use in hepatic impairment 224
    use in old age 246
    use in pregnancy 253
    use in renal impairment 270
Imipramine
    for depression 78
    for panic disorder 127
    see also tricyclics
Insomnia
    drug-induced 401
    treatment of 113
Interactions
    see drug interactions 275
Isocarboxazid
    for depression 81
    see also MAOIs
Lamotrigine
    for epilepsy 103
    interactions 332
    see also anticonvulsants
Levetiracetam
    for epilepsy 104
    interactions 334
    see also anticonvulsants
Levomepromazine
    for psychosis 137
    see also phenothiazines
Lewy body disease
    treatment of 58
Libido
    drug effects on 429
Lithium
    for aggression 6
    for bipolar disorder 34
    for depression 81
    for mania 41
    interactions 321
    use in breast-feeding 213
    use in cardiac disease 221
    use in diabetes 229
    use in ECT 177
    use in epilepsy 234

use in glaucoma 238
use in hepatic impairment 241
use in old age 246
use in pregnancy 253
use in renal impairment 270
weight changes with 211
Liver impairment
drugs in 241
Lofepramine
for depression 78
see also tricyclics
Loprazolam
for insomnia 114
see also benzodiazepines
Lorazepam
for acute psychiatric emergency 4
for anxiety 19
for status epilepticus 111
see also benzodiazepines
Lormetazepam
for insomnia 114
see also benzodiazepines
Loxapine
see also antipsychotics
L-tryptophan
see tryptophan
Mania
drug-induced 381
treatment of 40
Manic-depression
see bipolar mood disorder
MAOIs
for depression 81
interactions — drugs 316
interactions — food 320
patient information 319
relative side-effects 180
switching 180
use in breast-feeding 213
use in cardiac disease 221
use in diabetes 229
use in ECT 177
use in epilepsy 234
use in glaucoma 238
use in hepatic impairment 241
use in old age 246
use in pregnancy 253
use in renal impairment 270
weight changes with 210
Maprotiline
for depression 78
see also tricyclics
Memantine
for Alzheimer's disease 61
interactions 354
use in breast-feeding 213
use in cardiac disease 221
use in diabetes 229
use in epilepsy 234
use in glaucoma 238
use in hepatic impairment 241
use in old age 246
use in pregnancy 253

use in renal impairment 270
Methadone
interactions 355
Methotrimeprazine
see levomepromazine
Methylphenidate
for attention deficit disorder 25
interactions 356
Mianserin
for depression 79
interactions 308
see also antidepressants
Midazolam
for status epilepticus 111
see also antidepressants
Mirtazapine
for anxiety 21
for depression 79
for insomnia 117
for panic disorder 128
interactions 308
pharmacokinetics 183
relative side-effects 181
sexual side-effects 428–432
switching to and from 180
use in breast-feeding 213
use in cardiac disease 221
use in diabetes 229
use in ECT 177
use in epilepsy 234
use in glaucoma 238
use in hepatic impairment 241
use in old age 246
use in pregnancy 253
use in renal impairment 270
weight changes with 210
see also antidepressants
Moclobemide
for depression 79
interactions 309
pharmacokinetics 183
relative side-effects 181
sexual side-effects 428–429
switching to and from 181
use in breast-feeding 213
use in cardiac disease 221
use in diabetes 229
use in ECT 177
use in epilepsy 234
use in hepatic impairment 241
use in old age 246
use in pregnancy 253
use in renal impairment 270
weight changes with 210
Modafinil
for narcolepsy 119
interactions 357
use in breast-feedbing 213
use in cardiac disease 221
use in diabetes 229
use in epilepsy 234
use in glaucoma 238
use in hepatic impairment 241

use in old age 246
use in pregnancy 253
use in renal impairment 270
Movement disorders
drug-induced 384
management of side-effects 418
Naltrexone
for self-injurious behaviour 163
Narcolepsy
treatment of 118
Narcotics
equivalent doses 196
Nervousness
drug-induced 373
Neuroleptic malignant syndrome
drug-induced 390
management of side-effects 425
Neuroleptics
see antipsychotics
Nightmares
drug-induced 402
Nitrazepam
for insomnia 114
see also benzodiazepines
Nortriptyline
for depression 78
see also tricyclics
Obsessive-compulsive disorder
drug-induced 391
treatment of 120
Olanzapine
for acute psychiatric emergency 3
for bipolar 48
for mania 42
for psychosis and schizophrenia 145
interactions 288
see also antipsychotics
Old age
drug use in 246
Orphenadrine
for extra-pyramidal side-effects 422
see also anticholinergics
Oxazepam
for anxiety 19
see also benzodiazepines
Oxcarbazepine
for epilepsy 104
interactions 334
see also anticonvulsants
Oxprenolol
see also beta-blockers
P450 enzymes
see Cytochrome P450
Panic disorder
drug-induced 392
treatment of 125
Paraldehyde
for status epilepticus 111
use in breast-feeding 213
use in cardiac disease 221
use in diabetes 229
use in epilepsy 234
use in glaucoma 238

use in hepatic impairment 241
use in old age 246
use in pregnancy 253
use in renal impairment 270
Parkinsonian side-effects
drug-induced 385
management of side-effects 422
Paroxetine
for agoraphobia 9
for anxiety 20
for depression 76
for PTSD 129
for OCD 122
for panic disorder 126
for social anxiety 167
interactions 304
see also SSRIs
Pericyazine
for psychosis 137
see also phenothiazines
Perphenazine
for psychosis 137
see also phenothiazines
Phenelzine
for depression 81
see also MAOIs
Phenobarbital
for epilepsy 107
interactions 336
see also barbiturates
Phenobarbitone
see phenobarbital
Phenothiazines
for acute psychiatric emergency 3
for anxiety 21
for psychosis 137
relative side-effects 185
switching/equivalent doses 196
use in breast-feeding 213
use in cardiac disease 221
use in diabetes 229
use in epilepsy 234
use in glaucoma 238
use in hepatic impairment 241
use in old age 246
use in pregnancy 253
use in renal impairment 270
weight changes with 208
see also antipsychotics
Phenytoin
for epilepsy 105
for status epilepticus 111
interactions 338
see also anticonvulsants
Phobia
see panic disorder
Pimozide
for psychosis 141
see also diphenylbutylpiperidines
Pipothiazine
for psychosis 150
see also phenothiazines
Piracetam

for epilepsy 108
interactions 345
see also anticonvulsants
Post-traumatic stress disorder
treatment of 129
Potassium clorazepate
see clorazepate
Pregabalin
in epilepsy 108
interactions 345
see also anticonvulsants
Pregnancy
drug use in 253
Priapism 433
Primidone
for epilepsy 107
interactions 336
see also barbiturates
Prochlorperazine
for psychosis 137
see also phenothiazines
Procyclidine
for extra-pyramidal side-effects
422–423
see also anticholinergics
Promazine
for psychosis 137
see also phenothiazines
Promethazine
for insomnia 116
see also antihistamines
Propranolol
for anxiety 19
see also beta-blockers
Psychosis
drug-induced 392
treatment of 133
Quetiapine
for mania 42
for psychosis 146
interactions 290
see also antipsychotics
Rapid-cycling bipolar disorder 51
Rapid tranquillisation 1
Reboxetine
for depression 80
interactions 311
see also antidepressants
relative side-effects 179–187
Renal disease
drug use in 270
RIMAs
see moclobemide
Risperidone
for mania 43
for psychosis 146
long-acting injection 150
interactions 290
see also antipsychotics
Rivastigmine
for Alzheimer's disease 60
interactions 351
see also anticholinesterases

Schizophrenia
drug-induced 392
treatment of 133
Seasonal affective disorder
treatment of 161
Seizures
drug-induced 396
Self-injurious behaviour
treatment of 163
Serotonin syndrome
drug-induced 399
management of side-effects 427
Sertindole
for psychosis 147
interactions 291
see also antipsychotics
Sertraline
for depression 76
for OCD 122
for PTSD 130
interactions 305
see also SSRIs
Sexual deviancy disorders
treatment of 164
Sexual side-effects 428
Sleep disorders
drug-induced 401
treatment of 113
Smoking
interactions 362
Social anxiety (phobia) 166
Sodium oxybate
for narcolepsy 119
interactions 358
Sodium valproate see valproate
Somnolence
drug-induced 401
SSRIs
for agoraphobia 9
for anxiety 21
for bulimia 98
for depression 73
for OCD 122–123
for panic disorder 125, 129
for PTSD 131
for social phobia 166, 168
interactions 297
relative side-effects 180
sexual side-effects 428
switching or stopping 180
use in breast-feeding 213
use in cardiac disease 221
use in diabetes 229
use in ECT 177
use in epilepsy 234
use in glaucoma 238
use in hepatic impairment 241
use in old age 246
use in pregnancy 253
use in renal impairment 270
weight changes with 209
Status epilepticus
treatment of 110

Sulpiride
  for psychosis 141
  see also antipsychotics
Switching psychotropics
  anticholinergics 179
  antidepressants 199
  antipsychotics 190
  benzodiazepines 198
  narcotics etc 199
Tardive dyskinesia
  drug-induced 388
  management of side-effects 420
Tardive dystonia
  drug-induced 387
  management of side-effects 418
Temazepam
  for insomnia 114
  see also benzodiazepines
Tetrabenazine
  for tardive dyskinesia 421
  use in breast-feeding 213
  use in cardiac disease 221
  use in diabetes 229
  use in epilepsy 234
  use in glaucoma 238
  use in hepatic impairment 241
  use in old age 246
  use in pregnancy 253
  use in renal impairment 270
Thioridazine
  for psychosis 137
  see also phenothiazines
Thioxanthenes
  for psychosis 140
  interactions 280, 281
  relative side-effects 185
  relative receptor blockade 186
  switching/equivalent doses 196
  use in breast-feeding 213
  use in cardiac disease 221
  use in diabetes 229
  use in epilepsy 234
  use in hepatic impairment 241
  use in old age 246
  use in pregnancy 253
  use in renal impairment 270
  weight changes with 208
  see also antipsychotics
Tiagabine
  for epilepsy 108
  interactions 345
  see also anticonvulsants
Tics
  drug-induced 389
  management of side-effects 423
Topiramate
  for epilepsy 105
  interactions 346
  see also anticonvulsants
Tourette's syndrome
  drug-induced 389
  treatment of 169

Tranylcypromine
  for depression 81
  see also MAOIs
Trazodone
  for depression 80
  interactions 311
  use in ECT 178
  sexual side-effects 431
  switching or discontinuing 180
  see also antidepressants
Trichotillomania
  treatment of 172
Triclofos
  for insomnia 116
  see also hypnotics
Tricyclic antidepressants
  for depression 71, 77
  for panic disorder 113
  for eating disorders 96
  interactions 293
  pharmacokinetics 183
  relative side-effects 181
  sexual side-effects 428
  use in breast-feeding 213
  use in cardiac disease 221
  use in diabetes 229
  use in ECT 178
  use in epilepsy 234
  use in glaucoma 238
  use in hepatic impairment 241
  use in old age 246
  use in pregnancy 253
  use in renal impairment 270
  weight changes with 210
Trifluoperazine
  for acute psychiatric emergency 3
  for psychosis 140
  see also phenothiazines
Trihexyphenidyl
  for extra-pyramidal side-effects
    418, 422
  see also anticholinergics
Trimipramine
  for depression 78
  see also tricyclics
Tryptophan
  for depression 82
  interactions 312
  see also antidepressants
U&Es 440–441
Valproate
  for mania 40–43
  for epilepsy 106
  interactions 346
  see also anticonvulsants
Valproic acid
  see valproate
Valproate semisodium
  see valproate
Venlafaxine
  for anxiety 21
  for depression 80

  interactions 312
  pharmacokinetics 183
  relative side-effects 181
  sexual side-effects 431
  switching or discontinuing 199
  use in breast-feeding 213
  use in cardiac disease 221
  use in diabetes 229
  use in ECT 178
  use in epilepsy 234
  use in hepatic impairment 241
  use in old age 246
  use in pregnancy 253
  use in renal impairment 270
  weight changes with 209, 210
Vigabatrin
  for epilepsy 108
  interactions 348
  see also anticonvulsants
Vitamins
  for alcohol dependence 11
  for alcohol withdrawal 15–16
Zaleplon
  for insomnia 115
  interactions 280
  see also hypnotics
Ziprasidone
  for psychosis 133, 148
  interactions 292
  see also antipsychotics
Zolpidem
  for insomnia 115
  interactions 280
  see also hypnotics
Zonisamide
  for epilepsy 108
  interactions 348
Zopiclone
  for insomnia 116
  interactions 281
  use in ECT 178
  see also hypnotics
Zotepine
  for psychosis 148
  interactions 293
  see also antipsychotics
Zuclopenthixol
  for psychosis 140
  see also thioxanthenes
Zuclopenthixol acetate
  for acute psychiatric emergency 3
  for psychosis 150
  see also thioxanthenes
Zuclopenthixol decanoate
  for psychosis 150
  see also thioxanthenes

Abbreviations

FOR DETAILS OF STUDIES:

n = number of patients
RCT = randomised controlled trial
d/b = double-blind
c/o = cross-over
o/p = out-patient
s/b = single blind (trial)
p/c = placebo-controlled

OTHER ABBREVIATIONS:

AAPCD = American Academy of Pediatrics Committee on Drugs
ACh = acetylcholine
AD = Alzheimer's disease
ADHD = attention deficit hyperactivity disorder
ADD = attention deficit disorder
ADME = absorption, distribution, metabolism and excretion
ADR = adverse drug reaction
AED = anti-epileptic drug
AFP = alpha-fetoprotein
AIMS = abnormal involuntary movement scale
APE = acute psychiatric emergency
APA = American Psychiatric Association
AWS = alcohol withdrawal syndrome
BAP = British Association for Psychopharmacology
BDI = Beck Depression Inventory
BDZ = benzodiazepine(s)
BMA = British Medical Association
BMI = body mass index
BNF = British National Formulary
BPD = borderline psychiatric disorder
BPRS = Brief Psychiatric Rating Scale
BPSD = behavioural and psychological symptoms of dementia
bp = blood pressure
BP = British Pharmacopoeia
CBT = cognitive behavioural therapy
CBZ = carbamazepine
CBZ-E = carbamazepine-epoxide

CCK = cholecystokinin
CDSR = Cochrane Database Systematic Reviews
CGI = clinical global impression
CHD = coronary heart disease
CNS = central nervous system
CPK = creatinine phosphokinase
CSE = convulsive status epilepticus
CSM = Committee on the Safety of Medicines
D1 = dopamine-1 (receptor)
D2 = dopamine-2 (receptor)
DA = dopamine
DSM-IV = Diagnostic Statistical Manual IV
e/c = enteric-coated
ECG = electrocardiogram
ECT = electroconvulsive therapy
EBMH = Evidence-Based Mental Health (Journal)
EEG = electro-encephalogram
EPO = Evening primrose oil
EPSE = extra-pyramidal side-effects
FBC = full blood count
GABA = gamma-aminobutyric acid
GFR = glomerular filtration rate
GTC = generalised tonic-clonic (seizure)
5-HT = 5-hydroxytryptamine
HF = heart failure
IV = intravenous
IM = intramuscular
INR = international normalised ratio
ISE = ion-selective electrode
L/A = long-acting
LD = low dose
LFT = liver function tests
LTG = lamotrigine
MAOI = mono-amine oxidase inhibitor
MHA = Mental Health Act (1983)
MHRA = Medicines and Healthcare products Regulatory Agency (was CSM/MCA)
MI = manufacturers' information

MMSE = Mini-Mental State Examination
NA = noradrenaline
NE = norepinephrine
N/K = not known
NMDA = N-methyl-D-aspartate receptor
NMS = neuroleptic malignant syndrome
NNT = numbers needed to treat
OCD = obsessive-compulsive disorder
O/C = oral contraceptive
OD = overdose
OTC = over-the-counter (medicine)
PNBP = Progress in Neuropsycho-pharmacology and Biological Psychiatry
PD = personality disorder, Pro-drug
PMH = previous medical history
PMS = pre-menstrual syndrome
PT = prothrombin time
PTSD = post-traumtic stress disorder
REM = rapid eye movement
RIMA = reversible inhibitor of monoamine-A
RPSGB = Royal Pharmaceutical Society of Great Britain
RT = rapid tranquillisation
SA = short-acting
SAD = seasonal affective disorder
s/c = subcutaneous
SF = sugar-free
SIB = self-injurious behaviour
SJW = St John's wort
SPC = summary of product characteristics
SSRI = serotonin-selective reuptake inhibitor
t½ = half life
TCA = tricyclic antidepressant
TD = tardive dyskinesia
TDM = therapeutic drug monitoring
U&E = urea and electrolytes
USP = United States Pharmacopoeia